KT-152-753

ROSS AND WILSON

Anatomy
and
Physiology

in Health and Illness

For Churchill Livingstone:

Commissioning Editor: Ellen Green
Project Manager: Valerie Burgess
Design Direction: Judith Wright
Project Development Editor: Mairi McCubbin
Project Controller: Derek Robertson
Copy-editor: Sue Beasley
Indexer: Liza Weinkove
Sales Promotion Executive: Hilary Brown

ROSS AND WILSON

Anatomy and Physiology

in Health and Illness

Kathleen J. W. Wilson OBE BSc PhD RGN SCM RNT

Formerly: Senior Lecturer, Department of Nursing Studies, University of Edinburgh;
Nursing Research Liaison Officer, West Midlands Regional Health Authority/University
of Birmingham; Principal Tutor, Royal Infirmary, Edinburgh.

Anne Waugh BSc(Hons) MSc CertEd SRN RNT

Senior Nurse Teacher, Lothian College of Health Studies, Edinburgh

EIGHTH EDITION

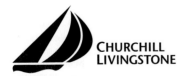
CHURCHILL
LIVINGSTONE

NEW YORK EDINBURGH LONDON MADRID MELBOURNE SAN FRANCISCO TOKYO 1996

CHURCHILL LIVINGSTONE
Medical Division of Pearson Professional Limited

Distributed in the United States of America by Churchill Livingstone Inc., 650 Avenue of the Americas, New York, N.Y. 10011, and by associated companies, branches and representatives throughout the world.

© E. & S. Livingstone Ltd 1963, 1966, 1968
© Longman Group Limited 1973, 1981, 1987, 1990
© Pearson Professional Limited 1996

All rights reserved. No part of this publication may be reproduced, stored in a retrieval system, or transmitted in any form or by any means, electronic, mechanical, photocopying, recording or otherwise, without either the prior permission of the publishers (Churchill Livingstone, Robert Stevenson House, 1–3 Baxter's Place, Leith Walk, Edinburgh EH1 3AF), or a licence permitting restricted copying in the United Kingdom issued by the Copyright Licensing Agency Ltd, 90 Tottenham Court Road, London, W1P 9HE.

First published 1963
Second edition 1966
Third edition 1968
Fourth edition 1973
Fifth edition 1981
Sixth edition 1987
Seventh edition 1990
Eighth edition 1996

ISBN 0 443 05156 9

British Library of Cataloguing in Publication Data
A catalogue record for this book is available from the British Library.

Library of Congress Cataloging in Publication Data
A catalogue record for this book is available from the Library of Congress

The
publisher's
policy is to use
**paper manufactured
from sustainable forests**

Printed in Hong Kong
SWT/01

Contents

Preface

The purpose of this book is to provide nurses and other health workers with knowledge of the structure and functions of the human body and the changes that take place when diseases disrupt normal processes. As in the seventh edition, the objective is to describe not to prescribe: diagnostic procedures, medical treatments and nursing care are not included.

In this edition large parts of the text have been revised and updated, and the material rearranged into sections, each containing a number of systems: the body as a whole and its constituents; internal communication; intake of raw materials and elimination of waste; protection and survival.

Chapter 1 continues to provide a brief overview of the interrelationships between the body systems, the stylised illustrations showing the links between the various parts. Later chapters provide anatomically accurate illustrations, more detailed physiological material and descriptions of the associated commonly occurring diseases. The latter includes abnormal physiology, the likely progress and the probable outcome of untreated disease. The pathophysiological material has been arranged in three columns and placed at the end of each chapter so that the abnormal follows the normal. Diseases of the skin and nutritional disorders have been added.

Some biological values have been extracted from the text and listed on pages 443 and 444 for easy reference. In some cases, slightly different 'normals' may be found in other texts and used by different medical practitioners.

We are grateful to readers of the seventh edition for their constructive comments, many of which have influenced the changes made to this edition.

We would like to express thanks to Ian Lennox for drawing the new illustrations and altering others, and to the staff of Churchill Livingstone for their assistance in the preparation of this edition.

1996   Kathleen J. W. Wilson
                                         Anne Waugh

Section 1
The body as a whole and its constituents

1
Introduction to the body as a whole

The human animal is a very complex multicellular organism in which the maintenance of life depends upon a vast number of physiological and biochemical activities. The sum of these activities enables human beings to live in and utilise their environment, and to maintain the species by reproducing.

There is considerable variation in the complexity of organisms. At one end of the continuum there is the *single cell organism* such as the amoeba, and at the other, the highly complex *multicellular human animal*. A cell is the smallest functional unit of an organism; thus a single cell organism is the simplest kind of organism that can exist independently.

In order to survive, each species, simple and complex, must be able to perform certain functions. A single cell organism can carry out all these functions because all its parts have easy access to its external environment. The inside of the single cell organism is separated from its environment by only one porous membrane, which is described as *semipermeable* because small particles can pass through it while large ones cannot (Fig. 1.1). It is not possible for all the cells of the multicellular human animal to be in close contact with the external environment so, in order to survive, *specialisation of cells* has evolved. Different types of cells have developed to carry out specific functions within the body, i.e. functional specialisation has taken place in parallel with structural specialisation. Figure 1.2 shows a multicellular structure.

The cells of the body are too small to be seen with the naked eye, but when magnified using a microscope, different types of cells can be distinguished by their size, shape and the types of dye they absorb when stained in the laboratory.

Groups of cells which have the same physical characteristics tend to have similar specialised functions, and a large number of cells that perform the same functions are described as *tissues. Organs* are made up of a number of different types of tissue, and *systems* consist of a number of organs and tissues. Each system contributes to one or more of the survival needs (vital functions) of the body. However, because of specialisation of cells, no system can exist in isolation.

In general the combined activities of the specialised systems provide the optimum environment for individual cells. This means the maintenance of a constant, or near constant, composition of the fluid that bathes the body cells. This situation is essential for health and is called *homeostasis*.

THE INTERNAL ENVIRONMENT AND HOMEOSTASIS

The *external environment* surrounds the body and provides the oxygen and nutritional materials required by all the cells of the body. Waste products of cell activity are eventually excreted into the external environment (Fig. 1.2).

The *internal environment* provides chemical substances produced by specialised cells. All living cells in the body are bathed in fluid called *interstitial* or *tissue fluid*. Oxygen, nutritional materials, chemicals produced by the body, and waste products, pass through the interstitial fluid between the cells and the internal transportation

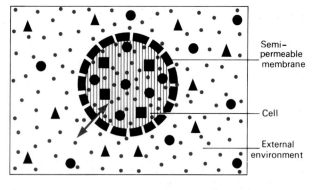

=Small particles able to pass through pores in the cell membrane

▲ =Large particles—outside—cannot pass into the cell

■ = Large particles—inside—cannot pass out of the cell

● = Large particles—inside and outside the cell which cannot pass through its membrane

Figure 1.1 Diagram of a single cell organism with a semipermeable membrane.

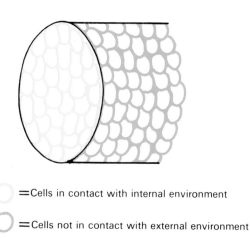

◯ =Cells in contact with internal environment

◯ =Cells not in contact with external environment

Figure 1.2 Diagram of a cylindrical multicellular structure.

systems. The composition of the internal environment is maintained within narrow limits, and this fairly constant state is called *homeostasis*. Literally, this term means 'unchanging', but in practice it describes a dynamic, ever-changing situation kept within narrow limits. When this balance is threatened or lost, there is a serious risk to the well-being of the individual. There are many factors in the internal environment which must be maintained within narrow limits, including:

- temperature
- water and electrolyte concentrations
- acidity (pH)
- glucose levels
- oxygen and carbon dioxide levels
- blood pressure.

Homeostasis is maintained by control systems which detect and respond to changes in the internal environment. A control system (Fig. 1.3) has three basic components: detector, control centre and effector. The *control centre* determines the limits within which the variable factor should be maintained. It receives an input from the *detector* or *sensor*, and integrates the incoming information. When the incoming signal indicates that an adjustment is needed the *effector* responds and the input is changed. This is a dynamic process that maintains homeostasis.

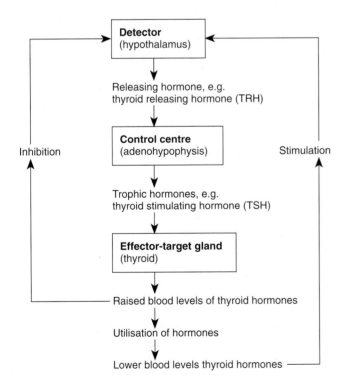

Figure 1.3 Example of negative feedback mechanism, i.e., regulation of the secretion of thyroid hormones.

Negative feedback mechanisms

In these mechanisms the effector response decreases or negates the effect of the original stimulus, restoring homeostasis (thus the term negative feedback). Control of body temperature is similar to the non-physiological example of a domestic central heating system. The thermometer (temperature detector) is sensitive to changes in room temperature (variable factor) and is connected to the boiler control unit (control centre). The heating control unit controls the boiler (effector). The thermostat constantly compares the information from the detector with the preset temperature and, when necessary, adjustments are made to raise the room temperature. When the preset temperature is reached the system is then reversed and the boiler is switched off. This series of events is a negative feedback mechanism and it enables continuous self-regulation or control of a variable within a narrow range.

Most of the homeostatic controls in the body utilise negative feedback mechanisms to prevent sudden and serious changes in the internal environment. Many of these negative feedback mechanisms are explained in the following chapters.

Positive feedback mechanisms

There are only a few of these *amplifier* or *cascade systems* in the body. They operate by the effector and its response further increasing the original stimulus, triggering off a cascade reaction. Examples include blood clotting and uterine contractions during labour.

Homeostatic imbalance

This arises when the fine control of a factor in the internal environment is inadequate and the level of the factor falls outside the normal range. If control cannot achieve homeostasis, an abnormal state develops that may be recognised as a specific illness.

SURVIVAL NEEDS OF THE BODY AND THEIR ASSOCIATED SYSTEMS

In this chapter a *brief* description of the various survival needs is provided, along with an overview of the body systems involved (Table 1.1). The illustrations are

Table 1.1 Survival needs of the body and their associated systems

Survival needs	System(s) involved
Internal transportation	Circulatory
	Lymphatic
Communication	
With the outside world	Nervous
	Special senses
	Respiratory (voice production)
	Skeletal
	Muscular
	Joints
Within the body	Nervous
	Endocrine
Intake of raw materials	
Food	Digestive
Oxygen	Respiratory
Elimination of waste	Respiratory
materials	Urinary
	Digestive
Protection against the	Skin
external environment	Membranes lining passages which open on to the surface of the body
Movement within the	Skeletal
external environment	Muscular
	Joints
	Nervous
	Special senses
Reproduction	Male and female reproductive
	Hormones

stylised representations of anatomy and of some functions. Anatomically accurate illustrations and more detailed descriptions of physiology and commonly occurring malfunctions of each system are provided in later chapters.

Some systems contribute to a number of survival needs but all are necessary to maintain homeostasis and health.

Internal transportation

This is described first, because all the systems depend upon the circulation of blood. Because of specialisation and the need to maintain homeostasis, a sophisticated transport system is required to ensure that all cells have access to the internal and external environments of the body. The systems involved are the *circulatory* and *lymphatic*.

Circulatory system (Chs 4, 5 and 6. Figs 1.4 and 1.5)

This system consists of the *blood*, the *blood vessels* and the *heart*.

Blood

Blood constitutes about 6 to 8% of body weight in adults and consists of two parts—a sticky fluid called *plasma*, and *cells* which float in the plasma. The adult body contains 5 to 6 litres of blood.

Plasma

This consists of water and chemical substances dissolved or suspended in it. These are:

- nutrient materials absorbed from the intestine
- oxygen absorbed from the lungs
- chemical substances synthesised by body cells
- waste materials produced by body cells to be eliminated from the body by excretion.

Blood cells (Fig. 1.4)

There are three distinct groups, classified according to their functions.

Erythrocytes (red blood cells) are concerned with the transport of oxygen and, to a lesser extent, carbon dioxide between the lungs and all body cells. They contain *haemoglobin* which combines with oxygen and carries it from the lungs to the cells. Both the amount of oxygen needed and of carbon dioxide to be removed increase as cell activity increases, e.g. during hard physical exercise the blood supply to the muscles involved increases.

Leukocytes (white blood cells) are mainly concerned with the protection of the body against microbes and other potentially damaging substances that gain entry to the body. They are also involved in the removal of cells at the end of their normal life span and those damaged by disease and injury. There are three types of leukocytes which carry out their protective functions in different ways: *neutrophils*, *basophils* and *eosinophils*. These cells are larger than erythrocytes and are less numerous.

Thrombocytes (platelets) are tiny cell fragments which play an essential part in the very complex process of blood clotting. A blood clot is a 'plug' consisting of blood cells and fibrous material which forms in the cut or torn ends of a blood vessel. It prevents excessive loss of blood.

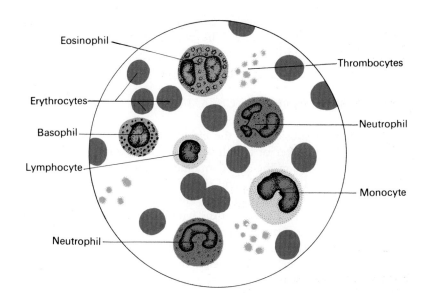

Figure 1.4 Blood cells after staining in the laboratory viewed through a microscope.

Blood vessels

There are three types:

- *arteries*, which convey blood away from the heart
- *veins*, which return blood to the heart
- *capillaries*, which link the arteries and veins. These are tiny blood vessels with very thin walls consisting of only one layer of cells. Between these cells there are very small openings or pores, which allow some of the constituents of blood to pass through, such as oxygen, nutritional materials, some chemical substances synthesised in the body and waste products from cells. Larger-sized substances, such as erythrocytes and large molecule proteins, cannot pass through the *semipermeable* capillary walls.

Heart

The heart is a muscular sac. It pumps the blood into the blood vessels which transport it to:

- the lungs (*pulmonary circulation*) where oxygen is absorbed from the air in the lungs and at the same time carbon dioxide is excreted from the blood into the air
- cells in all parts of the body (*general* or *systemic circulation*).

The muscle in the heart wall is not under the control of the will. At rest, the heart contracts between 65 and 75 times per minute. The rate may be greatly increased during physical exercise, when the oxygen and nutritional needs of the muscles moving the limbs are increased, and in some emotional states.

The rate at which the heart beats can be counted by taking the *pulse*. This is a wave of expansion of artery walls which occurs when the heart contracts and pushes blood into the *aorta*, the first artery of the general circulation. The pulse can be felt most easily where an

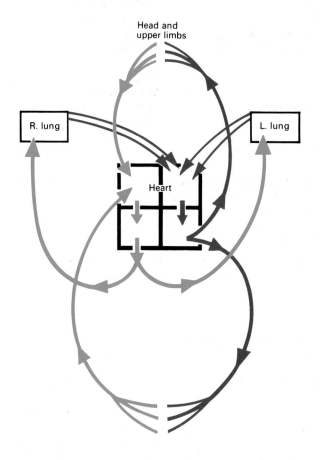

Figure 1.5 Diagram representing the circulatory system.

artery lies close to the surface of the body and can be pressed gently against a bone. The wrist is the site most commonly used for this purpose.

Lymphatic system (Ch. 6. Fig. 1.6)

This system is a subsidiary of the circulatory system. It consists of a number of lymph vessels which begin as blind-ended tubes in the area containing tissue fluid between the blood capillaries and the cells (Fig. 1.6). Structurally they are similar to veins and blood capillaries but the pores in the walls of the lymph capillaries are larger than those of the blood capillaries. This means that water containing large molecule substances, fragments of damaged cells and foreign matter such as microbes drains away by passing into the lymph vessels. The two largest lymph vessels empty lymph into large veins near the heart.

There are collections of tissue called *lymph nodes* situated at various points along the length of the lymph vessels. Lymph, derived from tissue fluid, is filtered as it passes through the lymph nodes, and microbes, noxious substances and some waste materials are removed.

Communication

In order to live in and be able to adapt to the external environment, the individual must be able to communicate with it. Similarly, communication is necessary for the stimulation, regulation and coordination of activities within the body, i.e. to maintain homeostasis. In both cases communication involves a cycle of receiving, collating and giving information.

With the outside world

Nervous system (Ch. 7. Figs 1.7 and 1.8)

The brain receives nerve impulses from outside the body through the five senses (Fig. 1.7). These senses and the special organs involved are:

Sight   — eyes
Hearing — ears
Smell   — nose
Taste   — tongue
Touch   — skin.

Although the senses are considered different and separate from each other, one sense is rarely used on its own. For example, when the smell of smoke is per-

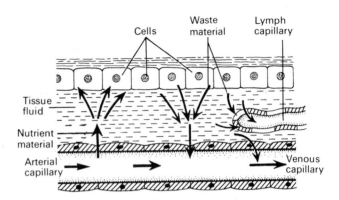

Figure 1.6 Diagram showing the beginning of a lymph capillary in the interstitial space.

ceived, other senses such as sight and hearing are likely to be used to try to locate the source of the smoke. Similarly, taste and smell are closely associated in the enjoyment, or otherwise, of food.

Nerve endings are stimulated by phenomena outside the body and the resultant nerve impulses are transmitted to the brain by nerve fibres for 'interpretation' or *perception*. The brain collates this material with information obtained from the memory, and the result is coordinated and regulated communication with the outside world. The nervous system consists of:

- the *brain*, situated inside the skull
- the *spinal cord*, which extends from the base of the brain to the lumbar region and is protected from injury by the bones of the vertebral column
- *nerve fibres*, of two types: *sensory* or *afferent nerves*, which provide the brain with 'input' from organs and tissues, and *motor* or *efferent nerves*, which convey nerve impulses from the brain to effector organs: muscles and glands.

Voice production

This mechanism provides a means of communication with the outside world. Sound is produced in the larynx as a result of blowing air through the space between the *vocal cords* during expiration. What is known as speech is the *manipulation* of *sound* by the contraction of the muscles of the throat and the cheeks and the movements of the tongue and lower jaw.

Skeletal and muscular systems (Chs 15, 16 and 17)

These systems combined produce the posture and movements associated with nonverbal communication

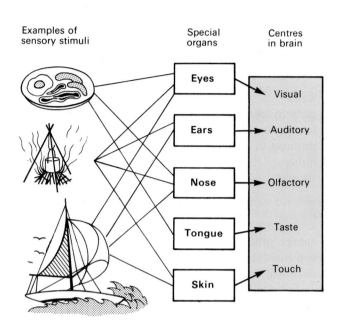

Figure 1.7 Diagram representing the special senses.

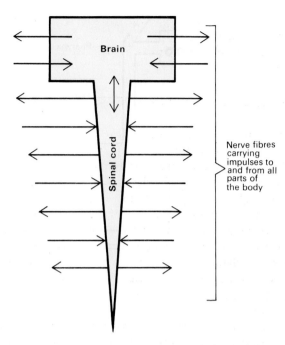

Figure 1.8 Diagram representing the nervous system.

with the outside world. The skeletal system provides the bony framework of the body, and movement takes place at joints between bones. The muscles which move the bones lie between them and the skin. They are stimulated by the part of the nervous system under the control of the will. Some nonverbal communication, e.g. changes in facial expression, may not involve the movement of bones.

Within the body

Nervous system

The brain receives information from inside the body by means of:

- nerve impulses transmitted by sensory nerve fibres
- chemical substances circulating in the blood supplying the brain.

The brain collates this information and responds by initiating efferent (motor) nerve impulses and secreting chemical substances. These pass from the brain to other parts of the body to stimulate, regulate and coordinate the activities of other organs and systems. Some of this activity is under the control of the will but much of it is involuntary, e.g. the individual cannot control the heart rate, emptying of the stomach or dilatation of the pupils of the eyes.

Endocrine system (Ch. 9)

This system consists of a number of *endocrine glands*, situated in different parts of the body. They communicate with each other, and with other organs and tissues of the body, by means of chemical substances, called *hormones*, which they synthesise. The glands are 'informed' about conditions within the body by variations in the concentration of chemical substances in the blood that supplies them and by nerve impulses. Changes in the amount of a hormone secreted result in stimulation or depression of activity in the organs and tissues they affect.

Intake of raw materials

Food (Chs 11 and 12)

Food is one of the sources of the raw materials that cells must obtain from the external environment, but it is seldom in a form that cells can use. A specialised system has developed to modify or *digest* food so that it can be absorbed and then used by body cells.

Digestive system (Ch. 12. Figs 1.9 and 1.10)

This system consists of the *alimentary canal* and *glands*.

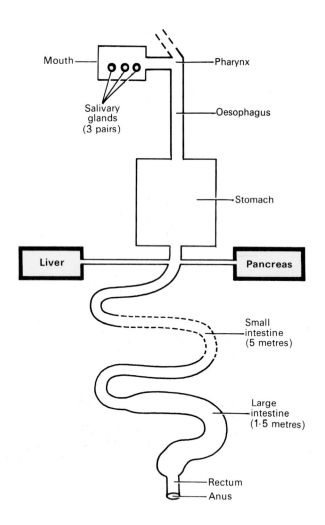

Figure 1.9 Diagram representing the digestive system.

Alimentary canal

This is a tube that begins at the mouth and continues through the pharynx, oesophagus, stomach, small and large intestines, rectum and anus.

Glands

These are aggregates of secretory cells enclosed in sheets, or membranes, of connective tissue. Most glands synthesise *digestive enzymes** and discharge them into the canal through ducts, or little tubes. Many glands are in the walls of the alimentary canal but those situated outside the canal with ducts leading into it are the *salivary glands*, the *pancreas* and the *liver*.

---

* *Enzymes are chemical compounds which cause, or speed up, chemical changes in substances with which they are in contact. They are organic catalysts.*

Food, which is chemically complex, is taken in at the mouth and broken down by *physical* and *chemical* means into forms in which it can pass through the walls of the alimentary canal into the blood to be transported around the body (Fig. 1.10). The substances absorbed are:

- water
- carbohydrates in the form of *monosaccharides*
- fats in the form of *fatty acids* and *glycerol*
- proteins in the form of *amino acids*
- mineral salts
- vitamins.

These substances provide the materials required by the body for:

- energy production—carbohydrates and fats
- cell building, growth and repair—proteins
- chemical synthesis—minerals, proteins, fats, carbohydrates, vitamins
- medium for all chemical activity—water.

Oxygen (Ch. 10)

Oxygen is a gas which makes up about 21% of the atmospheric air. It is essential for human life because most of the chemical activities which take place in the cells can only occur in its presence. Oxygen is involved in the series of chemical changes that result in the release of the energy from nutrient materials. It is essential for all cellular activities.

Metabolism

This is the sum total of the chemical activity in the body. It consists of two groups of processes:

- *anabolism*, building or synthesising new products
- *catabolism*, breaking down substances to provide energy and raw materials for anabolism, and substances for excretion as waste.

The sources of energy are mainly the dietary nutrients, carbohydrates and fats. If these are in short supply, proteins are used.

Respiratory system (Ch. 10. Fig. 1.11)

This is the system through which oxygen is taken into the body from the external environment and carbon dioxide, a waste product of cell metabolism, is excreted. It consists of a series of tubes or *respiratory passages* which carry air from the nose to the *lungs* and a network of *blood capillaries* in the lungs. The respiratory passages are continuous with each other. They are the

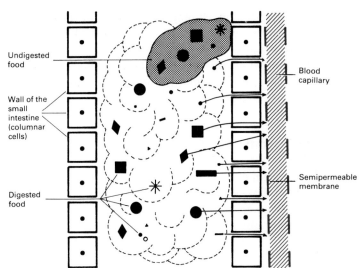

Figure 1.10 Diagram representing the digestion and absorption of food.

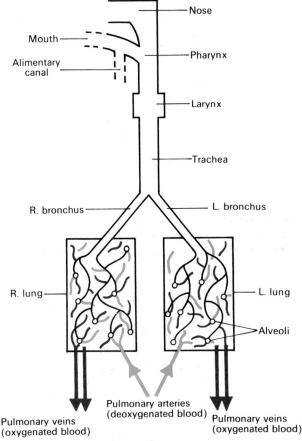

Figure 1.11 Diagram representing the respiratory system.

nose, the *pharynx* (also part of the alimentary canal), the *larynx* (voice box), the *trachea*, two *bronchi* (one bronchus to each lung) and a large number of *bronchial tubes* which subdivide and lead to millions of tiny air sacs called *alveoli*. Air may also enter the pharynx through the mouth.

The *lungs* are two in number and are situated one on each side of the heart in the thoracic cavity. They consist of bronchial tubes, alveoli, blood and lymph vessels and nerves, all of which are supported by connective tissue. Each alveolus is surrounded by a dense network of blood capillaries.

Respiration
Air containing oxygen and carbon dioxide is breathed into the lungs, filling the alveoli, and it is separated from the blood in the capillaries by two semipermeable membranes. These are the walls of the alveoli and the capillary walls, each of which is only one cell thick. Oxygen is in higher concentration in the alveoli so it passes from the alveoli to the blood; carbon dioxide is in higher concentration in blood so it passes in the opposite direction, from the blood to the alveoli (Fig. 1.12). Oxygen is carried in the blood in solution in the blood water and in chemical combination with haemoglobin in the red blood cells. The cells throughout the body obtain oxygen and get rid of carbon dioxide by the reverse process. Oxygen is in higher concentration in the blood than in the cells and the interstitial fluid around the cells, so it diffuses down the concentration gradient from the capillaries to the cells. Carbon dioxide, which is a waste product of cell metabolism, is in

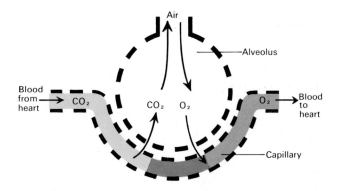

Figure 1.12 Diagram showing the interchange of gases between air in an alveolus and the blood in a capillary.

higher concentration in the cells and interstitial fluid and diffuses down the concentration gradient from the cells to the blood.

Breathing is the regular inflation and deflation of the lungs which maintains a steady concentration of atmospheric gases in the alveoli, i.e. the constant intake of oxygen and output of carbon dioxide.

Nitrogen, which is present in atmospheric air, is breathed in and out with oxygen and carbon dioxide but, in this gaseous form, it cannot be used by the body. The nitrogen needed by the body is present in protein foods, mainly meat and fish.

Elimination of waste materials

Substances in the body are regarded as waste materials if they cannot be used by the cells and if their accumulation will upset the fine balance needed to maintain homeostasis. One of the most important of these is the acidity / alkalinity balance for which the *scale of measurement* is pH. The scale extends from 0 to 14 with 7 the *neutral point*. From 7 to 0 represents *increasing acidity* and from 7 to 14, *increasing alkalinity* (Fig. 1.13).

Varying quantities of acids and alkalis are produced by metabolism. It is an important function of the sys-

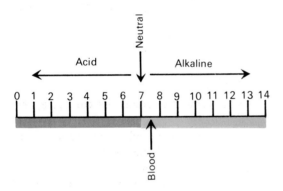

Figure 1.13 The pH scale.

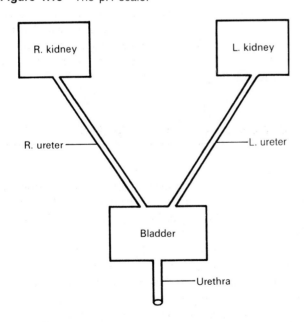

Figure 1.14 Diagram representing the urinary system.

tems involved in elimination to control excretion of these substances in order to maintain the optimum blood pH, i.e. about 7.4. In addition, other waste materials which do not affect the pH are also excreted, e.g. faeces. The *respiratory, urinary* and *digestive systems* are those involved in elimination.

Respiratory system

This system excretes carbon dioxide, as described above. Carbon dioxide dissolved in water forms an acid and it must be excreted in appropriate amounts to maintain the optimum pH of the blood at about 7.4.

Urinary system (Ch. 13. Fig. 1.14)

This system has an important role in the maintenance of homeostasis by:

- keeping the appropriate balance between water and substances dissolved in it, and between acids and alkalis
- eliminating the waste products resulting from the catabolism of cell protein (urea, creatinine and uric acid).

The organs of the urinary system are shown in Figure 1.14.

Digestive system

The large intestine excretes *faeces* which contain:

- food residue that remains in the alimentary canal because it cannot be digested and absorbed
- bile from the liver, which contains the waste products resulting from the catabolism (breakdown) of erythrocytes
- large numbers of microbes.

Protection against the external environment

All the living cells in the body are in a watery environment and the substances which enter and leave the cells are either dissolved or suspended in water.

The *skin* and the *mucous membrane* lining the passages which open to the surface of the body provide a barrier between the 'dry' external environment of the body and the watery environment of the body cells.

Skin (Ch. 13. Fig. 1.15)

The skin is described in two parts, the *epidermis* and the *dermis*.

The epidermis lies superficially and is composed of several layers of cells that grow towards the surface from its deepest layer. The surface layer consists of *dead cells* that are constantly being rubbed off by clothes etc. and replaced from below. The epidermis constitutes the barrier between the moist environment of the living cells of the body and the dry atmosphere of the external environment.

The dermis is composed of collagen and elastic fibres. It contains tiny *sweat glands* that have little canals or ducts, leading to the surface. When sweat from these glands reaches the surface it evaporates, cooling the body and thus playing a major part in the maintenance of temperature.

Hair is not living material. Hairs grow from *follicles* in the dermis, consisting of invaginated epidermal cells, which have groups of specialised cells called *sebaceous glands*. These glands secrete *sebum* into the follicles and so on to the skin surface. The oily materials present in sebum keep the skin soft, pliable and to a large extent waterproof.

Sebum and tears contain chemical substances which kill microbes. In this way sebum enhances the protective function of the skin and tears protect the eyes.

Sensory nerve endings present in the dermis are stimulated by pain, temperature and touch. If the finger touches a very hot plate, it is removed immediately. This cycle of events is called a *reflex action*, i.e. a very rapid motor response (contraction of muscles) to a sensory stimulus (stimulation of sensory nerve endings in the skin). This type of reflex action is an important protective mechanism.

Mucous membrane (Ch. 2)

This type of membrane consists of living cells. Their free surface is kept moist by the thick sticky fluid they secrete, called *mucus*. Mucus protects the mouth and the alimentary canal from mechanical injury by food and the respiratory passages from inhaled dust and microbes.

Movement within the external environment

The essential purposes of the physical movement of the whole, or parts, of the body within the environment are:

- to obtain food and water
- to avoid injury
- to reproduce.

Most body movement is under the control of the will and can be initiated consciously. The exceptions include protective movements which are carried out before the individual is aware of them, e.g. the reflex action of removing the finger from a very hot surface.

The skeleton provides the bony framework of the body and movement takes place at joints between two or more bones. *Skeletal muscles* move the *joints* and they are stimulated to contract by the *nervous system*. A brief description of the skeleton is given in Chapter 2 and a more detailed account of bones, muscles and joints is presented in Chapters 15, 16 and 17.

Reproduction (Ch. 18. Fig. 1.16)

Successful reproduction is essential in order to ensure the continuation of a species from one generation to the next. *Bisexual reproduction* results from the fertilisation of the female egg cell or *ovum* by the male sperm cell or *spermatozoon*. Ova are produced by two *ovaries* situated in the female pelvis. Usually only one ovum is released at a time and it travels towards the *uterus* in the *uterine tube*. The spermatozoa are produced in large numbers by the two *testes*, situated in the *scrotum*. From each testis spermatozoa pass through a duct called the *deferent duct (vas deferens)* to the *urethra*. During coitus the spermatozoa are deposited in the female *vagina*.

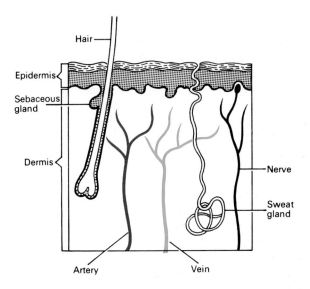

Figure 1.15 Diagram of the skin.

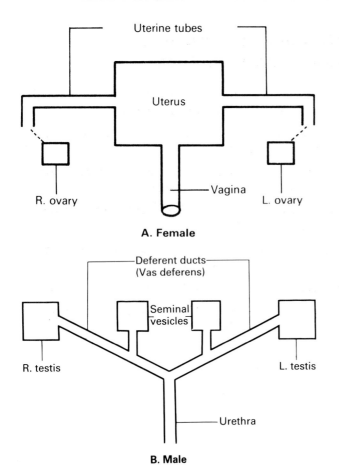

A. Female

B. Male

Figure 1.16 Diagram representing the female and male reproductive systems.

They then pass upwards through the uterus and fertilise the ovum in the uterine tube. The fertilised ovum (*zygote*) then passes into the uterus, embeds itself in the uterine wall and grows to maturity in about 40 weeks. The newborn baby is entirely dependent on others for food and protection that was provided by the mother's body before birth.

One ovum is produced about every 28 days during the child-bearing years, beginning at *puberty*, at about 13 years of age, and ending at the *menopause*, about 35 years later. When the ovum is not fertilised it passes out of the uterus accompanied by bleeding, called *menstruation*. The cycle in the female, called the *menstrual cycle*, has recognisable phases associated with changes in the concentration of hormones involving the endocrine system. There is no similar cycle in the male but hormones similar to those of the female are involved in the production and development to maturity of the spermatozoa.

INTRODUCTION TO THE STUDY OF ILLNESS

In order to understand the specific diseases described in later chapters, it is necessary to be familiar with the relevant anatomy and physiology and also the pathological processes outlined below.

Many different illnesses, disorders and diseases are known, and these vary from minor, but often very troublesome conditions, to the very serious. The study of abnormalities can be made much easier when a systematic approach is adopted. In order to achieve this in later chapters where specific diseases are explained, the following framework will be used:

- what is the cause? *aetiology*
- what is the nature of the disease process and its effect on normal body functioning? *pathogenesis*
- what other consequences might arise if the disease progresses? *complications*
- what is the likely outcome? *prognosis.*

Aetiology

Diseases are known to be caused by a limited number of factors which include:

- genetic abnormalities
- microbes and parasites, e.g. viruses, bacteria, worms
- chemicals
- ionising radiation
- failure of control mechanisms
- degeneration.

In some diseases more than one of the aetiological factors listed above is involved, while in others, no specific cause has been identified and these may be described as: *essential*, *idiopathic* or *spontaneous*. For some diseases where the precise cause is unknown, links may have been established with *predisposing factors*, or *risk factors*. *Iatrogenic* conditions are those that result from harm caused by members of the caring professions.

Pathogenesis

The main disease processes that cause illness or disease are:

- *Inflammation* (p. 69)—tissue response to damage by, e.g. trauma, invasion of microbes*.

Inflammatory conditions are recognised by the suffix -itis, e.g. appendicitis.

- *Tumours* (p. 42)—arise when the rate of cell production exceeds that of normal cell destruction causing a mass to develop. Tumours are recognised by the suffix -oma, e.g. carcinoma.
- *Abnormal immune mechanisms* (p. 67)—response of the normally protective immune system which causes undesirable effects.
- *Thrombosis, embolism and infarction* (p. 116)—are the effects and consequences of abnormal changes in the blood and/or blood vessel walls.
- *Degeneration*—often associated with normal ageing but also arises prematurely when structures deteriorate causing impaired function.
- *Metabolic abnormalities*—causing undesirable effects.
- *Genetic abnormalities*—either inherited or caused by environmental factors such as ionising radiation.

---

* The term **microbe**, used throughout the text, includes all types of organisms that can only be seen by using a microscope. Specific microbes are named where appropriate.

Glossary of terminology associated with disease

Acute: a disease with sudden onset often requiring urgent treatment (compare with chronic).

Acquired: a disorder which develops any time after birth (compare with congenital).

Chronic: a long-standing disorder which cannot usually be cured (compare with acute).

Congenital: a disorder which one is born with (compare with acquired).

Sign: an abnormality seen or measured by people other than the patient.

Symptom: an abnormality described by the patient.

Syndrome: a collection of signs and symptoms which tend to occur together.

2
The cells, tissues and organisation of the body

CELLS

Cells are the smallest functional units of the body. They are grouped together to form *tissues*, each of which has a specialised function, e.g. blood, muscle, bone. Different tissues are grouped together to form *organs*, e.g. heart, stomach, brain. Organs are grouped together to form *systems*, each of which performs a particular function, e.g. the digestive system is responsible for taking in, digesting and absorbing food and involves a number of organs, including the stomach and intestines.

The cell

The human body develops from a single cell called the *zygote* which results from the fusion of the ovum (female egg cell) and the spermatozoon (male germ cell). Cell multiplication follows and, as the fetus grows, cells with different structural and functional specialisations develop, all with the same genetic make-up as the zy-gote. Individual cells are too small to be seen with the naked eye. However, they can be seen when thin slices of *tissue*, consisting of millions of cells, are stained in the laboratory and magnified by a microscope. Different types of cell are distinguished by the dye they absorb and by their shape and size.

A cell consists of a *plasma membrane* inside which there are a number of *organelles* floating in a watery fluid called *cytosol* (Fig. 2.1). Organelles are small structures with highly specialised functions, many of which are contained within a membrane. They include: the *nucleus, mitochondria, ribosomes, endoplasmic reticulum, Golgi apparatus, lysosomes, microfilaments* and *microtubules*.

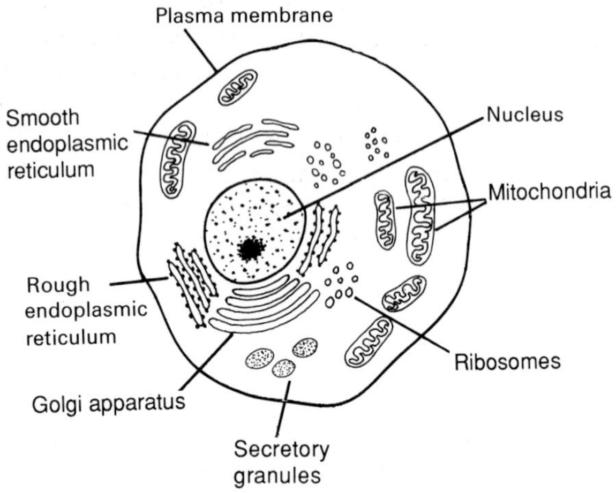

Plasma membrane

The plasma membrane (Fig. 2.2) consists of two layers of phospholipids (fatty substances) with some protein molecules embedded in them. Those that extend all the way through the membrane may provide channels that allow the passage of, e.g. electrolytes, non-lipid-soluble substances.

The phospholipid molecules have a head which is electrically charged and hydrophilic (attracting water) and a tail which has no charge and is hydrophobic (water repelling). The phospholipid bilayer is arranged like a sandwich with the hydrophilic heads aligned on the outer surfaces of the membrane and the hydrophobic tails forming a central water-repelling layer. These differences influence the transfer of substances across the membrane.

The membrane proteins perform several functions:

Figure 2.1 The simple cell.

Labels for Figure 2.1: Plasma membrane; Smooth endoplasmic reticulum; Nucleus; Mitochondria; Rough endoplasmic reticulum; Ribosomes; Golgi apparatus; Secretory granules

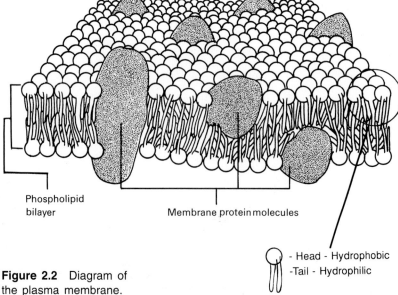

Phospholipid bilayer

Membrane protein molecules

- Head - Hydrophobic
-Tail - Hydrophilic

Figure 2.2 Diagram of the plasma membrane.

- they give the cell its immunological identity (p. 64)
- they can act as specific receptors for hormones and other chemical messengers
- some are enzymes
- some are involved in transport across the membrane.

Organelles

Nucleus

Every cell in the body has a nucleus, with the exception of mature erythrocytes (red blood cells). The nucleus is contained within a membrane similar to the plasma membrane but it has tiny pores through which some substances can pass between it and the *cytoplasm*,

i.e. the cell contents excluding the nucleus. The nucleus contains chromosomes, the body's genetic material in the form of large double chains of molecules of *deoxyribonucleic acid* (DNA), in a spiral (helical) arrangement which resembles a twisted ladder (Fig. 2.3). *Chromosomes* are clusters of DNA molecules.

The molecule of DNA is a sequence of *nucleotides*. Each nucleotide has three components: a sugar molecule, a phosphate group and a nitrogen-containing *base*. There are four bases in DNA: adenine [A], thiamine [T], guanine [G] and cytosine [C] and they occur in a set pattern: A in one chain is paired with T in the other, and G with C. In this way the nucleotides are arranged in a precisely ordered manner in which one chain is complementary to the other. DNA acts as the template for each protein synthesised within the cell. The functional subunits of chromosomes are called *genes*, each of which corresponds to about 1000 pairs of nucleotides. Each cell contains the total complement of genes required to synthesise all the proteins in the body but most cells only synthesise the defined range of proteins that are appropriate to their own specialised functions. This means that only part of the *genome* or *genetic code* is used by each cell. Metabolic processes occur in a series of steps, each of which is catalysed by a specific enzyme, and each enzyme can only be produced if the controlling gene is present. This is the 'one gene, one enzyme' concept. Therefore, when a gene is missing the associated enzyme is also missing and the chemical change it should catalyse does not occur (Fig. 2.4). This means that the intermediate metabolic product upon which the enzyme should act

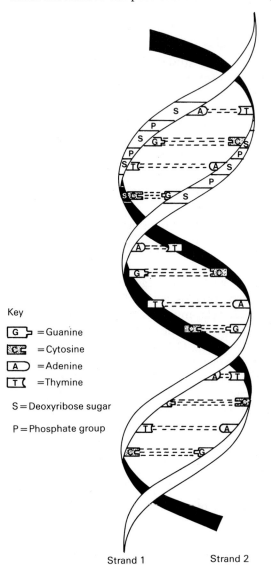

Key

[G] = Guanine

[C] = Cytosine

[A] = Adenine

[T] = Thymine

S = Deoxyribose sugar

P = Phosphate group

Strand 1   Strand 2

Figure 2.3 Diagram of deoxyribonucleic acid.

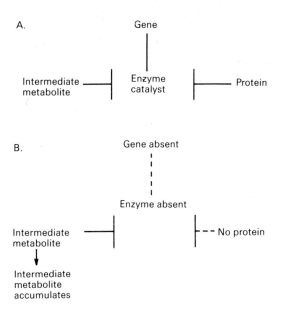

Figure 2.4 Diagram of the relationship between genes, enzymes and metabolism.

accumulates. In physiological quantities such metabolites are harmless but when they accumulate they may become toxic. There are a number of diseases caused by such inborn errors of metabolism, e.g. phenylketonuria, abnormal haemoglobin and some immune deficiencies (see later chapters).

The transfer of genetic information from nuclear DNA to the site where proteins are synthesised in the cytoplasm is the function of ribonucleic acid (RNA). The formation of RNA is controlled by genes in the DNA, i.e. genetic information passes from DNA in the nucleus to RNA promoting protein synthesis in the cytoplasm.

$$DNA \longrightarrow RNA \longrightarrow Protein$$

Mitochondria
These are sausage-shaped structures in the cytoplasm, sometimes described as the power house of the cell. They are involved in cellular respiration, the processes by which chemical energy is made available in the cell. This is in the form of adenosine triphosphate (ATP). ATP is a high energy unstable compound formed from the catabolism of carbohydrates, fats and, if these are in short supply, proteins. Synthesis of ATP is most efficient in the final stages of cellular respiration. This is called oxidative phosphorylation, requiring the presence of oxygen.

Ribosomes
These are tiny granules composed of RNA and protein. They synthesise proteins from amino acids, using RNA as the template. When present in free units or in small clusters in the cytoplasm, the ribosomes make proteins for use within the cell. Ribosomes are also found on the outer surface of rough endoplasmic reticulum.

Endoplasmic reticulum (ER)
This is a series of membranous canals in the cytoplasm. There are two types, smooth and rough. Smooth ER synthesises lipids and steroid hormones, and is also associated with the detoxification of some drugs. Rough ER is studded with *ribosomes*. It is the site of synthesis of proteins that are 'exported' (extruded) from cells, i.e. enzymes and hormones that pass out of their parent cell to be used by other cells in the body.

Golgi apparatus
This consists of stacks of closely folded flattened membranous sacs. It is present in all cells but is larger in

those that synthesise and export proteins. The proteins move from the endoplasmic reticulum to the Golgi apparatus where they are 'packaged' into *secretory vesicles*, sometimes called *secretory granules*. The vesicles are stored and, when needed, they move to the plasma membrane, through which the proteins are exported.

Lysosomes
These are oval or spherical membrane-bound bodies formed by the Golgi apparatus. They contain a variety of enzymes involved in breaking down fragments of organelles and large molecules (e.g. RNA, DNA, carbohydrates, proteins) inside the cell into smaller particles that are then extruded from the cell as waste material.

Lysosomes in white blood cells contain enzymes that digest foreign material such as microbes.

Microfilaments and microtubules
These are contractile structures in the cytoplasm involved in the movement of the cell and of organelles within the cell, the movement of cilia (small projections from the free border of some cells) and possibly the organisation of proteins in the plasma membrane. They also maintain the characteristic shape of the cell.

Cell division (multiplication) (Fig. 2.5)

There are two types of cell division, *mitosis* and *meiosis*.

Mitosis
Beginning with the fertilised egg, or zygote, cell division is an ongoing process. As the fetus develops in the mother's uterus, cells multiply and grow into all the specialities that provide the sum total of the body's physiological functions. The life span of most individual cells is limited. Many become worn out and die, and are replaced by identical cells by the process of mitosis.

Mitosis occurs in two stages: replication of DNA, in the form of 23 pairs of chromosomes, then division of the cytoplasm. DNA is the only type of molecule capable of independently forming a duplicate of itself. When the two identical sets of chromosomes have moved to the opposite poles of the parent cell, a 'waist' forms in the cytoplasm, and the cell divides. There is then a complete set of chromosomes in each daughter cell. The organelles in the cytoplasm of the daughter cells are incomplete at cell division but they develop as the cell grows to maturity.

The frequency with which cell division occurs varies with different types of cell.

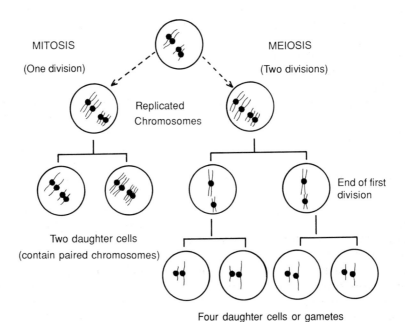

MOTHER CELL

(Before chromosomes
have replicated)

MITOSIS   MEIOSIS

(One division)   (Two divisions)

Replicated
Chromosomes

End of first
division

Two daughter cells
(contain paired chromosomes)

Four daughter cells or gametes

Figure 2.5 Cell division. Simplified diagram of mitosis and meiosis.

Meiosis

This is the process of cell division that occurs in the formation of reproductive cells (*gametes*—the ova and spermatozoa). The ova grow to maturity in the ovaries of the female and the spermatozoa in the testes of the male. In meiosis four daughter cells are formed after two divisions. During meiosis the pairs of chromosomes separate and one from each pair moves to opposite poles of the 'parent' cell. When it divides, each of the 'daughter' cells has only 23 chromosomes, i.e. the haploid number. This means that when the ovum is fertilised the resultant zygote has the full complement of 46 chomosomes, half from the father and half from the mother. Thus the child has some characteristics inherited from the mother and some from the father, such as colour of hair and eyes, height, facial features, and some diseases.

Determination of sex depends upon one pair of chromosomes, the *sex chromosomes*. In the female both sex chromosomes are the same size and shape and are called X chromosomes. In the male there is one X chromosome and a slightly smaller Y chromosome. When the ovum is fertilised by an X-bearing spermatozoon the child is female and when by a Y-bearing spermatozoon the child is male.

Sperm X + ovum X = child XX = female
Sperm Y + ovum X = child XY = male

Mutation

Cells are said to mutate when their genetic make-up is altered in any way. Mutation may cause:

- no significant change in cell function
- modification of cell function that may cause physiological abnormality but does not prevent cell growth and multiplication, e.g. inborn errors of metabolism, defective blood clotting
- the death of the cell.

Some mutations occur by chance, which may be accounted for by the countless millions of cell divisions and DNA replications that occur in the body throughout life. Others may be caused by extraneous factors, such as X-rays, ultraviolet rays, some chemicals.

The most important mutations are those that occur in the ova and spermatozoa. Genetic changes in these cells are passed on to subsequent generations although they do not affect the parent.

Transfer of substances across cell membranes

Some substances cross plasma and organelle membranes by passing from a higher concentration on one side to a lower concentration on the other, without the use of energy. These are said to pass *down the concentration gradient* (downhill). Other substances that pass *up the concentration gradient* (uphill), i.e. from a lower to a higher concentration, require the input of energy.

Diffusion

This is the physical process involved in the 'downhill' movement of substances (see also p. 51 and Fig. 2.6). The molecules in solution bombard and pass through the membrane in a random fashion, so that eventually the concentration is the same on both sides of the membrane. Substances are transferred by:

- dissolving in the lipid part of the membrane, e.g. lipid-soluble substances: oxygen, carbon dioxide, fatty acids, steroids
- passing through water-filled channels, or pores, that form in the protein molecules in the membrane, e.g. small, water-soluble substances: sodium, potassium, calcium
- binding to specialised protein 'carriers' on one side of the membrane which deposit the substance on the other, called *facilitated diffusion*, e.g. larger molecules: glucose, amino acids (Fig. 2.7). As there are a finite number of carriers, there is a limit to the amount of a substance which can be transported at any time. The limit is called the *transport maximum*.

Active transport

This is the 'uphill' transport of substances across membranes. It involves the input of energy derived from ATP, a high-energy molecule inside cells. In this way substances may be 'pumped' across membranes in either direction.

The mechanism of active transport is the same as in facilitated diffusion. The 'carrier' molecules have specific sites that attract and bind the substances to be transferred, like a lock and key mechanism. The carrier then changes its shape and deposits the substance on the other side of the membrane (Fig. 2.7). The carrier sites are specific and can be used by only one substance; therefore the rate at which a substance is transferred depends on the number of sites available.

The sodium pump. This active transport mechanism maintains homeostasis of the electrolytes sodium (Na^+) and potassium (K^+). It may utilise up to 30% of the ATP required for cellular metabolism.

The principal cations are: K^+ intracellularly and Na^+ extracellularly. There is a tendency for these ions to diffuse along their concentration gradients, K^+ outwards and Na^+ into the cell. Excess Na^+ is pumped out across the cell membrane in exchange for K^+.

Bulk transport (Fig. 2.8)

Transfer of particles too large to cross cell membranes occurs by *pinocytosis* or *phagocytosis*. These particles are engulfed by extensions of the cytoplasm which enclose

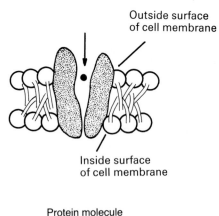
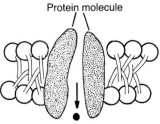

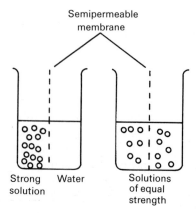

Figure 2.6 Diffusion.

Figure 2.7 Facilitated diffusion and active transport.

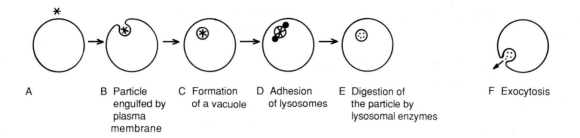

Figure 2.8 Bulk transport across plasma membranes: A.–E. phagocytosis; F. exocytosis.

them, forming a membrane-bound vacuole. When the vacuole is small, pinocytosis occurs. In phagocytosis, larger particles, e.g. cell fragments, foreign materials, microbes, are taken into the cell. Lysosomes then adhere to the vacuole membrane, releasing enzymes which digest the contents.

Extrusion of waste material by the reverse process through the plasma membrane is called *exocytosis*. Secretory packages formed by the Golgi apparatus usually leave the cell in this way, as do any indigestible residues of phagocytosis.

TISSUES

The tissues of the body consist of large numbers of cells and they are classified according to the size, shape and functions of these cells. There are four main types of tissue, each of which has subdivisions. They are:

- epithelial tissue or epithelium
- connective tissue
- muscle tissue
- nervous tissue.

Epithelial tissue

This group of tissues is found covering the body and lining cavities and tubes. It is also found in glands. The structure of epithelium is closely related to its functions which include:

- protection of underlying structures
- secretion
- absorption.

The cells are very closely packed and the intercellular substance, called the *matrix*, is minimal. The cells usually lie on a *basement membrane* which is an inert connective tissue.

Epithelial tissue may be:

- *simple*: a single layer of cells
- *stratified*: several layers of cells.

Simple epithelium

Simple epithelium consists of a single layer of identical cells and is divided into four types. It is usually found on absorptive or secretory surfaces where the single layer enhances these processes, but never on surfaces subject to stress. The types are named according to the shape of the cells, which differ according to their functions. The more active the tissue the taller the cells.

Squamous (pavement) epithelium

This is composed of a single layer of flattened cells (Fig. 2.9). The cells fit closely together like flat stones, forming a thin and very smooth membrane.

Diffusion takes place freely through this thin, smooth, inactive lining of the following structures:

- heart
- blood vessels   } where it is also known as
- lymph vessels   endothelium
- alveoli of the lungs.

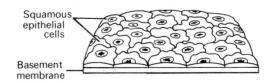

Figure 2.9 Squamous epithelium.

Cuboidal (cubical) epithelium

This consists of cube-shaped cells fitting closely together lying on a basement membrane (Fig. 2.10). It forms the tubules of the kidneys and is found in some glands. Cuboidal epithelium is actively involved in secretion, absorption and excretion.

Columnar epithelium

This is formed by a single layer of cells, rectangular in shape, on a basement membrane (Fig. 2.11). It is found lining the organs of the alimentary tract and consists of a mixture of cells; some absorb the products of digestion and others secrete *mucus*. Mucus is a thick sticky substance secreted by modified columnar cells called *goblet cells*.

Ciliated epithelium (Fig. 2.12)

This is formed by columnar cells which have fine, hair-like processes, called *cilia*. The cilia consist of microtubules inside the plasma membrane that extends from the free border (luminal border) of the columnar cells. The wave-like movement of many cilia propels the contents of the tubes which they line in one direction only.

Ciliated epithelium is found lining the uterine tubes and most of the respiratory passages. In the uterine tubes the cilia propel ova towards the uterus (Ch. 18) and in the respiratory passages they propel mucus towards the throat (Ch. 10).

Stratified epithelia

Stratified epithelia consist of several layers of cells of various shapes. The superficial layers grow up from below. Basement membranes are usually absent. The main function of compound epithelium is to protect underlying structures. There are two main types: stratified and transitional.

Stratified squamous epithelium (Fig. 2.13)

This is composed of a number of layers of cells of different shapes. In the deepest layers the cells are mainly columnar and, as they grow towards the surface, they become flattened.

Non-keratinised stratified epithelium is found on wet surfaces that may be subjected to wear and tear but are protected from drying, e.g. the conjunctiva of the eyes, the lining of the mouth, the pharynx, the oesophagus and the vagina.

Keratinised stratified epithelium is found on dry surfaces that are subjected to wear and tear, i.e. skin, hair and nails. The surface layer consists of dead epithelial cells to which the protein keratin has been added. This forms a tough, relatively waterproof protective layer

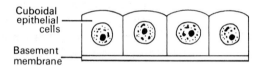

Figure 2.10 Cuboidal epithelium.

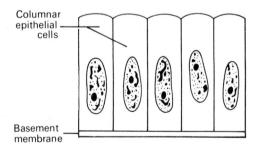

Figure 2.11 Columnar epithelium.

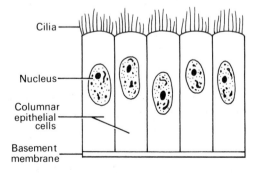

Figure 2.12 Ciliated columnar epithelium.

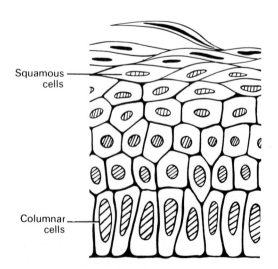

Figure 2.13 Stratified epithelium.

that prevents drying of the underlying live cells. The surface layer of skin is rubbed off and is replaced from below (Ch. 14).

Transitional epithelium (Fig. 2.14)
This is composed of several layers of pear-shaped cells and is found lining the urinary bladder. It allows for stretching as the bladder fills.

Connective tissue

The cells forming the connective tissues are more widely separated from each other than those forming the epithelium, and intercellular substance is present in considerably larger amounts. There may or may not be fibres present in the matrix, which may be of a semi-solid jelly-like consistency or dense and rigid, depending upon the position and function of the tissue. Major functions of connective tissue are:

- binding and support
- protection
- transport
- insulation.

Cells of connective tissue

Connective tissue, excluding blood (Ch. 4), is found in all organs supporting the specialised tissue. The different types of cell involved include:

- fibroblasts
- macrophages
- plasma cells
- mast cells
- fat cells.

Fibroblasts
These are large flat cells with irregular processes. They produce *collagen* and *elastic* fibres and a matrix of extracellular material. Very fine collagen fibres, sometimes called reticulin fibres, are found in very active tissue, such as the liver and lymphoid tissue. Fibroblasts are particularly active in tissue repair where they may bind together the cut surfaces of wounds or form *granulation tissue* following tissue destruction (see p. 366). The collagen fibres formed during healing shrink as they grow old, sometimes interfering with the functions of the organ involved and with adjacent structures.

In some glands a type of fibroblast called *reticular cells* produce fine fibrous strands called *reticulin* and are closely associated with phagocytosis.

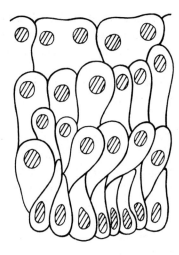

Figure 2.14
Transitional epithelium.

Macrophages
These are irregular-shaped cells with granules in the cytoplasm. Some are fixed, i.e. attached to connective tissue fibres, and others are *motile*. They are actively phagocytic, engulfing and digesting cell debris, bacteria and other foreign bodies. Their activities are typical of those of the macrophage/monocyte defence system, e.g. monocytes in blood, phagocytes in the alveoli of the lungs, Kupffer cells in liver sinusoids, fibroblasts in lymph nodes and spleen and microglial cells in the brain.

Plasma cells
Plasma cells are derived from B-lymphocytes (see p. 65). They synthesise and secrete specific antibodies into the blood in response to the presence of foreign material, such as microbes.

Mast cells
These cells are similar to basophil leukocytes (see p. 63). They are found in loose connective tissue and under the fibrous capsule of some organs, e.g. liver and spleen, and in considerable numbers round blood vessels. They produce granules containing *heparin*, *serotonin* (5-hydroxytryptamine) and *histamine* which are released when the cells are damaged by disease or injury. Histamine is involved in local and general inflammatory reactions, it stimulates the secretion of gastric juice and may be associated with the development of allergies and hypersensitivity (see p. 67). Heparin prevents coagulation of plasma which may aid the passage of protective substances from blood to affected tissues.

Fat cells
These cells occur singly or in groups in many types of connective tissue and are especially abundant in adipose

tissue. They vary in size and shape according to the amount of fat they contain.

Areolar tissue (Fig. 2.15)

This is the most generalised of all connective tissue. The matrix is described as semisolid with many *fibroblasts* widely separated by *elastic* and *collagen fibres*. It is found in almost every part of the body providing elasticity and tensile strength. It connects and supports other tissues, for example:

■ under the skin
■ between muscles
■ supporting blood vessels and nerves
■ in the alimentary canal
■ in glands supporting secretory cells.

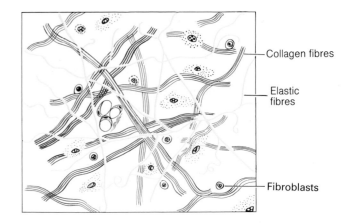

Figure 2.15   Areolar tissue.

Adipose tissue (Fig. 2.16)

Adipose tissue consists of fat cells, containing large fat globules, in a matrix of areolar tissue. There are two types: white and brown.

White adipose tissue makes up 20 to 25% of body weight in well-nourished adults. It is found supporting the kidneys and the eyes, between muscle fibres and under the skin, where it acts as a thermal insulator.

Brown adipose tissue is present in relatively small quantities situated mainly between the scapulae, in the nape of the neck and in the walls of the large blood vessels of the trunk. It has a more extensive capillary network than white adipose tissue. When brown tissue is metabolised, it produces less energy and considerably more heat than other fat, contributing to the maintenance of body temperature and preventing obesity.

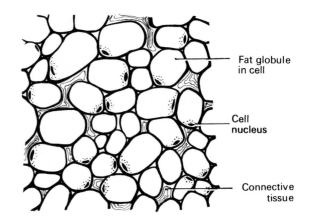

Figure 2.16   Adipose tissue.

Fibrous tissue (Fig. 2.17)

This is a dense fibrous connective tissue made up mainly of closely packed bundles of *collagen fibres* with very little matrix. There are very few cells, lying in rows between the bundles of fibres. Fibrous tissue is found:

■ forming the ligaments which bind bones together
■ as an outer protective covering for bone, called *periosteum*
■ as an outer protective covering of some organs, e.g. the kidneys, lymph nodes and the brain
■ forming muscle sheaths, called *muscle fascia*, which extend beyond the muscle to become the tendon that attaches the muscle to bone.

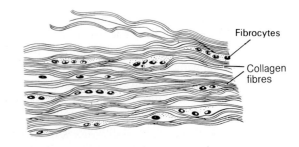

Figure 2.17   Fibrous tissue.

Elastic tissue (Fig. 2.18)

Elastic tissue is capable of considerable extension and recoil. There are few cells and the matrix consists mainly of masses of *elastic fibres* secreted by fibroblasts. It is found in organs where alteration of shape is required, e.g. in blood vessel walls and in the elastic cartilage of the epiglottis and the external ears.

Blood

This is a fluid connective tissue and is described in detail in Chapter 4.

Lymphoid tissue (Fig. 2.19)

This tissue has a semisolid matrix with fine branching reticulin fibres. The highly specialised cells are called *lymphocytes* (see p. 64). They are found in blood and in lymphoid tissue in the:

- lymph nodes
- spleen
- palatine and pharyngeal tonsils
- vermiform appendix
- solitary and aggregated nodes in the small intestine
- wall of the large intestine.

Cartilage

Cartilage is a much firmer tissue than any of the other connective tissues; the cells are called *chondrocytes* and are less numerous. They are embedded in matrix reinforced by collagen and elastic fibres. There are three types:

- hyaline
- fibrocartilage
- elastic fibrocartilage.

Hyaline cartilage (Fig. 2.20)

Hyaline cartilage appears as a smooth bluish-white tissue. The chondrocytes are in small groups and the matrix is solid and smooth. Hyaline cartilage is found:

- on the surface of the parts of the bones which form joints
- forming the costal cartilages which attach the ribs to the sternum
- forming part of the larynx, trachea and bronchi.

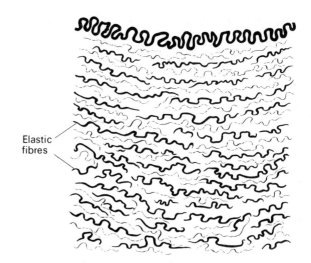

Figure 2.18 Elastic tissue.

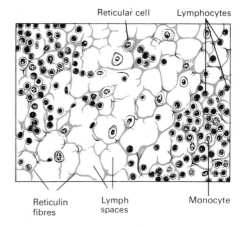

Figure 2.19 Lymphoid tissue.

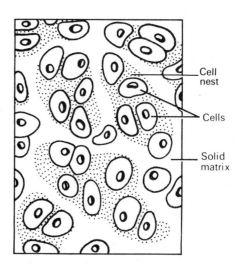

Figure 2.20 Hyaline cartilage.

Fibrocartilage (Fig. 2.21)

This consists of dense masses of white fibres in a matrix similar to that of hyaline cartilage with the cells widely dispersed. It is a tough, slightly flexible tissue found:

- as pads between the bodies of the vertebrae, called the intervertebral discs
- between the articulating surfaces of the bones of the knee joint, called semilunar cartilages
- on the rim of the bony sockets of the hip and shoulder joints, deepening the cavities without restricting movement
- as ligaments joining bones.

Elastic cartilage (Fig. 2.22)

This consists of elastic fibres lying in a solid matrix. The cells lie between the fibres. It forms the pinna or lobe of the ear, the epiglottis and part of the tunica media of blood vessel walls.

Bone

Bone is a connective tissue with cells (osteocytes) surrounded by a matrix of collagen fibres that is strengthened by inorganic salts, especially calcium and phosphate. This provides bones with their characteristic strength and rigidity. Bone also has considerable capacity for growth in the first two decades of life, and for regeneration throughout life. Two types of bone can be identified by the naked eye:

- compact bone—solid or dense appearance
- cancellous or spongy bone—spongy or fine honeycomb appearance.

These are described in detail in Chapter 15.

Muscle tissue

There are three types of muscle tissue:

- striated, skeletal or voluntary muscle
- non-striated, involuntary, visceral or smooth muscle
- cardiac muscle.

Striated muscle tissue (Fig. 2.23)

This may be described as *skeletal*, *striated*, *striped* or *voluntary* muscle. It is called voluntary because contraction is under the control of the will.

When voluntary muscle is examined microscopically the cells are found to be roughly cylindrical in shape and may be as long as 35 cm. Each cell, commonly

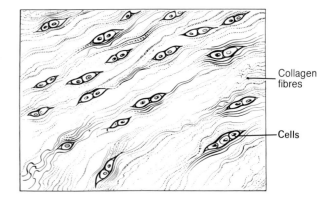

Figure 2.21   Fibrocartilage.

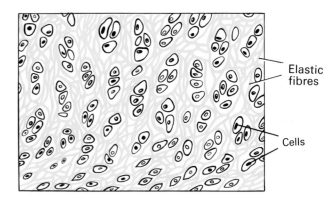

Figure 2.22   Elastic fibrocartilage.

called a fibre, has several nuclei situated just under the *sarcolemma*, or cell membrane of each muscle fibre. The muscle fibres lie parallel to one another and, when viewed under the microscope, they show well-marked transverse dark and light bands, hence the name striated or striped muscle.

Sarcoplasm, the cytoplasm of muscle fibres, contains:

- bundles of myofibrils which consist of filaments of contractile proteins including *actin* and *myosin*
- many mitochondria that generate chemical energy (ATP) from glucose and oxygen by cellular oxidation
- *glycogen*, a carbohydrate store which is broken down into glucose when required
- *myoglobin*, a unique oxygen-binding protein molecule, similar to haemoglobin in red blood cells (p. 59), that stores oxygen within muscle cells.

A myofibril has a repeating series of dark and light bands, consisting of units called *sarcomeres*. A sarcomere represents the smallest functional unit of a skeletal muscle fibre and consists of:

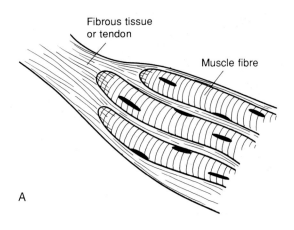

Fibrous tissue or tendon

Muscle fibre

A

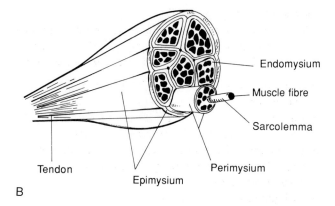

Endomysium

Muscle fibre

Sarcolemma

Perimysium

Tendon

Epimysium

B

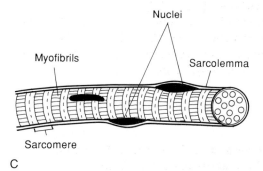

Nuclei

Myofibrils

Sarcolemma

Sarcomere

C

Figure 2.23 Striated muscle fibres and their connective tissue.
A. Longitudinal section with some connective tissue removed.
B. Cross section.
C. A single fibre.

- thin filaments of actin
- thick filaments of myosin.

The sliding filament theory explains the finding that sarcomeres shorten but the filaments remain the same length when skeletal muscle contracts. The thin actin filaments slide past the thick myosin filaments, increasing the overlap of the filaments when contraction takes place. The movement of filaments occurs as chemical cross-bridges are formed and broken, moving the actin filaments towards the centre of the sarcomere during contraction. As the sarcomeres shorten, so does the skeletal muscle involved. When the muscle relaxes, the cross-bridges break and the filaments slide apart and the sarcomeres return to their original length.

A muscle consists of a large number of muscle fibres. In addition to the sarcolemma mentioned previously, each fibre is enclosed in and attached to fine fibrous tissue called *endomysium*. Small bundles of fibres are enclosed in *perimysium*, and the whole muscle in *epimysium*. The fibrous tissue enclosing the fibres, the bundles and the whole muscle extends beyond the muscle fibres to become the *tendon* which attaches the muscle to bone or skin.

Non-striated (visceral) muscle tissue (Fig. 2.24)
Non-striated muscle may also be described as *smooth* or *involuntary*. It is not under the control of the will. It is found in the walls of hollow organs, i.e. blood and lymph vessels, ducts of glands, the alimentary tract, the respiratory tract, the urinary bladder, the biliary tract and the uterus.

When examined under a microscope, the cells are seen to be spindle-shaped with only one central nucleus. There is no distinct sarcolemma but a very fine membrane surrounds each fibre. Bundles of fibres form sheets of muscle, such as those found in the walls of the above structures.

Cardiac muscle tissue (Fig. 2.25)
This type of muscle tissue is found exclusively in the wall of the heart. It is not under the control of the will but, when viewed under a microscope, cross stripes characteristic of voluntary muscle can be seen. Each

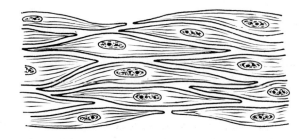

Figure 2.24 Smooth muscle fibres.

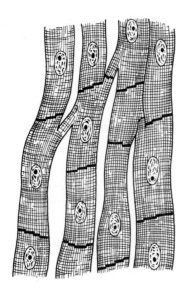

Figure 2.25
Cardiac muscle fibres.

fibre (cell) has a nucleus and one or more branches. The ends of the cells and their branches are in very close contact with the ends and branches of adjacent cells. Microscopically these 'joints', or *intercalated discs*, can be seen as lines which are thicker and darker than the ordinary cross stripes. This arrangement gives cardiac muscle the appearance of a sheet of muscle rather than a very large number of individual fibres. The end-to-end contiguity of cardiac muscle cells has significance in relation to the way the heart contracts. A wave of contraction spreads from cell to cell across the intercalated discs which means that cells do not need to be stimulated individually.

Function of muscle

Muscle functions by alternate phases of contraction and relaxation. When the fibres contract they become thicker and shorter. Skeletal muscle fibres are stimulated by *motor nerve impulses* originating in the brain or spinal cord (p. 151 and p. 159). Non-striated and cardiac muscle have the intrinsic ability to initiate contraction. In addition, contraction is stimulated by *autonomic nerve impulses*, some hormones and local metabolites (see p. 141). When muscle fibres contract they follow the *all or none law*, i.e. each fibre contracts to its full capacity. The *strength* of contraction, e.g. lifting a weight, depends on the *number* of fibres contracting at the same time. When effort is sustained, groups of fibres contract in series. Contraction of non-striated muscle is slower and more sustained than skeletal muscle.

In order to contract when it is stimulated, a muscle fibre must have an adequate blood supply to provide sufficient oxygen, calcium and nutritional materials and to remove waste products.

Muscle tone

This is a state of partial contraction of muscles. It is achieved by the contraction of a few muscle fibres at a time. Muscle tone in relation to striated muscle is associated with the maintenance of posture in the sitting and standing positions. The muscle is stimulated to contract through a system of *spinal reflexes*. Stretching a muscle or its tendon stimulates the reflex action (Ch. 7). A degree of muscle tone is also maintained by smooth and cardiac muscle.

Muscle fatigue

If a muscle is stimulated to contract at very frequent intervals, it gradually becomes depressed and will cease to respond. Fatigue is prevented during sustained muscular effort because the fibres usually contract in series. All the fibres of a muscle rarely contract at the same time but if maximum effort is made it can be sustained, if for only a short time.

Energy source for muscle contraction

The chemical energy (ATP) which muscles require is derived from the breakdown (catabolism) of carbohydrate and fat. Protein molecules inside the fibres are used to provide energy when supplies of carbohydrate and fat are deficient. Each molecule undergoes a series of changes and, with each change, small quantities of energy are released. For the complete breakdown of these molecules and the release of all the available energy, an adequate supply of oxygen is required. If the individual undertakes excessive exercise, the oxygen supply may be insufficient to meet the metabolic needs of the muscle fibres. This may result in the accumulation of intermediate metabolic products, such as lactic acid. Where the breakdown process and the release of energy are complete, the waste products are carbon dioxide and water (Ch. 12).

Not all the chemical energy (ATP) used by muscle fibres is converted into mechanical energy during contraction. Some is lost as heat.

Further features of striated muscle

The voluntary muscles are those which produce body movements. Each muscle consists of a *fleshy* part made up of striped fibres and *tendinous* parts consisting of fibrous tissue, usually at both ends of the fleshy part. The muscle is attached to bone or skin by these tendons. When the tendinous attachment of a muscle is broad and flat it is called an *aponeurosis*.

To be able to produce movement at a joint, a muscle or its tendon *must stretch across the joint*. When a muscle contracts, its fibres *shorten and it pulls* one bone towards another, e.g. bending the elbow.

The muscles of the skeleton are arranged in groups, some of which are *antagonistic* to each other. To produce movement at a joint, one muscle or group of muscles contracts while the antagonists relax, e.g. to bend the knee the muscles on the back of the thigh contract and those on the front relax. The constant adjustment of the contraction and relaxation of antagonistic groups of muscles is well demonstrated in the maintenance of balance and posture when sitting and standing. These adjustments usually occur without conscious effort.

Individual muscles and groups of muscles have been given names that reflect certain characteristics, e.g.:

- *the shape* of the muscle—the trapezius is shaped like a trapezium
- *the direction* in which the fibres run—the oblique muscles of the abdominal wall
- *the position* of the muscle—the tibialis in the leg is associated with the tibia
- *the movement* produced by contraction of the muscle—flexors, extensors, adductors.
- *the number of points of attachment* of a muscle—the biceps muscle has two tendons at one end.
- *the names of the bones to which the muscle is attached*—the carpi radialis muscles are attached to the carpal bones in the wrist and to the radius in the forearm.

A more detailed description of voluntary muscles is given in Chapters 16 and 17.

Nervous tissue

Two types of tissue are found in the nervous system:

- excitable cells—they are called neurones and they initiate, receive, conduct and transmit information
- non-excitable cells—they support the neurones.

These are described in detail in Chapter 7.

Cell regeneration

When cell regeneration occurs it is essential that some of the original cells are available to replicate by mitosis. The extent to which regeneration is possible depends on the normal rate of physiological turnover of particular types of cell. Those with a rapid turnover regenerate most effectively. There are three types.

Labile cells are those in which replication is normally a continuous process. They include cells in:

- epithelium of, e.g., skin, mucous membrane, secretory glands, ducts, uterus lining
- bone marrow
- blood
- spleen and lymphoid tissue.

Stable cells have retained the ability to replicate but do so infrequently. They include:

- liver, kidney and pancreatic cells
- fibroblasts
- smooth muscle cells
- osteoblasts and osteoclasts in bone.

Permanent cells are unable to replicate after normal growth is complete. They include:

- nerve cells (neurones)
- skeletal and cardiac muscle.

Membranes

Membranes are sheets of epithelial tissue and their basement membranes that cover or line internal structures or cavities. The main membranes are:

- mucous
- serous
- synovial.

Mucous membrane

This is the moist lining of the alimentary tract, respiratory tract and genito-urinary tracts and is sometimes referred to as the *mucosa*. The membrane consists of epithelial cells, some of which produce a secretion called *mucus*, a slimy tenacious fluid. As it accumulates the cells become distended and finally burst, discharging the mucus on to the free surface. As the cells fill up with mucus they have the appearance of a goblet or flask and are known as *goblet cells* (Fig. 2.26). Organs

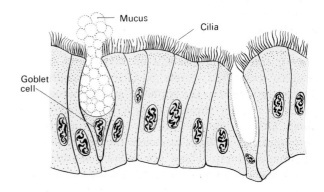

Figure 2.26 Ciliated columnar epithelium with goblet cells.

lined by mucous membrane have a moist slippery surface. Mucus protects the lining membrane from mechanical and chemical injury and in the respiratory tract it traps inhaled foreign particles, preventing them from entering the alveoli of the lungs.

Serous membrane

Serous membranes, or serosa, secrete serous watery fluid. They consist of a double layer of epithelial tissue. The *visceral* layer closely invests organs and the *parietal* layer lines the space that they occupy. The visceral layer is reflected off the organ to become the parietal layer and the two layers are separated by a watery or *serous fluid* secreted by the membrane.

There are three sites in which serous membranes are found. In the thoracic cavity the *pleura* surround the lungs and the *pericardium* surrounds the heart, and in the abdominal cavity the *peritoneum* surrounds the abdominal organs.

The serous fluid between the visceral and parietal layers enables an organ to move without being damaged by friction between it and adjacent organs. For example, the heart changes its shape and size during each beat and friction damage is prevented by the arrangement of pericardium and its serous fluid.

Synovial membrane

This membrane is found lining the joint cavities and surrounding tendons which could be injured by rubbing against bones, e.g. over the wrist joint. It is made up of a layer of fine, flattened epithelial cells on a layer of delicate connective tissue.

Synovial membrane secretes clear, sticky, oily *synovial fluid* which acts as a lubricant to the joints and helps to maintain their stability. Synovial fluid also helps to nourish the hyaline cartilage which covers the articular surfaces of the bones, and synovial cells remove damaging material from within the joint cavity (Ch. 16).

Glands

Some groups of epithelial cells are called *glands* and they produce specialised secretions. Glands that discharge their secretion on to the epithelial surface of an organ, either directly or through a *duct*, are called *exocrine glands*. Other groups of cells that have become isolated from epithelial surfaces discharge their secretions into blood and lymph. These are called *endocrine glands* (ductless glands) and their secretions are *hormones* (see Ch. 9).

Figure 2.27 shows the different lines of development of exocrine and endocrine glands. Exocrine glands

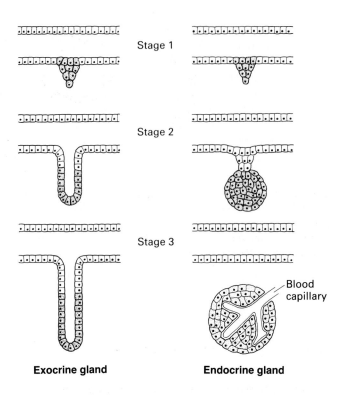

Figure 2.27 Stages of development of exocrine and endocrine glands.

vary considerably in size, shape and complexity as shown in Figure 2.28.

ORGANISATION OF THE BODY

In this part of the chapter a brief account is given of some anatomical terms and the names and positions of bones. A more detailed account of the bones, muscles and joints is given in Chapters 15, 16 and 17.

Anatomical terms

The anatomical position. This is the position assumed in all anatomical descriptions to ensure accuracy and consistency. The body is in the upright position with the head facing forward, the arms at the sides with the palms of the hands facing forward and the feet together.

Median plane. When the body, in the anatomical position, is divided *longitudinally* into right and left halves it has been divided in the median plane.

Medial and lateral. Any structure which is *medial* to another is nearer the midline and any structure *lateral*

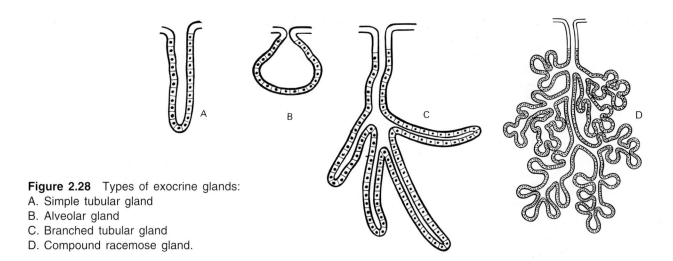

Figure 2.28 Types of exocrine glands:
A. Simple tubular gland
B. Alveolar gland
C. Branched tubular gland
D. Compound racemose gland.

to another is farther from the midline or at the side of the body.

Proximal and distal. These terms are used when describing the bones of the limbs. The proximal end of a bone is the one nearest the point of attachment of the limb, and the distal end is farthest away.

Anterior or ventral. This indicates that the part being described is nearer the front of the body.

Posterior or dorsal. This means that the part being described is nearer the back of the body.

Superior. This indicates a structure nearer the head.

Inferior. This indicates a structure farther away from the head.

Border. This is a ridge of bone which separates two surfaces.

Spine, spinous process or crest. This is a sharp ridge of bone.

Trochanter, tuberosity and tubercle. These are roughened bony projections, usually for the attachment of muscles or ligaments. The different names are used according to the size of the projection. Trochanters are the largest and tubercles the smallest.

Styloid process. This is a sharp downward projection of bone which gives attachment to muscles and ligaments.

Fossa (*plural:* ***fossae***). This is a hollow or depression.

Foramen (*plural:* ***foramina***). This is a hole in a structure.

Bony sinus. This is a hollow cavity within a bone.

Meatus. This indicates a tube-shaped cavity within a bone.

Articulation. This is a joint between two or more bones.

Suture. This is the name given to an immovable joint, e.g. between the bones of the skull.

Articulating surface. This is the part of the bone which enters into the formation of a joint.

Facet. This is a small, generally rather flat, articulating surface.

Condyle. This is a smooth rounded projection of bone which takes part in a joint.

Septum. This is a partition separating two cavities.

Fissure or cleft. This indicates a narrow slit.

Bones of the skeleton

The skeleton is the bony framework of the body. It forms the cavities and fossae that protect some structures, forms the joints and gives attachment to muscles. Bone marrow is involved in the formation of blood cells.

It is described in two parts: *axial* and *appendicular* (Fig. 2.29).

The axial skeleton (axis of the body) consists of:

- skull
- vertebral column
- sternum or breast bone
- ribs.

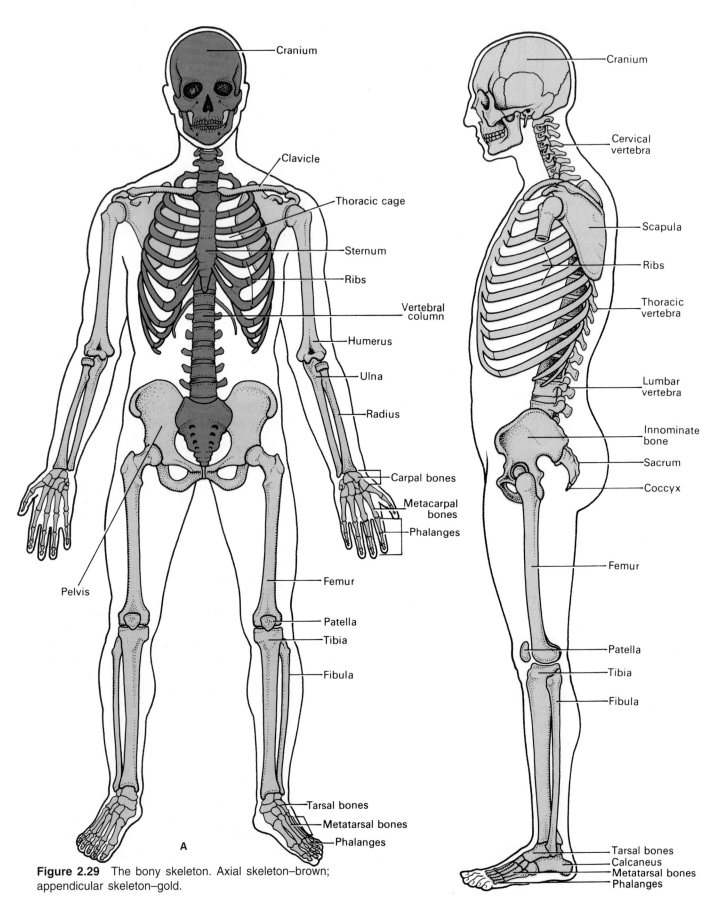

Cranium

Clavicle

Thoracic cage

Sternum

Ribs

Vertebral column

Humerus

Ulna

Radius

Carpal bones

Metacarpal bones

Phalanges

Femur

Patella

Tibia

Fibula

Pelvis

Tarsal bones

Metatarsal bones

Phalanges

A

Cranium

Cervical vertebra

Scapula

Ribs

Thoracic vertebra

Lumbar vertebra

Innominate bone

Sacrum

Coccyx

Femur

Patella

Tibia

Fibula

Tarsal bones
Calcaneus
Metatarsal bones
Phalanges

B

Figure 2.29   The bony skeleton. Axial skeleton–brown; appendicular skeleton–gold.

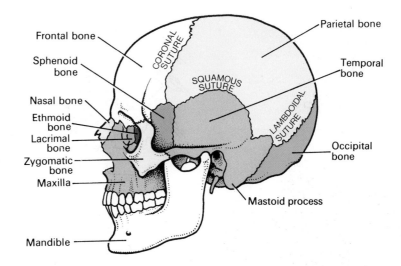

Figure 2.30
The bones of the skull and face.

The appendicular skeleton (appendages attached to the axis of the body) consists of:

- the bones of the upper limbs, the two clavicles and the two scapulae
- the bones of the lower limbs and the two innominate bones of the pelvis.

Axial skeleton (Figs 2.30, 2.31 and 2.32)

Skull

The skull is described in two parts, the *cranium* which contains the brain, and the *face*. It consists of a number of bones which develop separately but fuse together as they mature. The only movable bone is the mandible or lower jaw. The names and positions of the individual bones of the skull can be seen in Figure 2.30.

The various parts of the skull have specific and different functions:

- The cranium protects the delicate tissues of the brain.
- The bony eye sockets provide the eyes with some protection against injury and give attachment to the muscles which move the eyes.
- The temporal bone protects the delicate structures of the ear.
- Some bones of the face and the base of the skull give resonance to the voice because they have

cavities called *sinuses*, containing air. The sinuses have tiny openings into the nasal cavity.
- The bones of the face form the walls of the posterior part of the nasal cavities. They keep the air passage open, facilitating breathing.
- The maxilla and the mandible provide alveolar ridges in which the teeth are embedded.
- The mandible is the only movable bone of the skull and chewing food is the result of raising and lowering the mandible by contracting and relaxing some muscles of the face, the muscles of mastication.

Vertebral column

This consists of 24 movable bones (vertebrae) plus the sacrum and coccyx. The bodies of the bones are separated from each other by *intervertebral discs*, consisting of cartilage. The vertebral column is described in five parts and the bones of each part are numbered from above downwards (Figs 2.29 and 2.31):

- 7 cervical
- 12 thoracic
- 5 lumbar
- 1 sacrum (5 fused bones)
- 1 coccyx (4 fused bones).

The first cervical vertebra, called *the atlas*, articulates with the skull. Thereafter each vertebra forms a joint with the vertebrae immediately above and below. In the cervical and lumbar regions more movement is possible than in the thoracic region.

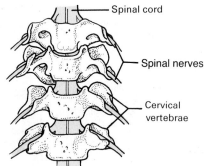

Figure 2.32 The lower cervical vertebrae separated to show the spinal cord and spinal nerves in yellow.

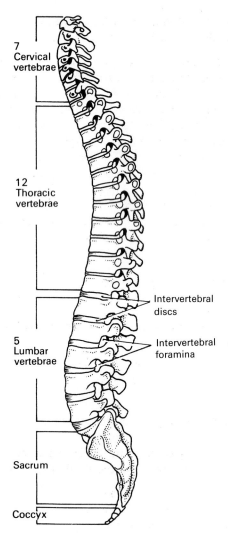

Figure 2.31 The vertebral column—lateral view.

The sacrum consists of five vertebrae fused into one bone which articulates with the 5th lumbar vertebra above, the coccyx below and an innominate (pelvic or hip) bone at each side.

The coccyx consists of the four terminal vertebrae fused into a small triangular bone which articulates with the sacrum above.

Functions of the vertebral column

The vertebral column has several important functions:

■ It protects the spinal cord. In each bone there is a hole or *foramen* and when the vertebrae are arranged one above the other, as shown in Figure 2.31, the foramina form a canal. The spinal cord, which is an extension of nerve tissue from the brain, lies in this canal (Fig. 2.32).

■ Adjacent vertebrae form openings (intervertebral foramina) through which spinal nerves pass from the spinal cord to all parts of the body (Fig. 2.32). There are 31 pairs of spinal nerves.
■ In the thoracic region the ribs articulate with the vertebrae forming joints which move during respiration.

Thoracic cage

The thoracic cage is formed by:

■ 12 thoracic vertebrae
■ 12 pairs of ribs
■ 1 sternum or breast bone.

The arrangement of the bones can be seen in Figure 2.33.

Functions of the thoracic cage

The functions of the thoracic cage are:

■ To protect the thoracic organs. The bony framework protects the heart, lungs, large blood vessels and other structures.
■ To form joints between the upper limbs and the axial skeleton. The upper part of the sternum, the *manubrium*, articulates with the clavicles forming the only joints between the upper limbs and the axial skeleton.
■ To give attachment to the muscles of respiration:
—intercostal muscles occupy the spaces between the ribs and when they contract the ribs move upwards and outwards, increasing the capacity of the thoracic cage, and inspiration (breathing in) occurs.
—the diaphragm is a dome-shaped muscle which separates the thoracic and abdominal cavities. It is attached to the bones of the thorax and when it contracts it assists with inspiration. Structures which extend from one cavity to the other pass through the diaphragm.

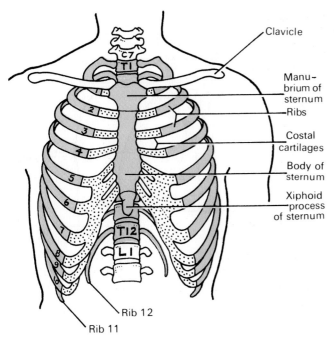

Figure 2.33 The structures forming the walls of the thoracic cage.

Appendicular skeleton

The appendages are:

- the upper limbs and the shoulder girdles
- the lower limbs and the innominate bones of the pelvis.

The names of the bones involved, their position and their relationship to other bones are shown in Figure 2.29.

Functions of the appendicular skeleton

The appendicular skeleton has two functions:

- Voluntary movement. The bones, muscles and joints of the limbs are involved in voluntary movement. This may range from the very fine movements of the fingers associated with writing, to the coordinated movement of all the limbs associated with running and jumping.
- Protection of delicate structures. Structures such as blood vessels and nerves lie along the length of bones of the limbs and are protected from injury by the muscles and skin. These structures are most vulnerable where they cross joints and where bones can be felt near the skin.

Cavities of the body

The organs that make up the systems of the body are contained in four *cavities*:

- cranial
- thoracic
- abdominal
- pelvic.

Cranial cavity

The cranial cavity contains the *brain*, and its *boundaries* are formed by the bones of the skull (Fig. 2.34).

Anteriorly — 1 frontal bone
Laterally — 2 temporal bones
Posteriorly — 1 occipital bone
Superiorly — 2 parietal bones
Inferiorly — 1 sphenoid and 1 ethmoid bone and parts of the frontal, temporal and occipital bones.

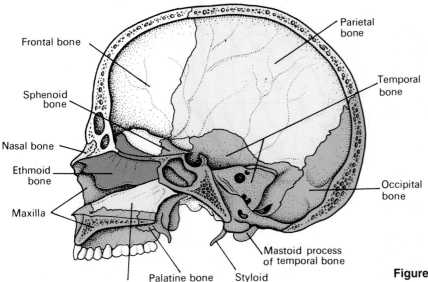

Figure 2.34 Bones forming the right half of the cranium and the face—viewed from the left.

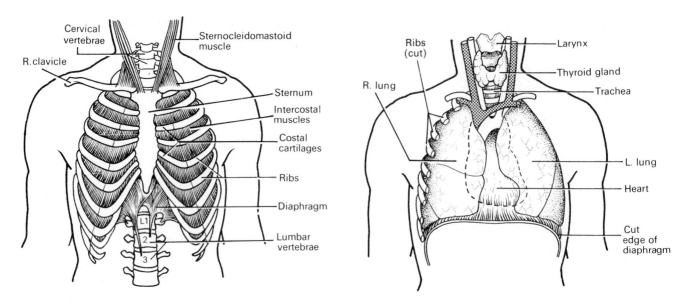

Figure 2.35 Structures forming the walls of the thoracic cavity and associated structures.

Figure 2.36 Main structures in the thoracic cavity and the root of the neck. Broken line shows the position of the heart.

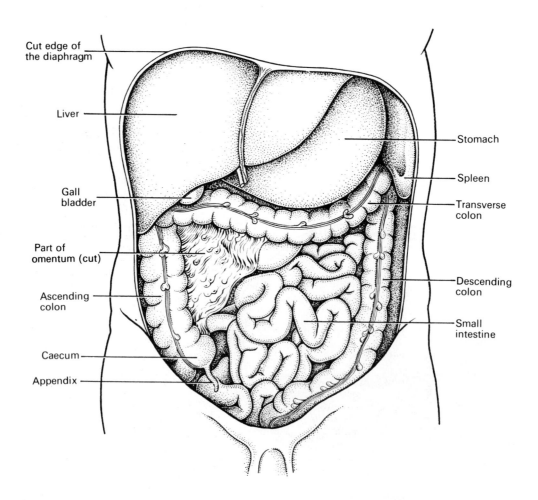

Figure 2.37 Organs occupying the anterior part of the abdominal cavity and the diaphragm (cut).

Thoracic cavity

This cavity is situated in the upper part of the trunk. Its *boundaries* are formed by a bony framework and supporting muscles (Fig. 2.35).

Anteriorly — the sternum and costal cartilages of the ribs

Laterally — 12 pairs of ribs and the intercostal muscles

Posteriorly — the thoracic vertebrae and the intervertebral discs between the bodies of the vertebrae

Superiorly — the structures forming the root of the neck

Inferiorly — the diaphragm, a dome-shaped muscle.

Contents

The main organs and structures contained in the thoracic cavity are (Fig. 2.36):

- the trachea, 2 bronchi, 2 lungs
- the heart, aorta, superior and inferior vena cava, numerous other blood vessels
- the oesophagus
- lymph vessels and lymph nodes
- nerves.

The *mediastinum* is the name given to the space between the lungs.

Abdominal cavity

This is the largest cavity in the body and is oval in shape (Figs 2.37 and 2.38). It is situated in the main part of the trunk and its *boundaries* are:

Superiorly — the diaphragm, which separates it from the thoracic cavity

Anteriorly — the muscles forming the anterior abdominal wall

Posteriorly — the lumbar vertebrae and muscles forming the posterior abdominal wall

Laterally — the lower ribs and parts of the muscles of the abdominal wall

Inferiorly — the pelvic cavity with which it is continuous.

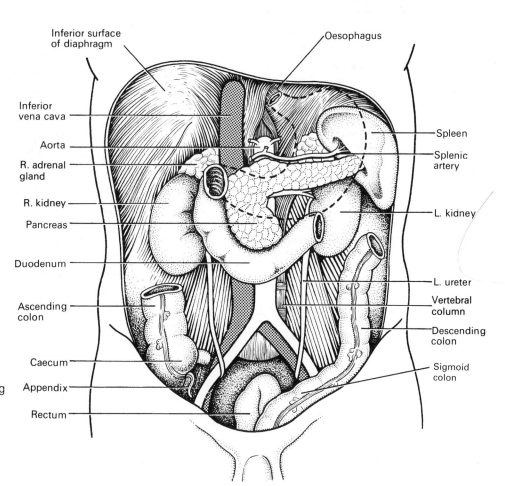

Figure 2.38 Organs occupying the posterior part of the abdominal cavity and the diaphragm (cut). Broken line shows the position of the stomach.

By convention, the abdominal cavity is divided into the nine regions shown in Figure 2.39. This facilitates the description of the positions of the organs and structures it contains.

Contents

Most of the space in the abdominal cavity is occupied by the organs and glands involved in the digestion and absorption of food. These are:

- the stomach, small intestine and most of the large intestine
- the liver, gall bladder, bile ducts and pancreas.

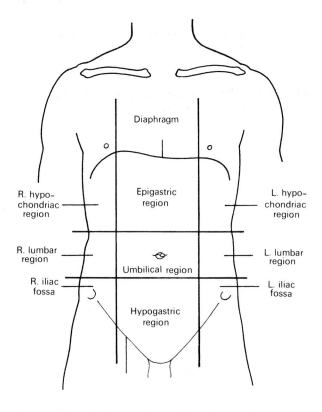

Figure 2.39 Regions of the abdominal cavity.

Other structures include:

- the spleen
- 2 kidneys and the upper part of the ureters
- 2 adrenal (suprarenal) glands
- numerous blood vessels, lymph vessels, nerves
- lymph nodes.

Pelvic cavity

The pelvic cavity is roughly funnel-shaped and extends from the lower end of the abdominal cavity (Figs 2.40 and 2.41). The *boundaries* are:

Superiorly — it is continuous with the abdominal cavity
Anteriorly — the pubic bones
Posteriorly — the sacrum and coccyx
Laterally — the innominate bones
Inferiorly — the muscles of the pelvic floor.

Contents

The pelvic cavity contains the following structures:

- sigmoid or pelvic colon, rectum and anus
- some loops of the small intestine
- urinary bladder, lower parts of the ureters and the urethra
- in the female, the organs of the reproductive system: the uterus, uterine tubes, ovaries and vagina (Fig. 2.40)
- in the male, some of the organs of the reproductive system: the prostate gland, seminal vesicles, spermatic cords, deferent ducts (vas deferens), ejaculatory ducts and the urethra (common to the reproductive and urinary systems) (Fig. 2.41).

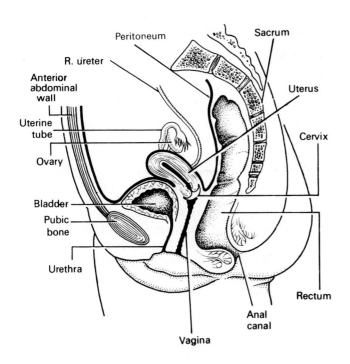

Figure 2.40   Female reproductive organs and other structures in the pelvic cavity.

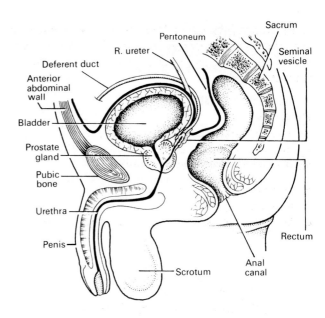

Figure 2.41   Male reproductive organs and other structures in the pelvic cavity.

DISORDERS OF CELLS AND TISSUES

Neoplasms or tumours

A tumour or *neoplasm* (literally meaning 'new growth') is a mass of tissue that grows in excess of normal in an uncoordinated manner, and continues to grow after the initial stimulus has ceased.

Tumours are classified as benign or malignant although a clear distinction is not always possible (see Table 2.1). Benign tumours only rarely change their character and become malignant.

Rate of growth

A tumour forms when the rate of cell multiplication is greater than that of cell death. Blood vessels grow with the proliferating cells, but in some malignant tumours the blood supply does not keep pace with growth and *ischaemia* (lack of blood supply) leads to tumour cell death, called *necrosis*. If the tumour is near the surface, this may result in skin

Table 2.1 Differences between benign and malignant tumours

Benign	Malignant
Slow growth	Rapid growth
Cells well differentiated	Cells poorly differentiated
Usually encapsulated	Not encapsulated
Does not spread	Spreads:
	—by local infiltration
	—via lymph and blood
Recurrence is rare	Recurrence is common

ulceration and infection. In deeper tissues there is fibrosis, e.g. retraction of the nipple in breast cancer is due to the shrinkage of fibrous tissue in a necrotic tumour. The mechanisms controlling the life span of tumour cells are not known.

Cell differentiation

Differentiation of cells into types with particular structural and functional characteristics occurs at an early stage in fetal development, e.g. epithelial cells develop different characteristics from lymphocytes. Later, when cell replacement occurs, daughter cells have the same appearance, functions and genetic make-up as the parent cell. In benign tumours the cells from which they originate are easily recognised, i.e. tumour cells are well differentiated. In malignant tumours there is a wide range of differentiation. In some cases most identifying features are retained, causing only a slight degree of *dysplasia*. At the other extreme, when the parent cells cannot be identified, the tumour is described as *anaplastic*. Tumours with well-differentiated cells are usually benign but some may be malignant.

Encapsulation and spread of tumours

Most benign tumours are contained within a fibrous capsule derived partly from the surrounding tissues and partly from the tumour. They neither infiltrate local tissues nor spread to other parts of the body, even when they are not encapsulated.

Malignant tumours are not encapsulated. They spread locally by infiltration, and tumour fragments may spread to other parts of the body in blood or lymph. Some spreading cells may be phagocytosed but others grow into *secondary (metastatic)* tumours.

Local spread

Benign tumours enlarge and may cause pressure damage to local structures. They do not spread to other parts of the body. *Malignant tumours* grow into and *infiltrate* surrounding tissues. They may:

- erode blood and lymph vessel walls, causing spread of tumour cells to other parts of the body
- damage nerves, causing pain and loss of nerve control of other tissues and organs supplied by the damaged nerves
- compress adjacent structures causing, e.g., ischaemia (lack of blood), necrosis (death of tissue), blockage of ducts, organ dysfunction or displacement, pain due to pressure on nerves.

Lymphatic spread

This occurs when malignant tumours grow into lymph channels. Groups of tumour cells break off and are carried to lymph nodes where they lodge and may grow into secondary tumours. There may be further spread through the lymphatic system, and to blood because lymph eventually enters the subclavian veins.

Blood spread

This occurs when the walls of a blood vessel are eroded by a malignant tumour. A *thrombus* (blood clot) may form at the site and *emboli*, consisting of fragments of tumour and blood clot, enter the bloodstream. These emboli block small blood vessels, cause *infarcts* (areas of dead tissue), and metastatic tumours develop. Phagocytosis of tumour cells in the emboli is unlikely to occur because they are protected by blood clot. Single tumour cells can also lodge in the capillaries of other body organs. Division and subsequent growth of secondary tumours, or *metastases*, may then occur. The sites of blood-spread metastases depend on the site of the original tumour and the anatomy of the circulatory system, although the reasons why some organs develop metastases more frequently than others are not always clear.

Body cavities spread

This occurs when a tumour penetrates the wall of a cavity. The peritoneal cavity is most frequently involved. If, for example, a malignant tumour in an abdominal organ penetrates the visceral peritoneum, tumour cells may metastasise to folds of peritoneum or any abdominal or pelvic organ. Where there is less scope for the movement of fragments within a cavity the tumour tends to bind layers of tissue together, e.g. a pleural tumour binds the visceral and parietal layers together, limiting expansion of the lung.

Table 2.2 shows common sites of primary tumours and their metastases.

Table 2.2 Common sites of primary tumours and their metastases	
Primary tumour	Metastatic tumours
Bronchi	Adrenal glands, brain
Alimentary tract	Abdominal and pelvic structures, especially liver
Prostate gland	Pelvic bones, vertebrae
Thyroid gland	Pelvic bones, vertebrae
Breast	Vertebrae, brain
Many organs	Lungs

Effects of tumours

Pressure effects

Both benign and malignant tumours may cause pressure damage to adjacent structures, especially if in a confined space. The effects depend on the site of the tumour but are most marked in areas where there is little space for expansion, e.g. inside the skull, under the periosteum of bones, in bony sinuses and respiratory passages. Compression of adjacent structures may cause ischaemia, necrosis, blockage of ducts, organ dysfunction or displacement, pain due to invasion of nerves or pressure on nerves.

Hormonal effects

Tumours of endocrine glands may secrete hormones, producing the effects of hypersecretion. The extent of cell dysplasia is an important factor. Well-differentiated benign tumours are more likely to secrete hormones than markedly dysplastic malignant tumours. High levels of hormones are found in the bloodstream as secretion occurs in the absence of the normal stimulus and homeostatic control mechanism. Some malignant tumours produce *uncharacteristic hormones*. The cells of the tumour do not appear to originate from the appropriate endocrine gland. There is evidence of this phenomenon but the reasons for it are unclear. Endocrine glands may be destroyed by invading tumours, causing hormone deficiency.

Cachexia

This is the severe weight loss accompanied by progressive weakness, loss of appetite, wasting and anaemia that is usually associated with advanced cancer. The severity is usually indicative of the stage of development of the disease. The causes are not clear.

Causes of death in malignant disease

Infection

Acute infection is a common cause of death when superimposed on advanced malignancy. Predisposition to infection is increased by prolonged bedrest, and by depression of the immune system by cytotoxic drugs and irradiation by X-rays or radioactive isotopes used in treatment. The most commonly occurring infections are pneumonia, septicaemia, peritonitis and pyelonephritis.

Organ failure

A tumour may destroy so much tissue that an organ cannot function. Severe damage to vital organs, such as lungs, brain, liver and kidneys, are common causes of death.

Carcinomatosis

When there is widespread metastatic disease associated with cachexia, severe physiological and biochemical disruption follows. In time, this results in loss of the homeostatic control mechanisms necessary to maintain life.

Haemorrhage

This may occur when a tumour grows into and ruptures the wall of a vein or artery. The most common sites are the gastrointestinal tract, brain, lungs and the peritoneal cavity.

Causes of neoplasms

Normally cells divide in an orderly manner. Neoplastic cells have escaped from the normal controls and multiply in a disorderly manner. In malignancy they grow beyond their normal boundaries and develop varying degrees of dysplasia. Some factors are known to precipitate the changes found in tumour cells but the reasons for the uncontrolled cell multiplication are not known. The process of change is *carcinogenesis* and the agents precipitating the change are *carcinogens*. Carcinogenesis may be of genetic and/or environmental origin and a clear-cut distinction is not always possible.

Carcinogens

Environmental agents known to cause malignant changes in cells do so by progressive irreversible disorganisation and modification of the chromosomes and genes. It is impossible to specify a maximum 'safe dose' of a carcinogen. A small dose may initiate change but this may not be enough to cause malignancy unless there are repeated doses within a limited period of time that have a cumulative effect. In addition there are widely varying latent periods between exposure and evidence of malignancy. There may also be other unknown factors. Environmental carcinogens include chemicals, irradiations and oncogenic viruses.

Chemical carcinogens

Some chemicals are carcinogens when absorbed, others are modified after absorption and become carcinogenic. Some known chemical carcinogens are:

■ aniline dyes
■ arsenic compounds
■ asbestos
■ benzene derivatives
■ cigarette smoke
■ nickel compounds
■ some fuel oils
■ vinyl chloride.

Radiation carcinogens

Exposure to ionising radiation including X-rays, radioactive isotopes, environmental radiations and ultraviolet rays in sunlight may cause malignant changes in some cells and kill others. The cells are affected during mitosis so those normally undergoing continuous controlled division are most susceptible. These labile tissues include skin, mucous membrane, bone marrow, lymphoid tissue and germ cells in the ovaries and testes.

Oncogenic viruses

Viruses, some consisting of DNA and some of RNA, are known to cause malignant changes in animals and there are indications of similar involvement in man. Viruses enter cells and the addition of DNA or RNA to the host cell's nucleus causes mutation. The mutant cells may be malignant.

Host factors

Internal body factors of the host can influence susceptibility to tumours. These include:

■ race
■ diet
■ age
■ inherited factors.

Tumours of individual structures are described in the appropriate chapters.

3
Electrolytes and body fluids

efore going on to consider the importance and nature of body fluids it is necessary to understand the meaning of such terms as electrolytes, isotopes, pH and buffer substances. To do so it is essential to survey some of the principles of the physics and chemistry of atoms, elements and compounds.

Before discussing the compounds found in solution in the water of the body, the atom and its main constituent parts have to be considered.

ATOMS, MOLECULES AND COMPOUNDS

The atom is described as the smallest particle of an element which can exist as a stable entity. All atoms of an element have the same number of charged particles, which confers unique chemical and electrical activity. This will be more clearly understood when the structure of the atom has been described.

There are 92 naturally occurring elements. The body structures are made up of a great variety of combinations of four elements: carbon, hydrogen, oxygen and nitrogen. In addition small amounts of others are present, collectively described as *mineral salts* (p. 274).

Atomic structure
Atoms are made up of a number of types of particles, but only three are considered here.

Protons are particles present in the nucleus or central part of the atom. Each proton has *one unit of positive electrical charge* and *one atomic mass unit*.

Neutrons are also found in the nucleus of the atom. They have *no electrical charge* and *one atomic mass unit*.

Electrons are particles which revolve in orbit around the nucleus of the atom at a distance from it, as the planets revolve round the sun. Each electron carries *one unit of negative electrical charge* and its mass is so small that it can be disregarded when compared with the mass of the other particles.

Table 3.1 summarises the characteristics of these subatomic particles.

Table 3.1	Characteristics of subatomic particles	
Particle	Mass	Electric charge
Proton	1 unit	1 positive
Neutron	1 unit	neutral
Electron	negligible	1 negative

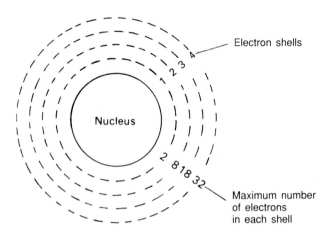

Figure 3.1 Diagram of the atom showing the nucleus and four electron shells.

In all atoms the number of positively charged protons in the nucleus is *equal to* the number of negatively charged electrons in orbit around the nucleus.

The difference between elements is in the *numbers* of these essential particles which make up their atoms.

The electrons are shown in Figure 3.1 to be in concentric rings round the nucleus. These shells diagrammatically represent the different energy levels of the electrons in relation to the nucleus, not their physical positions. The first energy level can hold only 2 electrons and is filled first. The second energy level can hold only 8 electrons and is filled next. The third and subsequent energy levels hold increased numbers of electrons, each containing more than the preceding level.

The *electron configuration* denotes the distribution of the electrons in each element, e.g. sodium is 2 8 1 (Fig. 3.2).

Atomic number
The atomic number of an element is the number of protons in the nuclei of the atoms of that element. For example, the atomic number of oxygen is 8 because it has 8 protons in its nucleus. Hydrogen is 1 and sodium 12 (Fig. 3.2).

Isotopes
These are atoms of an element in which there is a *different number of neutrons in the nucleus*. This does not affect the electrical activity of these atoms but it does affect their weight, e.g. there are three forms of the hydrogen atom. The most common form has one proton in the nucleus and one orbiting electron. Another form has one proton and *one neutron* in the nucleus. A third form has one proton and *two neutrons* in the nucleus and one orbiting electron. These three forms of hydrogen are called *isotopes* (Fig. 3.3).

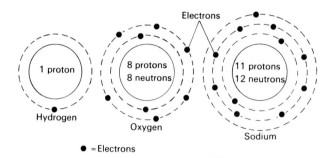

Figure 3.2 Diagram of the structure of atoms of different elements showing protons, neutrons and electrons.

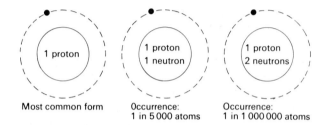

Figure 3.3 Diagram of the isotopes of hydrogen.

Atomic mass (weight)

The atomic weight of an element is the sum of the protons and neutrons in the nucleus of the atoms of the element. Taking into account the isotopes of hydrogen and the proportions in which they occur, the atomic weight of hydrogen is 1.008, although for many practical purposes it can be taken as 1.

Oxygen has an atomic weight of 16. This means that a specific number of atoms of oxygen weighs 16 times more than the same number of atoms of hydrogen.

Chlorine has an atomic weight of 35.5, because it exists in two forms; one isotope has an atomic weight of 35 (with 18 neutrons in the nucleus) and the other 37 (with 20 neutrons in the nucleus). Because the proportion of these two forms is not equal, the *average atomic weight* is 35.5.

Atomic weight is expressed simply as a number until a standard scale of measurement of weight is applied, e.g. grams, milligrams, micrograms.

Molecules and compounds

It was mentioned earlier that the atoms of each element have a specific number of electrons around the nucleus. When the number of electrons in the outer shell of an element is the optimum number (Fig. 3.1), the element is described as inert or chemically unreactive, i.e. it will not easily combine with other elements to form compounds. These elements are the inert or noble gases—helium, neon, argon, krypton, xenon and radon.

Molecules consist of two or more atoms which are chemically combined, e.g. a molecule of atmospheric oxygen (O_2) consists of two atoms of oxygen.

When two or more atoms of different elements are chemically combined the molecule formed may also be called a *compound*, e.g. a molecule of sodium chloride (NaCl) consists of one atom of chlorine and one atom of sodium.

Compounds which contain the element carbon are classified as *organic*, and all others as *inorganic*. The body fluids contain both.

Elements which have incomplete outer shells of electrons are reactive and will combine with other elements which also have incomplete outer electron shells. In the formation of *electrovalent* or *ionic compounds*, electrons are transferred from one element to another. For example, when sodium (Na) combines with chlorine (Cl) to form sodium chloride (NaCl) there is a transfer of the only electron in the outer shell of the sodium atom to the outer shell of the chlorine atom. This makes the outer shell (the third shell) of the chlorine up to its full capacity of 8 electrons and leaves the sodium part of the compound with a complete second shell and no electrons in the third shell (Fig. 3.4).

The number of electrons is the only change which occurs in the atoms in this type of reaction. There is no change in the number of protons or neutrons in the nuclei of the atoms. The chloride part now has *18*

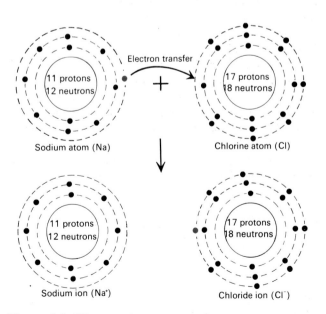

Figure 3.4 Diagram showing the formation of the ionic compound sodium chloride.

electrons, each with one negative electrical charge, and *17 protons*, each with one positive charge. The sodium part has lost one electron, leaving *10 electrons* orbiting round the nucleus with *11 protons*. When sodium chloride is dissolved in water the two atoms separate, i.e. they *ionise*, and the imbalance of protons and electrons leads to the formation of two *charged particles* called *ions*. Sodium, with the positive charge, is a *cation*, written Na^+, and chloride is an *anion*, written Cl^-. By convention the number of electrical charges carried by an ion is indicated by the superscript plus or minus signs.

An ionic compound, e.g. sodium chloride, in solution in water is called an *electrolyte* because it can conduct electricity. Non-ionising compounds are not electrolytes, e.g. carbohydrates.

In this discussion, sodium chloride has been used as an example of the formation of an ionic compound and to illustrate electrolyte activity. There are, however, many other electrolytes within the human body which, though in relatively small quantities, are equally important. Although these substances may enter the body in the form of compounds, such as sodium bicarbonate, they are usually discussed in the ionic form, that is, as sodium ions (Na^+) and bicarbonate ions (HCO_3^-).

The bicarbonate part of sodium bicarbonate is derived from carbonic acid (H_2CO_3). All inorganic acids contain hydrogen combined with another element, or with a group of elements called a *radical* which acts like a single element. Hydrogen combines with chlorine to form hydrochloric acid (HCl) and with the *phosphate radical* to form phosphoric acid (H_3PO_4). When these two acids ionise they do so thus:

$$HCl \rightarrow H^+ \; Cl^-$$
$$H_3PO_4 \rightarrow 3H^+ \; PO_4^{3-}$$

In the second example, three atoms of hydrogen have each lost one electron, all of which have been taken up by one unit, the phosphate radical, making a phosphate ion with three negative charges.

A large number of compounds present in the body are not ionic and therefore have no electrical properties when dissolved in water, e.g. carbohydrates.

Molecular weight

The molecular weight of a compound is the sum of the atomic weights of the elements which form its molecules, e.g.:

Water (H.OH)

2 hydrogen atoms	(atomic weight 1)	2
1 oxygen atom	(atomic weight 16)	16
	Molecular weight	= 18

Sodium bicarbonate ($NaHCO_3$)

1 sodium atom	(atomic weight 23)	23
1 hydrogen atom	(atomic weight 1)	1
1 carbon atom	(atomic weight 12)	12
3 oxygen atoms	(atomic weight 16)	48
	Molecular weight	= 84

Molecular weight, like atomic weight, is expressed simply as a figure until a scale of measurement of weight is applied.

Molar concentration

This is the term recommended in the *Système Internationale* for expressing the concentration of substances present in the body fluids (SI units).

The mole (mol) is the molecular weight in grams of a substance (formerly called 1 gram molecule). One mole of all substances contains 6.023×10^{23} molecules, or atoms.

A molar solution is a solution in which 1 mole of a substance is dissolved in 1 litre of solvent. In the human body the solvent is water or fat.

Molar concentration may be used to measure quantities of electrolytes, non-electrolytes, ions and atoms, e.g. molar solutions of the following substances mean:

1 mole of sodium chloride molecules = 58.5 g per litre (NaCl)

1 mole of sodium ions (Na^+)	= 23 g per litre
1 mole of carbon atoms (C)	= 12 g per litre
1 mole of atmospheric oxygen (O_2)	= 32 g per litre

In physiology this system has the advantage of being a measure of the number of particles (molecules, atoms, ions) of substances present because molar solutions of different substances contain the same number of particles. It has the advantage over the measure milliequivalents per litre* because it can be used for non-electrolytes, in fact for any substance of known molecular weight.

Many of the chemical substances present in the body are in very low concentrations so it is more convenient to use smaller metric measures, e.g. *millimoles per litre* (mmol/l) or micromoles per litre (μmol/l) as a biological measure (Table 3.2).

For substances of unknown molecular weight, e.g.

---

* Milliequivalents per litre (mEq/l)

$$\text{Equivalent weight} = \frac{\text{atomic weight}}{\text{number of electrical charges}}$$

Concentration is expressed:

$$\text{mEq/l} = \frac{\text{mg/l}}{\text{atomic weight}} \times \text{number of electrical charges}$$

Table 3.2	Examples of normal plasma levels	
Substance	Amount in SI units	Amount in other units
Chloride	97–106 mmol/l	97–106 mEq/l
Sodium	135–143 mmol/l	135–143 mEq/l
Glucose	3.5–5.5 mmol/l	60–100 mg/100 ml
Iron	14–35 μmol/l	90–196 μg/100 ml

insulin, concentration may be expressed in International Units per millilitre (IU/ml).

Hydrogen ion concentration (pH)

The number of hydrogen ions present in a solution is a measure of the acidity of the solution. The maintenance of the normal hydrogen ion concentration ([H$^+$]) within the body is an important factor in maintaining a stable environment, i.e. homeostasis.

A standard scale for the measurement of the hydrogen ion concentration in solution has been developed. Not all acids ionise completely when dissolved in water. The hydrogen ion concentration is a measure, therefore, of the amount of *dissociated acid* (ionised acid) rather than of the total amount of acid present. Strong acids dissociate more freely than weak acids, e.g. hydrochloric acid dissociates freely into H$^+$ and Cl$^-$, while carbonic acid dissociates much less freely into H$^+$ and HCO$_3^-$. The number of *free hydrogen ions* in a solution is a *measure of its acidity* rather than an indication of the type of molecule from which the hydrogen ions originated.

The alkalinity of a solution depends on the number of hydroxyl ions (OH$^-$). Water is a neutral solution because every molecule contains one hydrogen ion and one hydroxyl radical. For every molecule of water (H.OH) which dissociates, one hydrogen ion (H$^+$) and one hydroxyl ion (OH$^-$) are formed, neutralising each other.

The scale for measurement of pH was developed taking water as the standard. It was found that 1 molecule in 550 000 000 molecules of water ionises into a hydrogen ion and a hydroxyl ion. This is the same proportion as 1 gram of hydrogen ion in 10 000 000 litres of water. Therefore 1 litre of water contains $\dfrac{1}{10\,000\,000}$ of a gram of hydrogen ion. In order to make these figures more manageable this can be written:

1 litre of water contains $\dfrac{1}{10^7}$ g hydrogen ion

($10 = 10^1$; $100 = 10^2$; $10\,000 = 10^4$ and so on).

The fraction $\dfrac{1}{10^7}$ may be written 10^{-7}, the negative power indicating that this is a fraction.

For everyday use, only the '*power*' *figure* without the negative sign is used and the symbol pH placed before it.

Thus in a neutral solution such as water, where the number of hydrogen ions is balanced by the same number of hydroxyl ions, the pH = 7. The range of this scale is from 0 to 14. If the pH is 0 it means that 1 litre contains $\dfrac{1}{1}$ = 1 gram of hydrogen ion; or at the other end of the scale if there are no hydrogen ions present it may be written $\dfrac{1}{10^{14}}$ or pH 14. It will be noted that a change of pH of *one* at any level in the scale means an increase or decrease by a factor of 10 in hydrogen ion concentration.

A pH reading *below* 7 indicates an *acid solution*, while readings *above* 7 indicate *alkalinity* (Fig. 3.5).

Ordinary litmus paper indicates whether a solution is acid or alkaline by colouring blue for alkaline and red for acid. Other specially treated absorbent papers give an approximate measure of pH by a colour change. When accurate measurements of pH are required, sensitive pH meters are used.

pH values of the body fluids

Body fluids have pH values that must be maintained within relatively narrow limits for normal cell activity. The pH values are not the same in all parts of the body, e.g. the normal range of pH values of the following secretions are:

Blood	7.35 to 7.45
Saliva	5.4 to 7.5
Gastric juice	1.5 to 3.5
Bile	6 to 8.5
Urine	4.5 to 8.0

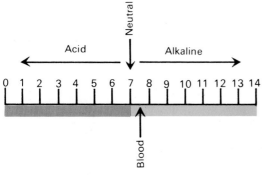

Figure 3.5 The pH scale.

The pH value in an organ is produced by its secretion of acids or alkalis which establishes the optimum level. The highly acid pH of the gastric juice is maintained by hydrochloric acid secreted by the parietal cells in the walls of the gastric glands. The low pH value in the stomach provides the environment best suited to the functioning of the enzyme pepsin that begins the digestion of dietary protein. Saliva has a pH of between 5.4 and 7.5 which is the optimum value for the action of salivary amylase, the enzyme present in saliva which initiates the digestion of carbohydrates. The action of salivary amylase is inhibited when food containing it reaches the stomach and is mixed with acid gastric juice.

The blood has a pH value of between 7.35 and 7.45. The range of pH of the blood compatible with life is 7.0 to 7.8. The metabolic activity of the body cells produces certain acids and alkalis which tend to alter the pH of the tissue fluid and blood. To maintain the pH within the normal range, there are substances present in blood that act as *buffers*.

Buffers

The optimum pH level is maintained by the balance between acids and bases produced by cells. Bases are substances that accept (or bind) hydrogen ions and when dissolved in water they are alkaline in reaction. Buffers are substances such as phosphates, bicarbonates and some proteins that maintain the [H$^+$] within normal, but narrow, limits. Some buffers 'bind' hydrogen ions and others 'bind' hydroxyl ions, reducing their circulating levels and preventing damaging changes. For example, if there is sodium hydroxide (NaOH) and carbonic acid (H$_2$CO$_3$) present, both will ionise to some extent, but they will also react together to form sodium bicarbonate (NaHCO$_3$) and water (H.OH). One of the hydrogen ions from the acid has been 'bound' in the formation of the bicarbonate radical and the other by combining with the hydroxyl radical to form water.

$$\text{NaOH} + \text{H}_2\text{CO}_3 \rightarrow \text{NaHCO}_3 + \text{H.OH}$$

sodium   carbonic   sodium   water
hydroxide   acid   bicarbonate

Acidosis and alkalosis

The substances in the complex buffer system that 'bind' hydrogen ions are called the *alkali reserve* of the blood. When the pH is below 7.35, and all the reserves of alkaline buffer are used up, the condition of *acidosis* (acidaemia) exists. When the reverse situation pertains and the pH is above 7.45, and the increased alkali uses up all the *acid reserve*, the state of *alkalosis* (alkalaemia) exists.

The buffer systems maintain *homeostasis* by preventing dramatic changes in the pH values in the blood, but can only function effectively if there is some means by which excess acid or alkali can be excreted from the body. The organs most active in this way are the *lungs* and the *kidneys*. When respiration is decreased there is an accumulation of carbon dioxide in the body. Carbon dioxide combines with water to form carbonic acid and when it dissociates hydrogen ions are released. If these are in excess of the alkaline reserve, acidosis develops. On the other hand, if there is 'over-breathing', which results in excessive excretion of carbon dioxide, the condition of alkalosis may develop.

The kidneys have the ability to form ammonia which combines with the acid products of protein metabolism which are then excreted in the urine.

The buffer and excretory systems of the body together maintain the *acid–base balance* so that the pH range of the blood remains within normal, but narrow, limits.

BODY FLUIDS

Intracellular and extracellular fluid

The total body water in adults of average build is about 60% of body weight. This proportion is higher in young people and in adults below average weight. It is lower in the elderly and in obesity in all age groups. About 22% of body weight is extracellular water and about 38% is intracellular water (Fig. 3.6).

The extracellular fluid consists of fluid in the blood and lymph vessels, cerebrospinal fluid and fluid in the interstitial spaces of the body. Interstitial fluid (tissue fluid) bathes all the cells of the body except the outer layers of skin. It is the medium through which substances pass from blood to the body cells, and from the cells to blood. The movement of substances dissolved or suspended in blood water is a passive process, depending on the size of the particles involved. Substances able to pass through include: electrolytes, enzymes, antibodies, nutrient materials, oxygen, carbon dioxide,

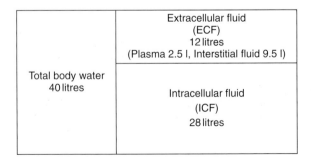

Figure 3.6 Distribution of body water in a 70 kg person.

cell waste materials. The concentration of these substances is not constant because cells take up substances selectively, according to their needs, and they extrude waste at different rates, depending on how active they are.

To maintain *homeostasis*, the concentration of the constituents of tissue fluid must be kept within narrow limits. This involves many of the body's organs and systems. Substances that remain in the blood because they are too large to pass through the pores in capillary walls are plasma proteins and blood cells, except those that are amoeboid.

Diffusion

Simple and facilitated diffusion are described in relation to the cell membrane on page 22.

Diffusion is the process by which *dissolved substances* (solutes) cross semipermeable membranes, establishing equal concentration on both sides (Fig. 3.7). Diffusible substances are those with molecules of smaller size than the pores in the membrane. Molecules of water and those of solute are constantly in random motion, called Brownian movement. In this random fashion the molecules collide with the semipermeable membrane and some pass through. Establishing equilibrium is a slow process but is speeded up when the temperature is raised and when the concentration of solute is increased. By diffusion, solutes move from the high concentration side of the membrane to the low side, i.e. down the concentration gradient, and when equilibrium is established the solutions are *isotonic*. The walls of capillaries are semipermeable membranes.

Osmosis

Osmosis is the process of the transfer of *water* across a semipermeable membrane when equilibrium cannot be achieved by diffusion of solute molecules, i.e. when they are too large to pass through the pores. The force with which this occurs is called the *osmotic pressure*.

It would be easier to understand this phenomenon if osmotic pressure was considered as *osmotic pull*, because water crosses the semipermeable membrane from the side of low solute concentration to that of high concentration. By taking water away from the side of lower concentration its concentration increases, and by adding it to the high concentration solution its concentration is reduced. The process will continue until the concentrations on each side of the membrane are equal. When equilibrium is established the solutions are called *isotonic*. The strength of osmotic pressure depends on the difference between the ratio of water molecules to non-diffusible particles on the two sides of the membrane.

Osmosis is demonstrated in the following example: a dilute solution of gelatine and water is prepared and placed in a beaker on one side of a semipermeable membrane and a more concentrated solution is placed on the other side (Fig. 3.7). Water passes from the *solution of lower concentration to the solution of higher concentration* and the number of molecules of gelatine on each side remains unchanged.

The processes of diffusion and osmosis have been described separately, but within the body they occur at the same time.

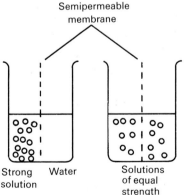
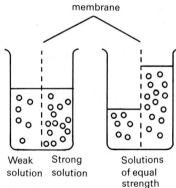
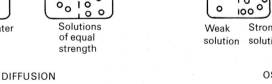

Figure 3.7
A. Before and after diffusion.
B. Before and after osmosis.

DIFFUSION
A

OSMOSIS
B

Section 2
Internal communication

4

The blood

lood is described as a connective tissue. It provides one of the means of communication between the cells of different parts of the body and the external environment, e.g. it carries:

- oxygen from the lungs to the tissues and carbon dioxide from the tissues to the lungs for excretion
- nutrient materials from the alimentary tract to the tissues and cell waste materials to the excretory organs, e.g. the kidneys
- hormones secreted by endocrine glands to their target glands and tissues
- heat produced in active tissues to other less active tissues
- protective substances, e.g. antibodies, to areas of infection
- Materials that clot blood, preventing its loss from a ruptured blood vessel.

Blood constitutes about 7% of body weight (about 5.6 litres in a 70 kg man). This proportion is less in women and considerably greater in children, gradually decreasing until the adult level is reached.

Blood in the blood vessels is always in motion. The flow is such that body cells have a fairly constant environment.

The volume and the concentration of many constituents are kept within narrow limits by control systems, maintaining homeostasis.

COMPOSITION OF BLOOD

Blood is composed of a straw-coloured transparent fluid, *plasma*, in which different types of *cells* are suspended. Plasma constitutes about 55% and cells about 45% of blood volume (Fig. 4.1).

Plasma

The constituents of plasma are water (90 to 92%) and dissolved substances, including:

- plasma proteins:
  —albumin, globulin, fibrinogen, clotting factors
- inorganic salts (mineral salts):
  —sodium chloride, sodium bicarbonate, potassium, magnesium, phosphorus, iron, calcium, copper, iodine, cobalt
- nutrient materials (from digested foods):
  —monosaccharides (mainly glucose) from

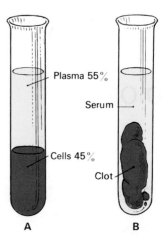

Figure 4.1 Blood in a test tube. A. Shows the proportions of plasma and cells. B. Shows the presence of a blood clot in serum.

carbohydrates, amino acids from proteins, fatty acids and glycerol from fats, vitamins from most foods
- organic waste materials:
  —urea, uric acid, creatinine
- hormones
- enzymes, e.g. various clotting factors
- antibodies (immunoglobulins)
- gases:
  —oxygen, carbon dioxide, nitrogen.

Plasma proteins

To a large extent plasma proteins remain in the blood vessels, although very small amounts may enter the tissues through the capillary wall.

Albumin. This is formed in the liver. It is the most abundant plasma protein and its main function is to maintain the plasma osmotic pressure at its normal level of about 25 mmHg (3.3 kPa).*

Globulins. Some are formed in the liver and some in lymphoid tissue. They are associated with a variety of activities:

- the immune response to the presence of antigens (p. 67).
- transportation of some hormones and mineral salts, e.g. thyroid hormone, iodine, iron, copper
- inhibition of some proteolytic enzymes, e.g. trypsin, chymotrypsin.

---

* 1 kilopascal (kPa) = 7.5 millimetres of mercury (mmHg)
   1 mmHg = 133.3 Pa = 1.3333 kPa

Clotting factors. These are substances essential for co-agulation of blood (p. 61).

Fibrinogen. This is synthesised in the liver and is essential for blood coagulation. *Serum* is plasma from which clotting factors have been removed.

Plasma viscosity (stickiness) is due to plasma proteins, mainly albumin and fibrinogen. Viscosity is used as a measure of the body's response to some diseases.

Inorganic salts (mineral salts)

These are involved in a wide variety of activities, including cell formation, contraction of muscles, transmission of nerve impulses, formation of secretions and maintenance of the balance between acids and alkalis. In health the blood is *slightly alkaline* in reaction. Alkalinity and acidity are expressed in terms of pH which is a measure of *hydrogen ion concentration*, or [H⁺] (p. 49 and Fig. 4.2). The pH of blood is maintained between 7.35 and 7.45 by an ongoing complicated series of chemical activities, involving buffering systems.

Nutrient materials

Food is digested in the alimentary tract and the resultant nutrient materials are absorbed, i.e. monosaccharides, amino acids, fatty acids, glycerol and vitamins. Together with mineral salts they are required by all body cells to provide energy, heat, materials for repair and replacement, and for the synthesis of other blood components and body secretions.

Organic waste products

Urea, creatinine and uric acid are the waste products of protein metabolism. They are formed in the liver and conveyed in blood to the kidneys for excretion. Carbon dioxide, excreted by all cells, is conveyed to the lungs for excretion.

Hormones

These are chemical compounds synthesised by endocrine glands. Hormones pass directly from the cells of the glands into the blood which transports them to their target tissues and organs elsewhere in the body, where they influence activity.

Antibodies (immunoglobins)

These are protective substances, consisting of complex protein molecules, produced by lymphoid tissue mainly in lymph nodes and in the spleen. Foreign materials, e.g. microbes, act as *antigens*, stimulating lymphoid cells to produce protective antibodies (p. 64).

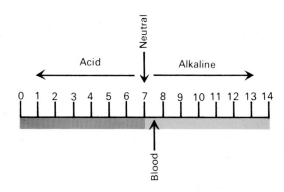

Figure 4.2 The pH scale.

Gases

Oxygen, carbon dioxide and nitrogen are transported round the body in solution in plasma. Oxygen and carbon dioxide are also transported in combination with haemoglobin in red blood cells (p. 59). Most oxygen is carried in combination with haemoglobin and most carbon dioxide as bicarbonate ions dissolved in plasma. Atmospheric nitrogen enters the body in the same way as other gases and is present in plasma but it has no physiological function (p. 255).

Cellular content of blood

There are three types of blood cells (Fig. 4.3).

- erythrocytes or red cells
- thrombocytes or platelets
- leukocytes or white cells.

All blood cells originate from stem cells (*haemocytoblasts*) and go through several developmental stages before entering the blood. Different types of blood cells follow separate lines of development. The process of blood cell formation is called *haemopoiesis* (Fig. 4.4) and takes place within red bone marrow. For the first few years, red marrow occupies the entire bone capacity and, over the next 20 years, is gradually replaced by fatty yellow marrow that has no erythropoietic function. In adults, erythropoiesis is confined to flat bones, irregular bones and the ends (*epiphyses*) of long bones.

Erythrocytes or red blood cells
(Fig. 4.3)

These are circular biconcave non-nucleated discs with a diameter of about 7 microns or 10⁻⁶ metre. There are

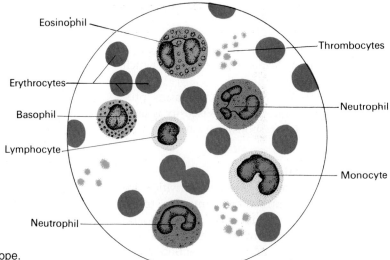

Figure 4.3 Blood cells, after staining in the laboratory, viewed through a microscope.

several other distinctive features, the measurements of which are used by physicians. The features are described below and normal values are shown in Table 4.1. The symbols in brackets are the abbreviations commonly used in laboratory reports.

Erythrocyte count is the number of erythrocytes per litre (l) or per cubic millimetre (mm^3) of blood.

Packed cell volume or haematocrit is the volume of red cells in l litre or 100 millilitres (ml) of whole blood.

Mean corpuscular volume is the average volume of cells, measured in femtolitres (fl = 10^{-15} litre).

Table 4.1 Erythrocytes—normal values	
Measure	Normal values
Erythrocyte count	
Male	4.5×10^{12}/l to 6.5×10^{12}/l (4.5 to 6.5 million/mm^3)
Female	4.5×10^{12}/l to 5×10^{12}/l (4.5 to 5 million/mm^3)
Packed cell volume (PCV)	0.4 to 0.5 l/l (40 to 50/mm^3)
Mean cell volume (MCV) Haemoglobin (Hb)	80 to 96 fl
Male	13 to 18 g/dl
Female	11.5 to 16.5 g/dl
Mean cell haemoglobin (MCH)	27 to 32 pg/cell
Mean cell haemoglobin concentration (MCHC)	30 to 35 g/dl of cells

Haemoglobin is the weight of haemoglobin in whole blood, measured in grams per decilitre (dl = 10^{-1} litre).

Mean corpuscular haemoglobin is the average amount of haemoglobin in each cell, measured in picograms (pg = 10^{-12} gram).

Mean corpuscular haemoglobin concentration is the amount of haemoglobin in 1 dl or 100 ml of red cells.

Development and life span of erythrocytes

Erythrocytes are formed in red bone marrow, which is present in the ends of long bones and in flat and irregular bones. They pass through several stages of development before entering the blood. Their life span in the circulation is about 120 days.

The process of development of red blood cells from *haemocytoblasts* takes about 7 days and is called *erythropoiesis* (Fig. 4.4). It is characterised by two main features:

- maturation of the cell
- formation of haemoglobin inside the cell (Fig. 4.5).

Maturation of the cell. During this process the cell decreases in size and loses its nucleus. These changes depend on a number of factors, especially the presence of *vitamin B_{12}* and *folic acid*. These are present in sufficient quantity in a normal diet containing dairy products, meat and green vegetables. If the diet contains more than is needed, it is stored in the liver. Absorption of vitamin B_{12} depends on a glycoprotein called *intrinsic factor* secreted by *parietal cells* in the *gastric glands*.

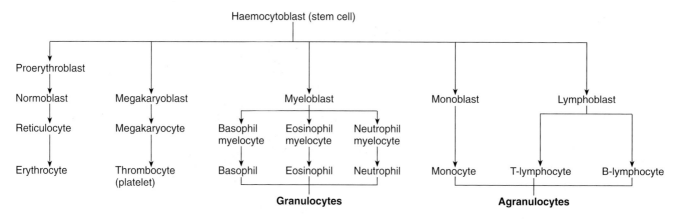

Figure 4.4 Haemopoiesis: stages in the development of blood cells.

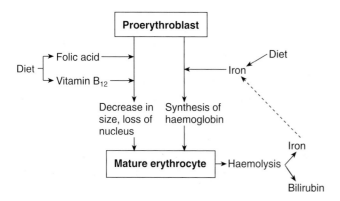

Figure 4.5 Maturation of the erythrocyte.

Together they form the *intrinsic factor–vitamin B₁₂ complex* (IF–B₁₂), absorbed by cells in the wall of the distal part of the ileum. Only the vitamin B₁₂ part enters blood to be transported to red bone marrow. The normal daily requirement of vitamin B₁₂ is about 1 to 2 μg. The effects of deficient intake do not appear for several years because there are large stores in the liver.

Folic acid is absorbed by cells in the walls of the duodenum and jejunum where it undergoes change before entering the blood. The normal daily requirement of folic acid is 100 to 200 μg. Signs of deficiency are apparent within a few months.

Formation of haemoglobin. Haemoglobin is a complex protein, consisting of *globin* and an iron-containing substance called *haem*, and is synthesised inside developing erythrocytes in red bone marrow. A normal diet containing meat, eggs, wholemeal bread and green vegetables contains more iron than the daily requirement. Women lose blood during menstruation and need more iron throughout the reproductive years and during pregnancy to supply the fetus.

Haemoglobin in erythrocytes combines with oxygen to form *oxyhaemoglobin*, giving blood its characteristic red colour. In this way the bulk of oxygen absorbed from the lungs is transported around the body to maintain a continuous oxygen supply to all cells. Haemoglobin is also involved, to a lesser extent, in the transport of carbon dioxide from the body cells to the lungs for excretion.

Control of erythropoiesis

The number of red cells remains fairly constant, which means that the bone marrow produces erythrocytes at the rate at which they are destroyed. This is due to a homeostatic negative feedback mechanism (Fig. 4.6).

The primary stimulus to increased erythropoiesis is *hypoxia*, i.e. deficient oxygen supply to body cells. This occurs when:

■ the oxygen-carrying power of blood is reduced by, e.g. haemorrhage or excessive erythrocyte breakdown (*haemolysis*) due to disease
■ the oxygen tension in the air is reduced, as at high altitudes.

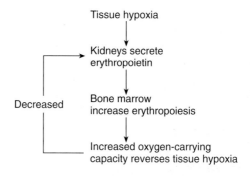

Figure 4.6 Control of erythropoiesis: a negative feedback mechanism.

Hypoxia stimulates the production of the hormone *erythropoietin*, mainly by the kidneys. Erythropoietin stimulates an increase in the production of pro-erythroblasts and the release of increased numbers of reticulocytes into the blood. These changes increase the oxygen-carrying capacity of the blood and reverse tissue hypoxia, the original stimulus. When the tissue hypoxia is overcome, erythropoietin production declines (Fig. 4.6). It is assumed that erythropoietin regulates normal red cell replacement, i.e. in the absence of hypoxia.

Destruction of erythrocytes

The life span of erythrocytes is about 120 days and their breakdown, or *haemolysis*, is carried out by *phagocytic reticuloendothelial cells*. These cells are found in many tissues but the main sites of haemolysis are the spleen, bone marrow and liver. As erythrocytes age, changes in their walls make them gradually more susceptible to haemolysis. Iron released by haemolysis is retained in the body and reused in the bone marrow to form haemoglobin (Fig. 4.5). *Biliverdin* is formed from the protein part of the erythrocytes. It is almost completely reduced to the yellow pigment *bilirubin*, before it is bound to plasma globulin and transported to the liver. In the liver it is changed from a fat-soluble to a water-soluble form before it is excreted as a constituent of bile.

Blood groups

Different blood groups are associated with genetically determined differences in antigens on red blood cell membranes and antibodies in blood serum. There are two main systems used to classify blood donated for administration by transfusion. If the donor's blood does not *match* that of the recipient the *incompatibility* results in agglutination and lysis of donated red cells after transfusion. The agglutinated cells block capillaries and the products of lysis, when in excessive amounts, damage the kidney tubules. The resultant condition is serious and may cause death.

ABO system

In some people there are *genetically determined antigens* on red cell membranes and *natural antibodies* in serum. The antibodies are inherited and are not associated with acquired immunity. Table 4.2 and Figure 4.7 summarise the system of compatibility and incompatibility.

Rhesus system

In over 80% of people the *rhesus factor* is present on red blood cell membranes, i.e. they are *rhesus positive* (Rh +ve). The rhesus factor consists of a number of antigens of which D is the most common. Individuals with D antigen are classified as rhesus positive. Administration of Rh +ve blood to Rh −ve recipients stimulates an immune response with the production of antibodies that cause haemolysis of the transfused red cells.

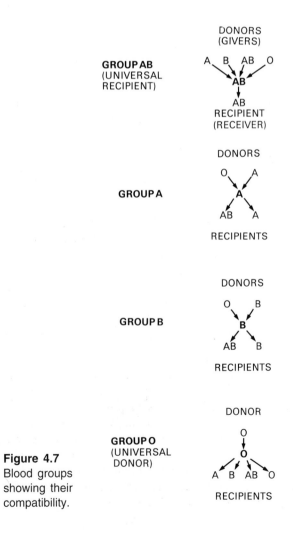

Figure 4.7 Blood groups showing their compatibility.

Table 4.2 Summary of the ABO system				
Blood group	Red cell antigens	Antibodies in serum	Can donate to groups	Can receive from groups
AB	A and B	None	AB	All groups
A	A	Anti-B	A and AB	A and O
B	B	Anti-A	B and AB	B and O
O	None	Anti-A and anti-B	All groups	O

As in active immunisation (p. 66), second and subsequent encounters with Rh +ve red cells lead to a sharp increase in antibody production.

Rhesus incompatibility of maternal and fetal blood is described on page 75.

Thrombocytes or platelets

These are very small non-nucleated discs, 2 to 4 μm in diameter, derived from the cytoplasm of megakaryocytes in red bone marrow (Fig. 4.4). They contain a variety of substances that promote blood clotting, which causes *haemostasis* (cessation of bleeding).

The normal blood platelet count is between 200×10^9/l and 350×10^9/l (200 000 to 350 000/mm^3). The control of platelet production is not yet entirely clear but it is believed that one stimulus is a fall in platelet count and that a substance called *thrombopoietin* is involved. The life span of platelets is between 8 and 11 days and those not used in the process of haemostasis are destroyed by macrophages, mainly in the spleen.

Haemostasis

When a blood vessel is damaged loss of blood is stopped and healing occurs in a series of overlapping processes, in which platelets play a vital part.

1. Vasoconstriction. When platelets come in contact with a damaged blood vessel, their surface becomes sticky and they adhere to the damaged wall. They then release *serotonin* (5-hydroxytryptamine), which constricts (narrows) the vessel, reducing blood flow through it. Other chemicals that cause vasoconstriction are released by the damaged vessel.

2. Platelet plug formation. The adherent platelets clump to each other and release other substances, including *adenosine diphosphate* (ADP), that attract more platelets to the site. Passing platelets stick to those already at the damaged vessel and they too release their chemicals. This is a positive feedback system by which many platelets rapidly arrive at the site of vascular damage and quickly form a temporary seal—the *platelet plug*.

3. Coagulation (blood clotting). This is a complex process that also involves a positive feedback system and only a few stages are included here. The factors involved are listed in Table 4.3. Their numbers represent the order in which they were discovered and not the order of participation in the clotting process. Blood clotting results in formation of an insoluble thread-like mesh of *fibrin* which traps blood cells and is much stronger than the rapidly formed platelet plug. In the final stages of this process *prothrombin activator* acts on the plasma

Table 4.3	Blood clotting factors
I	Fibrinogen
II	Prothrombin
III	Tissue factor
IV	Calcium
V	Labile factor, proaccelerin, Ac-globulin
VII	Stable factor, proconvertin
VIII	Antihaemophilic globulin (AHG), antihaemophilic factor A
IX	Christmas factor, plasma thromboplastin component (PTA), antihaemophilic factor B
X	Stuart-Power factor
XI	Plasma thromboplastin antecedent (PTA), antihaemophilic factor C
XII	Hageman factor
XIII	Fibrin stabilising factor

(There is no Factor VI)

Vitamin K is essential for synthesis of Factors II, VII, IX and X

protein *prothrombin* converting it to thrombin.

Thrombin then acts on another plasma protein *fibrinogen* and converts it to fibrin (Fig. 4.8).

Prothrombin activator can be formed by two processes which often occur together: the extrinsic and intrinsic pathways (Fig. 4.8). The *extrinsic pathway* occurs rapidly (within seconds) when there is tissue damage outside the circulation, and is initiated when chemicals secreted by damaged tissue enter the circulation. The *intrinsic pathway* is slower (3–6 minutes) and is confined to the circulation. It is triggered by

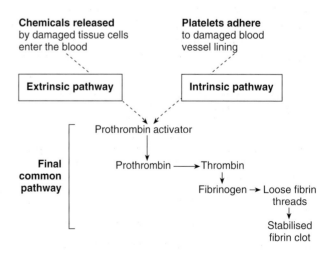

Figure 4.8 Stages of blood clotting (coagulation).

damage to a blood vessel lining (endothelium) and the effects of platelets adhering to it. After a time the clot shrinks, squeezing out *serum*, i.e. a clear sticky fluid that consists of plasma from which fibrinogen has been removed.

4. Fibrinolysis. After the clot has formed the process of removing it and healing the damaged blood vessel begins. The breakdown of the clot, or fibrinolysis, is the first stage. An inactive substance called *plasminogen* is present in the clot and is converted to the enzyme *plasmin* by activators released from the damaged endothelial cells. Plasmin initiates the breakdown of fibrin to soluble products and these are treated as waste material and removed by phagocytosis. As the clot is removed, the healing process restores the integrity of the blood vessel wall.

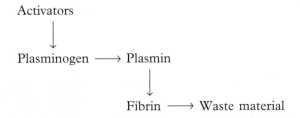

Activators

↓

Plasminogen ⟶ Plasmin

↓

Fibrin ⟶ Waste material

Leukocytes or white blood cells

These cells have an important function in defending the body against microbes and other foreign materials. Leukocytes are the largest blood cells and they account for about 1% of the blood volume. They contain nuclei and some have granules in their cytoplasm. There are two main types (Table 4.4):

- granulocytes (polymorphonuclear leukocytes)
  —neutrophils, eosinophils and basophils
- agranulocytes
  —monocytes and lymphocytes.

Granulocytes (polymorphonuclear leukocytes)

During their formation, *granulopoiesis*, they follow a common line of development through *myeloblast* to *myelocyte* before differentiating into the three types (Figs. 4.4 and 4.9). All granulocytes have multilobed nuclei in their cytoplasm. Their names represent the dyes they take up when stained in the laboratory. *Eosinophils* take up the red acid dye, eosin; *basophils* take up alkaline methylene blue; and *neutrophils* are purple because they take up both dyes.

Table 4.4 Numbers of different types of leukocyte in adult blood

Type of cell	Number x 10^9/l	Percentage of total
Granulocytes		
Neutrophils	2.5 to 7.5	40 to 75
Eosinophils	0.04 to 0.44	1 to 6
Basophils	0.015 to 0.1	<1
Agranulocytes		
Monocytes	0.2 to 0.8	2 to 10
Lymphocytes	1.5 to 3.5	20 to 50
Total	5 to 9	100

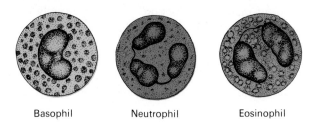

Basophil   Neutrophil   Eosinophil

Figure 4.9   The granulocytes (granular leukocytes).

Neutrophils

Their main function is to protect against any foreign material that gains entry to the body, mainly microbes,* and to remove waste materials, e.g. cell debris. They are attracted in large numbers to any area of infection by chemical substances, released by damaged cells, called *chemotaxins*. Neutrophils pass through the capillary walls in the affected area by *amoeboid movement* (Fig. 4.10). Thereafter they ingest and kill the microbes by *phagocytosis* (Fig. 4.11). Their granules are *lysosomes* that contain enzymes which degrade the ingested material. The pus that may form in the affected area consists of dead tissue cells, dead and live microbes, and phagocytes killed by microbes.

There is a physiological increase in circulating neutrophils following strenuous exercise and in the later stages of normal pregnancy. Numbers are also increased in:

- microbial infection
- tissue damage, e.g. inflammation, myocardial infarction, burns, crush injuries

---

* The term **microbe**, used throughout the text, includes all types of organisms that can only be seen by using a microscope. Specific microbes are named where appropriate.

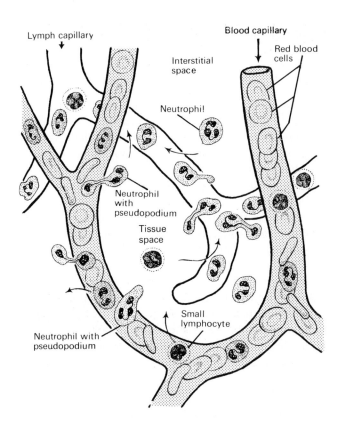

Figure 4.10 Amoeboid movement of leukocytes.

- metabolic disorders, e.g. diabetic ketoacidosis, acute gout
- leukaemia
- heavy smoking
- use of oral contraceptives.

Neutrophils stimulate the production of *interferons*, substances released by virus-infected tissue cells and lymphocytes. Interferons then diffuse in tissue fluid and protect adjacent cells from invasion by viruses.

Eosinophils

Many of these cells migrate out of the blood mainly to areas of the body exposed to the external environment, i.e. connective tissue just under the skin, in the mucous membrane of the respiratory and digestive systems and in the lining of the vagina and uterus. Their cytoplasmic granules are lysosomes. Eosinophils are believed to protect the body against foreign materials, especially invasion by parasites. They neutralise *histamine*, a chemical released during allergic reactions, and transport plasminogen which is the precursor of plasmin. Plasmin is involved in fibrinolysis and the later stage of wound healing. The number of eosinophils is increased in allergic conditions, such as asthma, hay fever, food and drug sensitivities and skin conditions.

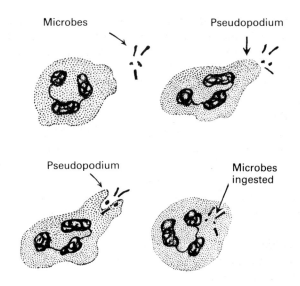

Figure 4.11 Phagocytic action of neutrophils.

Basophils

The cytoplasmic granules contain *heparin* (an anticoagulant) and *histamine* which causes vasodilatation and increases the permeability of small blood vessel walls. Histamine assists the movement of phagocytes and protective substances such as *antibodies*, into the tissue spaces. Together with *mast cells* they accumulate in the tissues in areas of local inflammation at the healing stage. Mast cells are very similar to basophils. They are found in the tissues, usually closely associated with small blood vessels, and they are involved in allergic reactions.

Agranulocytes

The types of leukocyte with a large nucleus and no granules in their cytoplasm are *monocytes* and *lymphocytes* and they make up 25% to 50% of all leukocytes (Fig. 4.12).

Monocytes

These are large mononuclear cells that originate in red bone marrow. Some circulate in the blood and are actively motile and phagocytic while others migrate into

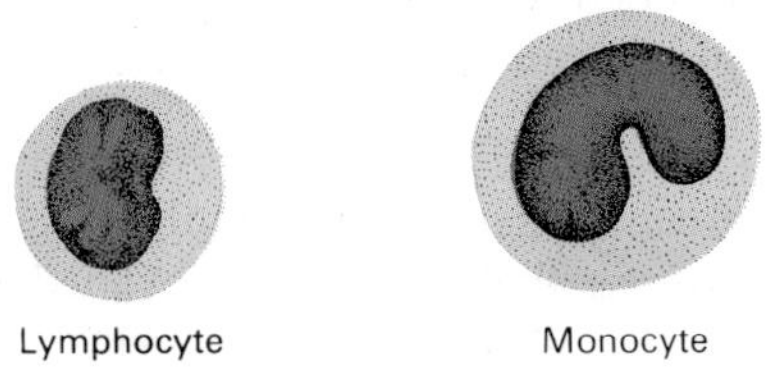

Figure 4.12
The agranulocytes.
    Lymphocyte   Monocyte

the tissues where they develop into *macrophages*. Both types of cell produce *interleukin 1* (endogenous pyrogen) which:

- acts on the hypothalamus, causing the rise in body temperature associated with microbial infections
- stimulates the production of some globulins by the liver
- enhances the production of activated T-lymphocytes.

Macrophages have important functions in inflammation (p. 69) and immunity.

The tissue macrophage system, sometimes called the *lymphoreticular system*, consists of fixed phagocytic cells which multiply in situ. These cells are found in a wide variety of tissues, e.g. as:

- *histiocytes* in connective tissues
- *microglia* in the brain
- *Kupffer cells* in the liver
- *alveolar macrophages* in the lungs
- *sinus-lining macrophages* (reticular cells) in the spleen, lymph nodes and thymus gland
- *mesangial cells* in the glomerulus of nephrons in the kidney
- *osteoclasts* in bone.

Macrophages function in close association with monocytes in the blood and with lymphocytes which influence their activity. They are actively phagocytic and if they encounter large amounts of foreign or waste material, they tend to multiply at the site and 'wall off' the area, isolating the material, e.g. in the lungs when foreign material has been inhaled. Their numbers are increased in microbial infections, collagen diseases and some non-infective bowel conditions.

Lymphocytes

Lymphocytes have large nuclei and there are two functionally distinct types: T-lymphocytes and B-lymphocytes. They circulate in the blood and are present in great numbers in lymphatic tissue such as lymph nodes and the spleen. Lymphocytes develop from haemocytoblasts (stem cells) in red bone marrow, then spread in the blood to lymphoid tissue elsewhere in the body where they are *activated*, i.e. they become immunocompetent which means they are able to respond to *antigens* (foreign material). Examples of antigens include:

- cells regarded by lymphocytes as abnormal, e.g. those that have been invaded by viruses, cancer cells, tissue transplant cells

- pollen from flowers and plants
- fungi
- bacteria
- some large molecule drugs, e.g. penicillin, aspirin.

The two types of lymphocyte sometimes function independently but usually in collaboration. *T-lymphocytes* are activated by *thymosin* in the thymus gland, and *B-lymphocytes* are activated in red bone marrow and in lymphoid tissue elsewhere in the body, possibly the walls of the intestine (Fig. 4.13). Thereafter some cells of both types circulate in the blood. Some settle in lymphoid tissue, mainly in lymph nodes, the spleen and the aggregated glands in the wall of the upper respiratory tract and the intestine.

When *activated lymphocytes* encounter antigens they develop specific protective capabilities. Each type divides into two groups: *effector cells* that promote destruction of their specific antigen; and *memory cells* that remain in lymphoid tissue and multiply, passing on their specific protective capabilities to subsequent generations of cells. The memory cells confer immunity, and subsequent encounters with the same antigen lead to proliferation of more sensitised lymphocytes.

Activated lymphocytes can respond to specific antigens by producing:

- *cell-mediated immunity*—mediated by T-lymphocytes and specialised T-cells that combat cells containing antigens
- *humoral immunity*—mediated by B-lymphocytes which involves the production of antibodies that neutralise antigens directly.

Immunity

Cell-mediated immunity

T-lymphocytes that have been activated in the thymus gland are *sensitised* when they encounter an antigen for the first time. The antigen is normally contained within a cell, either a macrophage which has ingested a microbe by phagocytosis or an abnormal cell which is recognised as foreign, or 'non-self'. In either case, the cell has unusual antigens on its membrane which the T-lymphocytes recognise as abnormal. Further development of the sensitised T-lymphocyte takes place in lymphatic tissue and several T-cells with different functions emerge (Figure 4.13):

Memory T-cells provide *cell-mediated immunity* by responding rapidly to another encounter with the same antigen.

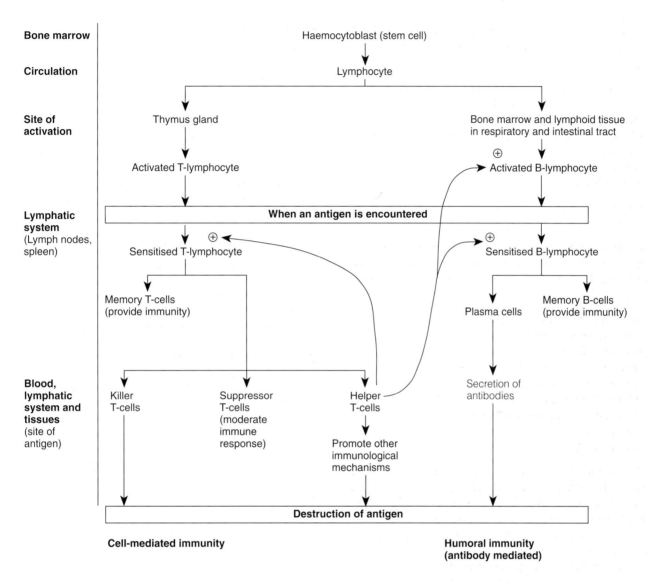

Figure 4.13 Summary of immunity (note that helper T-cells influence cell-mediated and humoral immunity).

Killer T-cells directly inactivate the cells carrying antigens.

Suppressor T-cells moderate the intensity of both humoral and cell-mediated immune responses, leading to *acquired immunological tolerance* which explains why individuals:

■ do not destroy their own cells and tissues
■ accept well-matched transplanted tissue, including blood transfusions.

Helper T-cells increase production of killer T-cells and are involved in activation of B-lymphocytes, thereby acting as amplifiers of the immune response, when this is required.

T-cell functions are mediated by chemicals they release, called *lymphokines*, including, e.g.:

■ *lymphotoxins*, which damage cell membranes and cause cell rupture
■ *interferons*, which protect cells from virus infection.

Humoral immunity

B-lymphocytes that have been activated are *sensitised* when they encounter specific antigens for the first time, e.g. microbes, bacterial toxins. They then migrate to lymphatic tissue for further processing where two types of cell develop (Fig 4.13).

Plasma cells. These are transient cells that secrete anti-bodies (immunoglobulins) that:

- kill bacteria
- neutralise bacterial toxins
- promote the phagocytosis of foreign particles
- form antibody–antigen complexes (immune complexes) that may be phagocytosed or accumulate and block small blood vessels, such as those in the kidneys that cause glomerulonephritis.

Small clusters of plasma cells that secrete the same antibodies are called *clones.*

Memory B-cells. These cells confer *humoral immunity* and rapidly respond to another encounter with the same antigen by stimulating the production of antibody-secreting plasma cells.

Helper T-cells. These are thought to be involved in the development of sensitised B-lymphocytes, highlighting the suggestion that both types of immune response are closely associated and occur simultaneously.

The fact that the body does not normally develop immunity to its own cells is due to the fine balance that exists between the immune reaction and its sup-pression. *Autoimmune diseases* are due to the distur-bance of this balance.

DEFENCE MECHANISMS

The body has many means of self-protection against invaders and they are divided into two categories:

- Specific defence mechanisms—result in an immune response to specific invaders. The body can destroy them conferring resistance to specific microbes by humoral and/or cell-mediated immune processes described above.
- Non-specific defence mechanisms—against any invaders.

Specific defence mechanisms

Antibody production following immunisation

When antigens, e.g. microbes, are encountered for the first time there is a *primary response* in which a low level of antibodies can be detected in the blood after about 2 weeks. Although the response may be sufficient to

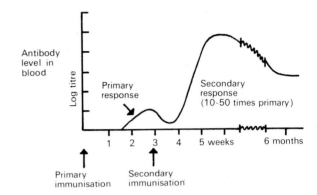

Figure 4.14   The antibody response to immunisation.

combat the antigen, the antibody levels then fall unless there is another encounter with the same antigen within a short period of time (2 to 4 weeks). The second encounter produces a *secondary response* in which there is a rapid response by memory B-cells resulting in a marked increase in antibody production (Fig. 4.14). Further increases can be achieved by later encounters but eventually a maximum is reached. This principle is used in active immunisation against infectious diseases.

Acquired immunity (Fig. 4.15)

Immunity may be acquired *naturally* or *artificially* and both forms may be *active* or *passive.* Active immunity means that the individual has responded to an antigen and produced his own antibodies, lymphocytes are activated and the memory cells formed provide long-lasting resistance. In passive immunity the individual is given antibodies produced by someone else. The anti-bodies are then destroyed and unless lymphocytes are stimulated, passive immunity is short lasting.

Active naturally acquired immunity
The body may be stimulated to produce its own anti-bodies in two ways.

1. By *having the disease.* During the course of the ill-ness, B-lymphocytes grow into plasma cells which

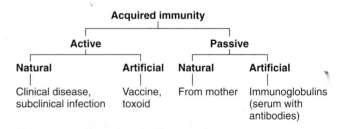

Figure 4.15   Summary of types of acquired immunity.

produce antibodies (immunoglobulins) in sufficient quantities to overcome the infecting microbes. After the individual recovers, the memory B-cells retain the ability to produce more plasma cells that produce the specific antibodies, conferring immunity to future infection by the same microbe or strain of microbe.

2. By *having a subclinical (subliminal) infection*. In this case the microbial infection is not sufficiently severe to cause clinical disease but stimulates sufficient memory B-cells to establish immunity.

Active artificially acquired immunity

This type of immunity develops in response to the administration of dead or live artificially weakened microbes (*vaccines*) or detoxicated toxins (*toxoids*). The vaccines and toxoids retain the antigenic properties that stimulate the development of immunity but they cannot cause the disease. Many microbial diseases can be prevented by artificial immunisation, e.g.:

- anthrax
- cholera
- diphtheria
- hepatitis B
- measles
- mumps
- poliomyelitis
- rubella
- smallpox
- tetanus
- tuberculosis
- typhoid
- whooping cough.

Active immunisation against some infectious disorders confers lifelong immunity, e.g. diphtheria, whooping cough, mumps. In other infections the immunity may last for a number of years or for only a few weeks before revaccination is necessary. Apparent loss of immunity may be due to infection with a different strain of the same microbe which has different antigenic properties but causes the same clinical illness, e.g. viruses that cause the common cold and influenza. In the elderly and when nutrition is poor the production of lymphocytes, especially B-lymphocytes, is reduced and the primary and secondary response may be inadequate.

Passive naturally acquired immunity

This type of immunity is acquired before birth by the passage of maternal antibodies across the placenta to the fetus and to the baby in breast milk. The variety of different antibodies provided depends on the mother's active immunity. The baby's lymphocytes are not stimulated and the immunity is short-lived.

Passive artificially acquired immunity

In this type, ready-made antibodies, in human or animal serum, are injected into the recipient. The source of the antibodies may be an individual who has recovered from the infection, or animals, commonly horses, that have been artificially actively immunised. Specific immunoglobulins (antiserum) may be administered *prophylactically* to prevent the development of disease in people who have been exposed to the infection, or *therapeutically* after the disease has developed. Proteins in serum sometimes cause sensitisation of lymphocytes that may be damaging if encountered a second time, causing an abnormal immune reaction.

Abnormal immune reactions

Allergic reactions (hypersensitivity)

These are harmful forms of immune reactions that occur in some people following second and subsequent encounters with the same antigen. They may be:

- antibody-mediated, i.e. immediate
- cell-mediated, i.e. delayed
- mixed antibody- and cell-mediated.

Antibody-mediated reactions

The antibodies formed by plasma cells combine with their antigens to form *antigen/antibody complexes* (Ag/Ab or immune complexes).

Anaphylactic reactions (Fig. 4.16). These occur within minutes of exposure to an *allergen* (antigen). In susceptible individuals, antibodies are formed following exposure to an allergen. The antibodies adhere to mast cell membranes and the mast cells are then referred to as *sensitised*. When re-exposure to the same allergen occurs, the allergen binds to the sensitised mast cells causing them to release their granules, which consist of several chemical substances, including histamine.

The most common manifestations of this type of allergic reaction include: food allergies, childhood eczema, hay fever (p. 258), extrinsic asthma (p. 261). In these conditions the released chemicals act locally, causing different effects that depend on the site:

- vasodilatation, leading to skin rashes
- increased permeability of small blood vessels, causing local swelling (*oedema*) and/or increased secretion by mucous membranes
- smooth muscle contraction, leading to difficulty in breathing or disturbance of intestinal function.

Acute systemic anaphylaxis (anaphylactic shock). This is a less common event that has very serious, and sometimes fatal, consequences. It is caused by the entry of an allergen into the blood, e.g. venom of a snake or

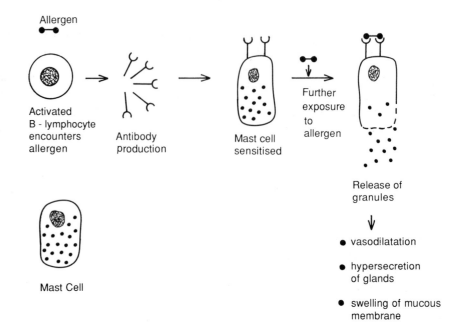

Figure 4.16 The sequence of events leading to an anaphylactic reaction.

insect, a large molecule therapeutic agent such as penicillin, usually administered by injection. There are profound effects throughout the body, including generalised vasodilatation, leading to severe hypotension and contraction of smooth muscle in the respiratory tract, causing acute breathing difficulties. A widespread skin rash may also occur.

Other antibody-mediated reactions. Reaction of antibodies with cells that have antigens on their cytoplasmic membranes may cause the cells to rupture, e.g. when incompatible blood is administered. Abnormal reactions to antibody/antibody complexes sometimes results in them adhering to the endothelium of blood vessels causing inflammation and local damage in, e.g. glomerulonephritis (p. 348), or rheumatoid arthritis (p. 409).

Cell-mediated reactions

These develop gradually over a period of 24 to 48 hours after the second encounter with an antigen. They are due to the activities of specifically activated T-lymphocytes and phagocytes. The lymphocytes release non-antibody substances called *lymphokines* that are believed to amplify the immune response, attract and retain macrophages in the affected area and promote phagocytosis. Local inflammation accompanies this process often causing skin rashes. The antigens include:

■ intracellular microbes, e.g. those causing tuberculosis, measles, mumps
■ some vaccines, e.g. against smallpox
■ some metals and chemical compounds that combine with protein in the skin and cause allergic contact dermatitis.

Immune response to tumours. There is increasing evidence to suggest that a cell-mediated immune response occurs when tumour cells form. This may either isolate and inactivate a single malignant cell, preventing tumour formation, or be on a larger scale, responding to established tumours.

Mixed reactions

Autoimmune diseases. These conditions are caused by an imbalance in the immune response and result in tissue damage and signs of disease as the body fails to recognise its own tissues. Destruction of the body's own cells may be either humoral due to the formation of antibodies or cell-mediated due to T-cell reactions.

When the self-antigen is limited to one type of cell, damage is limited to only one organ, e.g.:

■ thyroid—Hashimoto's thyroiditis (p. 230)
■ stomach—Addisonian pernicious anaemia (p. 74)
■ cortex of the adrenal gland—Addison's disease (p. 232)
■ pancreas—type 1 diabetes mellitus (p. 233).

In other cases the self-antigen is found in many locations throughout the body and tissue damage is widespread, e.g. synovial membranes, causing rheumatoid arthritis.

Organ transplantation and rejection. Tissue typing is carried out prior to tissue transplants from donors to minimise the possibility of rejection by the recipient. Transplant rejection occurs when the immune system of the host responds to the foreign tissue. It may be humoral or cell-mediated.

Non-specific defence mechanisms

These are the first lines of general defence; they prevent entry and minimise further passage of microbes and other foreign material into the body. The non-specific processes of dealing with successful invaders are: *phagocytosis* (p. 62) and *inflammation*.

Skin and mucous membrane

When skin and mucous membrane are intact and healthy they provide a physical barrier to invading microbes. The outer horny layer of skin can be penetrated by only a few microbes and the mucus secreted by mucous membrane traps microbes and other foreign material on its sticky surface. Sebum and sweat secreted on to the skin surface contain antibacterial and antifungal substances.

Hairs in the nose act as a coarse filter and the action of mucous membrane in the respiratory tract moves mucus and inhaled foreign materials towards the throat. Then it is expectorated or swallowed.

The one-way flow of urine from the bladder during micturition minimises the risk of microbes ascending through the urethra into the bladder.

Antimicrobial substances in body secretions

Hydrochloric acid, present in high concentrations in gastric juice, kills the majority of ingested microbes.

Lysozyme is a small molecule protein with antibacterial properties present in granulocytes, tears, and other body secretions. It is not present in sweat, urine and cerebrospinal fluid.

Immunoglobulins in nasal secretions and saliva are able to inactivate some viruses.

Saliva is secreted into the mouth and washes away food debris that may serve as culture medium for microbes. Its slightly acid reaction inhibits the growth of some microbes.

Interferons are substances produced by T-lymphocytes and by cells that have been invaded by viruses. They prevent viral replication within cells and spread of viruses to other cells.

Inflammation

This is the physiological response to tissue damage and is accompanied by a characteristic series of local changes. It most commonly takes place when microbes have overcome the non-specific defence mechanisms. Its purpose is protective: to isolate, inactivate and remove both the causative agent and damaged tissue so that healing can take place.

Inflammatory conditions are recognised by their Latin suffix -itis:

- appendicitis—inflammation of the appendix
- laryngitis—inflammation of the larynx.

Causes of inflammation

The agents that cause inflammation are very numerous but they may be classified as follows:

- microbes, e.g. bacteria, viruses, protozoa, fungi
- physical agents, e.g. heat, cold, mechanical injury, ultraviolet and ionising radiation
- chemical agents
  —organic, e.g. microbial toxins and organic poisons, such as weedkillers
  —inorganic, e.g. acids, alkalis
- antigens that stimulate immunological responses.

Acute inflammation

Episodes of acute inflammation are usually of short duration, e.g. days to a few weeks, and may range from mild to very severe. The cardinal signs of inflammation are:

- redness
- heat
- pain
- swelling
- loss of function.

The changes that take place in the tissues are active hyperaemia, exudation and migration of leukocytes.

Active hyperaemia

Following injury there is dilatation of arterioles and increased blood flow in the capillaries. This is caused by modification of the sympathetic nerve control of the arterioles and the secretion of a number of chemical mediators released by damaged cells, e.g. histamine, serotonin. Increased blood flow to the area of tissue damage provides more oxygen and nutrients for the increased cellular activity that accompanies inflammation. Redness and heat are caused by hyperaemia.

Exudation

In an area of inflammation the amount of interstitial fluid is increased and its composition changed. The amount depends on the net filtration pressure (hydrostatic and osmotic) across capillary walls, which is raised when arterioles dilate. Interstitial fluid normally consists of molecules of water and other substances small enough to pass through pores in the walls. The composition is changed because the permeability of small vessel walls is increased by basophils and by a number of powerful chemical mediators, e.g. histamine and serotonin produced by damaged cells. This enables large molecules, including antibodies and fibrinogen, to enter the tissue spaces. Some interstitial fluid returns to the capillaries at the venous end but most of the inflammatory exudate, phagocytes and cell debris are removed in lymph vessels because the pores of lymph vessels are larger, and the pressure inside is lower, than in blood capillaries.

Migration of leukocytes

The migrating cells are the phagocytic granulocytes and monocytes. The number involved and the duration of the migration depend on the severity of the inflammation and, to some extent, on the cause. Pyogenic (pus producing) microbes, such as *Streptococcus pyogenes*, *Staphylococcus aureus* and *Streptococcus pneumoniae*, are associated with large-scale migration. Exudation of fluid increases blood viscosity and slows the rate of flow. The leukocytes stick to the walls of small blood vessels, then pass between the endothelial cells into the interstitial spaces by amoeboid movement (Fig 4.10). The extra fluid dilutes toxins and fibrin walls off the site, preventing the local spread of the inflammation. Some microbes such as *Streptococcus pyogenes* secrete toxins that break down fibrin, enabling infection to spread.

Chemotaxis. This is the chemical attraction of leukocytes to an area of inflammation. The role of chemotaxins and the way in which they work is not fully understood. They increase the permeability of the walls of small blood vessels but their action also appears to be more specific. Large numbers of phagocytes accumulate in the inflamed area but substances of smaller size remain in the capillaries. The known chemotaxins include: microbial toxins, lymphokines from sensitised T-lymphocytes, products of immune complexes, prostaglandins from damaged cells.

Effects of acute inflammation

Most of these assist the body to overcome the cause of inflammation.

Phagocytosis (Fig. 4.11)

Neutrophils and macrophages in the tissue spaces engulf particles of biological and non-biological origin. Biological material includes dead and damaged cells, microbes, and damaged connective tissue fibres. Most biological material is digested by enzymes inside phagocytes. Some microbes resist digestion and provide a possible source of future infection, e.g. *Mycobacterium tuberculosis*. Non-biological materials which cannot be digested include inhaled dust particles, chemical substances and material contaminating wounds. Many phagocytes may die in an inflamed area if the material they ingest resists digestion, or if the number of particles is excessive. When this happens the phagocytes disintegrate and release material that may become fibrosed or cause further damage.

Immune response

When inflammation is caused by microbes, antibodies formed by lymphocytes following a previous encounter with a particular microbe or its toxin filter through the capillary walls in the inflammatory exudate. The antibodies may promote phagocytosis of the microbes and neutralise their toxins. Harmful immune responses include rejection of transplanted tissues and allergic reactions to normally innocuous substances, e.g. foods, pollen, talcum powder, clothing materials, feathers, dander from animal hair.

Toxin dilution

The water in inflammatory exudate dilutes damaging and waste materials in the area, and assists their removal from the site. This is of particular importance when injurious chemicals and bacterial toxins are involved.

Fibrin formation

Fibrinogen, secreted by fibroblasts present in inflammatory exudate, is acted upon by thromboplastin released from damaged cells and forms an insoluble fibrin network. This may:

- wall off the inflamed area, preventing the spread of the cause
- bind together the cut edges of a wound during primary healing.

Some microbes such as *Streptococcus pyogenes* secrete toxins that break down fibrin, enabling infection to spread.

Tissue swelling

This is the result of the increased blood flow and exudation and is often accompanied by loss of function. The effects can be harmful, depending on the site:

- in a joint—limitation of movement
- in the larynx—interference with breathing
- in a confined space, such as inside the skull or under the periosteum of bone—severe pain due to pressure on nerves.

Pain

This occurs when local swelling compresses sensory nerve endings. It is exacerbated by chemical mediators of the inflammatory process, e.g. bradykinin, prostaglandins that potentiate the sensitivity of the sensory nerve endings to painful stimuli.

Systemic effects

Body temperature rises when an endogenous pyrogen (interleukin 1) is released from macrophages and granulocytes in response to microbial toxins or immune complexes. Interleukin 1 is a chemical mediator that resets the temperature thermostat in the hypothalamus at a higher level causing pyrexia and other symptoms that may also accompany inflammation, e.g. fatigue and loss of appetite. Pyrexia increases the metabolic rate of cells in the inflamed area and, consequently, there is an increased need for oxygen and nutritional materials.

Outcomes of acute inflammation

Resolution

This occurs when the cause has been successfully overcome. The inflammatory process is reversed and:

- damaged cells are phagocytosed
- fibrin strands are broken down by fibrinolytic enzymes
- waste material is removed in lymph and blood vessels
- repair is complete leaving only a small scar.

Suppuration (pus formation)

Pus consists of dead phagocytes, dead cells, cell debris, fibrin, inflammatory exudate and living and dead microbes. It is contained within a membrane of new blood capillaries, phagocytes and fibroblasts. The most common causative pyogenic microbes are *Staphylococcus aureus* and *Streptococcus pyogenes*. Small amounts of pus form *boils* and larger amounts form *abscesses*. *Staphylococcus aureus* produces the enzyme coagulase which converts fibrinogen to fibrin, localising the pus. *Streptococcus pyogenes* produces streptolysins that promote the breakdown of connective tissue, causing spreading infection. Healing, following pus formation, is by granulation and fibrosis.

Superficial abscesses tend to rupture through the skin and discharge pus. Healing is usually complete unless there is extensive tissue damage.

Deep-seated abscesses may have a variety of outcomes. There may be:

- rupture with complete discharge of pus on to the surface, followed by healing
- rupture and limited discharge of pus on to the surface, followed by the development of a chronic abscess with an infected open channel or *sinus* (Fig. 4.17)
- rupture and discharge of pus into an adjacent organ or cavity, forming an infected channel open at both ends or *fistula* (Fig. 4.18)
- eventual removal of pus by phagocytes, followed by healing

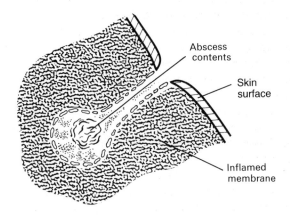

Figure 4.17 Sinus between an abscess and the surface of the body.

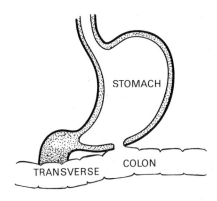

Figure 4.18 Fistula between the stomach and the colon.

- enclosure of pus by fibrous tissue that may become calcified, harbouring live organisms which may become a source of future infection
- formation of fibrous adhesions between adjacent membranes, e.g. pleura, peritoneum
- shrinkage of fibrous tissue as it ages that may reduce the lumen or obstruct a tube, e.g. oesophagus, bowel, blood vessel.

Chronic inflammation

The processes involved are very similar to those of acute inflammation. The main differences are:

- the inflammation is less severe and lasts longer, maybe weeks, months or years
- there is destruction of considerably more tissue
- more fibrous tissue is formed.

Chronic inflammation may either be a complication of acute inflammation or a primary condition of slow onset.

Following acute inflammation

Any form of acute inflammation may develop into the chronic form if resolution is not complete, e.g. if live microbes remain at the site, as in some deep-seated abscesses, wound infections and bone infections.

Slow onset of inflammation

This may be caused by:

- infection by low-virulence organisms in an area with a poor blood supply, e.g. endocarditis caused by non-haemolytic streptococci
- inorganic materials when:
  —an internal stitch has not dissolved
  —toxic silicic acid is formed when silicon, inhaled in dust, is dissolved

- hypersensitivity developed following repeated exposure to some chemicals, e.g. in contact dermatitis skin proteins are altered when some chemicals are absorbed, the altered proteins act as antigens, stimulating the production of antibodies and initiating the inflammatory process.

Fibrosis (scar formation)

Fibrous tissue is formed during healing when there is loss of tissue or the cells destroyed do not regenerate, e.g. following chronic inflammation, ischaemia, suppuration, large-scale trauma. The process begins with the formation of granulation tissue, then, over a period of time, the new capillaries and inflammatory material are removed leaving only the collagen fibres secreted by the fibroblasts. Fibrous tissue may have long-lasting damaging effects.

Adhesions consisting of fibrous tissue may limit movement, e.g. between the layers of pleura, preventing inflation of the lungs; between loops of bowel, interfering with peristalsis.

Fibrosis of infarcts. Blockage of an end-vessel by a thrombus or an embolus causes an infarct (area of dead tissue). Fibrosis of one large infarct or of numerous small infarcts may follow, leading to varying degrees of organ dysfunction, e.g. in heart, brain, kidneys, liver.

Tissue shrinkage occurs as fibrous tissue ages. The effects depend on the site and extent of the fibrosis, e.g.:

- small tubes, such as blood vessels, air passages, ureters, the urethra and ducts of glands may become narrow or obstructed and lose their elasticity
- contractures (bands of shrunken fibrous tissue) may extend across joints, e.g. in a limb or digit there may be limitation of movement or, following burns of the neck, the head may be pulled to one side.

ERYTHROCYTE DISORDERS

Anaemia

In anaemia there is not enough haemoglobin available to carry sufficient oxygen from the lungs to supply the needs of the tissues. It occurs when the rate of production of mature cells entering the blood from the red bone marrow does not keep pace with the rate of haemolysis. The classification of anaemia is based on the cause:

■ impaired erythrocyte production
—iron deficiency
—megaloblastic anaemias
—hypoplastic anaemia
■ increased erythrocyte loss
—haemolytic anaemias
—normocytic anaemia.

Red cells may appear abnormal when examined microscopically. Characteristic changes are listed in Table 4.5. Characteristics of severe anaemia include tachycardia, palpitations, angina and breathlessness on exertion.

Iron deficiency anaemia (hypochromic microcytic anaemia)

This is the most common form of anaemia in many parts of the world. The normal daily requirement of iron intake in men is about 1 to 2 mg derived from meat and highly coloured vegetables. The normal daily requirement in women is 3 mg. The increase is necessary to compensate for loss of blood during menstruation and to meet the needs of the growing fetus during pregnancy. Children, during their period of rapid growth, require more than adults.

The amount of haemoglobin in each cell is regarded as below normal when the MCH is less than 27 pg/cell. The anaemia is regarded as severe when the haemoglobin level is below 9 g/dl blood. It is caused by deficiency of iron in the bone marrow and may be due to dietary deficiency, excessively high requirement or malabsorption. Usually more than one factor is involved, e.g. loss of blood and malabsorption.

In this type of anaemia erythrocytes are small (microcytic) and paler than normal (hypochromic) as their haemoglobin content is low.

Dietary deficiency

Normal iron requirements with low intake
This occurs in babies fed only on milk because it contains very little iron. Until a mixed diet is established, the baby is dependent on iron stored in the liver before birth.

High iron requirements with normal or low intake
This type of anaemia occurs in pregnancy but is usually due to chronic blood loss and may be exacerbated by low iron intake. The causes include:

■ chronic peptic ulcers
■ menorrhagia
■ intestinal ulceration
■ haemorrhoids
■ carcinoma.

Malabsorption

Iron absorption is usually increased following haemorrhage but may be reduced in abnormalities of the stomach, duodenum or jejunum including:

■ resection of stomach or upper part of the small intestine
■ hypochlorhydria, e.g. in malignant disease, Addisonian pernicious anaemia.

Megaloblastic anaemias (macrocytic)

Maturation of erythrocytes is impaired when deficiency of Vitamin B_{12} and/or folic acid occurs (Fig. 4.5) and abnormally large erythrocytes (megaloblasts) are found in the

Table 4.5	Summary of the types of anaemia		
Type of anaemia	Bone marrow	Blood	Spleen
Normocytic	Erythropoiesis inadequate	Reduced numbers of normal cells	
Hypoplastic	Reduced erythropoiesis	Reduced number of normal cells	
Megaloblastic	Deficiency of vitamin B_{12} and/or folic acid	Large cells, some nucleated	
Hypochromic	Deficiency of iron	Reduced haemoglobin, pale coloured cells	
Haemolytic	Genetic abnormality	Normal or abnormal cells	Early lysis
	Immune reaction		Early lysis

blood. During normal erythropoiesis (Fig. 4.4) several cell divisions occur and the daughter cells at each stage are smaller than the parent cell because there is not much time for cell enlargement between divisions. When deficiency of Vitamin B_{12} and/or folic acid occurs, the rate of DNA and RNA synthesis is reduced, delaying cell division. The cells can therefore grow larger than normal between divisions. Circulating cells are immature, larger than normal and some are nucleated (MCV >94). The haemoglobin content of each cell is normal or raised. The cells are fragile and their life span is reduced to between 40 and 50 days. Depressed production and early lysis cause anaemia.

Vitamin B_{12} deficiency anaemia

Addisonian pernicious anaemia
This is the most common form of vitamin B_{12} deficiency anaemia. It occurs more often in females than males, usually between 45 and 65 years of age. It is an autoimmune disease in which auto-antibodies destroy intrinsic factor (IF) and parietal cells.

Dietary deficiency of vitamin B_{12}
Intake of less than the required 1 μg of vitamin B_{12} is rare, except in true vegans, i.e. when no animal products are included in the diet. The store of vitamin B_{12} is such that deficiency takes several years to appear.

Other causes of vitamin B_{12} deficiency
These include:

■ *gastrectomy*—leaves fewer cells available to produce IF after partial resection of the stomach.

■ *chronic gastritis, malignant disease, ionising radiation*—damage the gastric mucosa including the parietal cells that produce IF.
■ *blind loop syndrome*—occurs when the contents of the small intestine are slow moving or static allowing microbes to colonise the small intestine and use or destroy the intrinsic factor–vitamin B_{12} (IF–B_{12}) complex before it reaches the terminal ileum where it is absorbed. Blind loops of bowel occur in diverticular disease (p. 326) and are left after some surgical procedures.
■ *malabsorption of intrinsic factor–vitamin B_{12} complex*—may follow resection of terminal ileum or inflammation of the terminal ileum, e.g. Crohn's disease, tropical sprue.

Complications of vitamin B_{12} deficiency anaemia. These may appear before the signs of anaemia. They include:

■ subacute combined degeneration of the spinal cord in which nerve fibres in the posterior and lateral columns of white matter become demyelinated, causing ataxia, spastic paralysis, pain, loss of sensation and joint position sense. It usually begins in the lower thoracic region then extends upwards and outwards. Vitamin B_{12} is essential for the secretion and maintainance of myelin (p. 142 and p. 186).
■ atrophy and ulceration of the tongue and glossitis.

Folic acid deficiency anaemia

Deficiency in the bone marrow causes a form of megaloblastic anaemia not associated with degen-

eration of the spinal cord. It may be due to:

■ dietary deficiency, e.g. in infants if there is delay in establishing a mixed diet, in alcoholics, in anorexia and in pregnancy when the requirement is raised
■ malabsorption from the jejunum caused by, e.g. coeliac disease, tropical sprue, anticonvulsant drugs
■ interference with utilisation by, e.g. cytotoxic and anticonvulsant drugs.

Hypoplastic and aplastic anaemia

The degree of bone marrow depression varies from mild hypoplasia to aplasia when no erythrocytes enter the blood. Aplastic anaemia is usually accompanied by abnormal leukocyte and thrombocyte production when the condition is called *pancytopenia*. The condition is often idiopathic, but the known causes include:

■ drugs, e.g. cytotoxic drugs, some anti-inflammatory and anticonvulsant drugs, some sulphonamides and antibiotics
■ ionising radiation
■ some chemicals, e.g. benzene and its derivatives
■ chronic nephritis
■ virus disease, including hepatitis
■ invasion of bone marrow by, e.g., malignant disease, leukaemia, fibrosis.

Complications
These include the complications of severe anaemia and, in addition, leukopenia, leading to infection and thrombocytopenia, predisposing to bleeding.

Haemolytic anaemias

These occur when red cells are destroyed while in circulation or are removed prematurely from the circulation because the cells are abnormal or the spleen is overactive.

Congenital haemolytic anaemias

In these diseases genetic abnormality leads to the synthesis of abnormal haemoglobin and increased red cell membrane friability, reducing cell oxygen-carrying capacity and life span. The most common forms are sickle cell anaemia and thalassaemia.

Sickle cell anaemia
The abnormal haemoglobin molecules become misshapen when deoxygenated, making the erythrocytes sickle shaped. A high proportion of abnormal molecules makes the sickling permanent. The life span of cells is reduced by early haemolysis. Sickle cells do not move smoothly through the small blood vessels. This tends to increase the viscosity of the blood, reducing the rate of blood flow and leading to intravascular clotting, ischaemia and infarction. The anaemia is due to early haemolysis of irreversibly sickled cells.

Negroes are more affected than other races. Some affected individuals have a degree of immunity to malaria because the life span of the sickled cells is less than the time needed for the malaria parasite to mature inside the cells.

Complications. Pregnancy, infection and dehydration predispose to the development of 'crises' due to intravascular clotting and ischaemia, causing severe pain in, e.g. long bones, chest, abdomen. The formation of gallstones (cholelithiasis) and inflammation of the gall bladder (cholecystitis) also occurs (p. 334).

Thalassaemia
There is reduced globin synthesis with resultant reduced haemoglobin production and increased friability of the cell membrane, leading to early haemolysis. Severe cases may cause death in infants or young children. This condition is most common in Mediterranean countries.

Haemolytic disease of the newborn
This is caused by the presence of the *rhesus (Rh) factor* antigens on the fetal erythrocyte membrane. Incompatibility occurs when the Rh factor is absent from the mother's cells and the child has inherited it from the father. A small number of fetal erythrocytes cross the placental barrier and enter the mother's blood. Her immune system treats the fetal Rh factor as antigen and develops specific antibodies against it. These antibodies then pass from mother to fetus and haemolyse fetal erythrocytes before birth and for some time afterwards. It is believed that fetal erythrocytes are able to cross the placenta as it becomes more permeable near the end of pregnancy stimulating the immune reaction in the mother.

The severity of the condition depends on the concentration, or titre, of maternal antibodies. In second and subsequent pregnancies red cells from an Rh +ve fetus stimulate a dramatic increase in antibody production by the mother unless she is immunised with serum containing antibodies.

Acquired haemolytic anaemia

In this context acquired means haemolytic anaemia in which no familial or racial factors have been identified. There are several causes.

Chemical agents
These substances cause early or excessive haemolysis, e.g.:

- some drugs, especially when taken long term in large doses, e.g. phenacetin, primaquine, sulphonamides
- chemicals encountered in the general or work environment, e.g. lead, arsenic compounds
- toxins produced by microbes, e.g. *Streptococcus pyogenes*, *Clostridium welchii*.

Autoimmunity
In this disease antibodies are formed which react with red cell antigens, causing haemolysis. It may be acute or chronic and primary or secondary to other diseases, e.g. carcinoma, rheumatoid arthritis and other connective tissue diseases, virus infections, Raynaud's disease, other autoimmune conditions.

Cold antibody. The antibodies react with red cells at temperatures below 30°C, causing agglutination and haemolysis, usually in the blood vessels in hands and feet on exposure to cold.

Warm antibody type. The antibodies are active at normal temperature (37°C). The haemolysis is usually chronic but there may be fluctuations with periodic acute exacerbations.

Incompatible blood transfusions
In some people there are antigens on the erythrocyte cell membranes that react with natural antibodies in the plasma of others. Incompatibility of blood occurs when the antigens on the donor's red cells react with the antibodies in the recipient's plasma, causing erythrocyte agglutination and haemolysis (Table 4.2 and Fig. 4.7).

Complications In acute cases severe intravascular haemolysis occurs and is accompanied by severe loin pain and shock. This may then result in acute renal failure.

Other causes of haemolytic anaemia

These include:

- parasitic diseases, e.g. malaria
- ionising radiation, e.g. X-rays, radioactive isotopes
- destruction of blood trapped in tissues in, e.g. severe burns, crushing injuries
- physical damage to cells by, e.g. artificial heart valves, kidney dialysis machines.

Normocytic anaemia (normochromic)

In this type the cells are normal but the numbers are reduced and the proportion of reticulocytes in the blood may be increased. This occurs:

- in many chronic disease conditions, e.g. in chronic inflammation
- following severe haemorrhage
- in haemolytic disease.

Polycythaemia

There are an abnormally large number of erythrocytes in the blood. This increases blood viscosity, slows the rate of flow and increases the risk of intravascular clotting, ischaemia and infarction.

Relative increase in erythrocyte count

This occurs when the erythrocyte count is normal but the blood volume is reduced by fluid loss, e.g. excessive serum exudate from extensive superficial burns.

True increase in erythrocyte count

Physiological. Prolonged hypoxia stimulates erythropoiesis and the number of cells released into the normal volume of blood is increased. This occurs in people living at high altitudes where the oxygen tension in the air is low and the partial pressure of oxygen in the alveoli of the lungs is correspondingly low. Each cell carries less oxygen so more cells are needed to meet the body's oxygen needs.

Pathological. The reason for this increase in circulating red cells, sometimes to twice the normal number, is not known. It may be secondary to other factors that cause hypoxia of the red bone marrow e.g. cigarette smoking, pulmonary disease, bone marrow cancer.

Polycythaemia rubra vera

In this primary condition of unknown cause there is abnormal excessive production of the erythrocyte precursors, i.e. *myeloproliferation.* This raises the haemoglobin level and the haematocrit (relative proportion of cells to plasma). The blood viscosity is increased and may lead to: hypertension; cerebral, coronary and mesenteric thrombosis. Aplastic anaemia and leukaemia may also be present.

HAEMORRHAGIC DISEASES

Thrombocytopenia

This is defined as a blood platelet count below $150 \times 10^9/l$ (150 000/mm^3) but spontaneous capillary bleeding does not usually occur unless the count falls below $30 \times 10^9/l$ (30 000/mm^3). It may be due to a reduced rate of platelet production or increased rate of destruction.

Reduced platelet production. This is usually associated with pancytopenia, and accompanied by anaemia and leukopenia. It is often due to:

- platelets being crowded out of the bone marrow in bone marrow diseases, e.g. leukaemias, pernicious anaemia, malignant tumours
- ionising radiation, e.g. X-rays, radioactive isotopes
- drugs, e.g. cytotoxic drugs, chloramphenicol, chlorpromazine, phenylbutazone, sulphonamides.

Increased platelet destruction. A reduced platelet count occurs when production of new cells does not keep pace with destruction of damaged and worn out cells. This occurs in disseminated intravascular coagulation and autoimmune thrombocytopenic purpura.

Purpura

This is generalised bleeding due to increased capillary wall fragility and/or thrombocytopenia. It is seen either as small haemorrhagic spots on the skin and mucous membranes, called *petechiae*, or as large blotchy areas. Purpura occurs in scurvy due to vitamin C deficiency and as a complication of some diseases in which there is thrombocytopenia, e.g. leukaemia, aplastic anaemia, severe acute infections.

Autoimmune thrombocytopenic purpura

This usually affects children and young adults. It may be triggered by a virus infection in which anti-platelet antibodies are formed that lead to the destruction of platelets by phagocytosis. The severity of the disease varies from mild bleeding into the skin to severe haemorrhage. When the platelet count is very low there may be severe bruising, haematuria, gastrointestinal or cranial haemorrhages.

Secondary thrombocytopenic purpura

This may occur in association with red bone marrow diseases, excessive irradiation and some drugs, e.g. digoxin, chlorthiazides, quinine, sulphonamides. When the spleen is enlarged and congested, platelets are trapped in it and are destroyed by macrophages.

Vitamin K deficiency

Vitamin K is required by the liver for the synthesis of many clotting factors and therefore deficiency predisposes to impairment of haemostasis (p. 333).

Haemorrhagic disease of the newborn
Spontaneous haemorrhage from the umbilical cord and intestinal mucosa occurs in babies when the stored vitamin K obtained from the mother before birth has been used up and the intestinal bacteria needed for its synthesis in the infant's bowel are not yet established. This is most likely to occur when the baby is premature.

Deficient absorption in adults
Vitamin K is fat soluble and bile salts are required in the colon for its absorption. Deficiency may occur when there is liver disease, prolonged obstruction to the biliary tract or in any other disease where fat absorption is impaired, e.g. coeliac disease.

Dietary deficiency
This is rare because a sufficient supply of vitamin K is usually synthesised in the intestine by bacterial action. However, deficiency may occur during treatment with drugs that sterilise the bowel.

Disseminated intravascular coagulation (DIC)

In this disease the complex mechanisms that control haemostasis break down. Tiny intravascular clots form and fibrin is deposited in many small blood vessels in a wide range of internal organs. It occurs in association with a number of conditions in which substances that promote clotting are produced, e.g.:

- severe shock, especially when due to microbial infection
- septicaemia when endotoxins are released by Gram-negative bacteria
- severe trauma
- premature separation of placenta when amniotic fluid enters maternal blood
- acute pancreatitis when digestive enzymes are released into the blood
- malignant tumours with widely dispersed metastases.

Complications
The reduction of platelets and clotting factors predisposes to severe haemorrhage.

Genetic abnormalities

In each body cell, except gametes, there are 46 chromosomes arranged in 23 pairs of which one pair are sex chromosomes. In the female, the two sex chromosomes are identical and are called X chromosomes. In the male, each cell has one X chromosome and one Y chromosome.

Female—XX
Male—XY

Each gamete (ovum and spermatozoon) has only 23 chromosomes, one from each of the 23 pairs. This means that each ovum has an X chromosome and each spermatozoon has either an X *or* a Y chromosome.

The gene that promotes the antihaemophilic activity of factors VIII and IX in the clotting mechanism is carried on X chromosomes only. When this gene is abnormal or absent, *haemophilia* occurs in males. It is transmitted to the next generation by symptom-free females and by affected males.

Haemophilia A

In this disease, factor VIII is abnormal and is less biologically active. For descriptive purposes abnormal X chromosomes are designated X'. Thus the distribution of chromosomes is:

Female: XX' or XX
Ovum: X or X'
Male: X'Y or XY
Spermatozoon: X' or X or Y

The system of inheritance of haemophilia is as follows (Fig 4.19):

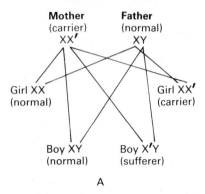

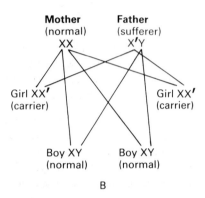

Figure 4.19 The pattern of inheritance of abnormal chromosomes in haemophilia.
A. Mother is a carrier.
B. Father is a sufferer.

- When an X′ ovum combines with a Y sperm the male child (X′Y) is a haemophiliac.
- When an X′ ovum combines with an X sperm the female child (X′X) is a carrier. The disease potential is present in her cells but the normal X chromosome provides the healthy gene that promotes clotting.
- When an X′ sperm combines with an X ovum the female child (X′X) is a carrier.

Sufferers from haemophilia may experience repeated episodes of severe and prolonged bleeding at any site, with little evidence of trauma. Recurrent bleeding into joints is common, causing severe pain and, in the long term, cartilage is damaged.

Haemophilia B (Christmas disease)

This is the less common sex-linked genetic haemorrhagic disease. Factor IX is not activated, resulting in deficiency of thromboplastin. The abnormal gene is on the X chromosome and the distribution and characteristics of the disease are the same as those in haemophilia A.

Von Willebrand's disease

In this disease a deficiency in the von Willebrand factor causes low levels of factor VIII. As the inheritance is not sex-linked, haemorrhages due to defective clotting occur in males and females.

LEUKOCYTE DISORDERS

Leukopenia

This is the name of the condition in which the total blood leukocyte count is less then $4 \times 10^9/l$ (4000/mm³).

Granulocytopenia (neutropenia)

This is a general term used to indicate an abnormal reduction in the numbers of circulating granulocytes (polymorphonuclear leukocytes), commonly called *neutropenia* because 40 to 75% of granulocytes are neutrophils. A reduction in the number of circulating granulocytes occurs when production does not keep pace with the normal removal of cells or when the life span of the cells is reduced. Extreme shortage or the absence of granulocytes is called *agranulocytosis*. A temporary reduction occurs in response to inflammation but the numbers are usually quickly restored. Inadequate granulopoiesis may be caused by:

- drugs, e.g. cytotoxic drugs, phenylbutazone, phenothiazines, some sulphonamides and antibiotics
- irradiation damage to granulocyte precursors in the bone marrow by, e.g. X-rays, radioactive isotopes
- diseases of red bone marrow, e.g. leukaemias, some anaemias
- severe microbial infections.

In conditions where the spleen is enlarged excessive numbers of granulocytes are trapped, reducing the number in circulation. Neutropenia predisposes to severe infections that can lead to tissue necrosis, septicaemia and death. Septicaemia is the presence of particles of inflammatory material in the blood. The infecting microbes are commonly *commensals*, i.e. microbes that are normally present in the body but do not usually cause infection, such as those in the bowel.

Lymphopenia

This relatively uncommon condition, in which there is a decrease in the number of lymphocytes in the blood, is associated with Hodgkin's disease, non-lymphocytic leukaemias, infection with human immunodeficiency virus (HIV) and treatment of patients with, e.g. ionising radiation, cytotoxic drugs and corticosteroids. It also occurs in children in some rare congenital diseases.

Leukocytosis

An increase in the number of circulating leukocytes occurs as a normal protective reaction in a variety of pathological conditions, especially in response to infections. When the infection subsides the leukocyte count returns to normal.

Pathological leukocytosis exists when a blood leukocyte count of more than $11 \times 10^9/l$ (11 000/mm^3) is sustained and is not consistent with the normal protective function. One or more of the different types of cell is involved.

Leukaemia

Leukaemia is a *malignant proliferation of white blood cell precursors* by the bone marrow. It results in the uncontrolled increase in the production of leukocytes and/or their precursors. As the tumour cells enter the blood the total leukocyte count is usually raised but in some cases it may be normal or even low. The proliferation of leukaemic cells crowds out other blood cells formed in bone marrow, causing anaemia, thrombocytopenia and leukopenia (pancytopenia).

Causes of leukaemia
Some causes of leukaemia are known but many cases cannot be accounted for. Some people may have a genetic predisposition that is triggered by environmental factors. Known causes include:

Ionising radiation produced by X-rays and radioactive isotopes is known to cause malignant changes in the precursors of white blood cells. The genetic material of the cells may be changed and some cells die while others reproduce at an abnormally rapid rate. Leukaemia may develop at any time after irradiation, even 20 or more years later.

Chemical substances. Some chemicals encountered in the general or work environment are known to change the genetic make-up of the white cell precursors in the bone

marrow. These include benzene and its derivatives, asbestos, cytotoxic drugs, chloramphenicol.

Dormant viruses. These may be activated by unknown factors.

Types of leukaemia

Leukaemias are usually classified according to the type of cell involved, the maturity of the cells and the rate at which the disease develops (Fig. 4.4 and Table 4.6).

Acute leukaemias
These types usually have a sudden onset and affect the poorly differentiated and immature 'blast' cells (Fig. 4.4). They are aggressive tumours that reach a climax within a few weeks or months. The rapid progress of bone marrow invasion impairs its function and culminates in anaemia, haemorrhage and susceptibility to infection. The mucous membranes of the mouth and upper gastrointestinal tract are most commonly affected.

Acute myeloblastic leukaemia. This occurs at any age, but most commonly between 25 and 60 years.

Acute lymphoblastic leukaemia. This disease is most common in children under 10 years, although a number of cases may occur up to about 40 years of age.

Chronic leukaemias
These conditions are less aggressive than the acute forms and the leukocytes are more differentiated, i.e. at the 'cyte' stage (Fig. 4.4).

Chronic granulocytic leukaemia. There is a gradual increase in the number of immature granulocytes in the blood. In the later stages, anaemia, secondary haemorrhages, infections and fever become increasingly severe. It is slightly more common in men than women and

Table 4.6 Types of leukaemia and the cells involved

Type of leukaemia	Type of cell involved
Myeloid (myelogenous myeloblastic)	Granulocytes, myelocytes, myeloblasts
Lymphocytic	Lymphocytes, lymphoblasts
Monocytic	Monocytes

usually occurs between the ages of 20 and 40 years. Although treatment may appear to be successful, death usually occurs within about 5 years.

Chronic lymphocytic leukaemia. There is enlargement of the lymph nodes and hyperplasia of lymphoid tissue throughout the body. The lymphocyte count is considerably higher than normal. Lymphocytes accumulate in the bone marrow and there is progressive anaemia and thrombocytopenia. It is three times more common in males than females and it occurs mainly between the ages of 50 and 70 years. Death is usually due to repeated infections of increasing severity, with great variations in survival times.

IMMUNODEFICIENCY

These conditions arise when the immune system is compromised. There is a tendency to recurrent infections, often by microbes not normally pathogenic in humans (*opportunistic infections*). They are classified as primary (usually occurring in infancy and genetically mediated) or secondary, that is, acquired in later life as the result of another disease, e.g. protein deficiency, acute infection, chronic renal failure, bone marrow diseases, following splenectomy, acquired immune deficiency syndrome (AIDS).

Acquired immune deficiency syndrome (AIDS)

This condition is caused by the human immunodeficiency virus (HIV), an RNA retrovirus which produces the enzyme *reverse transcriptase* inside the cells of the infected person (host cells). This enzyme transforms viral RNA to DNA and this new DNA, called the provirus, is incorporated into the host cell DNA. The host cell then produces new copies of the virus that pass out into tissue fluid and blood and infect other host cells. When infected host cells divide, copies of the provirus are integrated into the DNA of daughter cells, spreading the disease within the body.

HIV has an affinity for cells that have a protein receptor called CD_4 in their membrane, e.g. T-lymphocytes, monocytes, macrophages, some B-lymphocytes and, possibly, cells in the gastrointestinal tract and neuroglial cells in the brain. Helper T-cells (Fig. 4.13) are the main cells involved. When infected their number is reduced, causing suppression of both humoral and cell-mediated immunity with the consequent development of widespread opportunistic infections, often by microbes of relatively low pathogenicity.

HIV has been isolated from semen, cervical secretions, lymphocytes, plasma, cerebrospinal fluid, tears, saliva, urine and breast milk. The secretions known to be especially infectious are semen, cervical secretions, blood and blood products.

Infection is spread by:

- sexual intercourse, vaginal and anal
- contaminated needles used:
  —during treatment of patients
  —when drug abusers share needles
- an infected mother to her child:
  —across the placenta before birth
  —while the baby is passing through the birth canal
  —possibly by breast milk.

The presence of antibodies to HIV indicates that the individual has been exposed to the virus but *not* that a naturally acquired immunity has developed. Not all those who have antibodies in their blood develop AIDS although they may act as carriers and spread the infection to others.

A few weeks after infection there may be an acute influenza-like illness with no special features, followed by a period of two or more years without symptoms.

Chronic HIV infection may cause persistent generalised lymphadenopathy (PGL). Some patients may then develop AIDS-related complex (ARC) and experience chronic low-grade fever, diarrhoea, weight loss, anaemia and leukopenia.

When AIDS develops the main complications are widespread recurrent opportunistic infections and tumours. Outstanding features include:

- pneumonia, commonly caused by *Pneumocystis carinii*, but many other microbes may be involved
- persistent nausea, diarrhoea and loss of weight due to recurrent infections of the alimentary tract by a wide variety of microbes
- meningitis, encephalitis and brain abscesses, which may be recurrent, either caused by opportunistic microbes or possibly by HIV
- deterioration in neurological function characterised by forgetfulness, loss of concentration, confusion, apathy, dementia, limb weakness, ataxia, incontinence
- skin eruptions, often widespread, e.g. eczema, psoriasis, cellulitis, impetigo, warts, shingles, 'cold sores'
- generalised lymphadenopathy, i.e. non-infective enlargement of lymph nodes
- malignant tumours,
  —lymphomas, i.e. tumours of lymph nodes
  —Kaposi's sarcoma, consisting of tumours under the skin and in internal organs.

5
The circulatory system

The circulatory or vascular system is divided for descriptive purposes into two main parts.

1. *The blood circulatory system*, consisting of the *heart*, which acts as a pump, and the *blood vessels* through which the *blood* circulates.
2. *The lymphatic system*, consisting of *lymph nodes* and *lymph vessels* through which colourless *lymph* flows.

The two systems communicate with one another and are intimately associated.

Blood is transported (Fig. 5.1) to:

■ the lungs (pulmonary circulation) where oxygen is absorbed and carbon dioxide released
■ the rest of the body (systemic circulation) supplying oxygen and nutrients to the cells and removing waste products.

The circulatory system is involved in homeostasis as it ensures continuous supply of blood to all body cells. Control of this system enables rapid response to changes that affect delivery of adequate blood to the tissues. Should the supply of oxygen and nutrients to body cells become inadequate, homeostasis is threatened and tissue damage and death follows.

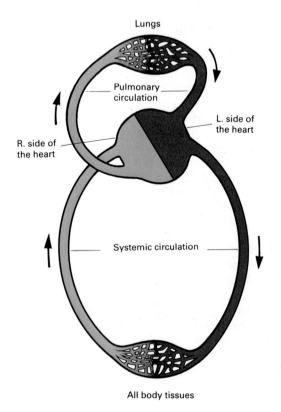

Figure 5.1 The relationship between the systemic and pulmonary circulations.

BLOOD VESSELS

These vary in size and function, and there are several types:

Arteries	Veins
Arterioles	Venules
Capillaries	

Arteries and arterioles

These are the blood vessels that transport blood away from the heart. They vary considerably in size and their walls consist of three layers of tissue (Fig. 5.2):

■ *tunica adventitia* or outer layer of fibrous tissue
■ *tunica media* or middle layer of smooth muscle and elastic tissue
■ *tunica intima* or inner lining of squamous epithelium called *endothelium*.

The amount of muscular and elastic tissue varies in the arteries depending upon their size. In the large arteries, sometimes called elastic arteries, the tunica media consists of more elastic tissue and less smooth muscle. These proportions gradually change as the arteries branch many times and become smaller until in the *arterioles* (the smallest arteries) the tunica media consists almost entirely of smooth muscle. Arteries have thicker walls than veins and this enables them to withstand the high pressure of arterial blood.

Anastomoses and end-arteries

Anastomoses are arteries that form a link between main arteries supplying an area, e.g. the arterial supply to the palms of the hand (p. 105) and soles of the feet, the brain, the joints and, to a limited extent, the heart muscle. If one artery supplying the area is occluded anastomotic arteries provide a *collateral circulation*. This is most likely to provide an adequate blood supply when the occlusion occurs gradually, giving the anastomotic arteries time to dilate.

End-arteries are the arteries with no anastomoses or those beyond the most distal anastomosis, e.g. the branches from the circle of Willis in the brain, the central artery to the retina of the eye. When an end-artery is occluded the tissues it supplies die because there is no alternative blood supply.

Veins and venules

The veins are the blood vessels that return blood at low pressure to the heart. The walls of the veins are thinner than those of arteries but have the same three layers of tissue (Fig. 5.2). They are thinner because there is less muscle and elastic tissue in the tunica media. When cut, the veins collapse while the thicker-walled arteries remain open.

When an artery is cut blood spurts at high pressure while a slower, steady flow of blood escapes from a vein.

Some veins possess *valves*, which prevent backflow of blood, ensuring that it flows towards the heart (Fig. 5.3). Valves are abundant in the veins of the limbs, especially the lower limbs where blood must travel a considerable distance against gravity when the individual is standing. Valves are absent in very small and very large veins in the thorax and abdomen. They are

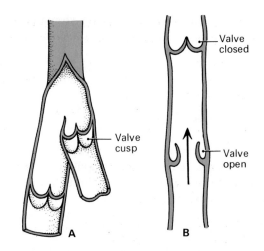

Figure 5.3 Interior of a vein. A. Showing the valves and cusps. B. Arrow showing the direction of blood flow through a valve.

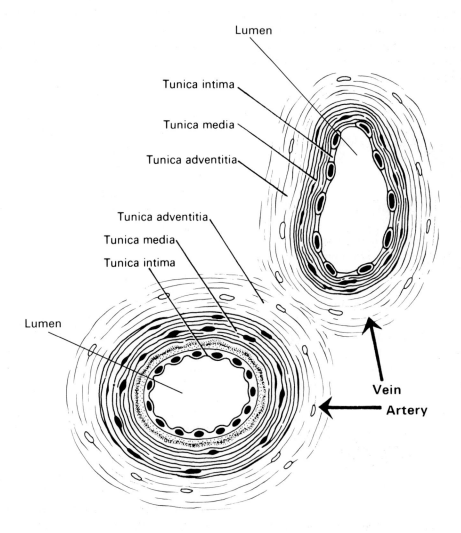

Figure 5.2 Structure of an artery and a vein.

formed by a fold of tunica intima strengthened by connective tissue. The cusps are *semilunar* in shape with the concavity towards the heart.

The smallest veins are called *venules*.

Capillaries and sinusoids

The smallest arterioles break up into a number of minute vessels called *capillaries*. Capillary walls consist of a single layer of endothelial cells through which water and other small-molecule substances can pass. Blood cells and large-molecule substances such as plasma proteins do not normally pass through capillary walls. The capillaries form a vast network of tiny vessels which link the smallest arterioles to the smallest venules. Their diameter is approximately that of an erythrocyte (7 μm). The capillary bed is the site of exchange of substances between the blood and the tissue fluid, thence to body cells.

Sinusoids are wider than capillaries and have extremely thin walls separating blood from the neighbouring cells. In some there are distinct spaces between the endothelial cells. Among the endothelial cells there may be many phagocytic macrophages, e.g. Kupffer cells in the liver. Sinusoids are found in bone marrow, endocrine glands, spleen and liver. Because of their larger lumen the blood pressure in sinusoids is lower than in capillaries and there is a slower rate of blood flow.

Control of blood vessel diameter

All blood vessels except capillaries have smooth muscle fibres in the tunica media which are supplied by nerves of the *autonomic nervous system*. These nerves arise from the *vasomotor centre* in the *medulla oblongata* and they change the diameter of the lumen of blood vessels, controlling the amount of blood they contain. Medium-sized and small arteries have more muscle than elastic tissue in their walls. In large arteries, such as the aorta, the middle layer is almost entirely elastic tissue. This means that small arteries and arterioles respond to nerve stimulation whereas the calibre of large arteries varies according to the amount of blood they contain.

Vasodilatation and vasoconstriction
Sympathetic nerves supply the smooth muscle of the tunica media of blood vessels. There is no parasympathetic nerve supply to most blood vessels and therefore the diameter of the vessel lumen and the tone of the smooth muscle is determined by the degree of sympa-

thetic nerve stimulation. There is always some nervous input to the smooth muscle in the vessel walls which can then be increased or decreased (Fig. 5.4). Decreased nerve stimulation causes the smooth muscle to relax, thinning the vessel wall and enlarging the lumen. This process is called *vasodilatation* and results in increased blood flow under less resistance. Conversely, when nervous activity is increased the smooth muscle of the tunica media contracts and thickens; this process is called *vasoconstriction*.

The blood vessels most susceptible to nerve control are the small arterioles, the walls of which consist mainly of smooth muscle. A small change in their lumen results in considerable alteration in blood flow to the part of the body they supply. Arterioles provide the *peripheral resistance* to the flow of blood and this is important in maintaining homeostasis of blood pressure (p. 95).

Resistance to flow of fluids along a tube is determined by three factors: the diameter of the tube; the length of the tube; and the viscosity of the fluid involved. The most important factor in relation to flow of blood along vessels is peripheral resistance. The length of the vessels and viscosity of blood could also contribute but in health these are constant and are therefore not significant determinants of changes in blood flow.

Autoregulation
The accumulation of metabolites in local tissues also influences the degree of dilatation of arterioles. This mechanism ensures that local blood flow is increased in:

- increased tissue activity, e.g. vasodilatation in muscles during exercise
- following decreased blood supply to a part, e.g. in response to temporary occlusion of local blood vessels
- in response to tissue damage, e.g. in inflammation (p. 69)
- situations where the circulation to vital organs, such as the brain and heart, is threatened.

Blood supply

The outer layers of tissue of thick-walled blood vessels receive their blood supply via a network of blood vessels called the *vasa vasorum*. Vessels with thin walls and the endothelium of the others receive oxygen and nutrients by diffusion from the blood passing through them.

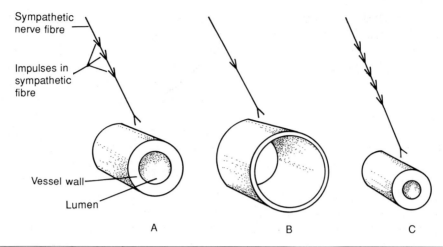

Figure 5.4 The relationship between sympathetic stimulation and blood vessel diameter. A. Resting situation. B. Vasodilatation. C. Vasoconstriction.

	Resting situation	Vasodilatation	Vasoconstriction
Sympathetic stimulation	Moderate	Decreased	Increased
Smooth muscle	Moderate Tone	Relaxes	Contracts
Thickness of vessel wall	Moderate	Thinner	Thicker
Diameter of lumen	Moderate	Increased	Decreased
Peripheral resistance in arterioles	Moderate	Decreased	Increased

Internal respiration (Fig. 5.5)

Internal respiration is the interchange of gases between the capillary blood and neighbouring body cells.

Oxygen is carried from the lungs to the tissues in chemical combination with haemoglobin as *oxy-haemoglobin*. The exchange in the tissues takes place between blood at the arterial end of the capillaries and the tissue fluid and then between the tissue fluid and the cells. The process involved is that of *diffusion from a higher concentration of oxygen in the blood to a lower concentration in the cells*, i.e. down the concentration gradient.

Oxyhaemoglobin is an unstable compound and breaks up (dissociates) easily to liberate oxygen. Factors that increase dissociation include raised carbon dioxide content of tissue fluid, raised temperature and a substance present in red blood cells. In active tissues there is an increased production of carbon dioxide and heat which leads to an increased availability of oxygen.

In this way oxygen is available to the tissues in greatest need.

Carbon dioxide is one of the waste products of cell metabolism and, towards the venous end of the capillary, it diffuses into the blood down the concentration

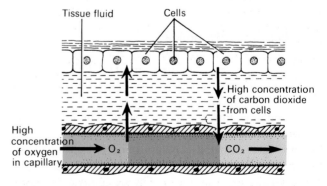

Figure 5.5 Direction of the exchange of gases in internal respiration.

gradient. Blood transports carbon dioxide to the lungs for excretion by three different mechanisms:

■ some dissolved in the water of the blood plasma
■ some in chemical combination with sodium in the form of sodium bicarbonate
■ the remainder in combination with haemoglobin.

Cell nutrition

The nutritive materials required by the cells of the body are transported round the body in the blood plasma. In the process of passing from the blood to the cells the nutritive materials pass through the semipermeable capillary walls into the tissue fluid which bathes the cells, then through the cell wall into the cell. The mechanism of the transfer of water and other substances from the blood capillaries depends mainly upon diffusion, osmosis and active transport.

Diffusion (p. 51)

The capillary walls consist of a single layer of epithelial cells that constitutes a *semipermeable membrane* which allows substances with small molecules to pass through into tissue fluid, and retains large molecules in the blood. Diffusible substances include dissolved oxygen and carbon dioxide, glucose, amino acids, fatty acids, glycerol, vitamins, mineral salts and water.

Osmosis (p. 51)

Osmotic pressure across a semipermeable membrane draws water from a dilute to a more concentrated solution in an attempt to establish a state of equilibrium. The force of the osmotic pressure depends on the *number of non-diffusible* particles in the solutions separated by the membrane. The main substances responsible for the osmotic pressure between blood and tissue fluid are the plasma proteins, especially albumin.

Capillary fluid dynamics

At the arterial end the capillary blood pressure, i.e. *hydrostatic pressure*, is about 35 mmHg. This causes the onward movement of blood and forces some water and solutes of small enough molecular size to pass out of the capillaries into the tissue spaces. The *osmotic pressure* in the capillaries is about 25 mmHg. This pressure draws water into the capillaries and is exerted mainly by plasma proteins of molecular size too large to pass through the capillary walls. The net outward pressure of 10 mmHg is the difference between the hydrostatic and osmotic pressures (Fig. 5.6 and Table 5.1).

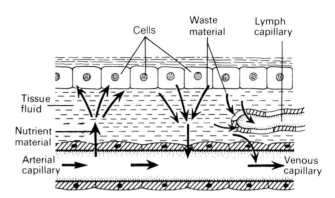

Figure 5.6 Direction of exchange of nutrients and waste products between capillaries and cells.

Table 5.1 Effects of capillary pressures		
	Arterial end	Venous end
Hydrostatic pressure (outward)	35mmHg	15mmHg
Osmotic pressure (inward)	25mmHg	25mmHg
Net movement of water	**Outwards**	**Inwards**

At the venous end of the capillaries hydrostatic pressure is reduced to about 15 mmHg and the osmotic pressure remains the same, at 25 mmHg. The net force moving water and solvents into the capillaries is again the difference between the two pressures, i.e. 10 mmHg.

This transfer of substances, including water, to the tissue spaces is a dynamic process. As blood flows slowly through the large network of capillaries from the arterial to the venous end, there is constant change. Not all the water and cell waste products return to the blood capillaries. The excess is drained away from the tissue spaces in the minute *lymph capillaries* which originate as blind-end tubes with walls similar to, but more permeable than, those of the blood capillaries (Fig 5.6). Extra tissue fluid and some cell waste materials enter the lymph capillaries and are eventually returned to the bloodstream (Ch. 6).

HEART

The heart is a roughly cone-shaped hollow muscular organ. It is about 10 cm long and is about the size of the owner's fist. It weighs about 225 g in women and is heavier in men (about 310 g).

Position (Fig. 5.7)

The heart is in the thoracic cavity in the mediastinum between the lungs. It lies obliquely, a little more to the

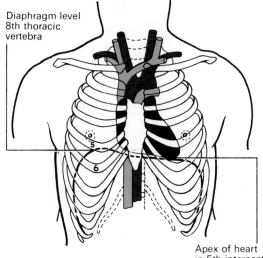

Figure 5.7 Position of the heart in the thorax.

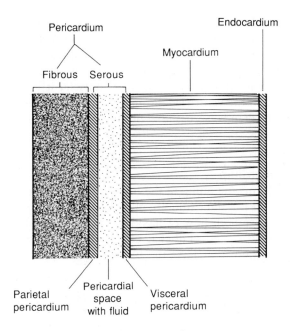

Figure 5.9 Layers of the heart wall.

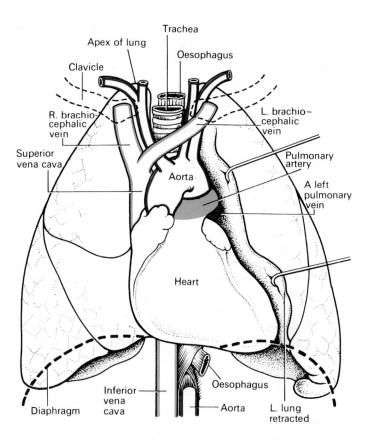

Figure 5.8 Organs associated with the heart.

left than the right, and presents a *base* above, and an *apex* below. The apex is about 9 cm to the left of the midline at the level of the 5th intercostal space, i.e. a little below the nipple and slightly nearer the midline. The base extends to the level of the 2nd rib.

Organs associated with the heart (Fig. 5.8)

Inferiorly — the apex rests on the central tendon of the diaphragm

Superiorly — the great blood vessels, i.e. the aorta, superior vena cava, pulmonary artery and pulmonary veins

Posteriorly — the oesophagus, trachea, left and right bronchus, descending aorta, inferior vena cava and thoracic vertebrae

Laterally — the lungs—the left lung overlaps the left side of the heart

Anteriorly — the sternum, ribs and intercostal muscles

Structure

The heart is composed of three layers of tissue (Fig. 5.9): pericardium, myocardium and endocardium.

Pericardium

The pericardium is made up of two sacs. The outer sac consists of fibrous tissue and the inner of a double layer of serous membrane.

The outer fibrous sac is continuous with the tunica adventitia of the great blood vessels above and is adherent to the diaphragm below. Its fibrous nature prevents overdistension of the heart.

The outer layer of the serous membrane, the *parietal pericardium*, lines the fibrous sac, and the inner layer, the *visceral pericardium*, or epicardium, is reflected on to the heart and is adherent to the heart muscle.

The serous membrane consists of flattened epithelial cells. It secretes serous fluid into the space between the visceral and parietal layers which allows smooth movement between them when the heart beats. The space between the parietal and visceral pericardium is only a *potential space*. In health the two layers are in close association, with only the thin film of serous fluid between them.

Myocardium

The myocardium is composed of specialised *cardiac muscle* tissue found only in the heart (Fig. 5.10). It is not under the control of the will but, like voluntary muscle, cross stripes can be seen on microscopic examination. Each fibre (cell) has a nucleus and one or more branches. The ends of the cells and their branches are in very close contact with the ends and branches of adjacent cells. Microscopically these 'joints', or *intercalated discs*, can be seen as thicker, darker lines than the ordinary cross stripes. This arrangement gives cardiac muscle the appearance of being a sheet of muscle rather than a very large number of individual cells. Because of the end-to-end contiguity of the fibres, each one does not need to have a separate nerve supply. When an impulse is initiated it spreads from cell to cell via the branches and intercalated discs over the whole 'sheet' of muscle, causing contraction. The 'sheet' arrangement of the myocardium enables the atria and ventricles to contract in a coordinated and efficient manner.

The myocardium is thickest at the apex and thins out towards the base (Fig. 5.11). This reflects the

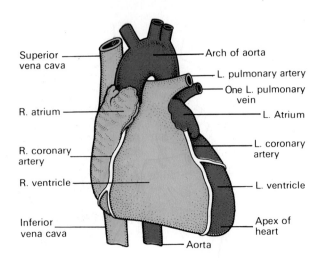

Figure 5.11 The heart and the great vessels viewed from the front.

amount of work each chamber contributes to the pumping of blood. It is thickest in the left ventricle.

The atria and the ventricles are separated by a *ring of fibrous tissue*. Consequently, when a wave of electrical activity passes over the atrial muscle, it can only spread to the ventricles through the conducting system which extends across the fibrous ring from atria to ventricles (p. 91).

Endocardium

This forms the lining of the myocardium and the heart valves. It is a thin, smooth, glistening membrane which permits smooth flow of blood inside the heart. It consists of flattened epithelial cells, continuous with the endothelium that lines the blood vessels.

Interior of the heart (Figs 5.12 and 5.13)

The heart is divided into a right and left side by the *septum*, a partition consisting of myocardium covered by endocardium. After birth blood cannot cross the septum from one side to the other. Each side is divided by an *atrioventricular valve* into an upper chamber, the *atrium*, and a lower chamber, the *ventricle*. The atrioventricular valves are formed by double folds of endocardium strengthened by a little fibrous tissue. The *right atrioventricular valve* (tricuspid valve) has three flaps or *cusps* and the *left atrioventricular valve* (mitral valve) has two cusps.

The valves between the atria and ventricles open and close passively according to changes in pressure in the chambers. They open when the pressure in the atria is greater than that in the ventricles. During

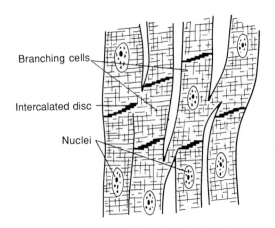

Figure 5.10 Cardiac muscle with fibres separated.

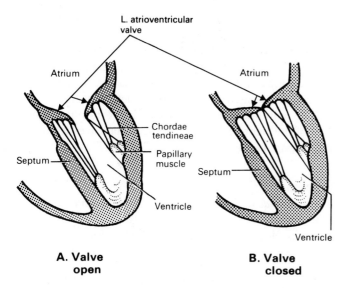

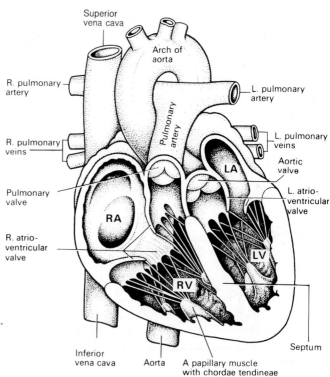

Figure 5.12 The left atrioventricular valve.

Figure 5.13 Interior of the heart.

ventricular systole (contraction) the pressure in the ventricles rises above that in the atria and the valves snap shut preventing backward flow of blood. The valves are prevented from opening upwards into the atria by tendinous cords, called *chordae tendineae*, which extend from the inferior surface of the cusps to little projections of myocardium covered with endothelium, called *papillary muscles* (Fig. 5.12).

Flow of blood through the heart
(Fig. 5.14)

The two largest veins of the body, the *superior* and *inferior venae cavae*, empty their contents into the right atrium. This blood passes via the right atrioventricular valve into the right ventricle, and from there it is pumped into the *pulmonary artery* or *trunk* (the only artery in the body which carries deoxygenated blood). The opening of the pulmonary artery is guarded by the *pulmonary valve*, formed by three *semilunar cusps*. This valve prevents the back flow of blood into the right ventricle when the ventricular muscle relaxes. After leaving the heart the pulmonary artery divides into *left* and *right pulmonary arteries* which carry the venous blood to the lungs where the interchange of gases takes place: carbon dioxide is excreted and oxygen is absorbed.

Two *pulmonary veins* from each lung carry *oxygenated blood* to the *left atrium*. It then passes through the left atrioventricular valve into the left ventricle, and from there it is pumped into the aorta, the first artery of the general circulation. The opening of the aorta is

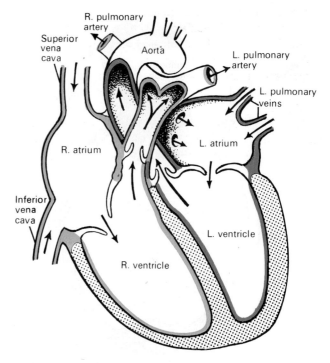

Figure 5.14 Direction of the flow of blood through the heart.

guarded by the *aortic valve*, formed by three *semilunar cusps* (Fig. 5.15).

From this sequence of events it can be seen that the blood passes from the right to the left side of the heart via the lungs, or pulmonary circulation (Fig. 5.16). However, it should be noted that both atria contract at the same time and this is followed by the simultaneous contraction of both ventricles.

The muscle layer of the walls of the atria is very thin in comparison with that of the ventricles (Fig. 5.14).

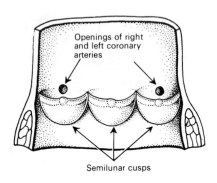

Figure 5.15 The aorta cut open to show the cusps of the semilunar valve.

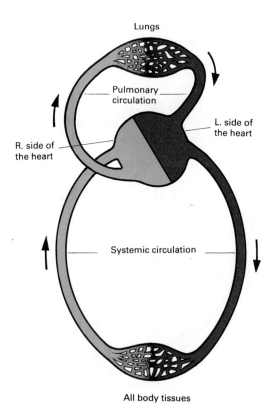

Figure 5.16 The relationship between the systemic and pulmonary circulations.

This is consistent with the amount of work it does. The atria, usually assisted by gravity, only propel the blood through the atrioventricular valve into the ventricles, whereas the ventricles actively pump the blood to the lungs and round the whole body. The muscle layer is thickest in the wall of the left ventricle.

The pulmonary trunk leaves the heart from the upper part of the right ventricle, and the aorta leaves from the upper part of the left ventricle.

Summary
The *right side* of the heart deals with *deoxygenated blood*.
The *left side* of the heart deals with *oxygenated blood*.
The vessels *carrying blood to* the heart are *veins*.
The vessels *carrying blood away* from the heart are *arteries*.

Blood supply to the heart (Fig. 5.17)

Arterial circulation. The heart is supplied with arterial blood by the *right and left coronary arteries* which branch from the aorta immediately distal to the aortic valve.

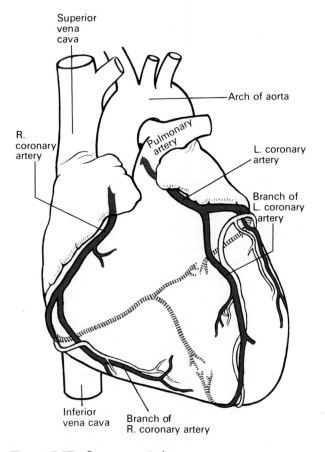

Figure 5.17 Coronary arteries.

The coronary arteries receive about 5% of the blood pumped from the heart, although the heart comprises a small proportion of body weight. This large blood supply, especially to the left ventricle, highlights the importance of the heart to body function. The coronary arteries traverse the heart, eventually forming a vast network of capillaries.

Venous drainage. Most of the venous blood is collected into several small veins that join to form the *coronary sinus* which opens into the right atrium. The remainder passes directly into the heart chambers through little venous channels.

Conducting system of the heart
(Fig. 5.18)

The heart has an intrinsic system whereby the cardiac muscle is automatically stimulated to contract without the need for a nerve supply from the brain. However, the intrinsic system can be stimulated or depressed by nerve impulses initiated in the brain and by circulating chemicals including hormones.

There are small groups of specialised neuromuscular cells in the myocardium which initiate and conduct impulses causing coordinated and synchronised contraction of the heart muscle.

Sinuatrial node (SA node)

This small mass of specialised cells is in the wall of the right atrium near the opening of the superior vena cava. The SA node is often described as the '*pace-maker*' of the heart because it normally initiates impulses more rapidly than other groups of neuromuscular cells.

Atrioventricular node (AV node)

This small mass of neuromuscular tissue is situated in the wall of the atrial septum near the atrioventricular valves. Normally the AV node is stimulated by impulses that sweep over the atrial myocardium. However, it too is capable of initiating impulses that cause contraction but at a slower rate than the SA node.

Atrioventricular bundle (AV bundle or bundle of His)

This consists of a mass of specialised fibres that originate from the AV node. The AV bundle crosses the fibrous ring that separates atria and ventricles then, at the upper end of the ventricular septum, it divides into

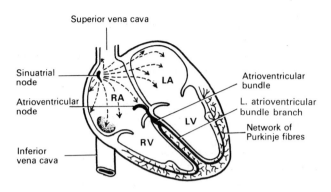

Figure 5.18 The conducting system in the heart.

right and left bundle branches. Within the ventricular myocardium the branches break up into fine fibres, called the *Purkinje fibres.* The AV bundle, bundle branches and Purkinje fibres convey impulses of contraction from the AV node to the apex of the myocardium where the wave of ventricular contraction begins, then sweeps upwards and outwards, pumping blood into the pulmonary artery and the aorta.

Nerve supply to the heart

In addition to the intrinsic impulses generated within the conducting system described above, the heart is influenced by autonomic nerves originating in the *cardiac centre* in the *medulla oblongata* which reach it through the autonomic nervous system. These are the *parasympathetic* and *sympathetic nerves* and they are antagonistic to one another.

The *vagus nerves* (parasympathetic) supply mainly the SA and AV nodes and atrial muscle. Parasympathetic stimulation reduces the rate at which impulses are produced, decreasing the rate and force of the heart beat.

The *sympathetic nerves* supply the SA and AV nodes and the myocardium of atria and ventricles. Sympathetic stimulation *increases* the rate and force of heart beat.

Factors affecting heart rate

Autonomic nervous system. As described above, the rate at which the heart beats is a balance of sympathetic and parasympathetic effects and this is the most important factor in determining heart rate.

Circulating chemicals. The catecholamines, adrenaline and noradrenaline (hormones secreted by the medulla of the adrenal glands) have the same effect as sympathetic stimulation, i.e. they increase the heart rate. Other hormones including thyroxine increase heart rate by their metabolic effect. Some drugs, dissolved gases and electrolytes in the blood may either increase or decrease the heart rate.

Exercise. Active muscles need more blood than resting muscles and this is achieved by an increased heart rate and selective vasodilatation.

Emotional states. During, e.g. excitement, fear and anxiety the heart rate is increased. Other effects mediated by the sympathetic nervous system may be present (p. 171 and Fig. 7.45).

Gender. The heart rate is faster in women than men.

Age. In babies and small children the heart rate is more rapid than in older children and adults.

Temperature. The heart rate rises and falls with body temperature.

Baroreceptor reflex. See p. 95.

The cardiac cycle

The function of the heart is to maintain a constant circulation of blood throughout the body. The heart acts as a pump and its action consists of a series of events known as the *cardiac cycle*.

During each heartbeat, or cardiac cycle, the heart contracts and then relaxes. The period of contraction is called *systole* and that of relaxation, *diastole*.

Stages of the cardiac cycle (Fig. 5.19)

The normal number of cardiac cycles per minute ranges from 60 to 80. Taking 74 as an example each cycle lasts about *0.8 of a second* and consists of:

- *atrial systole*—contraction of the atria
- *ventricular systole*—contraction of the ventricles
- *complete cardiac diastole*—relaxation of the atria and ventricles.

It does not matter at which stage of the cardiac cycle a description starts. For convenience the period when the atria are filling has been chosen.

The superior vena cava and the inferior vena cava transport deoxygenated blood into the right atrium *at the same time* as the four pulmonary veins convey oxygenated blood into the left atrium. The atrioventricular valves are open and blood flows through to the ventricles. The SA node emits an impulse which stimulates a wave of contraction that spreads over the myocardium of both atria, emptying the atria and com-

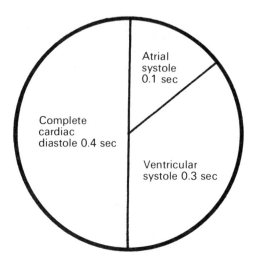

Total period of 1 cycle=0.8 sec

Figure 5.19   *The stages of one cardiac cycle.*

pleting ventricular filling (atrial systole 0.1 s). When the wave of contraction reaches the AV node it is stimulated to emit an impulse which quickly spreads to the ventricular muscle via the AV bundle, the bundle branches and Purkinje fibres. This results in a wave of contraction which sweeps upwards from the apex of the heart and across the walls of both ventricles pumping the blood into the pulmonary artery and the aorta (ventricular systole 0.3 s). The high pressure generated during ventricular contraction is greater than that in the aorta and forces the atrioventricular valves to close.

After contraction of the ventricles there is *complete cardiac diastole*, a period of *0.4 seconds*, when atria and ventricles are relaxed. During this time the myocardium recovers until it is able to contract again.

The valves of the heart and of the great vessels open and close according to the pressure within the chambers of the heart. The AV valves are open while the ventricular muscle is relaxed during atrial filling and systole. When the ventricles contract there is a gradual increase in the pressure in these chambers, and when it rises above atrial pressure the atrioventricular valves close. When the ventricular pressure rises above that in the pulmonary artery and in the aorta, the pulmonary and aortic valves open and blood flows into these vessels. When the ventricles relax and the pressure within them falls, the reverse process occurs. First the pulmonary and aortic valves close, then the atrioventricular valves open and the cycle begins again. This sequence of opening and closing valves ensures that the blood flows in only one direction (Fig. 5.20). This figure also shows how the walls of the aorta and other elastic arteries stretch and recoil in response to blood pumped into them.

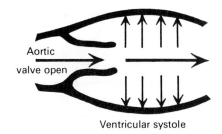

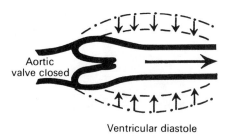

Figure 5.20 Diagram showing the elasticity of the walls of the aorta.

Heart sounds

The individual is not usually conscious of his heartbeat, but if the ear or the receiver of a stethoscope is placed on the chest wall a little below the left nipple and slightly nearer the midline the heartbeat can be heard.

Two sounds, separated by a short pause, can be clearly distinguished. They are described in words as '*lub dup*'. The first sound, '*lub*', is fairly loud and is due to the closure of the atrioventricular valves. The second sound, '*dup*', is softer and is due to the closure of the aortic and pulmonary valves.

Electrical changes in the heart

As the body fluids and tissues are good conductors of electricity, the electrical activity within the heart can be detected by attaching electrodes to the surface of the body. The pattern of electrical activity may be displayed on an oscilloscope screen or traced on paper. The apparatus used is an *electrocardiograph* and the tracing is an *electrocardiogram* (ECG).

The normal ECG tracing shows five waves which, by convention, have been named P, Q, R, S and T (Fig. 5.21).

The P wave arises when the impulse from the SA node sweeps over the atria.

The QRS complex represents the very rapid spread of the impulse from the AV node through the AV bundle

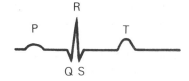

Figure 5.21 Electrocardiogram of one cardiac cycle.

and the Purkinje fibres and the electrical activity of the ventricular muscle.

The T wave represents the relaxation of the ventricular muscle.

The ECG described above originates from the SA node and is known as *sinus rhythm*. The rate of sinus rhythm is 60 to 100 beats per minute. A faster heart rate is called *tachycardia* and a slower heart rate, *bradycardia*.

By examining the pattern of waves and the time interval between cycles and parts of cycles the physician obtains valuable information about the state of the myocardium and the conducting system within the heart.

Cardiac output

The cardiac output is the amount of blood ejected from the heart. The amount expelled by each contraction of the ventricles is the *stroke volume*. Cardiac output is expressed in litres per minute (l/min) and is calculated by multiplying the stroke volume by the heart rate (measured in beats per minute):

Cardiac output = Stroke volume × Heart rate.

In a healthy adult at rest, the stroke volume is approximately 70 ml and if the heart rate is 72 per minute, the cardiac output is 5 l/minute. This can be greatly increased to meet the demands of exercise to around 25 l/minute, and in athletes up to 35 l/minute. This increase during exercise is called the *cardiac reserve*.

When increased blood supply is needed to meet increased tissue requirements of oxygen and nutrients, heart rate and/or stroke volume can be increased. Factors affecting heart rate include: the autonomic nervous supply, gender, age, body temperature.

Stroke volume

The stroke volume is determined by the volume of blood in the ventricles immediately before they contract, i.e. the ventricular end-diastolic volume (VEDV), sometimes called *preload*. This depends on the amount of blood returning to the heart through the superior and inferior venae cavae (the *venous return*). Increased

VEDV leads to stronger myocardial contraction, and more blood is expelled. In turn the stroke volume and cardiac output rise. This capacity to increase the stroke volume with increasing VEDV is finite, and when the limit is reached, the cardiac output cannot match the venous return, the cardiac output decreases and the heart begins to fail (p. 121). Other factors that increase myocardial contraction include:

■ increased stimulation of the sympathetic nerves innervating the heart
■ hormones, e.g. adrenaline, noradrenaline, thyroxine.

Arterial blood pressure affects the stroke volume as it creates resistance to blood being pumped from the ventricles into the great arteries. This resistance (sometimes called *afterload*) is determined by the distensibility, or *elasticity*, of the large arteries and the *peripheral resistance* of arterioles.

Blood volume is normally kept constant by the kidneys and if deficient the stroke volume, cardiac output and venous return decrease.

Venous return

Venous return is the major determinant of cardiac output and, normally, the heart pumps out all blood returned to it. The force of contraction of the left ventricle ejecting blood into the aorta is not sufficient to return the blood through the veins and back to the heart. Other factors are involved.

The position of the body
Gravity assists the venous return from the head and neck when standing or sitting and offers less resistance to venous return from the lower parts of the body when an individual is lying flat.

Muscular contraction
Back flow of blood in veins of the limbs, especially when standing, is prevented by valves. The contraction of skeletal muscles surrounding the deep veins puts pressure on them, pushing blood towards the heart (Fig. 5.22). In the lower limbs, this is called the *skeletal muscle pump*. When the pressure in deep veins is lowered during muscle relaxation, blood flows into them from superficial veins through *communicating veins*.

The respiratory pump
During inspiration the expansion of the chest creates a negative pressure within the thorax, assisting flow of

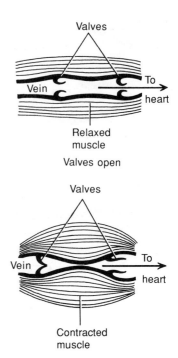

Figure 5.22 Diagram of the flow of blood through a vein aided by the contraction of skeletal muscle.

blood towards the heart. In addition, when the diaphragm descends during inspiration, the increased intra-abdominal pressure pushes blood towards the heart.

Summary of factors affecting cardiac output

Cardiac output = Stroke volume × Heart rate

Factors affecting stroke volume are:

■ VEDV (ventricular end-diastolic volume)
■ Venous return
 —position of the body
 —skeletal muscle pump
 —respiratory pump
■ Strength of myocardial contraction
■ Blood volume.

Factors affecting heart rate are:

■ Autonomic nerve stimulation
■ Circulating chemicals
■ Activity and exercise
■ Emotional states
■ Gender
■ Age
■ Body temperature
■ Baroreceptor reflex.

BLOOD PRESSURE

Blood pressure may be defined as the force or pressure which the blood exerts on the walls of the blood vessels.

The systemic arterial blood pressure, usually called simply arterial blood pressure, is the result of the discharge of blood from the left ventricle into the *already full aorta*.

When the left ventricle contracts and pushes blood into the aorta the pressure produced is called the *systolic blood pressure*. In adults it is about 120 mmHg (millimetres of mercury) or 16 kPa (kilopascals).

When *complete cardiac diastole* occurs and the heart is resting following the ejection of blood, the pressure within the arteries is called *diastolic blood pressure*. In an adult this is about 80 mmHg or 11 kPa. The difference between systolic and diastolic blood pressures is the *pulse pressure*.

These figures vary according to the time of day, the posture, gender and age of the individual. During bedrest at night the blood pressure tends to be lower. It increases with age and is usually higher in women than in men.

Arterial blood pressure is measured by the use of a sphygmomanometer and is usually expressed in the following manner:

$$\text{BP} = \frac{120}{80} \text{ mmHg or BP} = \frac{16}{11} \text{ kPa}$$

The elasticity of the artery walls. There is a considerable amount of elastic tissue in the arterial walls, especially in large arteries. Therefore, when the left ventricle ejects blood into the already full aorta, it distends, then the elastic recoil pushes the blood onwards. This distension and recoil occurs all through the arterial system. During cardiac diastole the elastic recoil of the arteries maintains the diastolic pressure (Fig. 5.20).

Systemic arterial blood pressure maintains the essential flow of substances into and out of the organs of the body. Control of blood pressure especially to the vital organs is essential to maintain homeostasis.

The blood pressure is maintained within normal limits by fine adjustments. Blood pressure is determined by cardiac output and peripheral resistance:

$$\text{Blood pressure} = \text{Cardiac output} \times \text{Peripheral resistance}$$

Cardiac output

The cardiac output is determined by the stroke volume and the heart rate. Factors that affect the heart rate and stroke volume are described above, and they may increase or decrease cardiac output and, in turn, blood pressure. An increase in cardiac output raises both the systolic and diastolic pressure. An increase in the stroke volume increases the systolic pressure more than it does the diastolic pressure.

Peripheral or arteriolar resistance

Arterioles are the smallest arteries and they have a tunica media composed almost entirely of smooth muscle which responds to nerve and chemical stimulation. Constriction and dilatation of the arterioles are the main determinants of peripheral resistance (p. 84). Vasoconstriction causes blood pressure to rise and vasodilatation causes it to fall.

When elastic tissue in the tunica media is replaced by fibrous tissue as part of the ageing process, blood pressure rises.

Dilatation and constriction of arterioles occurs selectively around the body, resulting in changes in the blood flow through organs according to their needs. The highest priorities are the blood supply to the brain and the heart muscle, and in an emergency, supplies to other parts of the body are reduced in order to ensure an adequate supply to these organs. Generally, changes in the amount of blood flowing to any organ depend on how active it is. A very active organ needs more oxygen and nutritional materials than a resting organ and it produces more waste materials for excretion.

Control of blood pressure (BP)

Homeostasis of blood pressure, i.e. normal BP, is achieved by the mechanisms described below.

The cardiovascular centre (CVC) is a collection of interconnected neurones in the brain and is situated within the medulla and pons. The CVC receives, integrates and coordinates inputs from:

■ baroreceptors (the primary mechanism)
■ chemoreceptors
■ higher centres in the brain.

The outputs of the CVC are via the autonomic nervous system to the heart and blood vessels, enabling rapid response to changes in blood pressure (Fig. 5.23).

Baroreceptors

These are nerve endings sensitive to stretch, situated in the arch of the aorta and in the carotid sinuses (Fig. 5.24). There is always some degree of stretch in the

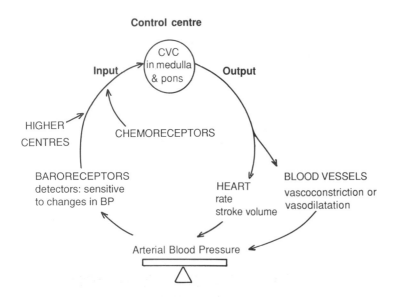

Figure 5.23 Relationships between structures involved in homeostasis of blood pressure.

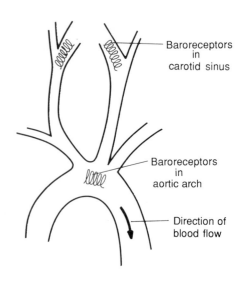

Figure 5.24 Location of baroreceptors.

baroreceptors which can be increased or decreased by changes in blood pressure. A rise in blood pressure in these arteries stretches the baroreceptors, increasing their input to the CVC. The CVC responds by adjusting its output to the heart and blood vessels. In this situation the stroke volume and heart rate decrease and the blood vessels become more dilated. The overall effect is a compensatory fall in blood pressure (Fig. 5.25B). The response to a decrease in blood pressure is shown in Figure 5.25C.

Chemoreceptors

These are nerve endings situated in the carotid and aortic bodies. They are primarily involved in control of respiration (p. 257). They are sensitive to changes in the levels of carbon dioxide, oxygen and the acidity of the blood (pH). Their input to the CVC influences its out-put only when severe disruption of respiratory function occurs. The effects are outlined in Figure 5.26.

Higher centres in the brain

Input to the CVC from the higher centres is influenced by emotional states such as fear, anxiety, pain, and anger that may stimulate changes in blood pressure.

The hypothalamus in the brain controls body temperature and influences the CVC which responds by adjusting the diameter of blood vessels in the skin—an important mechanism in determining heat loss and retention (p. 363).

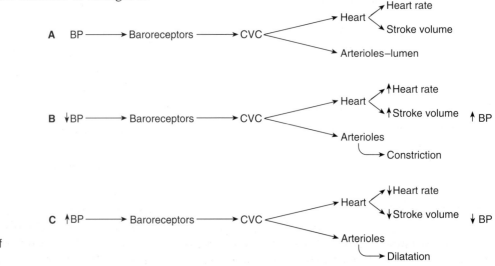

Figure 5.25 The role of baroreceptors in the control of arterial blood pressure.

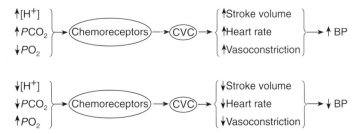

Figure 5.26 The relationship between stimulation of chemoreceptors and arterial blood pressure.

PULSE

The pulse is described as a wave of distension and elongation felt in an artery wall due to the contraction of the left ventricle forcing about 60 to 80 millilitres of blood into the already full aorta. When the aorta is distended, a wave passes along the walls of the arteries and can be felt at any point where an artery can be pressed gently against a bone. The number of pulse beats per minute represents the heart rate and varies considerably in different people and in the same person at different times. An average of 60 to 80 is common at rest. Information that may be obtained from the pulse includes:

- *The rate* at which the heart is beating.
- *The regularity* with which the heart beats occur, i.e. the length of time between beats should be the same.
- *The volume or strength* of the beat. It should be possible to compress the artery with moderate pressure, stopping the flow of blood. The compressibility of the blood vessel gives some indication of the blood pressure and the state of the blood vessel wall.
- *The tension.* The artery wall should feel soft and pliant under the fingers.

Factors affecting the pulse rate

Position. When the individual is standing up the pulse rate is usually more rapid than when he is lying down.

Age. The pulse rate in children is more rapid than in adults.

Gender. The pulse rate tends to be more rapid in females than in males.

Exercise. Any exercise—walking, running or playing games—will increase the rate of the pulse. The resting rate should be restored soon after exercise has stopped.

Emotion. In strong emotional states the pulse rate is increased, e.g. excitement, fear, anger, grief.

CIRCULATION OF THE BLOOD

Although circulation of blood round the body is continuous (Fig. 5.16) it is convenient to describe it in two parts:

- pulmonary circulation
- systemic or general circulation.

Pulmonary circulation

This consists of the circulation of blood from the right ventricle of the heart to the lungs and back to the left atrium. In the lungs, carbon dioxide is excreted and oxygen is absorbed.

The pulmonary artery or trunk, carrying *deoxygenated blood*, leaves the upper part of the right ventricle of the heart. It passes upwards and divides into left and right pulmonary arteries at the level of the 5th thoracic vertebra.

The left pulmonary artery runs to the root of the left lung where it divides into two branches, one passing into each lobe.

The right pulmonary artery passes to the root of the right lung and divides into two branches. The larger branch carries blood to the middle and lower lobes, and the smaller branch to the upper lobe.

Within the lung these arteries divide and subdivide into smaller arteries, arterioles and capillaries. The interchange of gases takes place between capillary blood and air in the alveoli of the lungs (p. 255). In each lung the capillaries containing oxygenated blood join up and eventually form two veins.

Two pulmonary veins leave each lung, returning oxygenated blood to the left atrium of the heart. During atrial systole this blood passes into the left ventricle, and during ventricular systole it is forced into the aorta, i.e. the first artery of the general circulation.

Systemic or general circulation

The blood pumped out from the left ventricle is carried by the *branches of the aorta* around the body and is returned to the right atrium of the heart by the *superior* and *inferior venae cavae*. Figure 5.30 gives a general impression of the positions of the aorta and the main arteries of the limbs. Figure 5.31 provides an overview of the venae cavae and the veins of the limbs.

The circulation of blood to the different parts of the body will be described in the order in which their arteries branch off the aorta.

Aorta (Fig. 5.27)

The aorta begins at the upper part of the left ventricle and, after passing upwards for a short way, it arches backwards and to the left. It then descends behind the heart through the thoracic cavity a little to the left of the thoracic vertebrae. At the level of the 12th thoracic vertebra it passes behind the diaphragm then downwards in the abdominal cavity to the level of the 4th lumbar vertebra, where it divides into the *right* and *left common iliac arteries*.

Throughout its length the aorta gives off numerous branches. Some of the branches are *paired*, i.e. there is a right and left branch of the same name, and some are single or *unpaired*.

Thoracic aorta

This part of the aorta is above the diaphragm and is described in three parts:

■ ascending aorta
■ arch of the aorta
■ descending aorta in the thorax.

Ascending aorta
This is about 5 cm long and lies behind the sternum.

The right and left coronary arteries are its only branches and they arise from the aorta just above the level of the aortic valve (Fig. 5.15).

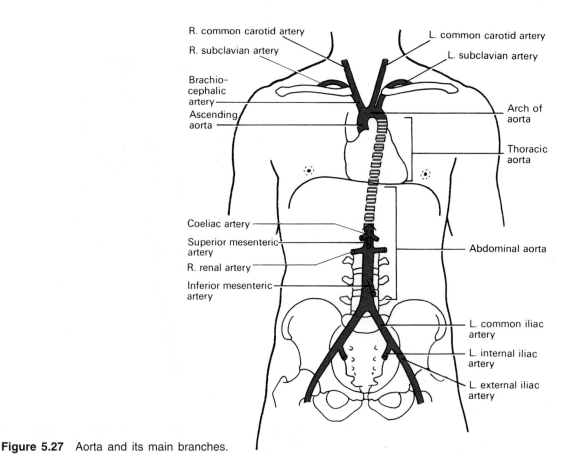

Figure 5.27 Aorta and its main branches.

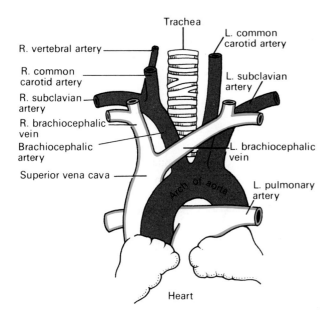

Figure 5.28 The arch of the aorta and its branches.

Arch of the aorta

The arch of the aorta is a continuation of the ascending aorta. It begins behind the manubrium of the sternum and runs upwards, backwards and to the left in front of the trachea. It then passes downwards to the left of the trachea and is continuous with the descending aorta.

Three branches are given off from its upper aspect (Fig. 5.28):

- brachiocephalic artery or trunk
- left common carotid artery
- left subclavian artery.

The brachiocephalic artery is about 4 to 5 cm long and passes obliquely upwards, backwards and to the right. At the level of the sternoclavicular joint it divides into the *right common carotid artery* and the *right subclavian artery.*

Circulation of blood to the head and neck

Arterial supply

The paired arteries supplying the head and neck are the *common carotid arteries* and the *vertebral arteries.*

Carotid arteries. The *right common carotid artery* is a branch of the brachiocephalic artery. The *left common carotid artery* arises directly from the arch of the aorta. They pass upwards on either side of the neck and have the same distribution on each side. The common ca-

rotid arteries are embedded in fascia, called the *carotid sheath.* At the level of the upper border of the thyroid cartilage they divide into:

- external carotid artery
- internal carotid artery.

The carotid sinuses are slight dilatations at the point of division (bifurcation) of the common carotid arteries into their internal and external branches. The walls of the sinuses are thin and contain numerous nerve endings of the glossopharyngeal nerves. These nerve endings, or *baroreceptors*, are stimulated by changes in *blood pressure* in the carotid sinuses. The resultant nerve impulses initiate reflex adjustments of blood pressure through the vasomotor centre in the medulla oblongata (p. 95).

The carotid bodies are two small groups of specialised cells, called *chemoreceptors*, one lying in close association with each common carotid artery at its bifurcation. They are supplied by the glossopharyngeal nerves and their cells are stimulated by changes in the carbon dioxide and oxygen content of blood. The resultant nerve impulses initiate reflex adjustments of respiration through the respiratory centre in the medulla oblongata.

External carotid artery (Fig. 5.29). This artery supplies the superficial tissues of the head and neck, via a number of branches.

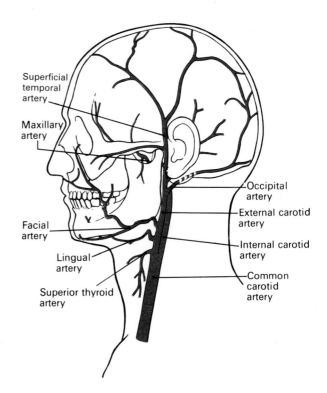

Figure 5.29 Main arteries of the left side of the head and neck.

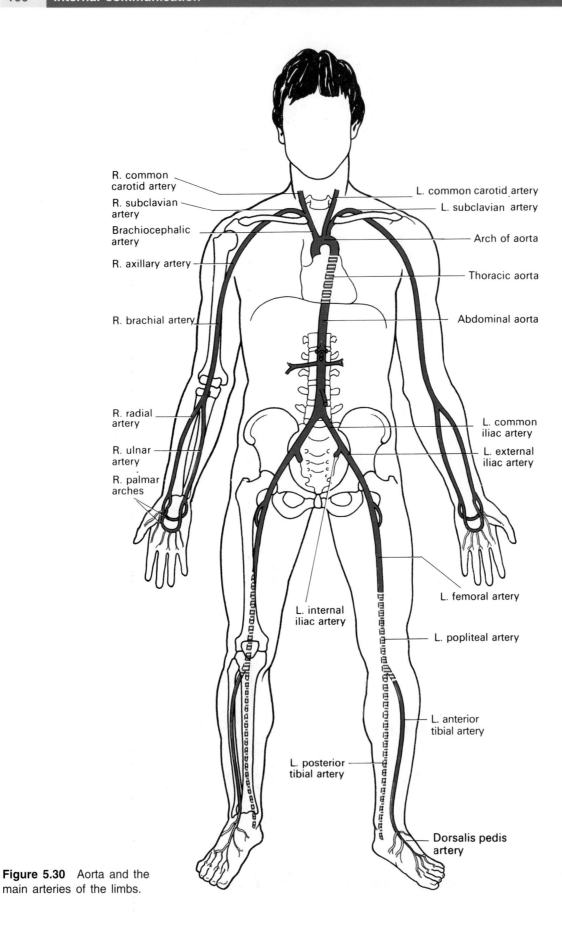

R. common
carotid artery

R. subclavian
artery

Brachiocephalic
artery

R. axillary artery

R. brachial artery

R. radial
artery

R. ulnar
artery

R. palmar
arches

L. common carotid artery

L. subclavian artery

Arch of aorta

Thoracic aorta

Abdominal aorta

L. common
iliac artery

L. external
iliac artery

L. femoral artery

L. internal
iliac artery

L. popliteal artery

L. anterior
tibial artery

L. posterior
tibial artery

Dorsalis pedis
artery

Figure 5.30 Aorta and the
main arteries of the limbs.

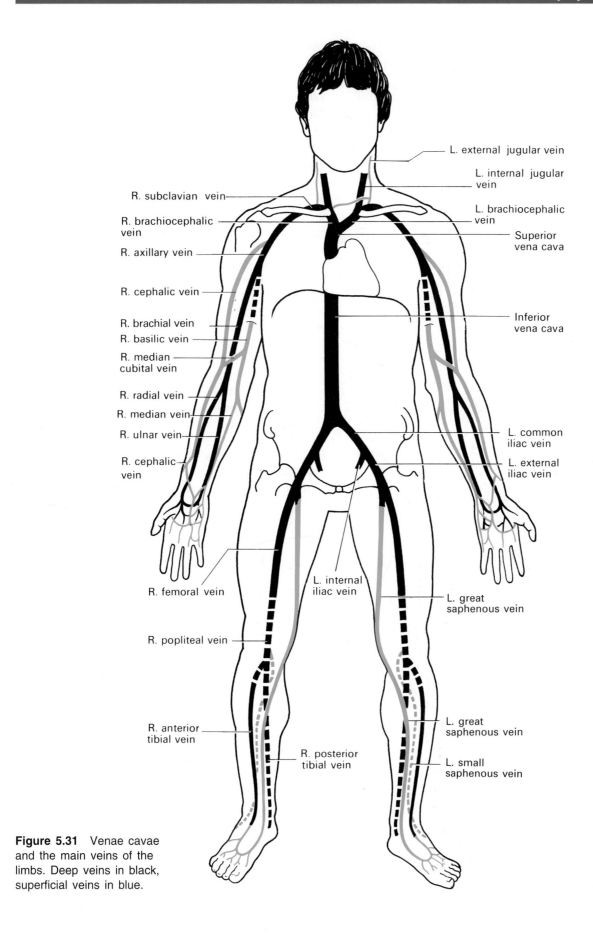

Figure 5.31 Venae cavae and the main veins of the limbs. Deep veins in black, superficial veins in blue.

The *superior thyroid artery* supplies the thyroid gland and adjacent muscles.

The *lingual artery* supplies the tongue, the lining membrane of the mouth, the structures in the floor of the mouth, the tonsil and the epiglottis.

The *facial artery* passes outwards over the mandible just in front of the angle of the jaw and supplies the muscles of facial expression and structures in the mouth. The pulse may be felt where the artery crosses the jaw bone.

The *occipital artery* supplies the posterior part of the scalp.

The *temporal artery* passes upwards over the zygomatic process in front of the ear and supplies the frontal, temporal and parietal parts of the scalp. The pulse may be felt in front of the upper part of the ear.

The *maxillary artery* supplies the muscles of mastication and a branch of this artery, the *middle meningeal artery*, runs deeply to supply structures in the interior of the skull.

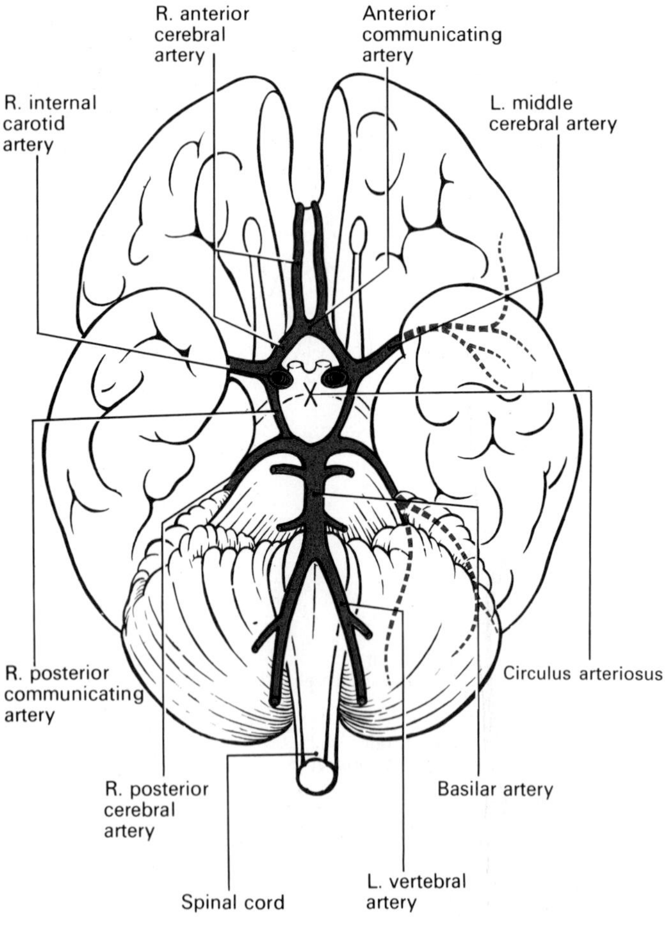

Internal carotid artery. The internal carotid artery is a major contributor to the *circle of Willis* which supplies the greater part of the brain. It also has branches that supply the eyes, forehead and nose. It ascends to the base of the skull and passes through the carotid foramen in the temporal bone.

Circulus arteriosus (circle of Willis). The greater part of the brain is supplied with arterial blood by an arrangement of arteries called the *circulus arteriosus* or the *circle of Willis* (Fig. 5.32). Four large arteries contribute to its formation: two *internal carotid arteries* and two *vertebral arteries* (Fig. 5.33). The vertebral arteries arise from the subclavian arteries, pass upwards through the foramina in the transverse processes of the cervical vertebrae, enter the skull through the foramen magnum, then join to form the *basilar artery*. The arrangement in the circle of Willis is such that the brain as a whole receives an adequate blood supply when a contributing artery is damaged and during extreme movements of the head and neck.

Anteriorly, *two anterior cerebral arteries* arise from the internal carotid arteries and are joined by the *anterior communicating artery*.

Posteriorly, *two vertebral arteries* join to form the *basilar artery*. After travelling for a short distance the basilar artery divides to form *two posterior cerebral arteries*, each of which is joined to the corresponding internal carotid artery by a *posterior communicating artery,*

Figure 5.32 Arteries forming the circulus arteriosus (circle of Willis) and its main branches to the brain.

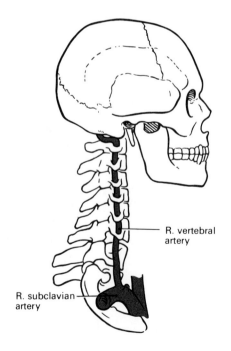

Figure 5.33 Right vertebral artery.

completing the circle. The *circulus arteriosus* is therefore formed by:

- 2 anterior cerebral arteries
- 2 internal carotid arteries
- 1 anterior communicating artery
- 2 posterior communicating arteries
- 2 posterior cerebral arteries
- 1 basilar artery.

From this circle, the *anterior cerebral arteries* pass forward to supply the anterior part of the brain, the *middle cerebral arteries* pass laterally to supply the sides of the brain, and the *posterior cerebral arteries* supply the posterior part of the brain.

Branches of the basilar artery supply parts of the brain stem.

Venous return from the head and neck (Figs 5.34, 5.35 and 5.36)

The venous blood from the head and neck is returned by *deep and superficial veins*.

Superficial veins with the same names as the branches of the external carotid artery return venous blood from the superficial structures of the face and scalp and unite to form the external jugular vein.

The *external jugular vein* begins in the neck at the level of the angle of the jaw. It passes downwards in front of the sternocleidomastoid muscle, then behind the clavicle before entering the *subclavian vein*.

The venous blood from the deep areas of the brain is collected into channels called the *dural venous sinuses*.

The *dural venous sinuses of the brain* (Fig 5.35) are formed by layers of *dura mater* lined with endothelium. The dura mater is the outer protective covering of the brain (p. 147). The main venous sinuses are:

- 1 superior sagittal sinus
- 1 inferior sagittal sinus
- 1 straight sinus
- 2 transverse or lateral sinuses
- 2 sigmoid sinuses.

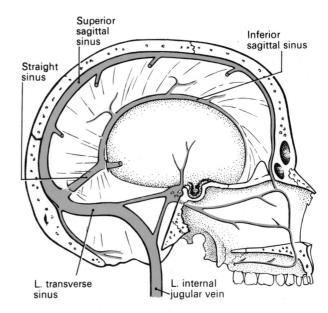

Figure 5.35 Venous sinuses of the brain viewed from the right side.

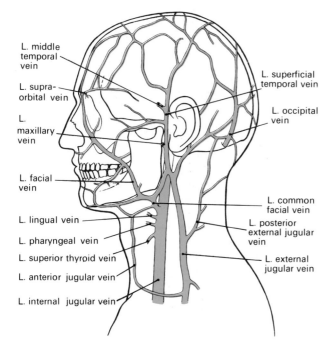

Figure 5.34 Veins of the left side of the head and neck.

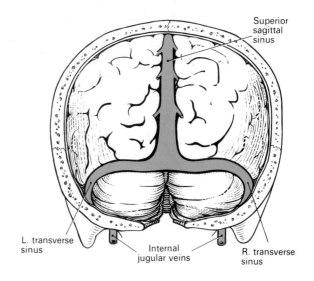

Figure 5.36 Venous sinuses of the brain viewed from above.

The *superior sagittal sinus* carries the venous blood from the superior part of the brain. It begins in the frontal region and passes directly backwards in the midline of the skull to the occipital region where it turns to the right side and continues as the *right transverse sinus*.

The *inferior sagittal sinus* lies deep within the brain and passes backwards to form the *straight sinus*.

The *straight sinus* runs backwards and downwards to become the *left transverse sinus*.

The *transverse sinuses* begin in the occipital region. They run forward and medially in a curved groove of the skull, to become continuous with the *sigmoid sinuses*.

The *sigmoid sinuses* are a continuation of the transverse sinuses. Each curves downwards and medially and lies in a groove in the mastoid process of the temporal bone. Anteriorly only a thin plate of bone separates the sinus from the air cells in the mastoid process of the temporal bone. Inferiorly it continues as the internal jugular vein.

The *internal jugular veins* begin at the jugular foramina in the middle cranial fossa and each is the continuation of a sigmoid sinus. They run downwards in the neck behind the sternocleidomastoid muscles. Behind the clavicle they unite with the *subclavian veins*, carrying blood from the upper limbs, to form the *brachiocephalic veins*.

The *brachiocephalic veins* are situated one on each side in the root of the neck. Each is formed by the union of the internal jugular and the subclavian veins. The left brachiocephalic vein is longer than the right and passes obliquely behind the manubrium of the sternum, where it joins the right brachiocephalic vein to form the *superior vena cava* (Fig. 5.37).

The *superior vena cava*, which drains all the venous blood from the head, neck and upper limbs, is about 7 cm long. It passes downwards along the right border of the sternum and ends in the right atrium of the heart.

Circulation of blood to the upper limb

Arterial supply (Figs 5.28 and 5.38)

The subclavian arteries. The right subclavian artery arises from the brachiocephalic artery; the left branches from the arch of the aorta. They are slightly arched and pass behind the clavicles and over the first ribs before entering the axillae, where they continue as the *axillary arteries*.

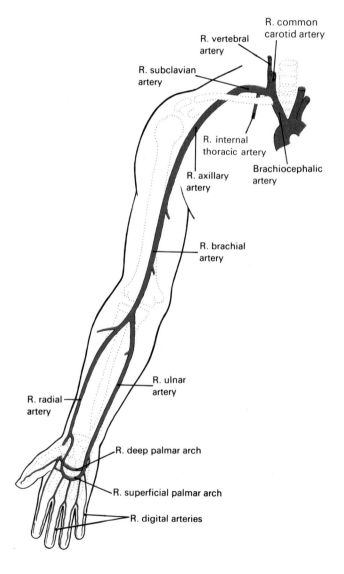

Figure 5.38 Main arteries of the right arm.

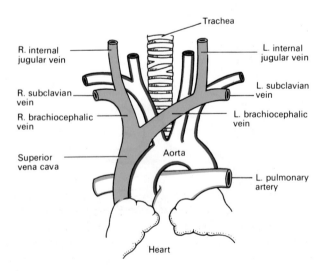

Figure 5.37 Superior vena cava and the veins which form it.

Before entering the axilla each subclavian artery gives off two branches: the *vertebral artery,* which passes upwards to supply the brain, and the *internal thoracic artery,* which supplies the breast and a number of structures in the thoracic cavity.

The *axillary artery* is a continuation of the subclavian artery and lies in the axilla. The first part lies deeply; then it runs more superficially to become the *brachial artery.*

The *brachial artery* is a continuation of the axillary artery. It runs down the medial aspect of the upper arm, passes to the front of the elbow and extends to about 1 cm below the joint, where it divides into *radial* and *ulnar arteries.*

The *radial artery* passes down the radial or lateral side of the forearm to the wrist. Just above the wrist it lies superficially and can be felt in front of the radius, where the radial pulse is palpable. The artery then passes between the first and second metacarpal bones and enters the palm of the hand.

The *ulnar artery* runs downwards on the ulnar or medial aspect of the forearm to cross the wrist and pass into the hand.

There are anastomoses between the radial and ulnar arteries, called the *deep* and *superficial palmar arches,* from which *palmar metacarpal* and *palmar digital arteries* arise to supply the structures in the hand and fingers.

Branches from the axillary, brachial, radial and ulnar arteries supply all the structures in the upper limb.

Venous return from the upper limb (Figs 5.29 and 5.39)

The veins of the upper limb are divided into two groups: deep and superficial veins.

The *deep veins* follow the course of the arteries and have the same names:

- palmar metacarpal veins
- deep palmar venous arch
- ulnar and radial veins
- brachial vein
- axillary vein
- subclavian vein.

The *superficial veins* begin in the hand and consist of the following:

- cephalic vein
- basilic vein
- median vein
- median cubital vein.

The *cephalic vein* begins at the back of the hand where it collects blood from a complex of superficial veins, many of which can be easily seen. It then winds round

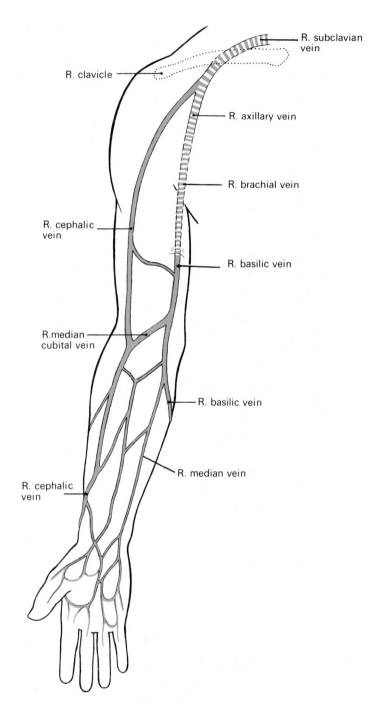

Figure 5.39 Main veins of the right arm. Broken line indicates deep veins.

the radial side to the anterior aspect of the forearm. In front of the elbow it gives off a large branch, the *median cubital vein,* which slants upwards and medially to join the *basilic vein.* After crossing the elbow joint the cephalic vein passes up the lateral aspect of the arm and in front of the shoulder joint to end in the axillary vein. Throughout its length it receives blood from the superficial tissues on the lateral aspects of the hand, forearm and arm.

The *basilic vein* begins at the back of the hand on the ulnar aspect. It ascends on the medial side of the forearm and upper arm then joins the axillary vein. It receives blood from the medial aspect of the hand, forearm and arm. There are many small veins which link the cephalic and basilic veins.

The *median vein* is a small vein that is not always present. It begins at the palmar surface of the hand, ascends on the front of the forearm and ends in the basilic vein or the median cubital vein.

The *brachiocephalic vein* is formed when the subclavian and internal jugular veins unite. There is one on each side.

The *superior vena cava* is formed when the two brachiocephalic veins unite. It drains all the venous blood from the head, neck and upper limbs and terminates in the right atrium. It is about 7 cm long and passes downwards along the right border of the sternum.

Descending aorta in the thorax
(Figs 5.27 and 5.40)

This part of the aorta is continuous with the arch of the aorta and begins at the level of the 4th thoracic vertebra. It extends downwards on the anterior surface of the bodies of the thoracic vertebrae to the level of the 12th thoracic vertebra, where it passes *behind* the diaphragm to become the abdominal aorta.

The descending aorta in the thorax gives off many *paired branches* which supply the walls of the thoracic cavity and the organs within the cavity, including:

- *bronchial arteries* that supply the bronchi and their branches, connective tissue in the lungs and the lymph nodes at the root of the lungs
- *oesophageal arteries* that supply the oesophagus
- *intercostal arteries* that run along the inferior border of the ribs and supply the intercostal muscles, some muscles of the thorax, the ribs, the skin and its underlying connective tissues.

Venous return from the thoracic cavity
(Fig. 5.41)

Most of the venous blood from the organs in the thoracic cavity is drained into the *azygos vein* and the *hemiazygos vein*. Some of the main veins which join them are the *bronchial, oesophageal* and *intercostal veins*. The azygos vein joins the superior vena cava and the hemiazygos vein joins the left brachiocephalic vein. At the distal end of the oesophagus some oesophageal veins

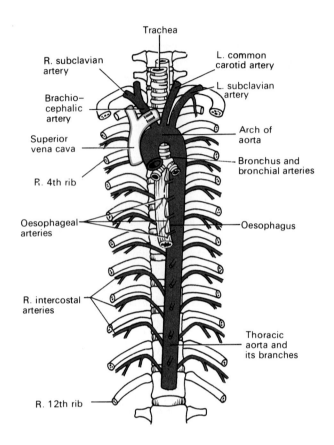

Figure 5.40   Aorta and its main branches in the thorax.

join the azygos vein and others, the left gastric vein. A venous plexus is formed by anastomoses between the veins joining the azygos vein and those joining the left gastric veins, linking the general and portal circulations.

Abdominal aorta (Fig. 5.42)

The abdominal aorta is a continuation of the thoracic aorta. The name changes when the aorta enters the abdominal cavity by passing behind the diaphragm at the level of the 12th thoracic vertebra. It descends in front of the bodies of the vertebrae to the level of the 4th lumbar vertebra, where it divides into the *right and left common iliac arteries.*

When a branch of the abdominal aorta supplies an organ it is only named here and is described in more detail in association with the organ. However, illustrations showing the distribution of blood from the coeliac, superior and inferior mesenteric arteries are presented here (Figs 5.43 and 5.44).

Many branches arise from the abdominal aorta, some of which are *paired* and some *unpaired*.

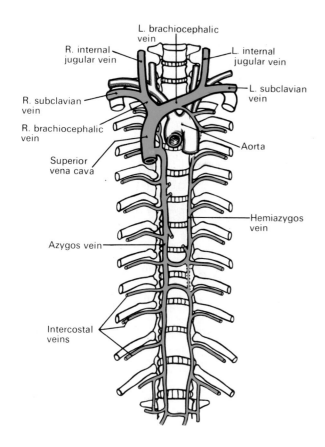

Figure 5.41 Superior vena cava and the main veins of the thorax.

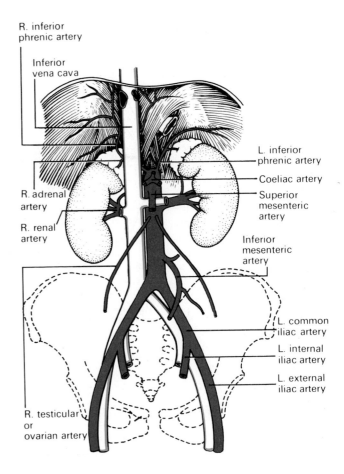

Figure 5.42 Abdominal aorta and its branches.

Paired branches

- *Inferior phrenic arteries* supply the diaphragm.
- *Renal arteries* supply the kidneys and give off branches, the *suprarenal arteries,* to supply the adrenal glands.
- *Testicular arteries* supply the testes in the male.
- *Ovarian arteries* supply the ovaries in the female.

The testicular and ovarian arteries are much longer than the other paired branches. This is because the testes and the ovaries begin their development in the region of the kidneys. As they grow they descend into the scrotum and the pelvis respectively and are accompanied by their blood vessels.

Unpaired branches (Figs 5.43 and 5.44)

The *coeliac artery* is a short thick artery about 1.25 cm long. It arises immediately below the diaphragm and divides into three branches:

- *left gastric artery*: supplies the stomach
- *splenic artery*: supplies the pancreas and the spleen

- *common hepatic artery*: supplies the liver, gall bladder and parts of the stomach, duodenum and pancreas.

The *superior mesenteric artery* branches from the aorta between the coeliac artery and the renal arteries. It supplies the whole of the small intestine and the proximal half of the large intestine.

The *inferior mesenteric artery* arises from the aorta about 4 cm above its division into the common iliac arteries. It supplies the distal half of the large intestine and part of the rectum.

Venous return from the abdominal organs (Fig. 5.45)

The *inferior vena cava* is formed when *right* and *left common iliac veins* join at the level of the body of the 5th lumbar vertebra. This is the largest vein in the body and it conveys blood from all parts of the body below the diaphragm to the right atrium of the heart. It passes through the central tendon of the diaphragm at the level of the 8th thoracic vertebra.

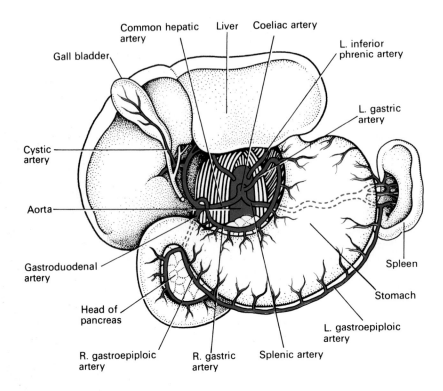

Figure 5.43   Coeliac artery and its branches and the inferior phrenic arteries.

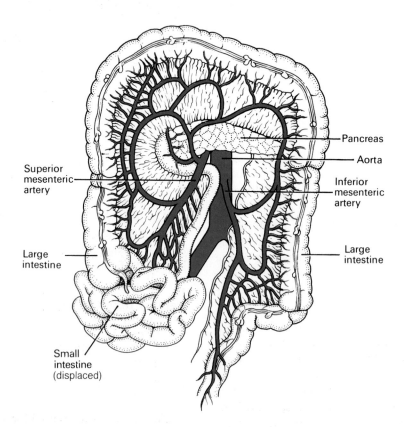

Figure 5.44   Superior and inferior mesenteric arteries and their branches.

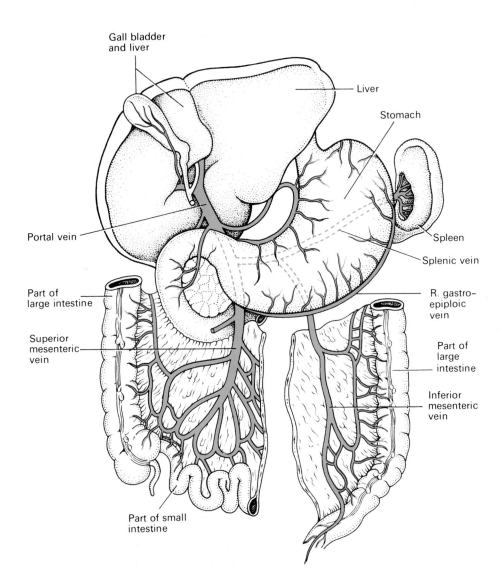

Figure 5.45 Venous drainage from the abdominal organs and the formation of the portal vein.

Paired testicular, ovarian, renal and adrenal veins join the inferior vena cava.

Blood from the remaining organs in the abdominal cavity passes through the liver via the *portal circulation* before entering the inferior vena cava.

Portal circulation

In all the parts of the circulation which have been described previously, venous blood passes from the tissues to the heart by the most direct route. In the portal circulation, venous blood passes from the capillary bed of the *abdominal part of the digestive system, the spleen and pancreas* to the *liver*. It passes through a second capillary bed, the hepatic sinusoids, in the liver before entering the general circulation via the inferior vena cava. In this way blood with a high concentration of nutrient materials, absorbed from the stomach and intestines, goes to the liver first. In the liver certain modifications take place, including the regulation of nutrient supply to other parts of the body.

Portal vein (Figs 5.45 and 5.46)
This is formed by the union of the following veins, each of which drains blood from the area supplied by the corresponding artery:

- splenic vein
- inferior mesenteric vein
- superior mesenteric vein
- gastric veins
- cystic vein.

The *splenic vein* drains blood from the spleen, the pancreas and part of the stomach.

The *inferior mesenteric vein* returns the venous blood from the rectum, pelvic and descending colon of the large intestine. It joins the splenic vein.

The *superior mesenteric vein* returns venous blood from the small intestine and the proximal parts of the large intestine, i.e. the caecum, ascending and transverse colon. It unites with the *splenic vein* to form the *portal vein*.

The *gastric veins* drain blood from the stomach and the distal end of the oesophagus, then join the portal vein.

The *cystic vein* which drains venous blood from the gall bladder joins the portal vein.

Hepatic veins

These are very short veins that leave the posterior surface of the liver and, almost immediately, enter the inferior vena cava.

Circulation of blood to the pelvis and lower limb (Figs 5.28, 5.47, 5.48 and 5.49)

Arterial supply

Common iliac arteries. The right and left common iliac arteries are formed when the abdominal aorta divides at the level of the 4th lumbar vertebra. In front of the sacroiliac joint each divides into:

- internal iliac artery
- external iliac artery.

The *internal iliac artery* runs medially to supply the organs within the pelvic cavity. In the female, one of the largest branches is the *uterine artery* which provides the main arterial blood supply to the reproductive organs.

The *external iliac artery* runs obliquely downwards and passes behind the inguinal ligament into the thigh where it becomes the *femoral artery*.

The *femoral artery* (Fig. 5.47) begins at the midpoint of the inguinal ligament and extends downwards in front of the thigh; then it turns medially and eventually passes round the medial aspect of the femur to enter the popliteal space where it becomes the *popliteal artery*. It supplies blood to the structures of the thigh and some superficial pelvic and inguinal structures.

The *popliteal artery* (Fig. 5.48) passes through the popliteal fossa behind the knee. It supplies the structures in this area, including the knee joint. At the lower border of the popliteal fossa it divides into the anterior and posterior tibial arteries.

The *anterior tibial artery* (Fig. 5.48) passes forwards

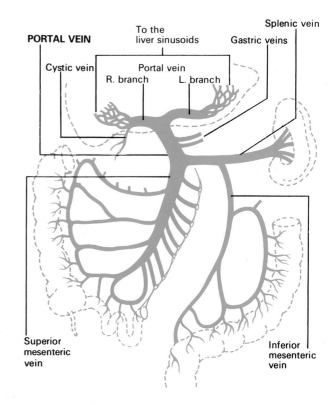

Figure 5.46 Portal vein—formation and termination.

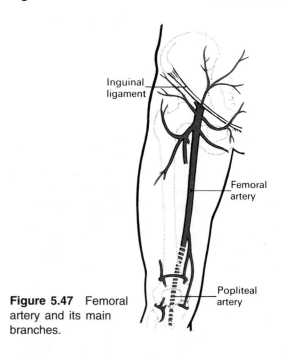

Figure 5.47 Femoral artery and its main branches.

between the tibia and fibula and supplies the structures in the front of the leg. It lies on the tibia, runs in front of the ankle joint and continues over the dorsum (top) of the foot as the *dorsalis pedis artery*.

The *dorsalis pedis artery* is a continuation of the anterior tibial artery and passes over the dorsum of the

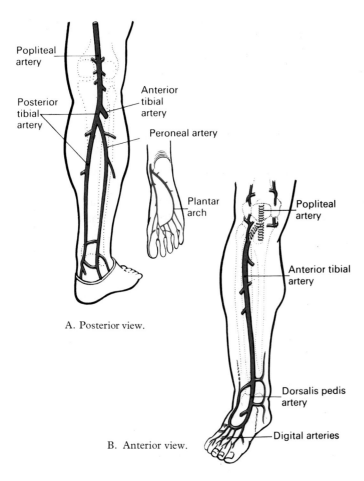

A. Posterior view.

B. Anterior view.

Figure 5.48 Right popliteal artery and its main branches.

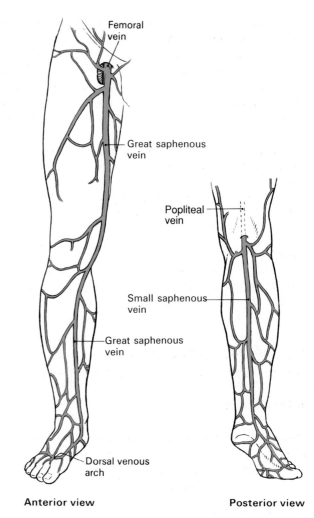

Anterior view

Posterior view

Figure 5.49 Superficial veins of the leg.

foot, supplying arterial blood to the structures in this area. It ends by passing between the first and second metatarsal bones into the sole of the foot where it contributes to the formation of the plantar arch.

The *posterior tibial artery* (Fig. 5.48) runs downwards and medially on the back of the leg. Near its origin it gives off a large branch called the *peroneal artery* which supplies the lateral aspect of the leg. In the lower part it becomes superficial and passes medial to the ankle joint to reach the sole of the foot where it continues as the *plantar artery*.

The *plantar artery* supplies the structures in the sole of the foot. This artery, its branches and the dorsalis pedis artery form the *plantar arch* from which the digital branches arise to supply the toes.

Venous return

There are some deep and some superficial veins in the lower limb (Fig. 5.29). Blood entering the superficial veins passes to the deep veins through *communicating*

veins. Movement of blood towards the heart is partly dependent on contraction of skeletal muscles. Backward flow is prevented by a large number of valves. Superficial veins receive less support by surrounding tissues than deep veins.

The deep veins. The deep veins accompany the arteries and their branches and have the same names. They are:

- digital veins
- plantar venous arch
- posterior tibial vein
- anterior tibial vein
- popliteal vein
- femoral vein
- external iliac vein
- internal iliac vein
- common iliac vein.

The *femoral vein* ascends in the thigh to the level of the inguinal ligament where it becomes the external iliac vein.

The *external iliac vein* is the continuation of the femoral vein where it enters the pelvis lying close to the femoral artery. It passes along the brim of the pelvis and at the level of the sacroiliac joint it is joined by the *internal iliac vein* to form the *common iliac vein*.

The *internal iliac vein* receives tributaries from several veins which drain the organs of the pelvic cavity.

The *two common iliac veins* begin at the level of the sacroiliac joints. They ascend obliquely and end a little to the right of the body of the 5th lumbar vertebra by uniting to form the *inferior vena cava*.

Superficial veins (Fig. 5.49). The two main superficial veins draining blood from the lower limbs are:

- small saphenous vein
- great saphenous vein.

The *small saphenous vein* begins behind the ankle joint where many small veins which drain the dorsum of the foot join together. It ascends superficially along the back of the leg and in the popliteal space it joins the *popliteal vein*—a deep vein.

The *great saphenous vein* is the longest vein in the body. It begins at the medial half of the dorsum of the foot and runs upwards, crossing the medial aspect of the tibia and up the inner side of the thigh. Just below the inguinal ligament it joins the *femoral vein*.

Many *communicating veins* join the superficial veins, and the superficial and deep veins of the lower limb.

SUMMARY OF THE SYSTEMIC CIRCULATION

Arteries supplying the trunk

Thoracic aorta

Ascending aorta
Coronary arteries—paired

Arch of aorta
Brachiocephalic { right common carotid artery / right subclavian artery
Left common carotid artery
Left subclavian artery

Descending aorta in the thorax
Bronchial arteries ⎫
Oesophageal arteries ⎬ paired
Intercostal arteries ⎭

Abdominal aorta

(branches in the order in which they leave the aorta)
Phrenic arteries—paired
Coeliac artery { gastric arteries / splenic artery / hepatic artery } unpaired
Superior mesenteric artery—unpaired
Renal arteries—paired
Ovarian or testicular arteries—paired
Inferior mesenteric artery—unpaired
Common iliac arteries { external iliac artery / internal iliac artery } paired

Venous drainage from the trunk

Internal iliac veins ⎫
External iliac veins ⎬ paired
Common iliac veins ⎭
Inferior vena cava—unpaired
Ovarian veins ⎫
Testicular veins ⎪
Renal veins ⎬ paired
Adrenal veins ⎪
Phrenic veins ⎭
Inferior mesenteric vein ⎫
Superior mesenteric vein ⎬ unpaired
Gastric veins ⎫
Splenic vein ⎬ unpaired
Portal vein ⎭
Hepatic veins—several
Oesophageal veins ⎫
Bronchial veins ⎬ paired
Intercostal veins ⎭
Azygos vein ⎫
Hemiazygos vein ⎬ unpaired
Brachiocephalic veins—paired
Superior vena cava—unpaired

Arteries supplying the head and neck

Common carotid arteries and branches—paired
External carotid artery:
   thyroid artery
   lingual artery
   facial artery
   occipital artery
   temporal artery
   maxillary artery

Internal carotid artery:
    ophthalmic artery
    anterior cerebral artery
    middle cerebral artery
    posterior communicating artery
Circulus arteriosus (circle of Willis):
    anterior cerebral arteries
    middle cerebral arteries
    posterior communicating arteries
    posterior cerebral arteries, which are branches
      from the basilar artery
Vertebral arteries—paired
Basilar artery—unpaired

Venous return from the head and neck

Superficial veins
  Thyroid vein ⎫
  Facial vein ⎬ paired
  Occipital vein ⎭
  External jugular veins—paired

Deep sinuses
  Superior sagittal sinus ⎫
  Inferior sagittal sinus ⎬ unpaired
  Straight sinus ⎭
  Transverse sinuses—paired
  Sigmoid sinuses—paired

Arteries supplying the upper extremity

Subclavian artery
Axillary artery
Brachial artery
Radial artery
Ulnar artery
Deep and superficial palmar arches
Palmar metacarpal arteries
Palmar digital arteries

Venous return from the upper extremity

Deep veins
  Palmar digital veins
  Palmar metacarpal veins
  Palmar venous arch
  Radial vein
  Ulnar vein
  Brachial vein
  Axillary vein
  Subclavian vein
  Brachiocephalic vein
  Superior vena cava

Superficial veins
  Digital veins
  Palmar venous arch
  Cephalic vein
  Basilic vein
  Median cubital vein
  Median vein

Arteries supplying the pelvis and lower extremity

Common iliac artery
Internal iliac artery
External iliac artery
Femoral artery
Popliteal artery
Anterior tibial artery
Posterior tibial artery
Plantar arch
Digital arteries

Venous return from the pelvis and lower extremity

Deep veins
  Digital veins
  Plantar veins
  Anterior tibial veins
  Posterior tibial veins
  Popliteal vein
  Femoral vein
  External iliac vein
  Internal iliac vein
  Common iliac vein
  Inferior vena cava

Superficial veins
  Great saphenous vein
  Small saphenous vein

SHOCK

Shock occurs when the metabolic needs of cells are not being met because of inadequate blood flow. In effect, there is a reduction in blood circulating, in blood pressure and in cardiac output. This causes tissue hypoxia, an inadequate supply of nutrients and the accumulation of waste products. A number of different types of shock are described:

■ hypovolaemic
■ cardiogenic
■ septic
■ neurogenic
■ anaphylactic.

Hypovolaemic shock

This occurs when the blood volume is reduced by 15 to 25%. Reduced venous return and, in turn, cardiac output may occur following:

■ severe haemorrhage—whole blood is lost
■ extensive superficial burns—serum is lost and blood cells at the site of the burn are destroyed
■ severe vomiting and diarrhoea—water and electrolytes are lost
■ perforation of an organ allowing its contents to enter the peritoneal cavity (peritonitis).

Cardiogenic shock

This occurs in acute heart disease when the damaged heart cannot maintain an adequate cardiac output, e.g. in myocardial infarction.

Septic shock (bacteraemic, endotoxic)

This is caused by severe infections in which endotoxins are released into the circulation from dead Gram-negative bacteria, e.g. *Enterobacteria, Pseudomonas*.

The mode of action of the toxins is not clearly understood. It may be that they cause an apparent reduction in the blood volume because of vasodilatation and pooling of blood in the large veins. This reduces the venous return to the heart and the cardiac output.

Neurogenic shock (vasovagal attack, fainting)

The causes include sudden acute pain, severe emotional experience, spinal anaesthesia and spinal cord damage. Nerve impulses reduce the heart rate, and in turn, the cardiac output. The venous return may also be reduced by the pooling of blood in dilated veins. These changes effectively reduce the blood supply to the brain, causing fainting. The period of unconsciousness is usually of short duration.

Anaphylactic shock

In allergic reactions an antigen interacts with an antibody and a variety of responses can occur (p. 67). In severe cases, the chemicals released, e.g. histamine, bradykinin, produce widespread vasodilatation and constriction of bronchiolar smooth muscle (bronchospasm). The vasodilatation profoundly reduces the venous return and cardiac output resulting in tissue hypoxia. Bronchospasm reduces the amount of air entering the lungs, increasing tissue hypoxia.

Physiological changes during shock

In the short term these are associated with physiological attempts to restore an adequate blood circulation. If the state of shock persists, the longer-term changes may be irreversible.

Immediate or reactive changes

As the blood pressure falls, a number of reflexes are stimulated and hormone secretions increased in an attempt to restore homeostasis. These raise the blood pressure by increasing peripheral resistance, the blood volume and the cardiac output. The changes include:

1. Vasoconstriction, following:
   a. stimulation of the baroreceptors in the aortic arch and carotid sinuses
   b. sympathetic stimulation of the adrenal glands which causes increased secretion of adrenaline and noradrenaline
   c. stimulation of the renin/angiotensin system by diminished blood flow to the kidneys (p. 343)
2. Increased heart rate, following sympathetic stimulation
3. Water retention by the kidney, following increased release of antidiuretic hormone by the posterior lobe of the pituitary gland, increasing salt and water retention

In shock of moderate severity the circulation to the heart and brain is maintained, in the short term. Restlessness, confusion and coma occur as circulation to the brain is impaired. If shock is very severe there may not be time for the above changes to be effective. The severe hypoxia that occurs disrupts cell metabolism. In the absence of adequate oxygen, cellular metabolism switches to less efficient anaerobic pathways, large amounts of lactic acid are formed and hydrogen ions accumulate, reaching dangerous levels in a few minutes. These are the changes that lead to the severe metabolic acidosis which occurs immediately prior to and following cardiac arrest.

Long-term changes associated with shock

If the state of shock is not reversed, hypoxia and low blood pressure cause irreversible brain damage and capillary dilatation and a vicious circle of events is established.

Hypoxia. When this persists there is cell damage and a release of chemical substances that increase the permeability of the capillaries. More fluid enters the interstitial spaces, leading to further hypovolaemia, further reduction in blood pressure and increased hypoxia.

Low blood pressure. As the blood pressure continues to fall, cerebral and myocardial hypoxia becomes progressively more marked and the reduced blood flow encourages the formation of thrombi and infarcts. There is acute renal failure and a marked reduction in the secretion of urine, leading to the retention of damaging metabolic waste products. If effective treatment is not possible these irreversible changes become progressively more severe and eventually may cause death.

ATHEROMA

Changes in arteries

Patchy changes (*atheromatous plaques*) develop in the tunica intima of large and medium-sized arteries. These consist of accumulations of cholesterol and other lipid compounds, excess smooth muscle and fibroelastic cells. As plaques grow they spread along the artery wall forming swellings that protrude into the lumen. Eventually the whole thickness of the wall and long sections of the vessel may be affected (Fig. 5.50).

Arteries most commonly involved are those in the heart, brain, kidneys, small intestine and lower limbs.

Causes of atheroma

The origin of atheromatous plaques is uncertain. *Fatty streaks* present in artery walls of infants are usually absorbed but their incomplete absorption may be the origin of atheromatous plaques in later life.

The incidence of atheroma is widespread in developed countries. Why atheromatous plaques develop is not yet clearly understood but the predisposing factors appear to exert their effects over a long period. This may mean that the development of atheroma can be delayed or even arrested by a change in lifestyle. Predisposing factors include:

- heredity—family history
- gender—males are more susceptible than females until after the menopause
- increasing age
- hypertension
- diabetes mellitus
- smoking, especially cigarettes
- excessive emotional stress in work or home environment
- diet, e.g. high intake of refined carbohydrates and/or cholesterol and saturated fatty acids (from animal fats)
- obesity
- sedentary lifestyle
- excessive alcohol consumption.

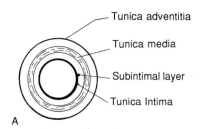
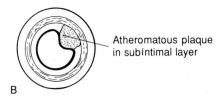
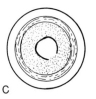
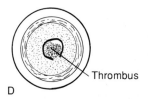

Figure 5.50 Development of atheroma.

Effects of atheroma

Arteries may be partially or completely blocked by atheromatous plaques alone, or by plaques combined with a thrombus. This may reduce or completely block the blood supply. The effects depend on the site and size of the artery involved and the extent of collateral circulation. Commonly the arteries affected are those in the heart, abdomen and pelvis.

Narrowing of artery

The tissues distal to the narrow point become ischaemic. The cells may receive enough blood to meet their minimum needs, but not enough to cope with an increase in metabolic rate, e.g. when muscle activity is increased. This causes acute cramp-like ischaemic pain. Heart muscle and skeletal muscles of the lower limb are most commonly affected. Ischaemic pain in the heart is called *angina pectoris* (p. 123), and in the lower limbs, *intermittent claudication*.

Occlusion of artery

When an artery is completely blocked, the tissues it supplies rapidly undergo degeneration and die from *ischaemia* which leads to *infarction*. The effect on the body depends on:

- the size of the artery occluded
- the amount and type of tissue involved
- the extent of collateral circulation, e.g. in the brain the circle of Willis provides extensive collateral blood vessels while in the heart there are very few.

When a coronary artery is occluded *myocardial infarction* (p. 123) occurs. Occlusion of arteries in the brain causes ischaemia and this leads to *cerebral infarction* (stroke).

Complications of atheroma

Thrombosis and infarction

If the epithelium lying over a plaque breaks down, platelets are stimulated by the damaged cells and a blood clot (thrombus) forms, blocking the artery and causing ischaemia and infarction. Pieces of the clot (emboli) may break off, travel in the bloodstream and lodge in small arteries distal to the clot, causing small infarcts (areas of dead tissue).

Haemorrhage

If calcium salts are deposited in the plaques, the artery walls become brittle, rigid and unresponsive to rises in blood pressure and may rupture, causing haemorrhage.

Aneurysm formation

If the artery wall is weakened by spread of the plaque between the layers of tissue, a local dilatation (aneurysm) may develop (p. 118). This may lead to thrombosis and embolism, or the aneurysm may rupture causing severe haemorrhage. The most common sites affected are the abdominal and pelvic arteries.

THROMBOSIS, EMBOLISM AND INFARCTION

A *thrombus* is an intravascular blood clot, causing *thrombosis*. It may partially or completely occlude an artery or vein, interfering with the circulation of blood.

Factors which predispose to thrombus formation include:

- an abnormality of the normally smooth endothelium, e.g. ulcerated atheromatous plaque
- abnormal blood flow in a vessel, especially venous stasis
- increased coagulability of the blood.

If a fragment of thrombus, called an *embolus*, becomes detached, it travels in the bloodstream until it lodges in and blocks a smaller vessel. The tissue supplied by the vessel becomes ischaemic and dies; this is *infarction*.

An *embolus* is a mass of any material carried in the bloodstream and large enough to block a blood vessel. Most emboli consist of fragments of thrombi but other materials include:

- fragments of atheromatous plaques
- fragments of vegetations from heart valves, e.g. infective endocarditis
- tumour fragments that may cause metastases
- amniotic fluid, during childbirth
- fat, from extensive bone fractures
- air, iatrogenic or following puncture of a blood vessel in the lung by a broken rib
- nitrogen in decompression sickness—'the bends'
- pus from an abscess
- clumps of platelets with adherent microbes.

Emboli in veins move towards the heart and lodge in the smaller vessels of the lungs or the liver (an important cause of metastases in tumours of the alimentary tract). Those in arteries travel away from the heart and lodge in smaller arteries or arterioles.

The effects of an embolus are determined by the site and size of the blood vessel occluded, not its composition. Common serious consequences include:

- myocardial infarction (p. 123)
- cerebral infarction (p. 181)
- pulmonary embolism (p. 119).

OEDEMA

In oedema there is excess tissue fluid, which causes swelling. It may occur in internal organs or in superficial tissues when there is disruption of the mechanisms that maintain homeostasis (p. 86).

Sites of oedema

When oedema is present in the superficial tissues *pitting* of the surface may be observed, i.e. an indentation in the skin remains after firm finger pressure has been applied. The sites at which superficial oedema is observed may be influenced by gravity and the position of the individual. When the individual is in the standing or sitting position the oedema is observed in the lower limbs, beginning in the feet and ankles. Patients on bedrest tend to develop oedema in the sacral area. This may be described as *dependent oedema*.

In *pulmonary oedema*, venous congestion in the lungs, or increased vessel permeability results in accumulation of fluid in the tissue spaces and in the alveoli. This reduces the area available for gaseous exchange and results in *dyspnoea* (breathlessness), cyanosis and expectoration of frothy sputum. The most common causes of pulmonary oedema are:

- cardiac failure
- inhalation of irritating gases
- inflammation
- intravenous infusion of excess fluid.

Causes of oedema

Increased venous hydrostatic pressure
Congestion of the venous circulation increases venous hydrostatic

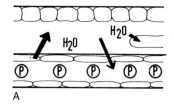

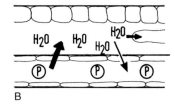

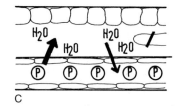

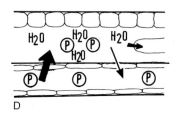

Figure 5.51 Mechanisms of oedema formation.
A. Normal formation of tissue fluid.
B., C. and D. Different mechanisms of oedema formation. Ⓟ = plasma protein. Arrows indicate direction of movement of water.

pressure, reducing the effect of osmotic pressure that draws fluid back into the capillary at the venous end. Excess fluid then remains in the tissues. This may be caused by:

- heart failure
- kidney disease
- external pressure on a limb due to, e.g. prolonged sitting, tight garments.

Decreased plasma osmotic pressure (Fig. 5.51B)
When there is depletion of plasma proteins, less fluid returns to the

circulation at the venous end of the capillary. Causes include:

- acute nephritis
- nephrotic syndrome (p. 350)
- liver failure (p. 333)
- famine, due to depleted intake of protein.

Impaired lymphatic drainage (Fig. 5.51C)
Some fluid returns to the circulation via the lymphatic system and when flow is impaired, oedema develops. Causes include:

- malignancy
- surgical removal of lymph nodes
- destruction of lymph nodes by chronic inflammation.

Increased small vessel permeability (Fig. 5.51D)
In inflammation (p. 69), chemical mediators increase small vessel permeability in the affected area. Plasma proteins then leave the circulation and the increased tissue osmotic pressure draws fluid into the area causing swelling of the affected tissue. This type of oedema also occurs in allergic reactions, e.g. anaphylaxis, asthma, hay fever.

Ascites and effusions

Ascites is the name given to the accumulation of excess fluid in the peritoneal cavity. The most common causes are:

- liver disease (p. 332)
- obstruction of lymph vessels in the abdominal cavity
- acute inflammation.

Pleural effusion means that excess serous fluid collects in the pleural cavity. The most common causes are:

- heart failure
- inflammation of the pleural membrane.

DISEASES OF BLOOD VESSELS

Arteriosclerosis

This is a progressive degenerative condition of the walls of arteries. It is associated with ageing and is accompanied by hypertension.

Large and medium arteries

The tunica media is infiltrated with fibrous tissue and calcium. This causes the vessels to lose their elasticity. The lumen dilates and they become tortuous (Fig. 5.52). Loss of elasticity increases systolic blood pressure, and the *pulse pressure* (the difference between systolic and diastolic pressure).

Small arteries and arterioles

Hyaline thickening of the tunica media and tunica intima causes narrowing of the lumen and they become tortuous (Fig. 5.52). These arteries are the main determinants of peripheral resistance (p. 84) and narrowing of their lumens increases peripheral resistance and blood pressure. Ischaemia of tissues supplied by affected arteries may occur. In the limbs, the resultant ischaemia predisposes to gangrene which is particularly serious in people with diabetes mellitus.

Senile arteriosclerosis is a condition affecting elderly people in which the progressive loss of elasticity and reduced arterial lumen leads to cerebral ischaemia and loss of mental function. There may or may not be evidence of hypertension.

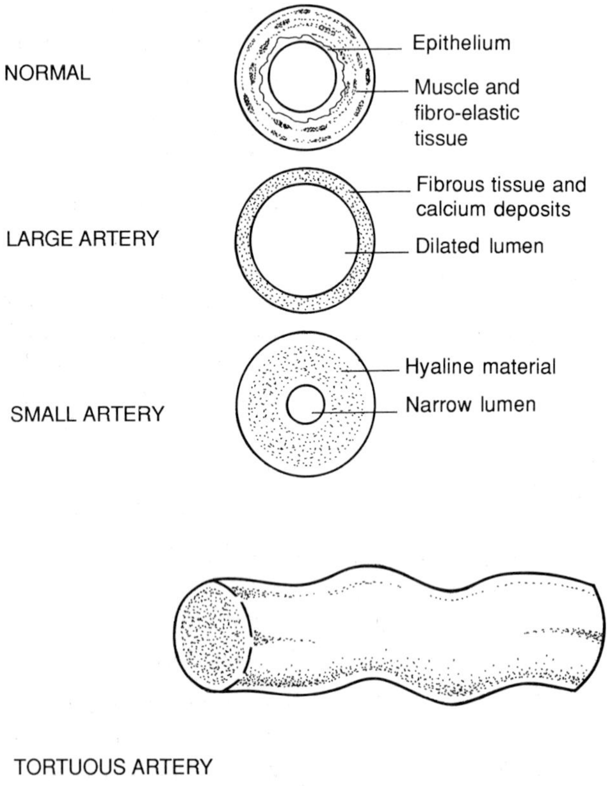

Figure 5.52 Arteriosclerotic arteries.

NORMAL — Epithelium; Muscle and fibro-elastic tissue

LARGE ARTERY — Fibrous tissue and calcium deposits; Dilated lumen

SMALL ARTERY — Hyaline material; Narrow lumen

TORTUOUS ARTERY

Thrombangitis obliterans (Buerger's disease)

In this condition there is acute inflammation with thrombosis of the small arteries mainly in the lower limbs. It occurs most commonly in men between the ages of 20 and 40 years and is associated with heavy cigarette smoking. The condition may be caused by an immune response to an antigen, possibly a tobacco protein. The condition may become chronic and the vessel walls become fibrosed, lose their elasticity and do not dilate during exercise. The individual suffers from acute ischaemic pain and, as the disease progresses, the distance walked with comfort is gradually reduced. In the long term the skin may ulcerate and, in extreme cases, gangrene may develop.

Polyarteritis nodosa

This is a connective tissue disorder associated with inflammation of the tunica media of medium-sized arteries in any part of the body. The most common sites are the heart, kidneys, alimentary tract, liver, pancreas and nervous system. It is acute at first but frequently becomes chronic. Necrosis and rupture of blood vessels may occur in the acute phase followed by thrombosis, ischaemia, infarction and death. It is believed to be caused by an immune reaction. In most cases the antigen is not known but it may be a virus or drug such as a sulphonamide or antibiotic.

Aneurysms (Fig. 5.53)

Aneurysms are abnormal local dilatations of arteries which vary considerably in size. The causes are not clear but predisposing factors

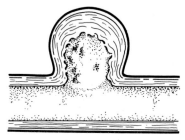

Saccular

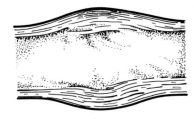

Fusiform

Dissecting

Figure 5.53 Types of aneurysm.

include atheroma, hypertension and defective formation of collagen in the blood vessel wall.

Fusiform or spindle-shaped distensions occur mainly in the abdominal aorta and less commonly in the iliac arteries. They are usually associated with atheromatous changes.

Saccular aneurysms bulge out on one side of the artery. When they occur in the relatively thin-walled arteries of the circle of Willis in the brain they are sometimes called 'berry' aneurysms. They may be associated with defective collagen production, with atheromatous changes or be congenital.

Dissecting aneurysms occur mainly in the arch of the aorta due to infiltration of blood between the endothelium and tunica media, beginning at a site of endothelial damage.

Micro-aneurysms are fusiform or saccular aneurysms, occurring in small arteries and arterioles in the

brain. They are associated with hypertension. Recurring small strokes (transient ischaemic attacks) are commonly due to thrombosis in the aneurysm or to haemorrhage when an aneurysm ruptures.

Complications of aneurysms

Haemorrhage
A ruptured aneurysm may cause sudden death or disability of varying severity, depending on the size and site of the artery.

Pressure
Localised swelling may cause pressure affecting adjacent tissues including organs, blood vessels and nerves.

Thrombosis and embolism
A blood clot (thrombus) may form in an artery where the endothelium has been damaged by an aneurysm. A piece of clot (embolus) may break off and travel in the bloodstream until it lodges in a small artery distal to the aneurysm and obstructs the blood flow, causing ischaemia and infarction.

Venous thrombosis

This may be *superficial thrombophlebitis* or *deep vein thrombosis*.

Superficial thrombophlebitis

In this acute inflammatory condition a thrombus forms in a superficial vein and the tissue around the affected vein becomes red and painful. The most common precursors are:

- intravenous infusion
- varicosities in the saphenous vein.

Deep vein thrombosis (DVT)

A thrombus forms in a deep vein commonly in the lower limb, pelvic or iliac veins, but occasionally in an upper limb. The thrombus may affect a long section of the vein and, after some days, fibrinolysis (p. 62) may enable recanalisation through the blockage. Deep vein thrombosis may be accompanied by pain and swelling, but is often asymptomatic. There are several predisposing factors.

Reduced rate of blood flow which may be caused by:

- immobility associated with prolonged bedrest
- pressure on veins in the popliteal region by, e.g. a pillow under the knees in bed or sitting in a chair for long periods, as in long journeys by air
- pressure on a vein by an adjacent tumour
- prolonged low blood pressure, as in shock.

Changes in the blood may trigger intravascular clotting, e.g.:

- increased blood viscosity in, e.g. dehydration, polycythaemia (p. 76)
- increased adhesiveness of platelets, e.g. associated with the use of some oral contraceptive drugs, and in some malignant diseases.

Damage to blood vessel wall can result in intravascular clotting, e.g.:

- accidental injury
- surgery.

Complication

Pulmonary embolism. This occurs when a large piece or several small fragments of a venous thrombus become detached and travel through the heart to lodge in the pulmonary artery or one of its branches. It causes infarction of lung tissue. A massive pulmonary embolism usually causes sudden collapse and death.

Varicose veins

A varicosed vein is one which is so dilated that the valves do not close to prevent backward flow of blood.

Such veins lose their elasticity, become elongated and tortuous and fibrous tissue replaces the tunica media.

Predisposing factors

Heredity. There appears to be a familial tendency but no abnormal genetic factor has been identified.

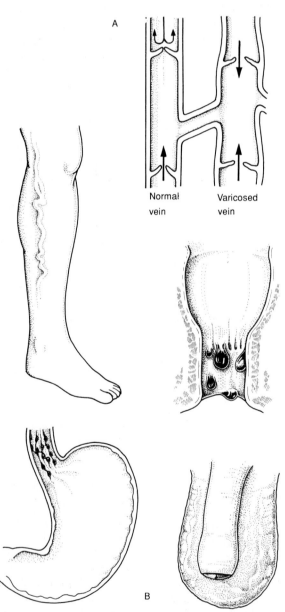

Gender. Females are affected more than males, especially following pregnancy.

Age. There is progressive loss of elasticity in the vein walls with increasing age so that elastic recoil is less efficient.

Obesity. Superficial veins in the limbs are supported by subcutaneous areolar tissue. Excess adipose tissue may not provide sufficient support.

Gravity. Standing for long periods with little muscle contraction tends to cause pooling of blood in the lower limbs and pelvis.

Pressure. Because of their thin walls, veins are easily compressed by surrounding structures, leading to increased venous pressure distal to the site of compression.

Sites and effects of varicose veins
(Fig. 5.54)

Varicose veins of the legs
When valves in the anastomosing veins between the deep and superficial veins in the legs become incompetent the venous pressure in the superficial veins rises. In the long term they stretch and become chronically dilated because the superficial veins are not supported by much tissue. Such areas are seen externally as *varicosities*. The great and small saphenous veins and the anterior tibial veins are most commonly affected causing aching and fatigue of the legs especially during long periods of standing. These dilated, inelastic veins rupture easily if injured, and haemorrhage occurs.

The skin over a varicose vein may become poorly nourished due to stasis of blood, leading to the formation of *varicose ulcers* usually on the medial aspects of the leg just above the ankle.

Figure 5.54 A. Normal and varicosed veins. B. Common sites of varicosities: the leg, oesophagus, scrotal varicocele, anal haemorrhoids.

Haemorrhoids

Sustained pressure on the veins at the junction of the rectum and anus leads to increased venous pressure, valvular incompetence and the development of haemorrhoids. The most common causes are chronic constipation, and the increased pressure in the pelvis towards the end of pregnancy. Slight bleeding may occur each time stools are passed and, in time, may cause anaemia. Severe haemorrhage is rare.

Oesophageal varices

The veins involved are at the lower end of the oesophagus. When the venous pressure in the liver rises, there is a rise in pressure in the anastomosing veins between the left gastric vein and the azygos vein. Sustained pressure causes varicosities to develop in the oesophagus. The commonest causes of increased portal vein pressure are cirrhosis of the liver and right-sided cardiac failure. If the pressure continues to rise, inelastic varicosed veins may rupture causing severe haemorrhage, and possibly death.

Scrotal varicocele

Each spermatic cord is surrounded by a plexus of veins that may become varicosed, especially in men whose work necessitates standing for long periods. If the varicocele is bilateral the increased temperature due to venous congestion may cause depressed spermatogenesis and result in infertility.

Tumours of blood and lymph vessels

Angiomas

Angiomas are benign tumours of either blood vessels (haemangiomas) or lymph vessels (lymphangiomas). The latter rarely occur, so angioma is usually taken to mean haemangioma.

Haemangiomas

These are not true tumours but are sufficiently similar to be classified as such. They consist of an excessive growth of blood vessels arranged in an uncharacteristic manner and interspersed with collagen fibres.

Capillary haemangiomas. Excess capillary growth interspersed with collagen in a localised area makes a dense, plexus-like network of tissue. Each haemangioma is supplied by only one blood vessel and if it thromboses the haemangioma atrophies and disappears.

Capillary haemangiomas are usually present at birth and are seen as a purple or red mole or birthmark. They may be quite small at birth but grow at an alarming rate in the first few months, keeping pace with the growth of the child. After 1 to 3 years, atrophy may begin and by the end of 5 years in about 80% of cases the tumours have disappeared.

Cavernous haemangiomas. Blood vessels larger than capillaries grow in excess of normal needs in a localised area and are interspersed with collagen fibres. They are dark red in colour and may be present in the skin, though more commonly in the liver. They grow slowly, do not regress and may become large and unsightly.

HEART DISEASES

Cardiac failure

The heart is described as failing when the cardiac output is unable to maintain the circulation of sufficient blood to meet the needs of the body. In mild cases, cardiac output is adequate at rest and becomes inadequate only when increased cardiac output is required, e.g. in exercise. Heart failure may involve either side of the heart, but as both sides pump in parallel, failure of one side usually results in failure of the other.

Acute cardiac failure

A sudden diminution in output of blood from both ventricles causes acute reduction in the oxygen supply to all the tissues. Recovery from the acute phase may be followed by chronic failure, or death may occur due to anoxia of vital centres in the brain. The commonest causes are:

- severe damage to an area of cardiac muscle due to ischaemia caused by sudden occlusion of one of the larger coronary arteries by atheroma or atheroma with thrombosis
- pulmonary embolism
- acute toxic myocarditis
- severe cardiac arrhythmia
- rupture of a heart chamber or valve cusp
- severe malignant hypertension.

Chronic cardiac failure

This develops gradually and in the early stages there may be no symptoms because the heart compensates by increasing the rate and force of contraction and the ventricles dilate. Myocardial cell hypertrophy increases the strength of the muscle. When further compensation is not possible there is a gradual decline in myocardial efficiency. During the development of chronic failure, hypoxia and venous congestion cause changes in other systems, making still greater demands on the heart, e.g. renal, endocrine, respiratory. Underlying causes include:

- chronic hypertension, myocardial fibrosis, valvular disease, lung diseases, anaemia
- previous acute cardiac failure
- degenerative changes of old age.

Right-sided or congestive cardiac failure

The right ventricle fails when pressure developed within it by the contracting myocardium is less than the force needed to push blood through the lungs.

When compensation has reached its limit, and the ventricle is not emptying completely, the right atrium and venae cavae become congested with blood and this is followed by congestion throughout the venous system. The organs affected first are the liver, spleen and kidneys. *Oedema* (p. 116) of the limbs and *ascites* (excess fluid in the peritoneal cavity) usually follow.

This discrepancy may be caused by increased resistance in the lungs, weakness of the myocardium and/ or stenosis and incompetence of valves in the heart or great vessels.

Resistance to the flow of blood through the lungs

When this is increased the right ventricle has more work to do. It may be caused by:

- the formation of fibrous tissue following inflammation or chronic disease of the lungs
- back pressure of blood from the left side of the heart, e.g. in left ventricular failure, when the mitral valve is stenosed and/or incompetent.

Weakness of the myocardium

This may be caused by ischaemia following numerous small myocardial infarcts.

Left-sided or left ventricular failure

This occurs when the pressure developed in the left ventricle by the contracting myocardium is less than the pressure in the aorta and the ventricle cannot then pump out all the blood it receives. Causes include:

- excessively high systemic blood pressure
- incompetence of the mitral and/ or the aortic valve
- aortic valve stenosis
- myocardial weakness.

Failure of the left ventricle leads to dilatation of the atrium and an increase in pulmonary blood pressure. This is followed by a rise in the blood pressure in the right side of the heart and eventually systemic venous congestion.

The congestion in the lungs leads to pulmonary oedema and dyspnoea, often most severe at night. This *paroxysmal nocturnal dyspnoea* may be due to raised blood volume as fluid from peripheral oedema is reabsorbed when the patient slips down in bed during sleep.

Disorders of heart valves

The heart valves prevent backflow of blood in the heart during the cardiac cycle. The atrioventricular and aortic valves in the left side of the heart are subject to greater pressures than those on the right side and are therefore more susceptible to damage.

Distinctive heart sounds arise when the valves close during the cardiac cycle (p. 93). Damaged valves generate abnormal heart sounds called *murmurs*. A severe valve disorder results in heart failure. The most common causes of valve defects are rheumatic fever, fibrosis

following inflammation and congenital abnormalities.

Stenosis

This is the narrowing of a valve opening impeding blood flow through the valve. It occurs when inflammation and encrustations roughen the edges of the cusps so that they stick together, narrowing the valve opening. When healing occurs fibrous tissue is formed which shrinks as it ages, increasing the stenosis and leading to incompetence.

Incompetence

Sometimes called *regurgitation*, this is a functional defect caused by failure of a valve to close completely, allowing blood to flow back into the ventricle when it relaxes.

Ischaemic heart disease

Ischaemic heart disease is due to the effects of atheroma, causing narrowing or occlusion of one or more branches of the coronary arteries. The narrowing is caused by atheromatous plaques. Occlusion may be by plaques alone, or plaques complicated by thrombosis. The overall effect depends on the size of the coronary artery involved and whether it is narrowed or occluded. Narrowing of the artery leads to *angina pectoris*, occlusion to *myocardial infarction*, i.e. an area of dead tissue.

When atheroma develops slowly, a *collateral arterial blood supply* may have time to develop and effectively supplement or replace the original. This consists of the dilatation of normally occurring anastomotic arteries joining adjacent branch arteries. When sudden severe narrowing or occlusion of an artery occurs the anastomotic arteries dilate but may not be able to supply enough blood to meet the needs of the myocardium.

Angina pectoris

This is sometimes called *angina of effort* because increased cardiac output required during extra physical effort causes severe ischaemic pain in the chest. The pain may also radiate to the arms, neck and jaw. Other factors which may precipitate angina include:

- cold weather
- exercising after a heavy meal
- strong emotions.

A narrowed artery may supply sufficient blood to the myocardium to meet its needs during rest or moderate exercise but not when increased cardiac output is needed, e.g. walking may be tolerated but not running. The thick, inflexible atheromatous artery wall is unable to dilate to allow for the increased blood flow needed by the more active myocardium which becomes ischaemic. In the early stages of development of the disease the pain stops when the cardiac output returns to its resting level soon after the extra effort stops.

Myocardial infarction

An *infarct* is an area of tissue that has died because of lack of oxygenated blood (p. 116). The myocardium is affected when a branch of a coronary artery is occluded. The commonest cause is an atheromatous plaque complicated by thrombosis. The extent of myocardial damage depends on the size of the blood vessel and site of the infarct. The damage is permanent because cardiac muscle cannot regenerate and the dead tissue is replaced with non-functional fibrous tissue. The effects and complications are great-est when the left ventricle is involved.

Myocardial infarction is usually accompanied by very severe crushing chest pain behind the sternum which, unlike angina pectoris, continues even when the individual is at rest.

Complications

These may be fatal and include:

- severe arrhythmias, especially ventricular fibrillation, due to disruption of the cardiac conducting system
- cardiac failure, caused by impaired contraction of the damaged myocardium and, in severe cases, cardiogenic shock
- rupture of a ventricle wall, usually within 2 weeks of the original episode
- pulmonary or cerebral embolism originating from a mural clot within a ventricle, i.e. a clot that forms inside the heart over the area of dead tissue
- pericarditis
- angina pectoris
- recurrence.

Rheumatic heart disease

Rheumatic fever

This autoimmune disease occurs 2 to 4 weeks after a throat infection, caused by *Streptococcus pyogenes* (beta-haemolytic Group A). The antibodies developed to combat the infection damage the heart. The microbes are not present in the heart lesion and the same infection in other parts of the body is very rarely followed by rheumatic fever. How the antibodies damage the heart is not yet understood. Children and young adults are most commonly affected.

Death rarely occurs in the acute phase but after recovery there may be permanent damage to the heart valves, eventually leading to disability and possibly cardiac failure.

Effects on the endocardium

The endocardium becomes inflamed and oedematous and tiny pale areas called *Aschoff's bodies* appear which, when they heal, leave thick fibrous tissue. Thrombotic fibrous nodules consisting of platelets and fibrin form on the free borders of the cusps of the heart valves. When healing occurs the fibrous tissue formed shrinks as it ages, distorting the shape of the cusps and causing stenosis and incompetence of the valve. The mitral and aortic valves are commonly affected, the tricuspid valve sometimes and the pulmonary valve rarely.

Effects on the myocardium

Aschoff's bodies form on the connective tissue between the cardiac muscle fibres. As in the endocardium, healing is accompanied by fibrosis which may interfere with myocardial contraction.

Effects on the pericardium

Inflammation leads to the accumulation of exudate in the pericardial cavity. Healing is accompanied by fibrous thickening of the pericardium and adhesions form between the two layers. In severe cases the layers may fuse, obliterating the cavity. Within this inelastic pericardium the heart may not be able to expand fully during diastole, leading to reduced cardiac output, generalised venous congestion and oedema.

Sydenham's chorea

This usually occurs between the ages of 5 and 15 years. The causes are unknown but it is commonly associated with streptococcal throat infection, rheumatic fever or endocarditis. There are rapid uncoordinated, involuntary muscle movements. In mild cases recovery takes place within about 4 weeks. In some cases the initial recovery may be followed by recurrences.

Choreiform movements may occasionally occur during pregnancy, in women taking contraceptive pills and following cerebrovascular lesions, especially in the elderly.

Subclinical rheumatic heart disease

Valvular incompetence developing in older people who have a history of rheumatic fever many years previously is believed to be due to repeated subclinical attacks. These attacks are not associated with repeated episodes of sore throat so it is assumed that the original disease has remained active in a subclinical form. In some cases there is no history of rheumatic fever.

Infective endocarditis

Infecting organisms in the blood may colonise any part of the endocardium but the most common sites are on or near the heart valves and round the margins of congenital heart defects. These areas are susceptible to infection because they are exposed to fast-flowing blood that may cause mild trauma.

The main predisposing factors are bacteraemia, depressed immune response and heart abnormalities.

Bacteraemia

Microbes may or may not multiply while in the bloodstream and, if not destroyed by phagocytes or antibodies, they tend to adhere to platelets and form tiny infected emboli. Inside the heart the emboli are most likely to settle on already damaged endocardium. Vegetations consisting of platelets and fibrin surround the microbes and seem to protect them from normal body defences and antibiotics. Because of this, infection may be caused by a wide range of microbes, including some of low pathogenicity, e.g.:

- non-haemolytic streptococci, e.g. following tooth extraction, tonsillectomy
- *Escherichia coli* and other normal bowel inhabitants, e.g. following intestinal surgery
- *Staphylococcus aureus*, e.g. from boils and carbuncles
- microbes from infections of, e.g. the biliary, urinary, respiratory tracts
- microbes accidentally introduced during medical and nursing procedures, e.g. cystoscopy, bladder catheterisation, arterial and venous catheterisation, surgery, wound dressing
- low-virulence microbes that cause infection in people with reduced immune response.

Depressed immune response

This enables low-virulence bacteria, viruses, yeasts and fungi to become established and cause infection. These are organisms always present in the body and the environment. Depression of the immune systems may be caused by:

- cytotoxic drugs
- ionising radiation, e.g. X-rays used in cancer treatment
- anti-inflammation drugs, e.g. corticosteroids
- malignant diseases, e.g. leukaemia, tumours of lymphoid tissue
- use of unsterile syringes by drug addicts, spreading human immuno deficiency virus (HIV).

Heart abnormalities

The sites most commonly infected are already abnormal in some way, e.g. valve cusps damaged by earlier attacks of rheumatic fever, endothelium damaged by the fast flow of blood through a narrow opening, such as a stenosed valve or congenital septal defect.

Acute infective endocarditis

This is a severe febrile illness usually caused by high-virulence microbes, commonly *Staphylococcus aureus*. Vegetations grow rapidly and pieces may break off, becoming infected emboli. These settle in other organs where the microbes grow, destroying tissue and forming pus. The effects depend on the organ involved, e.g. brain or kidney infection may cause death in a few days. The causative microbes rapidly destroy heart valves, impairing their function and resulting in acute heart failure.

Subacute infective endocarditis

This endocarditis is usually caused by low-virulence microbes, e.g. non-haemolytic streptococci, some staphylococci. Infected emboli may settle in any organ but do not cause suppuration and rarely cause death. Microbes in the vegetations seem to be protected by surrounding platelets and fibrin from normal body defences and antibiotics. Healing by fibrosis further distorts the shape of the valve cusps, increasing the original stenosis and incompetence. Heart failure may develop later.

Cardiac arrhythmias

The heart rate is normally initiated by intrinsic impulses generated in the SA node. The rhythm is determined by the route of impulse transmission through the conducting system. The heart rate is usually measured as the pulse, but to determine the rhythm, an electrocardiogram (ECG) is required. A *cardiac arrhythmia* is any disorder of heart rate or rhythm, and is the result of abnormal generation or conduction of impulses. The normal cardiac cycle (p. 92) gives rise to *normal sinus rhythm* which has a rate between 60 and 100 beats per minute.

Sinus bradycardia is sinus rhythm below 60 beats per minute. This may occur during sleep and is common in athletes. It is an abnormality when it follows myocardial infarction or accompanies raised intracranial pressure (p. 177).

Sinus tachycardia is sinus rhythm above 100 beats per minute when the individual is at rest. This accompanies exercise and anxiety; but is an indicator of some disorders, e.g. fever, hyperthyroidism, some cardiac conditions.

Asystole

This occurs when there is no electrical activity in the ventricles and therefore no cardiac output. Ventricular fibrillation and asystole cause sudden and complete loss of cardiac output, i.e. *cardiac arrest* and death.

Fibrillation

This is the contraction of the cardiac muscle fibres in a disorderly sequence. The chambers do not contract as a whole and the pumping action is disrupted.

In *atrial fibrillation* contraction of the atria is uncoordinated and rapid, pumping is ineffective and stimulation of the AV node is disorderly. Ventricular contraction becomes rapid and rhythm and force irregular; although an adequate cardiac output

and blood pressure may be maintained, the pulse is irregular. The causes of increased excitability and disorganised activity are not always clear but predisposing conditions include:

- ischaemic heart disease
- degenerative changes in the heart due to old age
- thyrotoxicosis
- rheumatic heart disease.

In *ventricular fibrillation* there is disorganised and very rapid contraction causing disruption of ventricular function. Blood is not pumped from the heart into either the pulmonary or the systemic circulation. No pulses can be felt, consciousness is lost and breathing stops. If normal heart action cannot be restored quickly, death follows due to cerebral anoxia.

Heart block

Heart block occurs when impulse formation is impaired or conduction is prevented, and the delay between atrial and ventricular contraction is increased. The severity depends on the extent of loss of stimulation of the AV node.

In *complete heart block*, ventricular contraction is entirely independent of impulses initiated by the SA node. Impulses generated by the AV node result in slow, regular ventricular contractions and a heart rate of about 30 to 40 beats per minute. In this state the heart is unable to respond quickly to a sudden increase in demand by, e.g. muscular exercise. The most common causes are:

- acute ischaemic heart disease
- myocardial fibrosis following repeated infarctions or myocarditis
- drugs used to treat heart disease, e.g. digitalis, propranolol.

When heart block develops gradually there is some degree of adjust-

ment in the body to reduced cardiac output but, if progressive, it eventually leads to death from cardiac failure and cerebral anoxia.

Congenital abnormalities

Abnormalities in the heart and great vessels at birth may be due to intrauterine developmental errors or to the failure of the heart and blood vessels to adapt to extrauterine life. In many cases there are no symptoms in early life and the abnormality is recognised only when complications appear.

Patent ductus arteriosus

Before birth the ductus arteriosus, joining the arch of the aorta and the pulmonary artery, allows blood to pass from the pulmonary artery to the aorta (Fig. 5.55). This is oxygenated blood from the placenta. At birth, when the pulmonary circulation is established, the ductus arteriosus should close completely. If it remains patent, blood regurgitates from the aorta to the pulmonary artery where the pressure is lower, reducing the volume entering the systemic circulation. This leads to pulmonary congestion and eventually cardiac failure.

Atrial septal defect

Before birth most oxygenated blood from the placenta enters the left atrium from the right atrium through the *foramen ovale* in the septum. There is a valve-like structure across the opening consisting of two partly overlapping membranes. The 'valve' is open when the pressure in the right atrium is higher than in the left. After birth, when

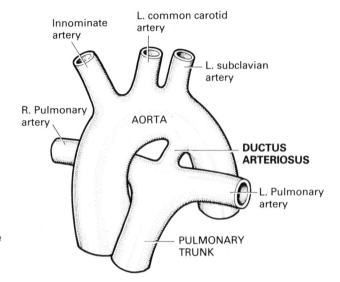

Figure 5.55
The position of the ductus arteriosus in the fetus.

the pulmonary circulation is established and the pressure in the left atrium is the higher, the two membranes come in contact, closing the 'valve'. Later the closure becomes permanent due to fibrosis (Fig. 5.56).

When the membranes do not overlap an opening between the atria remains patent after birth. In many cases it is too small to cause symptoms in early life but they may appear later. In severe cases blood flows back to the right atrium from the left. This increases the right ventricular and pulmonary pressure, causing hypertrophy of the myocardium and eventually cardiac failure. As pressure in the right atrium rises, blood flow through the defect

may be reversed, but this is not an improvement because deoxygenated blood gains access to the general circulation.

Coarctation of the aorta

The most common site of coarctation (narrowing) of the aorta is between the left subclavian artery and ductus arteriosus. This leads to hypertension in the upper body because increased force of contraction of the heart is needed to push the blood through the coarctation. There is hypotension in the rest of the body.

Fallot's tetralogy

Four concurrent abnormalities that interfere with the flow of blood from the left ventricle cause severe general hypoxia and heart failure. They are:

- stenosis of the pulmonary artery at its point of origin
- ventricular septal defect just below the atrioventricular valves
- aortic misplacement, i.e. the origin of the aorta is displaced to the right so that it is immediately above the septal defect
- right ventricular hypertrophy to counteract the pulmonary stenosis.

DISORDERS OF BLOOD PRESSURE

Hypertension

The term hypertension is used to describe blood pressure that is sustained at a higher than the generally accepted 'normal' maximum level for a particular age group, e.g.:

- at 20 years—140/90 mmHg
- at 50 years—160/95 mmHg
- at 75 years—170/105 mmHg.

Arteriosclerosis (p. 118) contributes to increasing blood pressure with age but is not the only factor involved.

Hypertension is described as *essential* (primary, idiopathic) or *secondary to other diseases*.

Essential hypertension

This means hypertension of unknown cause. It accounts for 85 to 90% of all cases and is subdivided according to the rate at which the disease progresses.

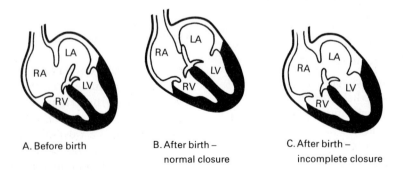

A. Before birth

B. After birth –
   normal closure

C. After birth –
   incomplete closure

Figure 5.56 Atrioseptal valve: normal and defective closure after birth.

Benign (chronic) hypertension

The rise in blood pressure is usually slight to moderate and continues to rise slowly over many years. Sometimes complications are the first indication of hypertension, e.g. heart failure, cerebrovascular accident, myocardial infarction. Occasionally the rate of progress increases and the hypertension becomes malignant. Predisposing factors include:

- inherited tendency
- obesity
- excessive alcohol intake
- cigarette smoking
- lack of exercise.

Malignant (accelerated) hypertension

The blood pressure is already elevated and continues to rise rapidly over a few months. Diastolic pressure in excess of 120 mmHg is common. The effects are serious and quickly become apparent, e.g. haemorrhages into the retina, papill-oedema (oedema around the optic disc), encephalopathy (cerebral oedema) and progressive renal disease, leading to cardiac failure.

Secondary hypertension

Hypertension resulting from other diseases accounts for 10 to 15% of all cases.

Kidney diseases

Raised blood pressure is a complication of many kidney diseases. The vasoconstrictor effect of excess *renin* released by damaged kidneys is one causative factor but there may be others, as yet unknown.

Endocrine disorders

Adrenal cortex diseases. Secretion of excess *aldosterone* and *cortisol* stimulates the retention of excess sodium and water by the kidneys, raising the blood volume and pressure. Oversecretion of aldosterone (Conn's syndrome) is due to a hormone-secreting tumour. Oversecretion of cortisol may be due to overstimulation of the gland by *adrenocorticotrophic hormone* secreted by the pituitary gland, or to a hormone-secreting tumour.

Adrenal medulla. Secretion of excess *adrenaline* and *noradrenaline* raises blood pressure, e.g. phaeochromocytoma (p. 233).

Stricture of the aorta

Hypertension develops in branching arteries proximal to the site of a stricture. In *congenital coarctation* the stricture is between the ductus arteriosus and the left subclavian artery causing hypertension in the head, neck and right arm. Compression of the aorta by an adjacent tumour may cause hypertension proximal to the stricture (Fig. 5.55).

Hypertension may be a complication of some drug treatment, e.g.:

- corticosteroids
- non-steroidal anti-inflammatory drugs
- oral contraceptives.

Effects and complications of hypertension

The effects of long-standing and progressively rising blood pressure are serious. Hypertension predisposes to atherosclerosis and has specific effects on particular organs.

Heart

The rate and force of cardiac contraction are increased to maintain the cardiac output against a sustained rise in arterial pressure. The left ventricle hypertrophies and begins to fail when compensation has reached its limit. This is followed by back pressure and accumulation of blood in the lungs, hypertrophy of the right ventricle and eventually to right ventricular failure. Hypertension also predisposes to ischaemic heart disease (p. 122) and aneurysm formation (p. 118).

Brain

Stroke, caused by cerebral haemorrhage, is common, the effects depending on the position and size of the ruptured vessel. When a series of small blood vessels rupture, e.g. microaneurysms, at different times, there is progressive disability. Rupture of a large vessel causes extensive loss of function or possibly death.

Kidneys

Essential hypertension causes kidney damage. If sustained for only a short time recovery may be complete. Otherwise the kidney damage causes further hypertension, progressive loss of kidney function and kidney failure.

Pulmonary hypertension

Raised blood pressure in the pulmonary circulation is secondary to:

- changes in blood vessels, described above
- chronic diseases of the respiratory system
- diseases of the heart, e.g. congenital defects of the septum, stenosis and incompetence of the mitral or aortic valve, heart failure
- diseases of other organs that cause raised pressure in the left side of the heart, e.g. cirrhosis of the liver, thrombosis of the portal vein.

Hypotension

This usually occurs as a complication of other conditions, e.g.:

- shock (p. 114)
- Addison's disease (p. 232).

Low blood pressure leads to inadequate blood supply to the brain. Depending on the cause, unconsciousness may be brief (fainting) or more prolonged, possibly causing death.

Postural hypotension syncope (fainting) is due to sudden reduction in blood pressure on standing up quickly from a sitting or lying position. It occurs most commonly in the elderly. It may be caused by delay in response of the baroreceptors in the carotid sinuses to the gravitational effects of standing up. It may also occur when patients are being treated with anti-hypertensive drugs, especially when the most suitable dose is being established.

6
The lymphatic system

All body tissues are bathed in tissue fluid, consisting of the diffusible constituents of blood and waste materials from cells. Some tissue fluid returns to the capillaries at their venous end and the remainder diffuses through the more permeable walls of the *lymph capillaries* and becomes *lymph*.

The composition of lymph is similar to that of plasma, but the concentrations of the constituents are different and there are some additional substances that are too large to pass through blood capillary walls, e.g. particles from areas of infection and cells damaged by disease. The lymphatic system returns plasma proteins and tissue fluid to the blood.

Lymph passes through vessels of increasing size and a varying number of *lymph nodes* before returning to the blood. The lymphatic system consists of:

- lymph vessels
- lymph nodes and other lymphatic tissue
- spleen
- thymus gland.

The lymphatic system is involved in the specific and non-specific defence mechanisms of the body, i.e. in phagocytosis and the development and maintenance of immunity (Ch. 4).

LYMPH VESSELS

Lymph capillaries

These originate as blind-end tubes in the interstitial spaces (Fig. 6.1). They have the same structure as blood capillaries, i.e. a single layer of endothelial cells, but their walls are more permeable to all interstitial fluid constituents, including proteins and cell debris. The tiny capillaries join up to form larger lymph vessels.

Larger lymph vessels

The walls of lymph vessels are about the same thickness as those of small veins and have the same layers of tissue, i.e. a fibrous covering, a middle layer of smooth muscle and elastic tissue and an inner lining of endothelium. Lymph vessels have numerous cup-shaped valves which ensure that lymph flows in one way only, i.e. towards the thorax (Fig. 6.2). There is no 'pump', like the heart, involved in the onward movement of lymph but the muscle tissue in the walls of the large lymph vessels has an intrinsic ability to contract rhythmically. Other factors believed to assist include:

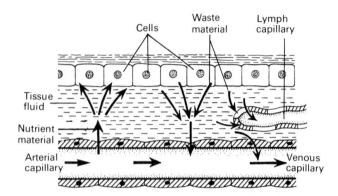

Figure 6.1 Diagram of the beginning of a lymph capillary.

- tissue fluid pressure
- contraction of surrounding muscles
- pressure caused by the pulsation of adjacent arteries
- negative pressure in the thorax during inspiration.

Lymph vessels become larger as they join together, eventually forming two large ducts, the *thoracic duct* and *right lymphatic duct*, that empty lymph into the *subclavian veins*.

Thoracic duct

This duct begins at the *cisterna chyli*, which is a lymph vessel dilatation situated in front of the bodies of the first two lumbar vertebrae. The duct is about 40 cm long and opens into the *left subclavian vein* in the root of the neck. It drains lymph from both legs, the pelvic and abdominal cavities, the left half of the thorax, head and neck and the left arm (Figs 6.3 and 6.4).

Right lymphatic duct

This is a dilated lymph vessel about 1 cm long. It lies in the root of the neck and opens into the *right subclavian vein*. It drains lymph from the right half of the thorax, head and neck and the right arm.

Functions of lymphatic vessels

- Return of excess tissue fluid to the blood (about 3 litres daily).
- Return of plasma proteins to the blood.
- Transport of other particulate material to lymph nodes for breakdown.
- Fat absorbed in the small intestine enters lymph capillaries called *lacteals* which transport the now milky fluid, called *chyle*, to the thoracic duct.

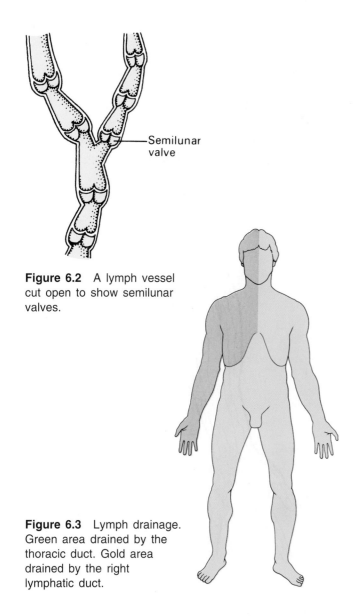

Figure 6.2 A lymph vessel cut open to show semilunar valves.

Figure 6.3 Lymph drainage. Green area drained by the thoracic duct. Gold area drained by the right lymphatic duct.

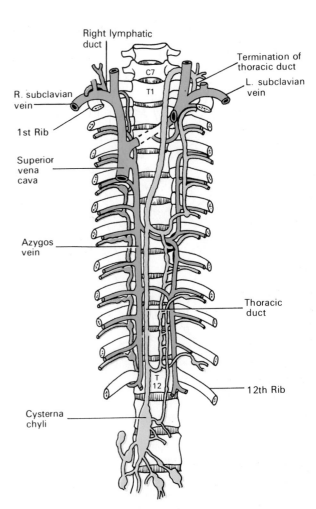

Figure 6.4 Origin and position of the thoracic duct and the right lymphatic duct.

LYMPH NODES

All the small and medium-sized lymph vessels open into *lymph nodes* which are situated in strategic positions throughout the body. The lymph drains through a number of nodes, usually 8 to 10, before returning to the blood. These nodes vary considerably in size: some are as small as a pin head and the largest are about the size of an almond.

Structure

Lymph nodes (Fig. 6.5) have a *surrounding capsule of fibrous tissue* which dips down into the node substance

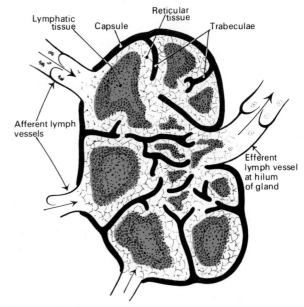

Figure 6.5 Section of a lymph node. Arrows show the direction of flow of lymph.

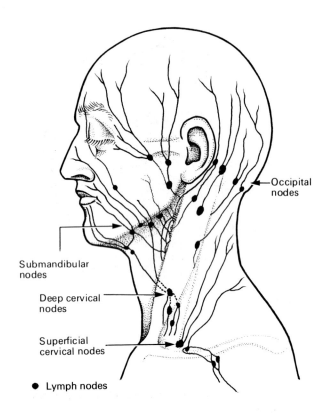

Figure 6.6 Some lymph nodes of the face and neck.

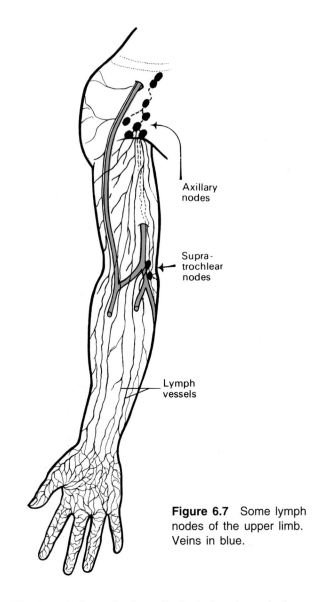

Figure 6.7 Some lymph nodes of the upper limb. Veins in blue.

forming partitions, or *trabeculae*. The main substance of the node consists of *reticular and lymphatic tissue* containing many *lymphocytes* and *macrophages*.

As many as four or five *afferent lymph vessels* may enter a lymph node while only one *efferent vessel* carries lymph away from the node. Each node has a concave surface called the hilum where an artery enters and a vein and the efferent lymph vessel leave.

The large numbers of lymph nodes situated in strategic positions throughout the body are arranged in *deep* and *superficial groups*.

Lymph from the head and neck passes through deep and superficial *cervical nodes* (Fig. 6.6).

Lymph from the *upper limbs* passes through nodes situated in the *elbow region* then through the deep and superficial *axillary nodes* (Fig. 6.7).

Lymph from organs and tissues in the *thoracic cavity* drains through groups of nodes, including: *parasternal, intercostal, brachiocephalic, mediastinal, tracheobronchial, bronchopulmonary* and *oesophageal nodes*. Most of the lymph from the breast passes through the *axillary nodes*.

Lymph from the *pelvic and abdominal cavities* passes through many lymph nodes before entering the cisterna chyli. The abdominal and pelvic nodes are situated mainly in association with the blood vessels supplying the organs and close to the main arteries, i.e. the aorta and the external and internal iliac arteries.

The lymph from the *lower limbs* drains through deep and superficial nodes including *popliteal nodes* and *inguinal nodes* (Fig. 6.8).

Functions of lymph nodes

Filtering and phagocytosis

Lymph is filtered by the reticular and lymphoid tissue as it passes through lymph nodes. Particulate matter may include microbes, dead and live phagocytes containing ingested microbes, cells from malignant tumours, worn-out and damaged tissue cells, inhaled particles. Organic material is destroyed in lymph nodes by macrophages and antibodies. Some inorganic inhaled particles cannot be destroyed by phagocytosis. These remain inside the macrophages, causing no damage or killing the cell. Material not filtered off and dealt with

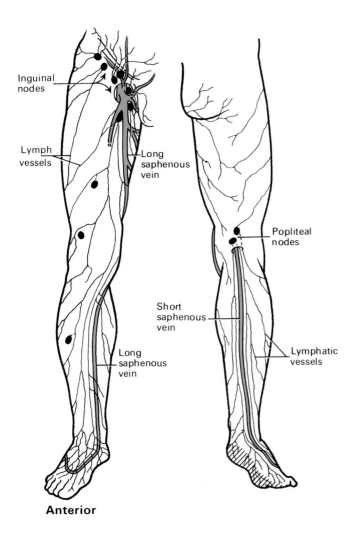

Anterior

Figure 6.8 Some lymph nodes of the lower limb. Veins in blue.

in one lymph node passes on to successive nodes and when lymph enters the blood, it has usually been cleared of foreign matter and cell debris. In some cases where phagocytosis of microbes is incomplete they may stimulate inflammation and enlargement of the node.

Proliferation of lymphocytes

Activated T- and B-lymphocytes multiply in lymph nodes (p. 65). Antibodies produced by sensitised B-lymphocytes enter lymph and blood draining the node.

OTHER LYMPHATIC TISSUE

Lymphatic tissue is found in a number of situations in the body in addition to the lymph nodes:

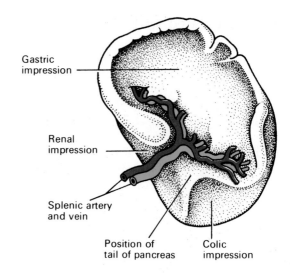

Figure 6.9 Spleen.

- palatine tonsil—between the mouth and the oral part of the pharynx
- pharyngeal tonsil—on the wall of the nasal part of the pharynx
- solitary lymphatic follicles
- aggregated lymphatic follicles (Peyer's patches)—in the wall of the small intestine
- vermiform appendix—an outgrowth from the caecum (first part of the large intestine).

These structures are discussed in the sections on the respiratory and digestive systems (Chs 10 and 12).

Collectively this tissue is referred to as *mucosa associated lymph tissue* (MALT) and along with the spleen and thymus it is involved in the development of immunity. However, unlike lymph nodes, MALT has no afferent lymph vessels and therefore does not filter lymph. MALT is strategically positioned to protect the respiratory and gastrointestinal tracts from microbes and other foreign material which has entered.

Spleen (Fig. 6.9)

The spleen is formed by reticular and lymphatic tissue and is the largest lymph organ.

The spleen lies in the *left hypochondriac region* of the abdominal cavity between the fundus of the stomach and the diaphragm. It is purplish in colour and varies in size in different individuals, but is usually about 12 cm long, 7 cm wide and 2.5 cm thick. It weighs about 200 g.

Organs associated with the spleen

Superiorly and posteriorly	— diaphragm
Inferiorly	— left colic flexure of the large intestine
Anteriorly	— fundus of the stomach
Medially	— pancreas and the left kidney
Laterally	— separated from the 9th, 10th and 11th ribs and the intercostal muscles by the diaphragm

Structure (Fig. 6.10)

The spleen is slightly oval in shape with the *hilum* on the lower medial border. The anterior surface is covered with peritoneum. It is enclosed in a *fibroelastic capsule* that dips into the organ, forming *trabeculae*. The cellular material, consisting of *lymphocytes* and *macrophages*, is called *splenic pulp*, and it lies between the trabeculae. *Red pulp* is the part suffused with blood and *white pulp* consists of areas of lymphatic tissue where there are sleeves of lymphocytes and macrophages around blood vessels.

The structures entering and leaving the spleen at the hilum are:

- splenic artery, a branch of the coeliac artery
- splenic vein, a branch of the portal vein
- lymph vessels (efferent only)
- nerves.

Blood passing through the spleen flows in sinuses which have distinct pores between the endothelial cells, allowing it to come into close association with splenic pulp.

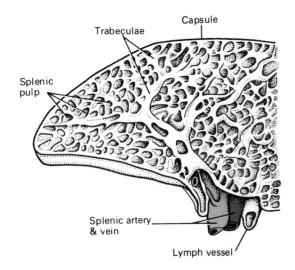

Figure 6.10 Diagram of a section of a spleen.

Functions

Phagocytosis

As described previously (p. 64), old and abnormal erythrocytes are destroyed in the spleen and the breakdown products, bilirubin and iron, are passed to the liver via the splenic and portal veins. Other cellular material, e.g. leukocytes, platelets and microbes, are phagocytosed in the spleen. Unlike lymph nodes, the spleen has no afferent lymphatics entering it, so it is not exposed to diseases spread by lymph.

Development of lymphocytes

The aggregates of lymphocytes respond to antigens by immune reactions. Sensitised B- and T-lymphocytes multiply and become immunocompetent (p. 65). Some B-lymphocytes develop into plasma cells and produce antibodies. The spleen provides many of the lymphocytes in the blood.

Erythropoeisis

The spleen and liver are important sites of fetal blood cell production, and the spleen can also fulfil this function in adults in times of great need.

Thymus gland

The thymus gland lies in the upper part of the mediastinum behind the sternum and extends upwards into the root of the neck. It weighs about 10 to 15 g at birth and grows until the individual reaches puberty, when it begins to atrophy. Its maximum weight, at puberty, is between 30 and 40 g and by middle age it has returned to approximately its weight at birth (Fig. 6.11).

Organs associated with the thymus

Anteriorly	— sternum and upper four costal cartilages
Posteriorly	— aortic arch and its branches, brachiocephalic veins, trachea
Laterally	— lungs
Superiorly	— structures in the root of the neck
Inferiorly	— heart

Structure

The thymus consists of two lobes joined by areolar tissue. The lobes are enclosed by a fibrous capsule

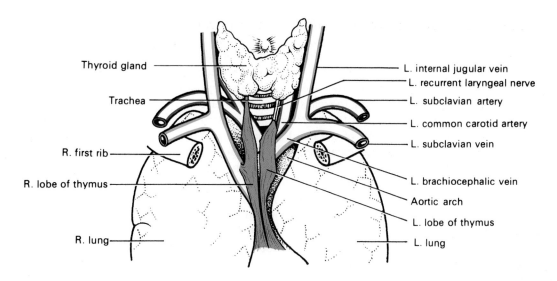

Figure 6.11 Thymus gland in the adult, and related structures.

which dips into their substance, dividing them into lobules that consist of an irregular branching framework of epithelial cells and lymphocytes.

Function

Lymphocytes originate from haemocytoblasts (stem cells) in red bone marrow. Those that enter the thymus mature and develop into activated T-lymphocytes, i.e. able to respond to antigens encountered elsewhere in the body (p. 65). They then divide into two groups:

- those that enter the blood, some of which remain in circulation and some lodge in other lymphoid tissue
- those that remain in the thymus gland and are the source of future generations of T-lymphocytes.

The maturation of the thymus and other lymphoid tissue is stimulated by *thymosin*, a hormone secreted by the epithelial cells that form the framework of the thymus gland. Involution of the gland begins in adolescence and, with increasing age, the effectiveness of T-lymphocyte response to antigens declines.

DISORDERS ASSOCIATED WITH LYMPH VESSELS

The main involvements of lymph vessels are in relation to:

- the spread of disease in the body
- the effects of lymphatic obstruction.

Spread of disease

The materials most commonly spread via the lymph vessels from their original site to the circulating blood are fragments of tumours and infected material.

Fragments of tumours

Tumour cells may enter a lymph capillary draining a tumour, or a larger vessel when a tumour has eroded its wall. Cells from a malignant tumour, if not phagocytosed, settle and multiply in the first lymph node they encounter. Later, there may be further spread to other lymph nodes, to the blood and to other parts of the body via the blood. In this sequence of events, each new metastatic tumour becomes a source of malignant cells that may spread by the same routes.

Infected material

Infected material may enter lymph vessels either at their origin in the interstitial spaces, or through the walls of larger vessels invaded by microbes when infection spreads locally. If phagocytosis is not effective the infection may spread from node to node, and eventually reach the blood stream.

Lymphangitis (infection of lymph vessel walls). This occurs in some acute pyogenic infections in which the microbes in the lymph draining from the area infect and spread along the walls of lymph vessels, e.g. in acute *Streptococcus pyogenes* infection of the hand, a red line may be seen extending from the hand to the axilla. This is caused by an inflamed superficial lymph vessel and adjacent tissues. The infection may be stopped at the first lymph node or spread through the lymph drainage network to the blood.

Lymphatic obstruction

When a lymph vessel is obstructed there is an accumulation of lymph distal to the obstruction, called *lymphoedema*. The amount of resultant swelling and the size of the area affected depend on the size of the vessel involved. Lymphoedema usually leads to low-grade inflammation and fibrosis of the lymph vessel and further lymphoedema. The most common causes are tumours and surgery.

Tumours

A tumour may grow into, and include, a lymph vessel or node, and obstruct the flow of lymph. A large tumour outside the lymphatic system may cause sufficient pressure to stop the flow of lymph.

Surgery

In some surgical procedures lymph nodes are removed because cancer cells may have already spread to them. This is done to prevent growth of secondary tumours in local lymph nodes and further spread of the disease via the lymphatic system, e.g. axillary nodes may be removed during mastectomy.

DISEASES OF LYMPH NODES

Enlarged lymph nodes

Lymph nodes become enlarged, *lymphadenopathy*, when their workload is increased by infection. They usually return to normal when the infection subsides but if there is chronic infection or repeated acute episodes they may become fibrosed and remain enlarged. Other causes include tumours (lymphomas) and excess abnormal material in lymph, especially if present for a long time, e.g. coal dust from the lungs, necrotic material from a tumour.

Lymphadenitis

Acute lymphadenitis is usually caused by microbes transported in lymph from other areas of infection. The nodes become inflamed, enlarged and congested with blood, and chemotaxis attracts large numbers of phagocytes. When phagocytic and antibody activity are not effective the infection may lead to:

- abscess formation in the node
- infection of adjacent tissues
- spread of infected material to other nodes and then to the blood, causing septicaemia or bacteraemia.

Acute lymphadenitis is secondary to a number of conditions.

Infectious mononucleosis (Glandular fever)

This is a highly contagious virus infection, usually of young adults, spread by direct contact. During the incubation period of 7 to 10 days viruses multiply in the epithelial cells of the pharynx. They subsequently spread to cervical nodes, then to lymphoid tissue throughout the body.

Clinical features include tonsillitis, lymphadenopathy and splenomegaly. A common complication is chronic fatigue syndrome. Clinical or subclinical infection confers lifelong immunity.

Other diseases

Minor lymphadenitis accompanies many infections and indicates the mobilisation of normal protective resources. More serious infection occurs in:

- measles
- anthrax
- typhoid fever
- wound and skin infections
- cat-scratch fever
- lymphogranuloma venereum
- bubonic plague.

Chronic lymphadenitis occurs following unresolved acute infections, in tuberculosis, syphilis and some low-grade infections.

Lymphomas

These are malignant tumours of lymphoid tissue that are classified as Hodgkin's or non-Hodgkin lymphomas.

Hodgkin's disease

In this disease there is progressive painless enlargement of lymph nodes throughout the body, often noticed first in the neck. The disease is malignant and the cause is unknown. The rate of progress varies considerably but the pattern of spread is predictable. The effectiveness of treatment depends largely on the stage of the disease at which it begins. Complications include deficiency of cell-mediated immunity (conferred by T-lymphocytes), some microbial infections, pressure on other structures by enlarged nodes.

Non-Hodgkin lymphomas

These tumours, e.g. multiple myeloma and Burkitt's lymphoma, may occur in any lymphoid tissue and in bone marrow. They are classified according to the type of cell involved and the degree of malignancy, i.e. low, intermediate or high grade. Low-grade tumours consist of well-differentiated cells and slow progress of the disease, death occurring after a period of years. High-grade lymphomas consist of poorly differentiated cells and rapid progress of the disease, death occurring in weeks or months. Some low- or intermediate-grade tumours change their status to high grade with increased rate of progress. Complications include:

- damage to adjacent structures due to pressure
- anaemia and possibly pancytopenia due to infiltration of bone marrow and spleen
- infection due to depression of the immune system.

Malignant neoplastic metastases

Metastatic tumours develop in lymph nodes in any part of the body. Lymph from a tumour may contain cancer cells that are filtered off by the lymph nodes. If not phagocytosed they multiply, forming metastatic tumours. Nodes nearest the primary tumour are affected first but there may be further spread through the sequence of nodes, eventually reaching the bloodstream.

DISORDERS OF THE SPLEEN

Splenomegaly (enlargement of spleen)

Enlargement of the spleen is usually secondary to other conditions, e.g. infections, circulatory disorders, blood diseases, malignant neoplasms.

Infections

The spleen may be infected by blood-borne microbes or by local spread of infection. The red pulp becomes congested with blood and there is an accumulation of phagocytes and plasma cells. *Acute infections* are rare.

Chronic infections. Some chronic non-pyogenic infections cause splenomegaly, but this is usually less severe than in the case of acute infections. The most commonly occurring primary infections include:

- tuberculosis
- typhoid fever
- malaria
- brucellosis (undulant fever)
- infectious mononucleosis.

Circulatory disorders

Splenomegaly due to congestion of blood occurs when the flow of blood through the liver is impeded by, e.g. fibrosis in cirrhosis of liver, portal venous congestion in right-sided heart failure.

Blood diseases

Splenomegaly may *be caused by blood diseases*. The spleen enlarges to deal with the extra workload associated with removing damaged, worn out and abnormal blood cells in, e.g. haemolytic and macrocytic anaemia, polycythaemia, chronic myeloid leukaemia.

Splenomegaly may *cause blood disease*. When the spleen is enlarged for any reason, especially in portal hypertension, excessive and premature haemolysis of red cells or phagocytosis of normal white cells and platelets leads to marked anaemia, leukopenia, thrombocytopenia.

Tumours

Benign and primary malignant tumours of the spleen are rare but blood-spread tumour fragments from elsewhere in the body may cause metastatic tumours. Splenomegaly caused by infiltration of malignant cells is characteristic of some conditions, especially: chronic leukaemia, Hodgkin's disease and non-Hodgkin lymphoma.

DISEASES OF THE THYMUS GLAND

Enlargement of the gland is associated with some auto-immune diseases, such as thyrotoxicosis and Addison's disease. Autoimmune conditions are those in which the immune system treats normal body cells or secretions as antigens and destroys them.

Tumours are rare and seldom metastasise. Pressure caused by enlargement of the gland may damage or interfere with the functions of adjacent structures, e.g. the trachea, oesophagus, veins in the neck.

In myasthenia gravis, a disease in which there is skeletal muscle weakness (p. 420), most patients have either thymic hyperplasia (majority) or thymoma (minority).

7
The nervous system

In a systematic study of anatomy and physiology the systems of the body are described separately but they are all interdependent. The nervous system detects and responds to changes inside and outside the body. Together with the endocrine system it controls important aspects of body function and maintains homeostasis. Nervous system stimulation provides an immediate response while endocrine activity is, in the main, slower and more prolonged (Ch. 8).

The nervous system consists of the brain, the spinal cord and peripheral nerves (Fig. 7.1). Organisation of nervous tissue within the body enables rapid communication between different parts of the body.

Response to changes in the internal environment maintains homeostasis and involuntary functions, e.g. blood pressure and the composition of the blood. Response to changes in the external environment maintains posture and other voluntary activities.

For descriptive purposes the parts of the nervous system are grouped as follows:

- the central nervous system (CNS), consisting of the brain and the spinal cord
- the peripheral nervous system (PNS), consisting of the 31 pairs of spinal nerves
- the autonomic nervous system (ANS) consisting of 12 pairs of cranial nerves; some are sensory (afferent), some are motor (efferent) and some mixed.

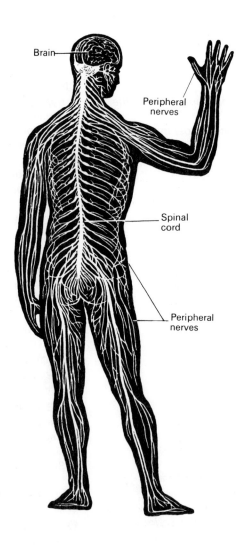

Figure 7.1 General view of the brain, spinal cord and spinal nerves.

NEURONES

The nervous system consists of a vast number of units called *neurones* (Fig. 7.2), supported by a special type of connective tissue, *neuroglia*. Each neurone consists of a *cell body* and its processes, *axons* and *dendrites*. Neurones are commonly referred to simply as nerves. They cannot divide and they need a continuous supply of oxygen and glucose. Unlike many other cells, neurones can only synthesise chemical energy (ATP) from glucose.

The physiological 'units' of the nervous system are *nerve impulses*, or *action potentials*, which are akin to tiny electrical charges. However, unlike ordinary electrical wires, the neurones are actively involved in conducting nerve impulses. In effect the strength of the impulse is maintained throughout the length of the neurone.

The cells of some neurones initiate nerve impulses while others act as 'relay stations' where impulses are passed on and sometimes redirected.

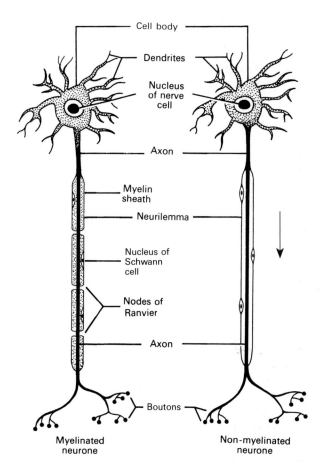

Figure 7.2 A neurone. Arrow indicates direction of impulse conduction.

Properties of neurones

Neurones have the characteristics of *irritability* and *conductivity*.

Irritability is the ability to initiate nerve impulses in response to stimuli from:

■ outside the body, e.g. touch, light waves
■ inside the body, e.g. a change in the concentration of carbon dioxide in the blood alters respiration; a thought may result in voluntary movement.

In the body this stimulation may be described as partly electrical and partly chemical—electrical in that motor nerve cells and sensory nerve endings initiate nerve impulses, and chemical in the transmission of impulses across synapses and at neuromuscular junctions.

Conductivity means the ability to transmit an impulse from:

■ one part of the brain to another
■ the brain to striated muscle, resulting in voluntary muscle contraction
■ muscles and joints to the brain, contributing to the maintenance of balance and posture
■ the brain to organs of the body, resulting in the contraction of muscle or secretion by glands
■ organs of the body to the brain in association with the regulation of body functions
■ the outside world to the brain through sensory nerve endings in the skin which are stimulated by temperature, touch, pain
■ the outside world to the brain through the special sense organs, i.e. eyes, ears, nose, tongue.

Cell bodies

The nerve cells vary considerably in size and shape but they are all too small to be seen by the naked eye. Cell bodies form the grey matter of the nervous system and are found at the periphery of the brain, in the centre of the spinal cord. Groups of cell bodies are called *nuclei* in the central nervous system and *ganglia* in the peripheral nervous system.

Axons and dendrites

Axons and dendrites are extensions of the cell bodies and form the *white matter* of the nervous system. They are found deep in the brain and in groups, called *tracts*, at the periphery of the spinal cord. They are referred to as *nerves* or *nerve fibres* outside the brain and spinal cord.

Axons

Each nerve cell has only one axon, carrying nerve impulses away from the cell body. They are usually longer than the dendrites, sometimes as long as 100 cm.

Structure of an axon

The membrane of the axon is called *axolemma* and it encloses the cytoplasmic extension of the nerve cell.

Large axons and those of peripheral nerves are surrounded by a *myelin sheath* (Fig. 7.3). This consists of a series of *Schwann cells* arranged along the length of the axon. Each one is wrapped around the axon so that it is covered by a number of concentric layers of Schwann cell plasma membrane. Between the layers of

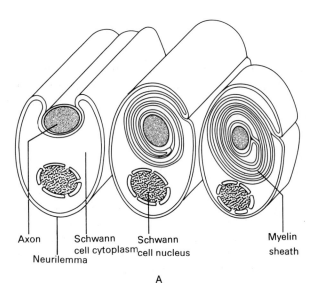

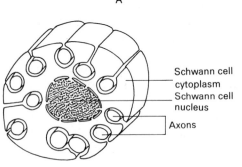

Figure 7.3 A. Myelinated nerve fibre. B. Non-myelinated nerve fibre.

plasma membrane there is a small amount of fatty substance called *myelin*. The outermost layer of Schwann cell plasma membrane is sometimes called *neurilemma*. There are tiny areas of exposed sarcolemma between adjacent Schwann cells, called *nodes of Ranvier*, which assist the rapid transmission of nerve impulses. Post-ganglionic fibres and some small fibres in the central nervous system are *non-myelinated*. In this type a number of axons are invaginated into a series of Schwann cell plasma membranes. The adjacent Schwann cells are in close association and there is no exposed sarcolemma.

Dendrites

The dendrites are the processes or nerve fibres which carry impulses towards cell bodies. They have the same structure as axons but they are usually shorter and branching. Each neurone has many dendrites. They form synapses with dendrites of other neurones or terminate in specialised sensory receptors, such as those in the skin.

The nerve impulse (action potential)

An impulse is initiated by stimulation of sensory nerve endings or by the passage of an impulse from another nerve. Transmission of the impulse, or action potential, is due to movement of ions across the nerve cell membrane. In the resting state the nerve cell membrane is *polarised* due to differences in the concentrations of ions across the plasma membrane. This means that there is a different electrical charge on each side of the membrane that is called the *resting membrane potential*. At rest the charge on the outside is positive and inside it is negative. The principal ions involved are:

- sodium (Na^+) the main extracellular cation
- potassium (K^+) the main intracellular cation.

In the *resting state* there is a continual tendency for these ions to diffuse along their concentration gradients, i.e. K^+ outwards and Na^+ into cells. When stimulated, the permeability of the nerve cell membrane to these ions changes. Initially Na^+ floods into the neurone from the ECF, then K^+ floods outwards, causing *depolarisation*, creating a *nerve impulse* or *action potential*. Depolarisation is very rapid, enabling the conduction of a nerve impulse along the entire length of a neurone in a few milliseconds (ms). It passes from the point of stimula-

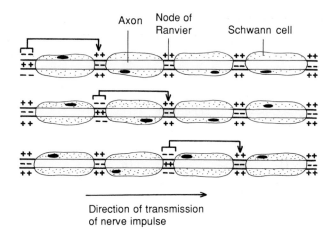

Figure 7.4 Saltatory conduction of an impulse in a myelinated nerve fibre.

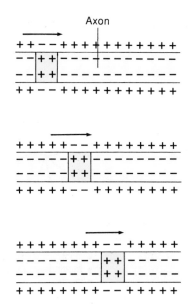

Figure 7.5 Simple propagation of an action potential in a non-myelinated nerve fibre.

tion in one direction only, i.e. away from the point of stimulation towards the area of resting potential. The direction of transmission is ensured because following depolarisation it takes time for *repolarisation* to occur. This is called the *refractory period* during which restimulation is not possible. As the neurone returns to its original resting state, the action of the *sodium pump* expels Na$^+$ from the cell in exchange for K$^+$ (p. 22).

In myelinated neurones, the insulating properties of the myelin sheath prevent the movement of ions. Therefore electrical changes across the membrane can only occur at the gaps in the myelin sheath, i.e. at the nodes of Ranvier. When an impulse occurs at one node, depolarisation passes along the myelin sheath to the next node so that the flow of current appears to 'leap' from one node to the next. This is called *saltatory conduction* (Fig. 7.4).

The speed of conduction depends on the diameter of the neurone: the larger the diameter, the faster the conduction. Myelinated fibres conduct impulses faster than unmyelinated fibres because saltatory conduction is faster than the complete conduction, or *simple propagation* (Fig. 7.5). The fastest fibres can conduct impulses to, e.g. skeletal muscles at a rate of 130 metres per second while the slowest impulses travel at 0.5 metres per second.

Types of nerves (Fig. 7.6)

Sensory or afferent nerves

When action potentials are generated by sensory receptors on the dendrites of these neurones, they are transmitted to the spinal cord by the sensory nerve fibres. The impulses may then pass to the brain or to connector neurones of reflex arcs in the spinal cord (p. 159).

Sensory receptors

Specialised endings of these neurones respond to different changes inside and outside the body. The *somatic*, *cutaneous* or *common senses*, originating in the skin, are pain, touch, heat and cold. *Proprioceptor senses* originate in muscles and joints and contribute to the maintenance of balance and posture. *Special senses* are sight, hearing, smell, touch and taste. *Autonomic afferent nerves* originate in internal organs, glands and tissues, e.g. baroreceptors, chemoreceptors, and are associated with reflex regulation of involuntary activity and visceral pain.

Motor or efferent nerves

Motor nerves originate in the brain, spinal cord and autonomic ganglia. They transmit impulses to the effector organs: muscles and glands. There are two types:

- somatic nerves—involved in voluntary and reflex skeletal muscle contraction
- autonomic nerves—involved in involuntary, or smooth, muscle contraction and glandular secretion.

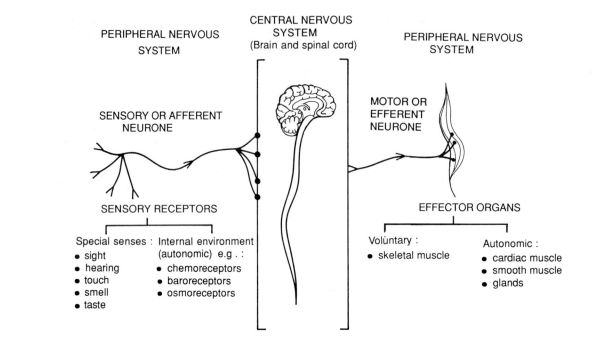

Figure 7.6
Functional
components of
the nervous
system.

PERIPHERAL NERVOUS SYSTEM

CENTRAL NERVOUS SYSTEM (Brain and spinal cord)

PERIPHERAL NERVOUS SYSTEM

SENSORY OR AFFERENT NEURONE

MOTOR OR EFFERENT NEURONE

SENSORY RECEPTORS

EFFECTOR ORGANS

Special senses :
• sight
• hearing
• touch
• smell
• taste

Internal environment (autonomic) e.g. :
• chemoreceptors
• baroreceptors
• osmoreceptors

Voluntary :
• skeletal muscle

Autonomic :
• cardiac muscle
• smooth muscle
• glands

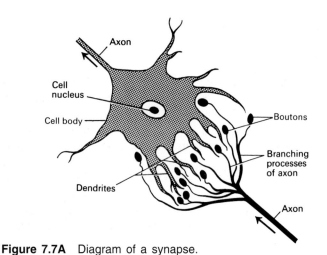

Figure 7.7A Diagram of a synapse.

Axon

Cell nucleus

Cell body

Boutons

Branching processes of axon

Dendrites

Axon

Vesicles containing chemical transmitter

Axon

Synaptic knob

Synaptic cleft

Dendrite

Nerve cell body

Figure 7.7B Section of a synapse, greatly enlarged.

Mixed nerves

In the spinal cord, sensory and motor nerves are arranged in separate groups, or *tracts*. Outside the spinal cord, when sensory and motor nerves are enclosed within the same sheath of connective tissue they are called *mixed nerves*.

Synapse and chemical transmitters

There is always more than one neurone involved in the transmission of a nerve impulse from its origin to its destination, whether it is sensory or motor. There is no anatomical continuity between these neurones. The point at which the nerve impulse passes from one to another is the *synapse* (Fig. 7.7A and B). At its free end the axon of one neurone breaks up into minute branches which terminate in small swellings called *synaptic knobs*, or boutons. These are in close proximity to the dendrites and the cell body of the next neurone. The space between them is the *synaptic cleft*. At the ends of synaptic knobs there are spherical *synaptic vesicles*, containing *chemical transmitters* which are released into synaptic clefts. Chemical transmitters are secreted by nerve cells, actively transported along the nerve fibres and stored in the synaptic vesicles. They are released by exocytosis, diffuse across the synaptic cleft and act on specific receptor sites on the postsynaptic membranes. Their action is short-lived as immediately they have stimu-

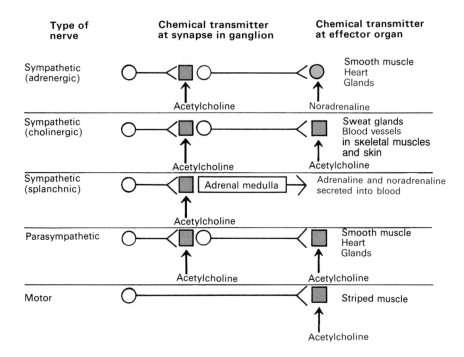

Type of nerve	Chemical transmitter at synapse in ganglion	Chemical transmitter at effector organ

Figure 7.8 Chemical transmitters of nerve impulses at synapses outside the brain and spinal cord.

lated the next neurone or effector organ, such as a muscle fibre, they are either inactivated by enzymes or taken back into the synaptic knob. A knowledge of the action of different chemical transmitters is important because drugs are available which neutralise or prolong their effect. Usually chemical transmitters have an excitatory effect at the synapse but they are sometimes inhibitory.

The chemical transmitters and their modes of action in the brain and spinal cord are not yet fully understood. It is believed however that *noradrenaline, gamma aminobutyric acid (GABA)* and *acetylcholine* act as chemical transmitters. Other substances, such as dopamine, serotonin (5-hydroxytryptamine), enkephalins, endorphins and substance P, have similar functions.

Figure 7.8 summarises the chemical transmitters known to function outside the brain and spinal cord.

Termination of nerves

The *sensory nerves*, e.g. in the skin, lose their myelin sheath and divide into fine branching filaments, the *sensory nerve endings* (Fig. 7.9). These are stimulated in the skin by touch, pain, heat and cold. The impulse generated is then transmitted by *sensory nerves* to the brain where the sensation is perceived.

The *motor nerves*, conveying impulses to skeletal muscle to produce contraction, divide into fine fila-

ments terminating in minute pads called *motor end-plates* (Fig. 7.10). At the point where the nerve reaches the muscle, the myelin sheath is absent and the fine filament passes to a sensitive area on the surface of the muscle fibre. Each muscle fibre is stimulated through a single motor end-plate, and one motor nerve has many motor end-plates. The motor end-plate and the sensitive area of muscle fibre through which it is stimulated is analogous to the synapse between neurones and is known as the *neuromuscular junction*. The nerve

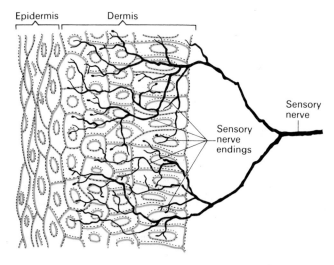

Figure 7.9 Sensory nerve endings in the skin.

impulse is passed across the gap between the motor end-plate and the muscle fibre by the neurotransmitter, *acetylcholine*. The group of muscle fibres and the motor end-plates of the nerve fibre that supplies them constitute a *motor unit*. Nerve impulses cause serial contraction of motor units in a muscle and each unit contracts

to its full capacity. The *strength* of the contraction depends on the *number* of motor units in action at a particular time.

The endings of *autonomic nerves* supplying smooth muscle and glands branch near their effector structure and release a transmitter substance which stimulates or depresses the activity of the structure.

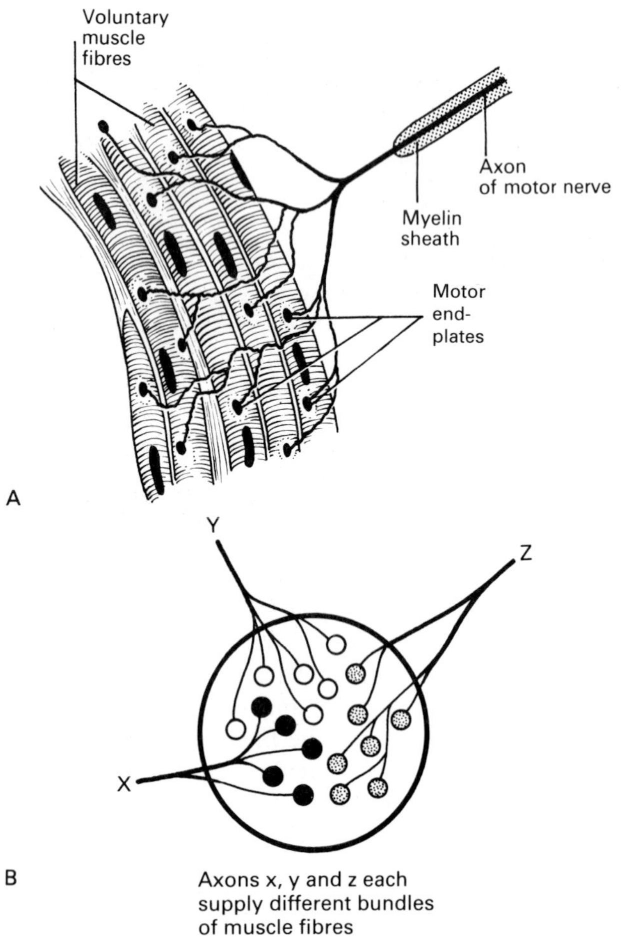

Figure 7.10 Motor unit. A. Longitudinal section. B. Cross-section.

CENTRAL NERVOUS SYSTEM

The central nervous system consists of the brain and the spinal cord.

Neuroglia

The neurones of the central nervous system are supported by three types of non-excitable *glial cells* that make up a quarter to a half of the volume of brain tissue. Unlike nerve cells these continue to replicate throughout life. They are *astrocytes, oligodendrocytes* and *microglia*.

Astrocytes

These cells form the main supporting tissue of the central nervous system. They are star-shaped with fine branching processes and they lie in a mucopolysaccharide ground substance. At the free ends of some of the processes there are small swellings called *foot processes*. Astrocytes are found in large numbers adjacent to blood vessels with their foot processes forming a sleeve round them. This means that the blood is separated from the neurones by the capillary wall and a layer of astrocyte foot processes which together constitute the *blood–brain barrier* (Fig. 7.11). Their functions are analogous to those of fibroblasts elsewhere in the body.

The blood–brain barrier is a selective barrier that protects the brain from chemical variations in the blood, e.g. after a meal. Oxygen, carbon dioxide, alcohol, barbiturates, glucose and lipophilic substances quickly cross the barrier into the brain. Some large molecules, drugs, inorganic ions and amino acids pass slowly from the blood to the brain.

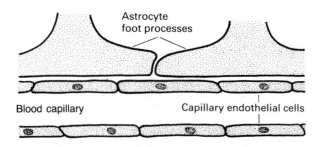

Figure 7.11 Blood–brain barrier.

Oligodendrocytes

These cells are smaller than astrocytes and are found:

Figure 7.12 The meninges covering the brain and spinal cord.

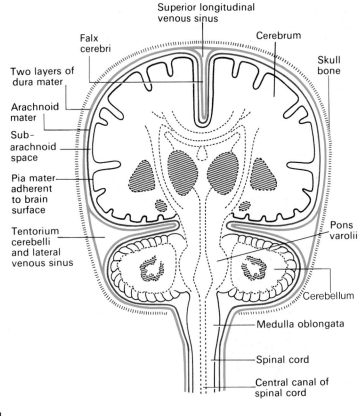

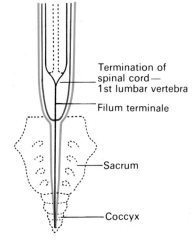

- in clusters round the neurone cell walls in grey matter
- adjacent to, and along the length of, myelinated nerve fibres.

The oligodendrocytes form and maintain myelin, having the same functions as Schwann cells in peripheral nerves.

Microglia

These cells are derived from monocytes that migrate from the blood into the nervous system before birth. They are found mainly in the area of blood vessels. They enlarge and become phagocytic in areas of inflammation and cell destruction.

Membranes covering the brain and spinal cord (the meninges)

The brain and spinal cord are completely surrounded by three membranes, the *meninges*, lying between the skull and the brain and between the vertebrae and the spinal cord (Fig. 7.12). Named from without inwards they are:

- dura mater
- arachnoid mater
- pia mater.

The dura and arachnoid maters are separated by a potential space, the *subdural space*. The arachnoid and pia maters are separated by the *subarachnoid space*, containing *cerebrospinal fluid*.

Dura mater

The cerebral dura mater consists of two layers of dense fibrous tissue. The outer layer takes the place of the periosteum on the inner surface of the skull bones and the inner layer provides a protective covering for the brain. There is only a potential space between the two layers except where the inner layer sweeps inwards between the cerebral hemispheres to form the *falx cerebri*; between the cerebellar hemispheres to form the *falx cerebelli*; and between the cerebrum and cerebellum to form the *tentorium cerebelli*.

Venous blood from the brain drains into venous sinuses between the layers of dura mater. The *superior sagittal sinus* is formed by the falx cerebri, and the tentorium cerebelli forms the *straight* and *transverse sinuses* (see Figs 5.35 and 5.36).

Spinal dura mater forms a loose sheath round the spinal cord, extending from the foramen magnum to the second sacral vertebra. Thereafter it invests the *filum terminale* and fuses with the periosteum of the coccyx. It is an extension of the inner layer of cerebral dura mater and is separated from the periosteum of the vertebrae and ligaments within the neural canal by the *epidural* or *extradural* space, containing blood vessels and areolar tissue. It is attached to the foramen magnum and, by a number of fibrous slips, to the posterior longitudinal ligament at intervals along its length. Nerves entering and leaving the spinal cord pass through the epidural space. These attachments stabilise the spinal cord in the neural canal. Dyes, used for diagnostic purposes, and local anaesthetics to relieve pain, may be injected into the epidural space.

Arachnoid mater

This delicate serous membrane lies between the dura and pia maters. It is separated from the dura mater by the *subdural space*, and from the pia mater by the *subarachnoid space*, containing *cerebrospinal fluid*. The arachnoid mater passes over the convolutions of the brain and accompanies the inner layer of dura mater in the formation of the falx cerebri, tentorium cerebelli and falx cerebelli. It continues downwards to envelop the spinal cord and ends by merging with the dura mater at the level of the 2nd sacral vertebra.

Pia mater

This is a fine connective tissue containing many minute blood vessels. It closely invests the brain, completely covering the convolutions and dipping into each fissure. It continues downwards to invest the spinal cord. Beyond the end of the cord it continues as the *filum terminale*, pierces the arachnoid tube and goes on, with the dura mater, to fuse with the periosteum of the coccyx.

Ventricles of the brain and the cerebrospinal fluid

Within the brain there are four irregular-shaped cavities, or *ventricles*, containing *cerebrospinal fluid* (CSF) (Fig. 7.13). They are:

- right and left lateral ventricles
- third ventricle
- fourth ventricle.

The lateral ventricles
These cavities lie within the cerebral hemispheres, one on each side of the median plane just below the *corpus callosum*. They are separated from each other by a thin membrane, the *septum lucidum*, and are lined with ciliated epithelium. They communicate with the third ventricle by *interventricular foramina*.

The third ventricle
The third ventricle is a cavity situated below the lateral ventricles between the two parts of the *thalamus*. It communicates with the fourth ventricle by a canal, the *cerebral aqueduct* or *aqueduct of the midbrain*.

The fourth ventricle
The fourth ventricle is a lozenge-shaped cavity situated below and behind the third ventricle, between the *cerebellum* and *pons varolii*. It is continuous below with

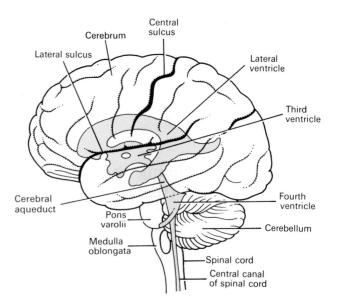

Figure 7.13 The positions of the ventricles of the brain (in yellow) superimposed on its surface. Viewed from the left side.

the *central canal* of the spinal cord and communicates with the subarachnoid space by foramina in its roof. Cerebrospinal fluid enters the subarachnoid space through these openings and through the open distal end of the central canal of the spinal cord.

Cerebrospinal fluid (CSF) (Fig. 7.14)

Cerebrospinal fluid is secreted into each ventricle of the brain by *choroid plexuses*, consisting of areas where the lining membrane of the ventricle walls is thin and has a profusion of blood capillaries. It passes back into blood through tiny diverticula of arachnoid mater, called *arachnoid villi* (arachnoid granulations), that project into the venous sinuses. The movement of CSF from the subarachnoid space to venous sinuses depends upon the difference in pressure on each side of the walls of the villi. When CSF pressure is higher than venous pressure CSF passes into the blood and when the venous pressure is higher the arachnoid villi collapse, preventing the passage of blood constituents into the CSF. There may also be some reabsorption of CSF by cells in the walls of the ventricles.

From the roof of the 4th ventricle CSF flows through foramina into the subarachnoid space and completely surrounds the brain and spinal cord. There is no intrinsic system of CSF circulation but its movement is aided by pulsating blood vessels, respiration and changes of posture.

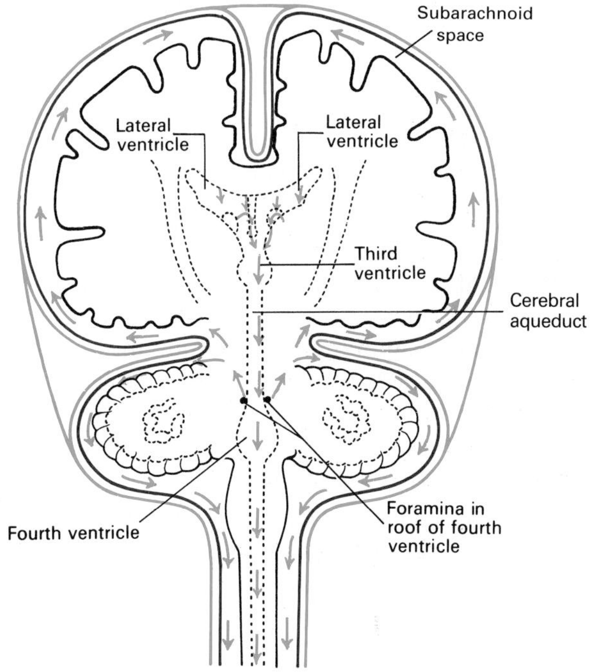

CSF is secreted continuously at a rate of about 0.5 ml per minute, i.e. 720 ml per day. The amount around the brain and spinal cord remains fairly constant at about 120 ml which means that absorption keeps pace with secretion. CSF pressure may be measured using a vertical tube attached to a lumbar puncture needle. It remains fairly constant at about 10 cmH$_2$O when the individual is lying on his side and about 30 cmH$_2$O when sitting up. If the brain is enlarged by, e.g. haemorrhage or tumour, some compensation is made by a reduction in the amount of CSF. When the volume of brain tissue is reduced, such as in degeneration or atrophy, the volume of CSF is increased. CSF is a clear, slightly alkaline fluid with a specific gravity of 1.005, consisting of:

- water
- mineral salts
- glucose
- plasma proteins: small amounts of albumin and globulin
- creatinine ⎫
- urea ⎭ small amounts.

Functions of the cerebrospinal fluid

- It supports and protects the brain and spinal cord.
- It maintains a uniform pressure around these delicate structures.
- It acts as a cushion and shock absorber between the brain and the cranial bones.
- It keeps the brain and spinal cord moist and there may be interchange of substances between CSF and nerve cells, such as nutrients and waste products.

Figure 7.14 Arrows showing the flow of cerebrospinal fluid.

BRAIN

The brain constitutes about one-fiftieth of the body weight and lies within the cranial cavity. The parts are (Fig. 7.15):

- cerebrum or forebrain
- midbrain ⎫
- pons varolii ⎬ the brain stem
- medulla oblongata ⎭
- cerebellum or hindbrain.

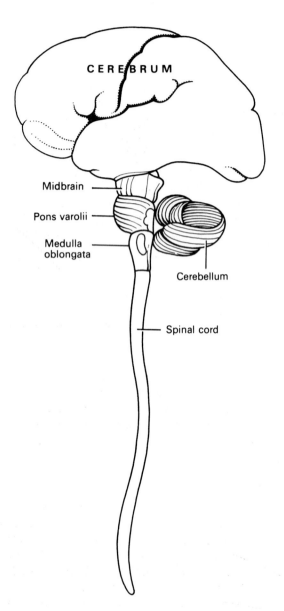

Figure 7.15 The parts of the central nervous system.

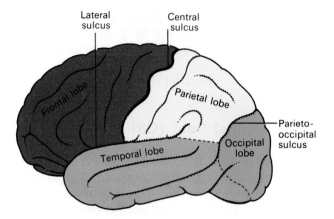

Figure 7.16 The lobes and sulci of the cerebrum.

Cerebrum

This is the largest part of the brain and it occupies the anterior and middle cranial fossae (see Fig. 15.8, p. 377). It is divided by a deep cleft, the *longitudinal cerebral fissure*, into *right* and *left cerebral hemispheres*, each containing one of the lateral ventricles. Deep within the brain the hemispheres are connected by a mass of white matter (nerve fibres) called the *corpus callosum*. The falx cerebri separates the two hemispheres and penetrates to the depth of the corpus callosum. The superficial (peripheral) part of the cerebrum is composed of nerve cell bodies or grey matter, forming the *cerebral cortex*, and the deeper layers consist of nerve fibres or white matter.

The cerebral cortex shows many infoldings or furrows of varying depth. The exposed areas of the folds are the *gyri* or *convolutions* and these are separated by *sulci* or *fissures*. These convolutions greatly increase the surface area of the cerebrum.

For descriptive purposes each hemisphere of the cerebrum is divided into *lobes* which take the names of the bones of the cranium under which they lie:

- frontal
- parietal
- temporal
- occipital.

The boundaries of the lobes are marked by deep sulci (fissures). These are the *central*, *lateral* and *parieto-occipital sulci* (Fig. 7.16).

Interior of the cerebrum (Fig. 7.17)

The cerebral cortex is composed of nerve cell bodies on the surface. Within the cerebrum the lobes are connected by masses of nerve fibres, or tracts, which make up the white matter of the brain. The afferent and efferent fibres linking the different parts of the brain and spinal cord are:

- *arcuate (association) fibres* which connect different parts of a cerebral hemisphere by extending from one gyrus to another, some of which are adjacent and some distant
- *commissural fibres* which connect corresponding areas of the two cerebral hemispheres; the largest and most important commissure is the corpus callosum

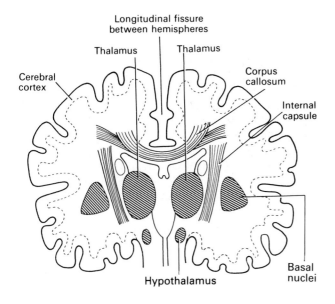

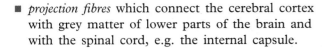

Figure 7.17 A section of the cerebrum showing some connecting nerve fibres.

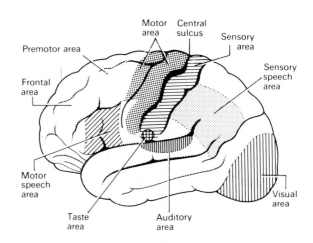

Figure 7.18 The cerebrum showing the functional areas.

- *projection fibres* which connect the cerebral cortex with grey matter of lower parts of the brain and with the spinal cord, e.g. the internal capsule.

The *internal capsule* is an important area consisting of projection fibres. It lies deep within the brain between the basal nuclei (ganglia) and the thalamus. All nerve impulses passing to and from the cerebral cortex are carried by fibres that form the internal capsule. Motor fibres within the internal capsule form the *pyramidal tracts* (corticospinal tracts) that decussate at the medulla oblongata.

Functions of the cerebrum

There are three main varieties of activity associated with the cerebral cortex:

- mental activities involved in memory, intelligence, sense of responsibility, thinking, reasoning, moral sense and learning are attributed to the *higher centres*
- sensory perception, including the perception of pain, temperature, touch, sight, hearing, taste and smell
- initiation and control of voluntary muscle contraction.

Functional areas of the cerebrum
(Fig. 7.18)

The main areas of the cerebrum associated with sensory perception and voluntary motor activity are known but it is unlikely that any area is associated exclusively with only one function. Except where specially mentioned, the different areas are active in both hemispheres.

Motor areas

The precentral (motor) area lies in the frontal lobe immediately anterior to the *central sulcus*. The nerve cells are pyramid-shaped (Betz's cells) and they initiate the contraction of voluntary muscles. A nerve fibre from a Betz's cell passes downwards through the internal capsule to the medulla oblongata where it crosses to the opposite side then descends in the spinal cord. At the appropriate level in the spinal cord the nerve impulse crosses a synapse to stimulate a second neurone which terminates at the motor end-plate of a muscle fibre. This means that the motor area of the *right hemisphere* of the cerebrum controls voluntary muscle movement on the left side of the body and vice versa. The neurone with its cell body in the cerebrum is the *upper motor neurone* and the other, with its cell body in the spinal cord, is the *lower motor neurone* (Fig. 7.19). Damage to either of these neurones may result in paralysis.

In the motor area of the cerebrum the body is represented upside down, i.e. the cells nearest the vertex control the feet and those in the lowest part control the head, neck, face and fingers (Fig. 7.20A). The sizes of the areas of cortex representing different parts of the body are proportional to the *complexity of movement* of the part, not to its size. Figure 7.20A shows that, in

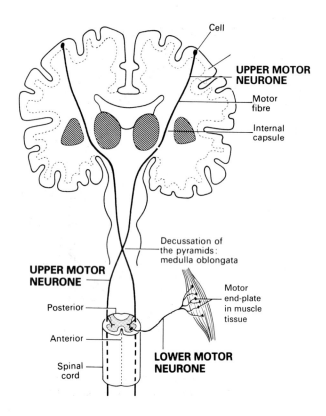

Figure 7.19 The motor nerve pathways: upper and lower motor neurones.

comparison with the trunk, the hand, foot, tongue and lips are represented by large cortical areas.

The premotor area lies in the frontal lobe immediately anterior to the motor area. The cells are thought to exert a controlling influence over the motor area, ensuring an orderly series of movements. For example, in tying a shoe lace or writing, many muscles contract but the movements must be coordinated and carried out in a particular sequence. Such a pattern of movement, when established, is described as *manual dexterity*.

In the lower part of this area just above the lateral sulcus there is a group of nerve cells known as the *motor speech (Broca's) area* which controls the movements necessary for speech. It is dominant in the *left hemisphere* in *right-handed people* and vice versa.

The frontal area or *pole* extends anteriorly from the premotor area to include the remainder of the frontal lobe. It is a large area and is more highly developed in humans than in other animals. It is thought that communications between this and the other regions in the cerebrum are responsible for the behaviour, character and emotional state of the individual. No particular behaviour, character or intellectual trait has, so far, been attributed to the activity of any one group of

cells.

Sensory areas

The postcentral (sensory) area is the area behind the central sulcus. Here sensations of pain, temperature, pressure and touch, knowledge of muscular movement and the position of joints are perceived. The sensory area of the *right hemisphere* receives impulses from the *left side of the body* and vice versa. The size of the areas representing different parts of the body (Fig. 7.20B) is proportional to the *extent of sensory innervation*, e.g. the large area for the face is consistent with the extensive sensory nerve supply by the three branches of the trigeminal nerve (5th cranial nerve).

The parietal area lies behind the postcentral area and includes the greater part of the parietal lobe of the cerebrum. Its functions are believed to be associated with obtaining and retaining accurate knowledge of objects. It has been suggested that objects can be recognised by touch alone because of the knowledge from past experience retained in this area.

The sensory speech area is situated in the lower part of the parietal lobe and extends into the temporal lobe. It is here that the spoken word is perceived. There is a dominant area in the *left hemisphere* in *right-handed* people and vice versa.

The auditory (hearing) area lies immediately below the lateral sulcus within the temporal lobe. The cells receive and interpret impulses transmitted from the inner ear by the vestibulocochlear (auditory) nerves.

The olfactory (smell) area lies deep within the temporal lobe where impulses from the nose via the olfactory nerves are received and interpreted.

The taste area is thought to lie just above the lateral sulcus in the deep layers of the sensory area. This is the area where impulses from special nerve endings in taste buds in the tongue and in the lining of the cheeks, palate and pharynx are perceived as taste.

The visual area lies behind the parieto-occipital sulcus and includes the greater part of the occipital lobe. The optic nerves (nerves of the sense of sight) pass from the eye to this area which receives and interprets the impulses as visual impressions.

Other areas

Deep within the cerebral hemispheres there are groups of cell bodies called *nuclei* (previously called ganglia) which act as relay stations where impulses are passed from one neurone to the next in a chain (Fig. 7.17).

Important masses of grey matter include:

■ basal nuclei
■ thalamus
■ hypothalamus.

Basal nuclei. This area of grey matter, lying deep within the cerebral hemispheres, is thought to influence skeletal muscle tone. If control is inadequate or absent, movements are jerky, clumsy and uncoordinated.

Thalamus. The thalamus consists of two masses of nerve cells and fibres situated within the cerebral hemispheres just below the corpus callosum, one on each side of the third ventricle. Sensory input from the skin, viscera and special sense organs is transmitted to the thalamus before redistribution to the cerebrum.

Hypothalamus. The hypothalamus is composed of a number of groups of nerve cells. It is situated below and in front of the thalamus, immediately above the pituitary gland. The hypothalamus is linked to the posterior lobe of the pituitary gland by nerve fibres and to the anterior lobe by a complex system of blood vessels. Through these connections the hypothalamus controls the output of hormones from both lobes of the gland (see p. 217).

Other functions with which the hypothalamus is concerned include maintenance of homeostasis, e.g. control of:

■ autonomic nervous system (p. 170)
■ hunger and thirst
■ body temperature (p. 363)
■ emotional reactions, e.g. pleasure, fear, rage
■ sexual behaviour including mating and child rearing
■ biological clocks or circadian rhythms, e.g. sleeping and waking cycles, body temperature and secretion of some hormones.

Brain stem

Midbrain

The midbrain is the area of the brain situated around the cerebral aqueduct between the cerebrum above and the *pons varolii* below. It consists of groups of nerve cells and nerve fibres which connect the cerebrum with lower parts of the brain and with the spinal cord. The nerve cells act as relay stations for the ascending and descending nerve fibres.

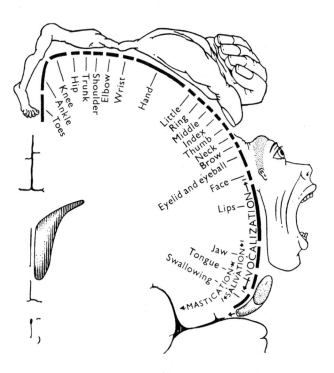

Figure 7.20A The *motor homunculus* showing how the body is represented in the motor area of the cerebrum.

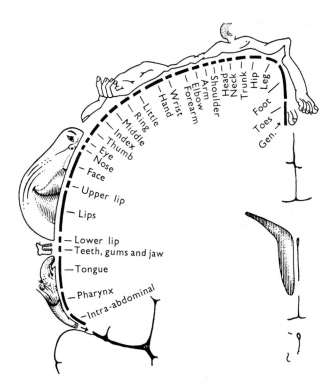

Figure 7.20B The *sensory homunculus* showing how the body is represented in the sensory area of the cerebrum. (Both A and B are from Penfield W, Rasmussen T 1950 The cerebral cortex of man. Macmillan, New York. © 1950 Macmillan Publishing Co., renewed 1978 Theodore Rasmussen.)

Pons varolii

The pons varolii is situated in front of the cerebellum, below the midbrain and above the medulla oblongata. It consists mainly of nerve fibres which form a bridge between the two hemispheres of the cerebellum, and of fibres passing between the higher levels of the brain and the spinal cord. There are groups of cells within the pons which act as relay stations and some of these are associated with the cranial nerves.

The anatomical structure of the pons varolii differs from that of the cerebrum in that the nerve cells lie deeply and the nerve fibres are on the surface.

Medulla oblongata

The medulla oblongata extends from the pons varolii above and is continuous with the spinal cord below. It is about 2.5 cm long, is shaped like a pyramid with its base upwards and it lies just within the cranium above the foramen magnum. Its anterior and posterior surfaces are marked by central fissures. The outer aspect is composed of *white matter* which passes between the brain and the spinal cord, and *grey matter* lies centrally. Some cells constitute relay stations for sensory nerves passing from the spinal cord to the cerebrum.

The vital centres, consisting of groups of cells associated with autonomic reflex activity, lie in its deeper structure. These are the:

- cardiac centre
- respiratory centre
- vasomotor centre
- reflex centres of vomiting, coughing, sneezing and swallowing.

The medulla oblongata has several special features:

- *Decussation of the pyramids.* In the medulla *motor nerves* descending from the motor area in the cerebrum to the spinal cord in the pyramidal (corticospinal) tracts cross from one side to the other. This means that the left hemisphere of the cerebrum controls the right half of the body, and vice versa. These tracts are the main pathway for impulses to voluntary (skeletal) muscles.
- *Sensory decussation.* Some of the *sensory nerves* ascending to the cerebrum from the spinal cord cross from one side to the other in the medulla. Others decussate at lower levels, i.e. in the spinal cord.
- *The cardiac centre* controls the rate and force of cardiac contraction. Sympathetic and parasympathetic nerve fibres originating in the medulla pass to the heart. Sympathetic stimulation increases the rate and force of the heart beat and parasympathetic stimulation has the opposite effect.
- *The respiratory centre* controls the rate and depth of respiration. From this centre, nerve impulses pass to the phrenic and intercostal nerves which stimulate contraction of the diaphragm and intercostal muscles, thus initiating inspiration. The respiratory centre is stimulated by excess carbon dioxide and, to a lesser extent, by deficiency of oxygen in its blood supply and by nerve impulses from the chemoreceptors in the carotid bodies.
- *The vasomotor centre* controls the diameter of the blood vessels, especially the small arteries and arterioles which have a large proportion of smooth muscle fibres in their walls. Vasomotor impulses reach the blood vessels through the autonomic nervous system. Stimulation may cause either constriction or dilatation of blood vessels depending on the site (Figs 7.45 and 7.46).

  The sources of stimulation of the vasomotor centre are the arterial baroreceptors, body temperature and emotions such as sexual excitement and anger. Pain usually causes vasoconstriction although severe pain may cause vasodilatation, a fall in blood pressure and fainting.
- *Reflex centres.* When irritating substances are present in the stomach or respiratory tract, nerve impulses pass to the medulla oblongata, stimulating the reflex centres which initiate the reflex actions of vomiting, coughing and sneezing.

Reticular formation

The reticular formation is a collection of neurones in the core of the brain stem, surrounded by neural pathways which pass nerve impulses between the brain and the spinal cord. It has a vast number of synaptic links with other parts of the brain and is therefore constantly receiving 'information' being transmitted in ascending and descending tracts.

Functions
The reticular formation is involved in:

- coordination of skeletal muscle activity associated with voluntary motor movement and the maintenance of balance
- coordination of activity controlled by the autonomic nervous system, e.g. cardiovascular, respiratory and gastrointestinal activity

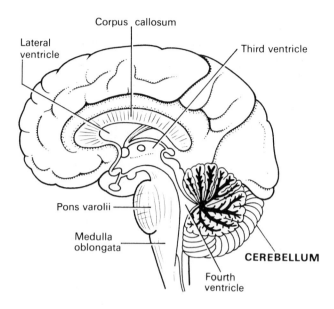

Figure 7.21 The cerebellum and associated structures.

■ selective awareness that functions through the *reticular activating system* (RAS) which selectively blocks or passes sensory information to the cerebral cortex, e.g. the slight sound made by a sick child moving in bed may arouse his mother but the noise of regularly passing trains may be suppressed.

Cerebellum

The cerebellum is situated behind the pons varolii and immediately below the posterior portion of the cerebrum occupying the posterior cranial fossa (Fig. 7.21). It is ovoid in shape and has two hemispheres, separated by a narrow median strip called the *vermis*. Grey matter forms the surface of the cerebellum, and the white matter lies deeply.

Functions

The cerebellum is concerned with the coordination of voluntary muscular movement, posture and balance. Cerebellar activities are carried out below the level of consciousness, i.e. not under voluntary control. The cerebellum controls and coordinates the movements of various groups of muscles ensuring smooth, even, precise actions. It coordinates activities associated with the *maintenance of the balance and equilibrium* of the body. The sensory input for these functions is derived from the muscles and joints, the eyes and the ears.

Proprioceptor impulses from the muscles and joints indicate their position in relation to the body as a whole and those impulses from the eyes and the semicircular canals in the ears provide information about the position of the head in space. Impulses from the cerebellum influence the contraction of skeletal muscle so that balance and posture are maintained.

Damage to the cerebellum results in clumsy unco-ordinated muscular movement, staggering gait and inability to carry out smooth, steady, precise movements.

SPINAL CORD

The spinal cord is the elongated, almost cylindrical part of the central nervous system, which is suspended in the vertebral canal surrounded by the meninges and cerebrospinal fluid (Fig. 7.22). It is continuous above with the medulla oblongata and extends from the *upper border of the atlas* to the lower border of the *1st lumbar vertebra* (Fig. 7.23). It is approximately 45 cm long in an adult Caucasian male, and is about the thickness of the little finger. When a specimen of cerebrospinal fluid is required it is taken from a point beyond the end of the cord, i.e. below the level of the 2nd lumbar vertebra. This procedure is called *lumbar puncture*.

Except for the cranial nerves, the spinal cord is the nervous tissue link between the brain and the rest of

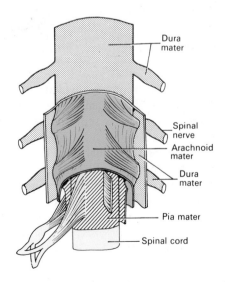

Figure 7.22 The meninges covering the spinal cord. Each cut away to show the underlying layers.

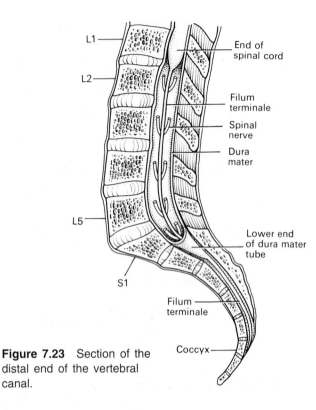

Figure 7.23 Section of the distal end of the vertebral canal.

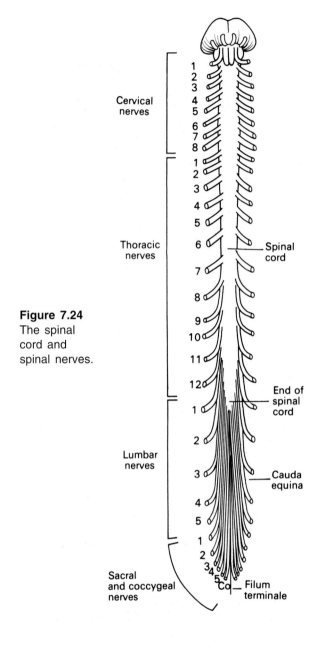

Figure 7.24 The spinal cord and spinal nerves.

through the spinal cord. At the appropriate level they leave the cord and pass to the structure they supply. Similarly, sensory nerves from organs and tissues enter and pass upwards in the spinal cord to the brain.

Some activities of the spinal cord are independent of the brain, i.e. *spinal reflexes*. To facilitate these there are extensive neurone connections between sensory and motor neurones at the same or different levels in the cord.

Structure

The spinal cord is incompletely divided into two equal parts, anteriorly by a short, shallow *median fissure* and posteriorly by a deep narrow septum, the *posterior median septum*.

A cross-section of the spinal cord shows that it is composed of grey matter in the centre surrounded by white matter supported by neuroglia. Figure 7.25 shows the parts of the spinal cord and the nerve roots on one side. The other side is the same.

Grey matter

The arrangement of grey matter in the spinal cord resembles the shape of the letter H, having *two poste-*

rior, two anterior and *two lateral columns*. The area of grey matter lying transversely is the *transverse commissure* and it is pierced by the central canal, an extension from the fourth ventricle, containing cerebrospinal fluid (Fig. 7.25). The cell bodies may be:

■ *sensory cells* which receive impulses from the periphery of the body
■ *lower motor neurones* which transmit impulses to the skeletal muscles
■ *connector neurones*, linking sensory and motor neurones, at the same or different levels, which form spinal reflex arcs.

At each point where nerve impulses are passed from

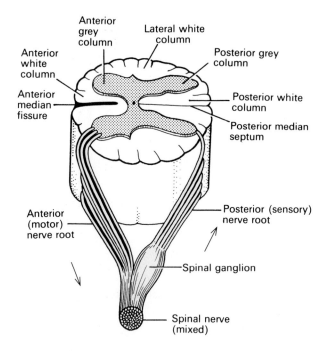

Figure 7.25 A section of the spinal cord showing nerve roots on one side.

one neurone to another there is a synaptic cleft and a chemical transmitter (Fig. 7.7).

Posterior columns of grey matter

These are composed of cell bodies which are stimulated by *sensory impulses* from the periphery of the body. The nerve fibres of these cells contribute to the formation of the white matter of the cord and transmit the sensory impulses to the brain.

Anterior columns of grey matter

These are composed of the *cell bodies of the lower motor neurones* which are stimulated by the axons of the upper motor neurones or by the *cell bodies of connector neurones* linking the anterior and posterior columns to form reflex arcs.

The posterior root (spinal) ganglia are composed of cell bodies which lie just outside the spinal cord on the pathway of the sensory nerves. All sensory nerve fibres pass through these ganglia. The only function of the cells is to promote the onward movement of nerve impulses.

White matter

The white matter of the spinal cord is arranged in three *columns* or *tracts*; anterior, posterior and lateral.

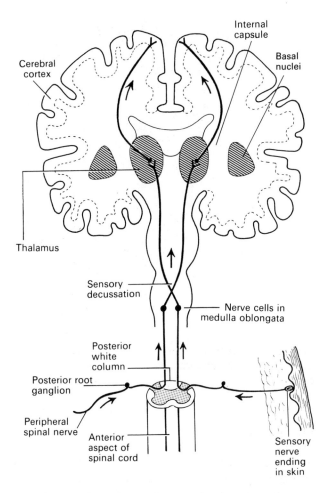

Figure 7.26 One of the sensory nerve pathways from the skin to the cerebrum.

These tracts are formed by *sensory nerve fibres* ascending to the brain, *motor nerve fibres* descending from the brain and fibres of *connector neurones*.

Sensory nerve tracts (afferent or ascending) in the spinal cord

There are two main sources of sensation transmitted to the brain via the spinal cord.

1. *The skin.* Sensory nerve endings in the skin, called *cutaneous receptors*, are stimulated by *pain, heat, cold* and *touch*, including pressure. The nerve impulses are passed by three neurones to the sensory area in the *opposite hemisphere of the cerebrum* where the sensation and its location are perceived (Fig. 7.26). Crossing to the other side, or *decussation*, occurs either at the level of entry into the cord or in the medulla.

Table 7.1 Sensory nerve impulses: origins, routes, destinations

Receptor	Route	Destination
Pain, touch, temperature	Neurone 1—to spinal cord by posterior root Neurone 2—decussation on entering spinal cord then in anterolateral spinothalamic tract to thalamus Neurone 3—	 to parietal lobe of cerebrum
Touch, proprioceptors	Neurone 1—to medulla in posterior spinothalamic tract Neurone 2—decussation in medulla, transmission to thalamus Neurone 3—	 to parietal lobe of cerebrum
Proprioceptors	Neurone 1—to spinal cord Neurone 2—	 no decussation, to cerebellum in posterior spinocerebellar tract

2. *The tendons, muscles and joints*. Sensory nerve endings in these structures, called *proprioceptors*, are stimulated by stretch. Together with impulses from the eyes and the ears they are associated with the maintenance of balance and posture and with perception of the position of the body in space. These nerve impulses have two destinations:
   a. by a three-neurone system the impulses reach the sensory area of the *opposite hemisphere of the cerebrum*
   b. by a two-neurone system the nerve impulses reach the *cerebellar hemisphere on the same side*.

Table 7.1 provides further information about the origins, routes of transmission and the destinations of sensory nerve impulses.

Motor nerve tracts (efferent or descending) in the spinal cord

Neurones which transmit nerve impulses away from the brain are motor (efferent or descending) neurones. Motor neurone stimulation results in:

■ contraction of voluntary (striated, skeletal) muscle

■ contraction of smooth (involuntary) muscle and the secretion by glands controlled by nerves of the *autonomic nervous system* (p. 170).

Voluntary muscle movement

The contraction of the muscles which move the joints is, in the main, under the control of the will, which means that the stimulus to contract originates at the level of consciousness in the cerebrum. However, some nerve impulses which affect skeletal muscle contraction are initiated in the midbrain, brain stem and cerebellum. This activity occurs below the level of consciousness and is associated with coordination of muscle activity, e.g. when very fine movement is required and in the maintenance of posture and balance.

Efferent nerve impulses are transmitted from the brain to the body via bundles of nerve fibres or *tracts* in the spinal cord. The *motor pathways* from the brain to the muscles are made up of two *neurones* (Fig. 7.19). These tracts are either pyramidal (corticospinal) or extrapyramidal. The motor fibres that form the pyramidal tracts travel through the internal capsule and are the main pathway for impulses to voluntary (skeletal) muscles. Those motor fibres that do not pass through the internal capsule form the extrapyramidal tracts and

Table 7.2 Extrapyramidal upper motor neurones: origins and tracts

Origin	Name of tract	Site in spinal cord	Functions
Midbrain and pons	Rubrospinal tract decussates in brain stem	Lateral column	Control of skilled muscle movement
Reticular formation	Reticulospinal tract does not decussate	Lateral column	Coordination of muscle movement Maintenance of posture and balance
Midbrain and pons	Tectospinal tract decussates in midbrain	Anterior column	
Midbrain and pons	Vestibulospinal tract, some fibres decussate in the cord	Anterior column	

have connections with many parts of the brain including the basal nuclei and the thalamus.

The upper motor neurone has its cell (Betz's cell) in the *precentral sulcus area* of the cerebrum. The axons pass through the internal capsule, pons and medulla. In the spinal cord they form the *lateral corticospinal tracts* of white matter and the fibres terminate in close association with the cells of the *lower motor neurones* in the anterior columns of grey matter. The axons of these upper motor neurones make up the pyramidal tracts and decussate in the medulla oblongata, forming the pyramids.

The lower motor neurone has its cell in the *anterior horn of grey matter* in the spinal cord. Its axon emerges from the spinal cord by the *anterior root*, joins with the incoming sensory fibres and forms the *mixed spinal nerve* which passes through the *intervertebral foramen*. Near its termination in muscle the axon branches into a variable number of tiny fibres which form *motor end-plates*, each of which is in close association with a sensitive area on the wall of a muscle fibre. The motor end-plates of each nerve and the muscle fibres they supply form a *motor unit* (Fig. 7.10). The chemical transmitter that conveys the nerve impulse across the gap to stimulate the muscle fibre is *acetylcholine*. Motor units contract as a whole and the strength of contraction of a muscle depends on the number of motor units in action at a time.

The lower motor neurone has been described as the *final common pathway* for the transmission of nerve impulses to striated muscles. The cell of this neurone is influenced by a number of upper motor neurones originating from various sites in the brain and by some neurones which begin and end in the spinal cord. Some of these neurones stimulate the cells of the lower motor neurone while others have an inhibiting effect. The

outcome of these influences is smooth, coordinated muscle movement, some of which is voluntary and some involuntary.

Involuntary muscle movement

Upper motor neurones which have their cells in the brain at a level *below* the cerebrum, i.e. in the midbrain, brain stem, cerebellum or spinal cord, influence muscle activity in relation to the maintenance of posture and balance, the coordination of muscle movement and the control of muscle tone.

Table 7.2 shows details of the area of origin of these neurones and the tracts which their axons form before reaching the cell of the lower motor neurone in the spinal cord.

Spinal reflexes. These consist of three elements: sensory neurones, connector neurones in the spinal cord and lower motor neurones. In the simplest *reflex arc* there is only one of each (Fig. 7.27). A *reflex action* is an immediate motor response to a sensory stimulus. Many connector and motor neurones may be stimulated by afferent impulses from a small area of skin, e.g. the pain impulses initiated by touching a very hot surface with the finger are transmitted to the spinal cord by sensory nerves. These stimulate many connector and lower motor neurones in the cord which results in the contraction of many skeletal muscles of the hand, arm and shoulder, and the removal of the finger. Reflex action takes place very quickly, in fact, the motor response may have occurred simultaneously with the perception of the pain in the cerebrum. Reflexes of this type are invariably protective but they can on occasion be inhibited. For example, if it is a precious plate that is very hot when lifted every effort will be made to overcome the pain to prevent dropping it!

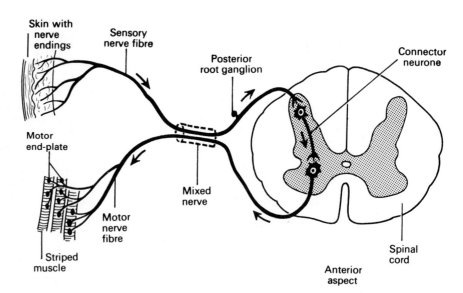

Figure 7.27 A single reflex arc involving one side only.

Stretch reflexes. Only two neurones are involved. The cell of the lower motor neurone is stimulated by the sensory neurone. There is no connector neurone involved. The *knee jerk* is one example, but this type of reflex can be demonstrated at any point where a stretched tendon crosses a joint. By tapping the tendon just below the knee when it is bent, the sensory nerve endings in the tendon and in the thigh muscles are stretched. This initiates a nerve impulse which passes into the spinal cord to the cell of the lower motor neurone in the anterior column of grey matter on the same side. As a result the thigh muscles suddenly contract and the foot kicks forward. This is used as a test of the integrity of the reflex arc. This type of reflex has a protective function—it prevents excessive joint movement that may damage tendons, ligaments and muscles.

Autonomic reflexes. See page 170.

PERIPHERAL NERVOUS SYSTEM

This part of the nervous system consists of:

- 31 pairs of spinal nerves
- 12 pairs of cranial nerves
- the autonomic part of the nervous system.

Most of the nerves of the peripheral nervous system are composed of *sensory nerve fibres* conveying impulses from sensory end organs to the brain, and *motor nerve fibres* conveying impulses from the brain through the spinal cord to the effector organs, e.g. skeletal muscles, smooth muscle and glands.

Each nerve consists of numerous nerve fibres col-

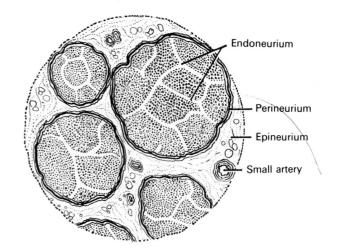

Figure 7.28 Transverse section of a peripheral nerve showing the protective coverings.

lected into bundles. Each bundle has several coverings of protective connective tissue (Fig. 7.28):

- *Endoneurium* is a delicate tissue, surrounding each individual fibre, which is continuous with the septa that pass inwards from the perineurium.
- *Perineurium* is a smooth tissue, surrounding each *bundle* of fibres.
- *Epineurium* is the tissue which surrounds and encloses a number of bundles of nerve fibres. Most large nerves are covered by epineurium.

Spinal nerves

There are *31 pairs of spinal nerves* that leave the vertebral canal by passing through the intervertebral foramina

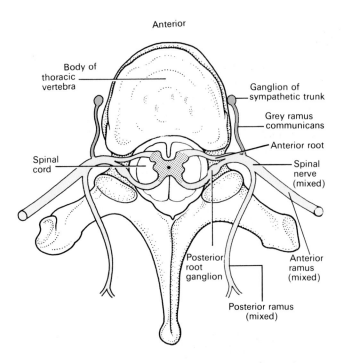

Figure 7.29 Diagram showing the relationship between sympathetic and mixed spinal nerves. Sympathetic part in green.

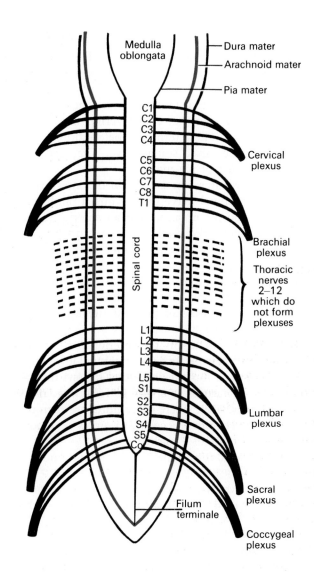

Figure 7.30 Diagram showing the membranes covering the spinal cord; spinal nerves and the plexuses they form.

formed by adjacent vertebrae. They are named and grouped according to the vertebrae with which they are associated (Fig. 7.24):

- 8 cervical
- 12 thoracic
- 5 lumbar
- 5 sacral
- 1 coccygeal.

Although there are only seven cervical vertebrae, there are eight nerves because the first pair leave the vertebral canal between the occipital bone and the atlas and the eighth pair leave below the last cervical vertebra. Thereafter the nerves are given the name and number of the vertebra immediately *above*.

The lumbar, sacral and coccygeal nerves leave the *spinal cord* near its termination at the level of the first lumbar vertebra, and extend downwards inside the vertebral canal in the subarachnoid space, forming a sheaf of nerves which resembles a horse's tail, the *cauda equina*. These nerves leave the vertebral canal at the appropriate lumbar, sacral or coccygeal level, depending on their destination.

The spinal nerves arise from both sides of the spinal cord and emerge through the intervertebral foramina. Each nerve is formed by the union of a *motor and a sensory nerve root* and is, therefore, a *mixed nerve*. Each spinal nerve has a contribution from the sympathetic part of the autonomic nervous system in the form of a *preganglionic fibre* (Fig. 7.45).

For details of the bones and muscles mentioned in the following section see Chapters 15 to 17. Bones and joints are supplied by adjacent nerves.

Nerve roots (Fig. 7.30)

The anterior nerve root consists of *motor nerve fibres* which are the axons of the nerve cells in the anterior column of grey matter in the spinal cord and, in the thoracic and lumbar regions, *sympathetic nerve fibres* which are the axons of cells in the lateral columns of grey matter.

The posterior nerve root consists of *sensory nerve fibres*. Just outside the spinal cord there is a *spinal ganglion* (posterior root ganglion), consisting of a little cluster of nerve cells. Sensory nerve fibres pass through these ganglia before entering the spinal cord. The area of skin supplied by each nerve is called a *dermatome* (Figs 7.34 and 7.38).

For a very short distance after leaving the spinal cord the nerve roots have a covering of *dura* and *arachnoid maters*. These terminate before the two roots join to form the mixed spinal nerve. The nerve roots have no covering of pia mater.

Immediately after emerging from the intervertebral foramen each spinal nerve divides into a ramus communicans, a posterior ramus and an anterior ramus.

The rami communicans are part of preganglionic sympathetic neurones of the autonomic nervous system (p. 171).

The posterior rami pass backwards and divide into medial and lateral branches to supply skin and muscles of relatively small areas of the posterior aspect of the head, neck and trunk.

The anterior rami supply the anterior and lateral aspects of the neck, trunk and the upper and lower limbs.

In the cervical, lumbar and sacral regions the anterior rami unite near their origins to form large masses of nerves, or *plexuses*, where nerve fibres are regrouped and rearranged before proceeding to supply skin, bones, muscles and joints of a particular area.

In the thoracic region the anterior rami do not form plexuses.

There are five large plexuses of mixed nerves formed on each side of the vertebral column. They are the:

- cervical plexuses
- brachial plexuses
- lumbar plexuses
- sacral plexuses
- coccygeal plexuses.

Cervical plexus (Fig. 7.31)

This is formed by the anterior rami of the first four cervical nerves. It lies opposite the 1st, 2nd, 3rd and 4th cervical vertebrae under the protection of the sternocleidomastoid muscle.

The superficial branches supply the structures at the back and side of the head and the skin of the front of the neck to the level of the sternum.

The deep branches supply muscles of the neck, e.g. the sternocleidomastoid and the trapezius.

The phrenic nerve originates from cervical roots 3, 4 and 5 and passes downwards through the thoracic cavity in front of the root of the lung to supply the muscle of the diaphragm with impulses which stimulate contraction.

Brachial plexus

The anterior rami of the lower four cervical nerves and

a large part of the first thoracic nerve form the brachial plexus. Figure 7.32 shows its formation and the nerves which emerge from it. The plexus is situated above and behind the subclavian vessels and in the axilla.

The branches of the brachial plexus supply the skin and muscles of the upper limbs and some of the chest muscles. Five large nerves and a number of smaller

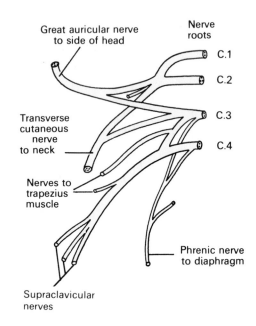

Figure 7.31   The cervical plexus.

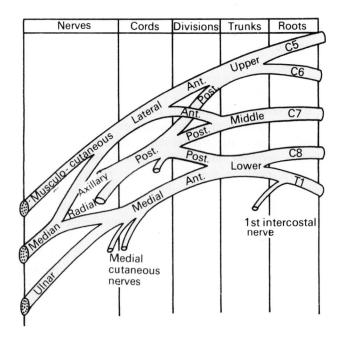

Figure 7.32   The brachial plexus.

ones emerge from this plexus, each with a contribution from more than one nerve root, containing sensory, motor and autonomic fibres:

- axillary (circumflex) nerve: C5, 6
- radial nerve: C5, 6, 7, 8, T1
- musculocutaneous nerve: C5, 6, 7
- median nerve: C5, 6, 7, 8, T1
- ulnar nerve: C7, 8, T1
- medial cutaneous nerve: C8, T1.

The axillary (circumflex) nerve winds round the humerus at the level of the surgical neck. It then breaks up into minute branches to supply the deltoid muscle, shoulder joint and overlying skin.

The radial nerve is the largest branch of the brachial plexus. It supplies the triceps muscle behind the humerus, crosses in front of the elbow joint then winds round to the back of the forearm to supply extensors of the wrist and finger joints. It continues into the back of the hand to supply the skin of the thumb, the first two fingers and the lateral half of the third finger.

The musculocutaneous nerve passes downwards to the lateral aspect of the forearm. It supplies the muscles of the upper arm and the skin of the forearm.

The median nerve passes down the midline of the arm in close association with the brachial artery. It passes in front of the elbow joint then down to supply the muscles of the front of the forearm. It continues into the hand where it supplies small muscles and the skin of the front of the thumb, the first two fingers and the lateral half of the third finger. It gives off no branches above the elbow.

The ulnar nerve descends through the upper arm lying medial to the brachial artery. It passes behind the medial epicondyle of the humerus to supply the muscles on the ulnar aspect of the forearm. It continues downwards to supply the muscles in the palm of the hand and the skin of the whole of the little finger and the medial half of the third finger. It gives off no branches above the elbow.

The main nerves of the arm are presented in Figure 7.33. The distribution and origins of the cutaneous sensory nerves of the arm are shown in Figure 7.34, i.e. the dermatomes.

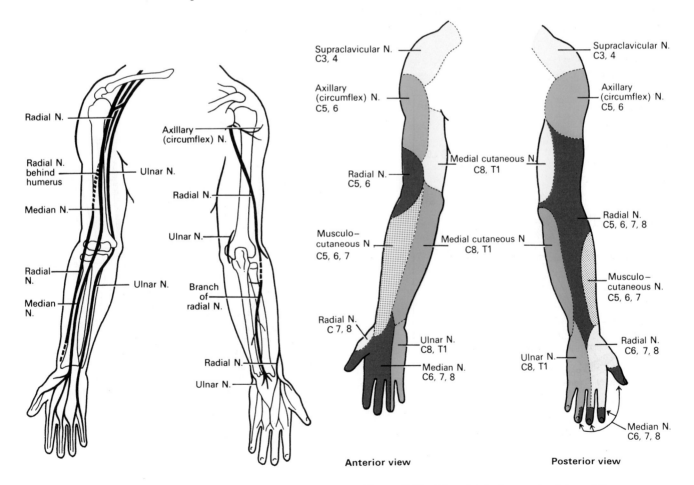

Figure 7.33   The main nerves of the arm.

Figure 7.34   The distribution and origins of the cutaneous nerves of the arm.

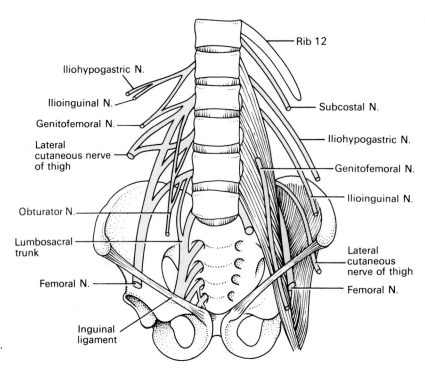

Iliohypogastric N.

Ilioinguinal N.

Genitofemoral N.

Lateral cutaneous nerve of thigh

Obturator N.

Lumbosacral trunk

Femoral N.

Inguinal ligament

Rib 12

Subcostal N.

Iliohypogastric N.

Genitofemoral N.

Ilioinguinal N.

Lateral cutaneous nerve of thigh

Femoral N.

Figure 7.35 The lumbar plexus.

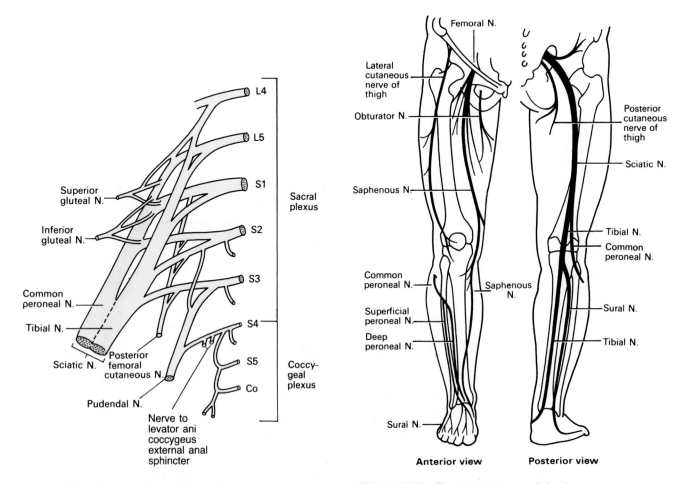

Superior gluteal N.

Inferior gluteal N.

Common peroneal N.

Tibial N.

Sciatic N.

Posterior femoral cutaneous N.

Pudendal N.

Nerve to levator ani coccygeus external anal sphincter

L4

L5

S1

S2

S3

S4

S5

Co

Sacral plexus

Coccygeal plexus

Figure 7.36 Sacral and coccygeal plexuses.

Femoral N.

Lateral cutaneous nerve of thigh

Obturator N.

Saphenous N.

Common peroneal N.

Superficial peroneal N.

Deep peroneal N.

Sural N.

Saphenous N.

Posterior cutaneous nerve of thigh

Sciatic N.

Tibial N.

Common peroneal N.

Sural N.

Tibial N.

Anterior view

Posterior view

Figure 7.37 The main nerves of the leg.

Lumbar plexus (Figs 7.35, 7.37 and 7.38)

The lumbar plexus is formed by the anterior rami of the first three and part of the fourth lumbar nerves. The plexus is situated in front of the transverse processes of the lumbar vertebrae and behind the psoas muscle. The main branches, and their nerve roots are:

- iliohypogastric nerve: L1
- ilioinguinal nerve: L1
- genitofemoral: L1, 2
- lateral cutaneous nerve of thigh: L2, 3
- femoral nerve: L2, 3, 4
- obturator nerve: L2, 3, 4
- lumbosacral trunk: L4, (5).

The iliohypogastric, ilioinguinal and *genitofemoral nerves* supply muscles and the skin in the area of the lower abdomen, upper and medial aspects of the thigh and the inguinal region.

The lateral cutaneous nerve of the thigh supplies the skin of the lateral aspect of the thigh including part of the anterior and posterior surfaces.

The femoral nerve is one of the larger branches. It passes behind the inguinal ligament to enter the thigh in close association with the femoral artery. It divides into cutaneous and muscular branches to supply the skin and the muscles of the front of the thigh. One branch, the *saphenous nerve*, supplies the medial aspect of the leg, ankle and foot.

The obturator nerve supplies the adductor muscles of the thigh and skin of the medial aspect of the thigh. It ends just above the level of the knee joint.

The lumbosacral trunk descends into the pelvis and makes a contribution to the sacral plexus.

Sacral plexus (Figs 7.36, 7.37 and 7.38)

The sacral plexus is formed by the anterior rami of the lumbosacral trunk and the first, second and third sacral nerves. The lumbosacral trunk is formed by the fifth and part of the fourth lumbar nerves. It lies in the posterior wall of the pelvic cavity.

The sacral plexus divides into a number of branches,

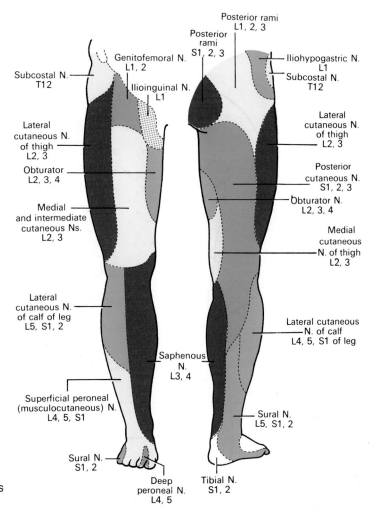

Figure 7.38 Distribution and origins of the cutaneous nerves of the leg.

supplying the muscles and skin of the pelvic floor, muscles around the hip joint and the pelvic organs. In addition to these it provides the *sciatic nerve* which contains fibres from L4, 5, S1, 2, 3.

The sciatic nerve is the largest nerve in the body. It is about 2 cm wide at its origin. It passes through the greater sciatic foramen into the buttock then descends through the posterior aspect of the thigh supplying the hamstring muscles. At the level of the middle of the femur it divides to form the *tibial* and the *common peroneal nerves*.

The tibial nerve descends through the popliteal fossa to the posterior aspect of the leg where it supplies muscles and skin. It passes under the medial malleolus to supply muscles and skin of the sole of the foot and toes. One of the main branches is the *sural nerve* which supplies the tissues in the area of the heel, the lateral aspect of the ankle and a part of the dorsum of the foot.

The common peroneal nerve descends obliquely along the lateral aspect of the popliteal fossa, winds round the neck of the fibula into the front of the leg where it divides into the *deep peroneal* (anterior tibial) and the *superficial peroneal* (musculocutaneous) nerves. These nerves supply the skin and muscles of the anterior aspect of the leg and the dorsum of the foot and toes.

The pudendal nerve (S2, 3, 4). The perineal branch supplies the external anal sphincter, the external urethral sphincter and adjacent skin. Figures 7.37 and 7.38 show the main nerves of the leg the dermatomes and the origins of the main nerves.

Coccygeal plexus (Fig. 7.36)
The coccygeal plexus is a very small plexus formed by part of the fourth and fifth sacral and the coccygeal nerves. The nerves from this plexus supply the skin in the area of the coccyx and the levators ani and coccygeus muscles of the pelvic floor and the external anal sphincter.

Thoracic nerves
The thoracic nerves *do not* intermingle to form plexuses. There are 12 pairs and the first 11 are the *intercostal nerves*. They pass between the ribs supplying them, the intercostal muscles and overlying skin. The 12th pair are the *subcostal nerves*. The 7th to the 12th thoracic nerves also supply the muscles and the skin of the posterior and anterior abdominal walls (Fig. 7.39).

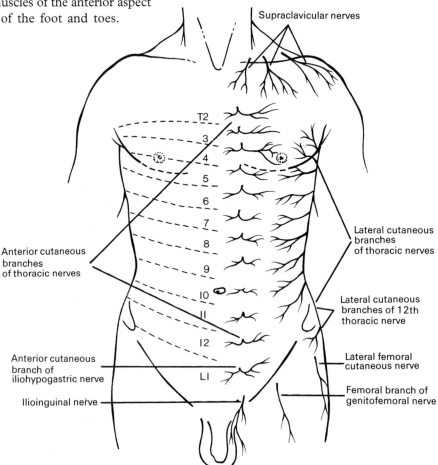

Figure 7.39 Distribution of the thoracic cutaneous nerves.

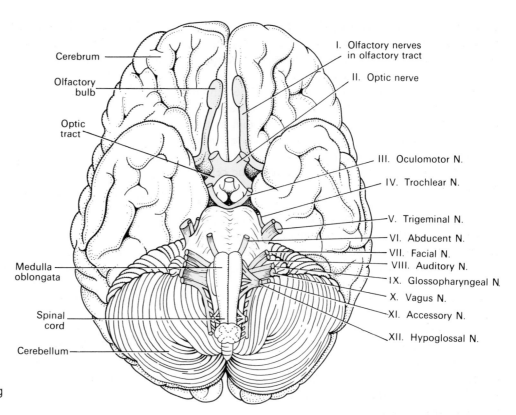

Figure 7.40 The inferior surface of the brain showing the cranial nerves.

Cranial nerves (Fig. 7.40)

There are 12 pairs of cranial nerves originating from nuclei in the inferior surface of the brain, some sensory, some motor and some mixed. Their names and numbers are:

- I. Olfactory: sensory
- II. Optic: sensory
- III. Oculomotor: motor
- IV. Trochlear: motor
- V. Trigeminal: mixed
- VI. Abducent: motor
- VII. Facial: mixed
- VIII. Vestibulocochlear (auditory): sensory
- IX. Glossopharyngeal: mixed
- X. Vagus: mixed:
- XI. Accessory: motor
- XII. Hypoglossal: motor

I. Olfactory nerves (sensory)

These are the nerves of the *sense of smell*. Their nerve endings and fibres arise in the upper part of the mucous membrane of the nose and pass upwards through the cribriform plate of the ethmoid bone (Fig. 7.41). These

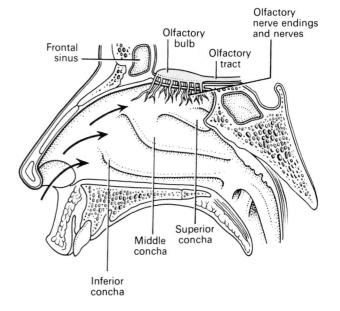

Figure 7.41 The olfactory nerve.

nerves pass to the *olfactory bulb*, a group of nerve cell bodies of the second neurones. The nerves then proceed backwards as the olfactory tract, to the area for the perception of smell in the temporal lobe of the cerebrum.

II. Optic nerves (sensory) (Fig. 7.42)

These are the nerves of the *sense of sight*. The fibres originate in the retinae of the eyes and they combine to form the optic nerves. They are directed backwards and medially through the posterior part of the orbital cavity. They then pass through the *optic foramina* of the sphenoid bone into the cranial cavity and join at the *optic chiasma* just above the pituitary gland. The nerves proceed backwards as the *optic tracts* to the *lateral geniculate body*. Impulses pass from these to the centre for sight in the occipital lobes of the cerebrum and to the cerebellum. In the occipital lobe sight is perceived, and in the cerebellum the impulses from the eyes contribute to the maintenance of balance, posture and orientation of the head in space (p. 152 and Ch. 8).

The central retinal artery and vein enter the eye enveloped by the fibres of the optic nerve.

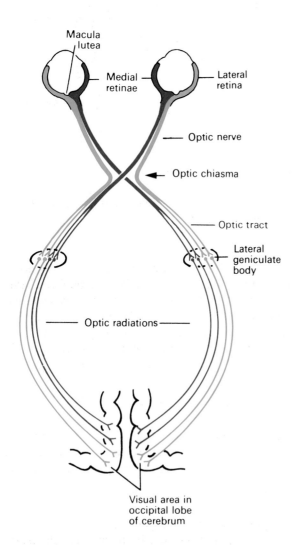

Figure 7.42 The visual pathway.

III. Oculomotor nerves (motor)

These nerves arise from nerve cells near the cerebral aqueduct. They supply:

- four extraocular muscles, i.e. the *superior, medial* and *inferior recti* and the *inferior oblique muscle*
- intraocular muscles:
  —*ciliary muscles* which alter the shape of the lens, changing its refractive power
  —*circular muscles of the iris* which constrict the pupil
- the *levator palpebrae* muscle which raises the upper eyelid.

IV. Trochlear nerves (motor)

These nerves arise from nerve cells near the cerebral aqueduct. They supply the *superior oblique muscles* of the eyes.

V. Trigeminal nerves (mixed)

These nerves contain motor and sensory fibres and are among the largest of the cranial nerves. They are the chief sensory nerves for the face and head, receiving impulses of *pain, temperature* and *touch*. The motor fibres stimulate the *muscles of mastication*.

There are three main branches of the trigeminal nerves. The dermatomes supplied by the sensory fibres on the right side are shown in Figure 7.43.

The ophthalmic nerves are sensory only and supply the *lacrimal glands, conjunctiva of the eyes, forehead, eyelids, anterior aspect of the scalp* and *mucous membrane of the nose.*

The maxillary nerves are sensory only and supply the *cheeks, upper gums, upper teeth* and *lower eyelids.*

The mandibular nerves contain both sensory and motor fibres. These are the largest of the three divisions and they supply the *teeth* and *gums of the lower jaw, pinnae of the ears, lower lip* and *tongue.* The motor fibres supply the *muscles of mastication.*

VI. Abducent nerves (motor)

These nerves arise from a group of nerve cells lying under the floor of the fourth ventricle. They supply the *lateral rectus muscles* of the eyeballs.

VII. Facial nerves (mixed)

These nerves are composed of both motor and sensory nerve fibres, arising from nerve cells in the lower part of the pons varolii. The motor fibres supply the *muscles of facial expression.* The sensory fibres convey impulses from the *taste buds* in the anterior two-thirds of the tongue to the taste perception area in the cerebral cortex.

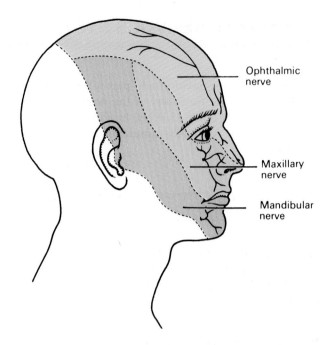

Figure 7.43 The cutaneous distribution of the main branches of the right trigeminal nerve.

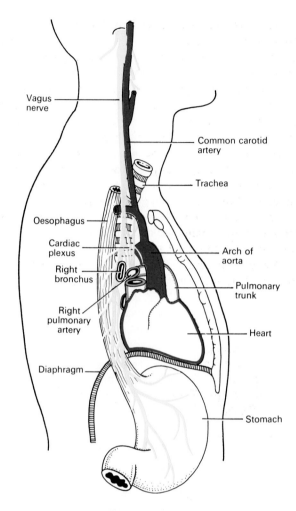

Figure 7.44 The position of the vagus nerve in the thorax viewed from the side.

VIII. Vestibulocochlear (auditory) nerves (sensory)

These nerves are composed of two distinct sets of fibres, vestibular nerves and cochlear nerves.

The vestibular nerves arise from the semicircular canals of the inner ear and convey impulses to the cerebellum. They are associated with the *maintenance of posture and balance.*

The cochlear nerves originate in the organ of Corti in the inner ear and convey impulses to the hearing areas in the cerebral cortex where *sound is perceived.*

IX. Glossopharyngeal nerves (mixed)

These nerves arise from nuclei in the medulla oblongata. The motor fibres stimulate the *muscles of the tongue and pharynx* and the *secretory cells of the parotid* (salivary) glands.

The sensory fibres convey impulses to the cerebral cortex from the posterior third of the tongue, the tonsils and pharynx and from *taste buds* in the tongue and pharynx.

X. Vagus nerves (mixed) (Fig. 7.44)

These nerves have a more extensive distribution than any other cranial nerves. They arise from nerve cells in the medulla oblongata and other nuclei, and pass down through the neck into the thorax and the abdomen.

The motor fibres supply the *smooth muscles* and *secretory glands* of the pharynx, larynx, trachea, heart, oesophagus, stomach, intestines, pancreas, gall bladder, bile ducts, spleen, kidneys, ureter and blood vessels in the thoracic and abdominal cavities.

The sensory fibres convey impulses from the *lining membranes* of the same structures to the brain.

XI. Accessory nerves (motor)

These nerves arise from nerve cells in the medulla oblongata and in the spinal cord. The fibres supply the *sternocleidomastoid* and *trapezius muscles.* Branches join the vagus nerves and supply the *pharyngeal* and *laryngeal muscles.*

XII. Hypoglossal nerves (motor)

These nerves arise from cells in the medulla oblongata. They supply the *muscles of the tongue* and *muscles sur-*

rounding the hyoid bone and contribute to swallowing and speech.

A summary of the cranial nerves is given in Table 7.3.

AUTONOMIC NERVOUS SYSTEM

The autonomic or involuntary part of the nervous system controls the functions of the body carried out automatically, i.e. initiated in the brain below the level of the cerebrum. Although stimulation does not occur

Table 7.3 Summary of the cranial nerves

Name and no.	Central connection	Peripheral connection	Function
I. Olfactory (sensory)	Smell area in temporal lobe of cerebrum through olfactory bulb	Mucous membrane in roof of nose	Sense of smell
II. Optic (sensory)	Sight area in occipital lobe of cerebrum	Retina of the eye	Sense of sight
	Cerebellum		Balance
III. Oculomotor (motor)	Nerve cells near floor of aqueduct of midbrain	Superior, inferior and medial rectus muscles of the eye	Moving the eyeball
		Ciliary muscles of the eye	Focusing
		Circular muscle fibres of the iris	Regulating the size of the pupil
IV. Trochlear (motor)	Nerve cells near floor of aqueduct of midbrain	Superior oblique muscles of the eye	Movement of the eyeball
V. Trigeminal (mixed)	Motor fibres from the pons varolii		Chewing
		Muscles of mastication	Sensation from the face
	Sensory fibres from the trigeminal ganglion	Sensory to gums, cheek, lower jaw, iris, cornea	
VI. Abducent (motor)	Floor of fourth ventricle		Movement of the eye
		Lateral rectus muscle of the eye	
VII. Facial (mixed)	Pons varolii		Sense of taste
		Sensory fibres to the tongue	Movements of facial expression
VIII. Vestibulocochlear (sensory) (a) Vestibular (b) Cochlear		Motor fibres to the muscles of the face	
	Cerebellum		Maintenance of balance
	Hearing area of cerebrum	Semicircular canals in the inner ear	Sense of hearing
IX. Glossopharyngeal (mixed)		Organ of Corti in cochlea	
	Medulla oblongata		Secretion of saliva
X. Vagus (mixed)		Parotid gland	Sense of taste
		Back of tongue and pharynx	Movement of pharynx
XI. Accessory (motor)	Medulla oblongata		Movement and secretion
		Pharynx, larynx; organs, glands, ducts, blood vessels in the thorax and abdomen	
XII. Hypoglossal (motor)	Medulla oblongata		Movement of the head, shoulders, pharynx and larynx
		Sternocleidomastoid, trapezius, laryngeal and pharyngeal muscles	
	Medulla oblongata		Movement of tongue
		Tongue	

voluntarily the individual may be conscious of its effects, e.g. an increase in the heart rate.

The effects of autonomic control are essential for homeostasis and include stimulation or depression of glandular secretion and contraction of cardiac and smooth muscle tissue, e.g.:

- rate and force of the heartbeat
- secretion of the glands of the alimentary tract
- vasoconstriction or dilatation
- change in the size of the pupils of the eyes.

The *efferent (motor) nerves* of the autonomic nervous system arise from nerve cells in the brain and emerge at various levels between the midbrain and the sacral region of the spinal cord. Many of them travel within the same nerve sheath as the peripheral nerves of the central nervous system to reach the organs which they innervate.

The autonomic nervous system is divided into two parts:

- *sympathetic* (thoracolumbar outflow)
- *parasympathetic* (craniosacral outflow).

The two parts have both structural and functional differences. They normally work in an opposing manner, enabling or restoring balance of involuntary functions, maintaining homeostasis. The sympathetic part tends to predominate in stressful situations, and the parasympathetic part during rest.

Sympathetic nervous system (thoracolumbar outflow)

Three neurones are involved in conveying impulses from their origin in the *hypothalamus, reticular formation* and *medulla oblongata* to effector organs and tissues (Fig. 7.45).

Neurone 1 has its cell body in the *brain* and its fibre extends into the *spinal cord*.

Neurone 2 has its cell body in the *lateral column of grey matter* in the spinal cord between the levels of the 1st thoracic and 2nd or 3rd lumbar vertebrae. The nerve fibre of this cell leaves the cord by the anterior root and terminates in one of the ganglia either in the *lateral chain of sympathetic ganglia* or passes through it to one of the *prevertebral ganglia*. Acetylcholine is the chemical transmitter.

Neurone 3 has its cell body in a ganglion and terminates in the organ or tissue supplied. Noradrenaline is the chemical transmitter.

Sympathetic ganglia

The lateral chains of sympathetic ganglia. These are chains of ganglia which extend from the upper cervical level to the sacrum, one chain lying on each side of the bodies of the vertebrae. The ganglia are attached to each other by nerve fibres. *Preganglionic fibres* that emerge from the cord may synapse with the cell body of the neurone 3 at the same level or they may pass up or down the chain through one or more ganglia before synapsing. For example, the nerve which dilates the pupil of the eye leaves the cord at the level of the 1st thoracic vertebra and passes up the chain to the superior cervical ganglion before it synapses with the cell body of neurone 3. The *postganglionic fibres* then pass to the eyes. The major exception is that there is no parasympathetic supply to the sweat glands, the skin and blood vessels of skeletal muscles. These structures are supplied by only sympathetic fibres, some of which have acetylcholine and some adrenaline and noradrenaline as their chemical transmitter. They have, therefore, the effects of both sympathetic and parasympathetic nerve supply (Fig. 7.45).

Prevertebral ganglia. There are three prevertebral ganglia situated in the abdominal cavity close to the origins of arteries of the same names:

- coeliac ganglion
- superior mesenteric ganglion
- inferior mesenteric ganglion.

The ganglia consist of nerve cells rather diffusely distributed among a network of nerve fibres which form plexuses. Second neurone sympathetic fibres pass *through* the lateral chain to reach these ganglia.

Parasympathetic nervous system (craniosacral outflow)

Two neurones are involved in the transmission of impulses from their source to the effector organ (Fig. 7.46). The chemical transmitter at both synapses is acetylcholine.

Neurone 1 has its cell body either in the brain or in the spinal cord. Those originating in the brain are the *cranial nerves* III, VII, IX and X, arising from nuclei in the midbrain and brain stem, and their nerve fibres terminate outside the brain. The cell bodies of the *sacral outflow* are in the lateral columns of grey matter at the distal end of the spinal cord. Their fibres leave the cord in sacral segments 2, 3 and 4 and synapse with second neurone cells in the walls of pelvic organs.

Neurone 2 has its cell body either in a ganglion or in the wall of the organ supplied.

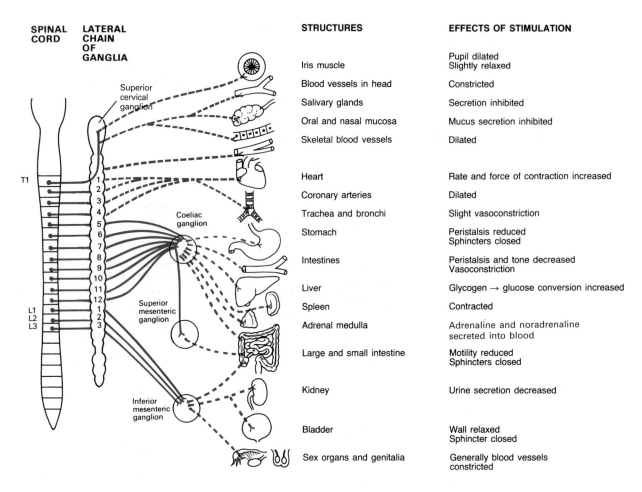

SPINAL CORD	LATERAL CHAIN OF GANGLIA	STRUCTURES	EFFECTS OF STIMULATION
	Superior cervical ganglion	Iris muscle	Pupil dilated Slightly relaxed
		Blood vessels in head	Constricted
		Salivary glands	Secretion inhibited
		Oral and nasal mucosa	Mucus secretion inhibited
		Skeletal blood vessels	Dilated
T1	1 2 3 4	Heart	Rate and force of contraction increased
	5	Coronary arteries	Dilated
	6	Coeliac ganglion Trachea and bronchi	Slight vasoconstriction
	7 8	Stomach	Peristalsis reduced Sphincters closed
	9 10	Intestines	Peristalsis and tone decreased Vasoconstriction
	11 12	Liver	Glycogen → glucose conversion increased
L1 L2 L3	Superior mesenteric ganglion 1 2 3	Spleen	Contracted
		Adrenal medulla	Adrenaline and noradrenaline secreted into blood
		Large and small intestine	Motility reduced Sphincters closed
	Inferior mesenteric ganglion	Kidney	Urine secretion decreased
		Bladder	Wall relaxed Sphincter closed
		Sex organs and genitalia	Generally blood vessels constricted

Figure 7.45 The sympathetic outflow, the main structures supplied and the effects of stimulation. Solid red lines— preganglionic fibres; broken lines—postganglionic fibres. There is a right and left lateral chain of ganglia.

Functions of the autonomic nervous system

The autonomic nervous system is involved in a complex of reflex activities which, like the reflexes described previously, depend on sensory input to the brain or spinal cord, and on motor output. In this case the reflex action is contraction, or inhibition of contraction, of involuntary (smooth and cardiac) muscle or glandular secretion. These reflexes are coordinated in the brain below the level of consciousness, i.e. below the level of the cerebrum. Some sensory input does reach consciousness and may result in temporary inhibition of the reflex action, e.g. reflex micturition can be inhibited temporarily.

The majority of the organs of the body are supplied by both sympathetic and parasympathetic nerves which have opposite effects that are finely balanced to ensure the optimum functioning of the organ.

Sympathetic stimulation as a whole has similar effects on the body to those produced by the hormones *adrenaline* and *noradrenaline* secreted by the medulla of the adrenal glands. It prepares the body to deal with exciting and stressful situations, e.g. strengthening its defences in danger and in extremes of environmental temperature. It is sometimes said that sympathetic stimulation mobilises the body for 'fight or flight'.

Parasympathetic stimulation has a tendency to slow down body processes except digestion and absorption of food and the functions of the genitourinary systems. Its general effect is that of a 'peace maker' allowing restoration processes to occur quietly and peacefully.

Normally the two systems function simultaneously producing a regular heartbeat, normal temperature and an internal environment compatible with the immediate external surroundings.

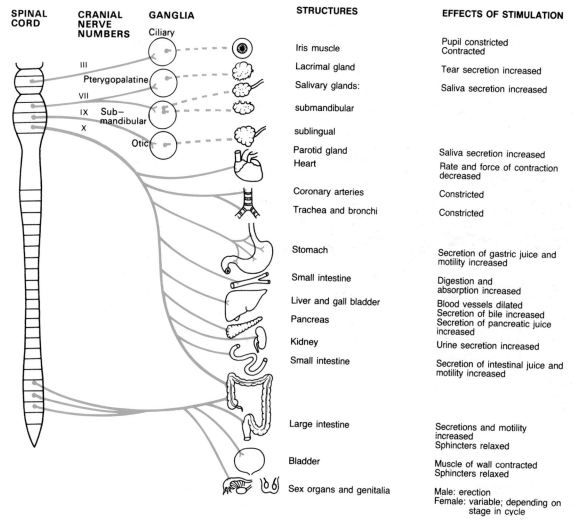

Figure 7.46 The parasympathetic outflow, the main structures supplied and the effects of stimulation. Solid blue lines—preganglionic fibres; broken lines—postganglionic fibres. Where there are no broken lines, the 2nd neurone is in the wall of the structure.

Effects of autonomic stimulation on the various body systems

Cardiovascular system

Sympathetic stimulation

- Exerts an accelerating effect upon the sinuatrial node in the heart, increasing the rate and force of the heart beat.
- Causes dilatation of the coronary arteries, increasing the blood supply to heart muscle.
- Causes dilatation of the blood vessels supplying skeletal muscle, increasing the supply of oxygen and nutritional materials and the removal of metabolic waste products, thus increasing the capacity of the muscle to do work.

- Raises peripheral resistance and blood pressure by constricting the small arteries and arterioles in the skin. In this way an increased blood supply is available for highly active tissue, such as skeletal muscle, heart, brain.
- Constricts the blood vessels in the secretory glands of the digestive system, reducing the flow of digestive juices. This raises the volume of blood available for circulation in dilated blood vessels.
- Blood coagulation occurs more quickly because of vasoconstriction.

Parasympathetic stimulation

This has effects opposite to those of sympathetic stimulation on the heart and blood vessels.

Respiratory system

Sympathetic stimulation

This causes dilatation of the bronchi allowing a greater amount of air to enter the lungs at each inspiration. In conjunction with the increased heart rate, the oxygen intake and carbon dioxide output of the body are increased.

Parasympathetic stimulation

Produces constriction of the bronchi.

Digestive and urinary systems

Sympathetic stimulation

- *The liver* converts an increased amount of glycogen to glucose, making more carbohydrate immediately available to provide energy.
- *The adrenal (suprarenal) glands* are stimulated to secrete adrenaline and noradrenaline which potentiate and sustain the effects of sympathetic stimulation.
- *The stomach* and *small intestine*. Smooth muscle contraction and secretion of digestive juices are inhibited, delaying digestion, onward movement and absorption of food and the tone of sphincter muscles is increased.
- *Urethral* and *anal sphincters*. The muscle tone of the sphincters is increased, inhibiting micturition and defaecation.
- *The bladder wall* relaxes.
- *The metabolic rate* is greatly increased.

Parasympathetic stimulation

- *The stomach* and *small intestine*. The rate of digestion and absorption of food is increased.
- *The pancreas*. There is an increase in the secretion of pancreatic juice and the hormone insulin.
- *Urethral* and *anal sphincters*. Relaxation of the internal urethral sphincter is accompanied by contraction of the muscle of the bladder wall and micturition occurs. Similar relaxation of the internal anal sphincter is accompanied by contraction of the muscle of the rectum and defaecation occurs. In both cases there is voluntary relaxation of the external sphincters.

Eye

Sympathetic stimulation

This causes contraction of the radiating muscle fibres of the iris, *dilating* the pupil. Retraction of the levator palpebral muscles occurs, opening the eyes wide and giving the appearance of alertness and excitement. The ciliary muscle that adjusts the thickness of the lens is slightly relaxed.

Parasympathetic stimulation

This causes contraction of the circular muscle fibres of the iris, constricting the pupil. The eyelids tend to close, giving the appearance of sleepiness.

Skin

Sympathetic stimulation

- Causes increased secretion of sweat, leading to increased heat loss from the body.
- Produces contraction of the arrectores pilorum (the muscles in the skin), giving the appearance of 'goose flesh'.
- Causes constriction of the blood vessels preventing heat loss.

There is no parasympathetic nerve supply to the skin. Some sympathetic fibres are adrenergic, causing vasoconstriction, and some are cholinergic, causing vasodilatation.

Genitalia

Sympathetic stimulation

This causes ejaculation in males.

Parasympathetic stimulation

This causes generalised vasodilatation, with erection of the penis in the male.

Afferent impulses from viscera

Sensory fibres from the viscera travel with autonomic fibres and are sometimes called *autonomic afferents*. The impulses they transmit are associated with:

- visceral reflexes, usually at an unconscious level, e.g. cough
- sensation of, e.g. hunger, thirst, nausea, sexual sensation, rectal and bladder distension
- visceral pain.

Visceral pain

Normally the viscera are insensitive to cutting, burning and crushing. However, a sensation of dull, poorly located pain is experienced when:

- visceral nerves are stretched
- a large number of fibres are stimulated
- there is ischaemia and the accumulation of metabolites
- the sensitivity of nerve endings to painful stimuli is increased, e.g. during inflammation.

If the cause of the pain, e.g. inflammation, affects the parietal layer of a serous membrane (pleura, peritoneum) the pain is acute and easily located over the site of inflammation. This is because the peripheral spinal (somatic) nerves supplying the superficial tissues also supply the parietal layer of serous membrane. They transmit the impulses to the cerebral cortex where *somatic pain* is perceived and accurately located. Ap-

pendicitis is an example of this type of pain. Initially it is dull and vaguely located around the midline of the abdomen. As the condition progresses the parietal peritoneum becomes involved and acute pain is clearly located in the right iliac fossa, i.e. over the appendix.

Referred pain (Fig. 7.47)

In some cases of visceral disease pain may be perceived to occur in superficial tissues remote from the viscus, i.e. referred pain. This occurs when sensory fibres from the viscus enter the same segment of the spinal cord as somatic nerves, i.e. those from the superficial tissues. It is believed that the sensory nerve from the viscus stimulates the closely associated nerve in the spinal cord and it transmits the impulses to the sensory area in the cerebral cortex where the pain is perceived as originating in the area supplied by the somatic nerve. Examples of referred pain are given in Table 7.4.

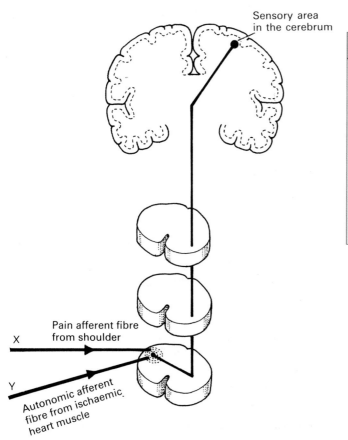

Figure 7.47 Referred pain. Pain perceived to originate from the tissues supplied by the damaged nerve. Y stimulates X and pain is perceived in the shoulder.

Table 7.4 Referred pain

Tissue of origin of pain	Site of referred pain
Heart	Left shoulder
Liver	
Biliary tract	Right shoulder
Kidney	
Ureter	Loin and groin
Uterus	Low back
Male genitalia	Low abdomen
Prolapsed intervertebral disc	Leg

RESPONSE OF NERVOUS TISSUE TO INJURY

Neurone damage

Damage to the nerve cells or their processes can lead to rapid necrosis with sudden acute functional failure, or to slow atrophy with gradually increasing dysfunction. These changes are associated with:

- anoxia
- hypoglycaemia
- nutritional deficiencies
- poisons, e.g. organic lead
- trauma
- infections
- ageing.

Neurone regeneration
(Fig. 7.48)

Neurones of the brain, spinal cord and ganglia reach maturity a few weeks after birth and are not replaced when they are damaged or die. The axons of *peripheral nerves* may regenerate if the cell body remains intact. Distal to the damage the axon and myelin sheath disintegrate and are removed by macrophages, but the Schwann cells survive and proliferate within the neurilemma. The live proximal part of the axon grows along the original track (about 3 mm per day), provided the two parts of neurilemma are correctly positioned and in close apposition. Restoration of function depends on the re-establishment of satisfactory connections with the end organ. When the neurilemma is out of position or destroyed the sprouting axons and Schwann cells form a tumour-like cluster (*traumatic neuroma*), e.g. following some fractures and amputation of limbs.

Neuroglia damage

Astrocytes
When severely damaged, astrocytes undergo necrosis and disintegrate. In less severe and chronic conditions there is proliferation of astrocyte processes and later cell atrophy (*gliosis*). This process occurs in many diseases and is analagous to fibrosis in other tissues.

Oligodendrocytes
These cells form and maintain myelin, having the same functions as Schwann cells in peripheral nerves. They increase in number around degenerating neurones and are

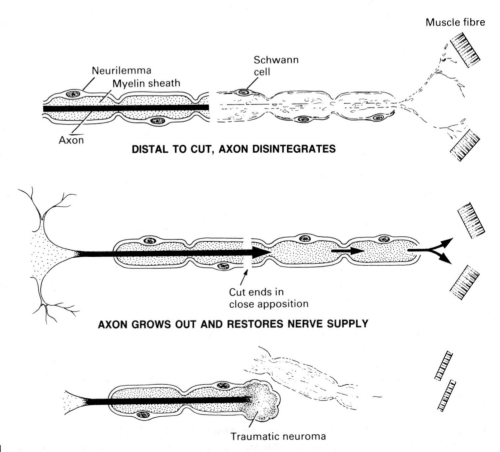

Figure 7.48 Regrowth of peripheral nerves following injury.

destroyed in demyelinating diseases such as *multiple sclerosis* (p. 184).

Microglia

Microglia are derived from monocytes that migrate from the blood into the nervous system before birth, and are found mainly around blood vessels. Where there is inflammation and cell destruction the microglia increase in size and become phagocytic.

DISEASES OF THE BRAIN

Increased intracranial pressure

This is not a disease in itself but it is a very important complication of many conditions. As the cranium forms a rigid cavity enclosing the brain, its blood supply and cerebrospinal fluid (CSF), an increase in volume of any one of these will lead to raised intracranial pressure. Sometimes its effects are more serious than the condition causing it, e.g. by disrupting the blood supply or distorting the shape of the brain especially if the intracranial pressure (ICP) rises rapidly. A slow rise in ICP allows time for compensatory adjustment to be made, i.e. a slight reduction in the volume of circulating blood and of CSF. The slower the rise in ICP, the more effective the compensation. As it reaches its limit a further small increase in pressure is followed by a sudden and possibly serious reduction in the cerebral blood flow, hypoxia and a rise in carbon dioxide level, causing arteriolar dilatation which further increases the ICP. This leads to progressive loss of functioning neurones, vasomotor paralysis (bradycardia and hypertension), further cerebral hypoxia and possibly death.

The causes of increased ICP are:

- expanding lesions, e.g. haematoma, tumour
- cerebral oedema
- hydrocephalus, i.e. accumulation of excess CSF.

Expanding lesions and their effects

These lesions may occur in the brain or in the meninges and they may damage the brain in various ways (Fig. 7.49).

Displacement of the brain

Lesions causing displacement are usually one-sided but may affect both sides. Such lesions may cause:

- herniation of the cerebral hemisphere between the corpus callosum and the free border of the falx cerebri on the same side
- herniation of the midbrain between the pons and the free border of the tentorium cerebelli on the same side
- compression of the subarachnoid space and flattening of the cerebral convolutions
- distortion of the shape of the ventricles and their ducts
- herniation of the cerebellum through the foramen magnum
- protrusion of the medulla oblongata through the foramen magnum ('coning').

Obstruction of the flow of cerebrospinal fluid

The ventricles or their ducts may be pushed out of position or a duct obstructed. The effects depend on the position of the lesion, e.g. compression of the aqueduct of the midbrain causes dilatation of the lateral ventricles and the third ventricle, further increasing the ICP.

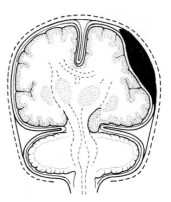

A. Subdural haematoma

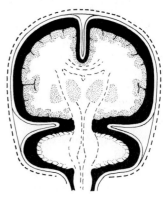

B. Subarachnoid haemorrhage

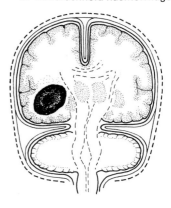

C. Tumour or intracerebral haemorrhage

Figure 7.49 Effects of different types of expanding lesions inside the skull.

Vascular damage

There may be stretching or compression of blood vessels, causing:

- haemorrhage when stretched blood vessels rupture
- ischaemia and infarction due to compression of blood vessels

- papilloedema (oedema round the optic disc) due to compression of the retinal vein in the optic nerve sheath where it crosses the subarachnoid space.

Neural damage
The vital centres in the medulla oblongata may be damaged when the increased ICP causes 'coning'. Stretching may damage cranial nerves, especially the oculomotor (III) and the abducent (VI), causing disturbances of eye movement and accommodation.

Bone changes
Prolonged increase of ICP causes bony changes, e.g.:

- erosion, especially of the sphenoid
- stretching and thinning before ossification is complete.

Cerebral oedema

In this condition there is excess water in brain cells and/or in the interstitial spaces, causing increased intracranial pressure. It is associated with:

- traumatic injury
- hypoglycaemia
- haemorrhage
- infections, abscesses
- hypoxia
- local ischaemia, infarcts
- tumours
- inflammation.

Cytotoxic oedema
The neurones and neuroglial cells contain excess water due to disturbances of their osmotic pressure caused by retention of excess electrolytes. The permeability of the capillary walls is normal.

Vasogenic oedema
Excess fluid collects in the interstitial spaces, especially round nerve fibres. The permeability of the capillary walls is increased and plasma proteins pass out of the capillaries, increasing the osmotic pressure in the interstitial spaces which causes oedema.

Hydrocephalus

In this condition the volume of CSF is abnormally high and is usually accompanied by increased ICP. An obstruction to CSF flow (Fig. 7.14) is the most common cause. It is described as *communicating* when there is free flow of CSF from the ventricular system to the subarachnoid space and *non-communicating* when there is not, i.e. there is obstruction in the system of ventricles, foramina or ducts.

Enlargement of the head occurs in children when ossification of the cranial bones is incomplete but, in spite of this, the ventricles dilate and cause stretching and thinning of the brain. After ossification is complete, hydrocephalus leads to a marked increase in ICP and destruction of neural tissue.

Primary hydrocephalus
This is usually caused by obstruction to the flow of CSF and may be communicating or non-communicating. Occasionally it is caused by malabsorption of CSF by the arachnoid villi.

Congenital primary hydrocephalus is due to malformation of the ventricles, foramina or ducts, usually at a narrow point.

Acquired primary hydrocephalus is caused by lesions that obstruct the circulation of the CSF, usually expanding lesions, e.g. tumours, haematomas or adhesions between arachnoid and pia maters, following meningitis.

Secondary hydrocephalus
Compensatory increases in the amount of CSF and ventricle capacity occur when there is atrophy of brain tissue, e.g. in senile dementia and following cerebral infarcts. There may not be a rise in ICP.

Head injuries

The brain may be injured by a blow to the head or movement of the brain during sudden acceleration or deceleration of the head. The damage to the brain may be serious even when there is no outward sign of injury.

Blow to the head

At the site of injury there may be:

- scalp wound, with haemorrhage between scalp and skull bones
- damage to the underlying meninges and/or brain with local haemorrhage inside the skull
- depressed fracture of the skull, causing local damage to the underlying meninges and brain tissue
- temporal bone fracture, making an opening between the middle ear and the meninges
- fracture involving the air sinuses of the sphenoid, ethmoid or frontal bones, making an opening between the nose and the meninges.

Acceleration–deceleration injuries

Because the brain floats relatively freely in 'a cushion' of CSF, sudden acceleration or deceleration has an inertia effect, i.e. there is delay between the movement of the head and the corresponding movement of the brain. During this period the brain may be compressed and damaged at the site of impact. In 'contre coup' injuries, brain damage is more severe on the side opposite to the site of impact. Other injuries include:

- nerve cell damage, usually to the frontal and parietal lobes, due to movement of the brain over the rough surface of bones of the base of the skull
- nerve fibre damage due to stretching, especially following rotational movement
- haemorrhage due to rupture of blood vessels in the subarachnoid space *on the side opposite* the impact or more diffuse small haemorrhages, following rotational movement.

Complications of head injury

If the individual survives the immediate effects, complications may develop hours or days later. Sometimes they are the first indication of serious damage caused by a seemingly trivial injury. Their effects may be to increase ICP, damage brain tissue or provide a route of entry for microbes.

Traumatic intracranial haemorrhage

Haemorrhage may occur causing secondary brain damage at the site of injury, on the opposite side of the brain or diffusely throughout the brain. If bleeding continues, the expanding haematoma damages the brain and increases the ICP.

Extradural haemorrhage
This may follow a direct blow that may or may not cause a fracture. The individual may recover quickly

and indications of increased ICP only appear several hours later as the haematoma grows and the outer layer of dura mater (periosteum) is stripped off the bone. The haematoma grows rapidly when arterial blood vessels are damaged. In children there is rarely a fracture because the skull bones are still soft and the joints have not fused. The haematoma usually remains localised.

Acute subdural haemorrhage
This is due to haemorrhage from small veins in the dura mater or from larger veins between the layers of dura mater before they enter the venous sinuses. The blood may spread in the subdural space over one or both hemispheres. There may be concurrent subarachnoid haemorrhage, especially when there are extensive brain contusions and lacerations.

Chronic subdural haemorrhage
This may occur weeks or months after minor injuries and sometimes there is no history of injury. It occurs most commonly in people in whom there is some cerebral atrophy, e.g. the elderly and alcoholics. Evidence of increased ICP may be delayed when brain volume is reduced. The haematoma formed gradually increases in size due to repeated small haemorrhages and causes mild chronic inflammation and the accumulation of inflammatory exudate. In time it is isolated by a wall of fibrous tissue.

Intracerebral haemorrhage and cerebral oedema
These occur following contusions, lacerations and shearing injuries associated with acceleration and deceleration, especially rotational movements.

Cerebral oedema is a common complication of contusions of the

brain, leading to increased ICP, hypoxia and further brain damage.

Meningitis

Inflammation of the meninges may occur following a compound fracture of the skull that is accompanied by leakage of CSF and blood from the site, providing a route of entry for microbes. The escape of CSF and blood may be through:

- skin, in compound fractures of the skull
- middle ear, in fractures of the temporal bone (CSF otorrhoea)
- nose, in fractures of sphenoid, ethmoid or frontal bones when the air sinuses are involved (CSF rhinorrhoea).

Post-traumatic epilepsy

This is usually characterised by seizures and may develop in the first week or several months after injury. Early development is most common after severe injuries, although in children the injury itself may have appeared trivial. After depressed fractures or large haematomas epilepsy tends to develop later.

Persistent vegetative state

In this condition there is severe brain damage that results in unconsciousness but the vital centres that control homeostasis remain intact, e.g. breathing, blood pressure.

Circulatory disturbances affecting the brain

A number of abnormalities of the circulation, not associated with head injuries, affect the brain.

Hypoxia

Hypoxia may be due to:

- disturbances in the autoregulation of blood supply to the brain
- conditions affecting cerebral blood vessels.

When the systolic blood pressure falls below about 50 mmHg there is failure of the autoregulating mechanisms that control the blood flow to the brain by adjusting the diameter of the arterioles. The consequent rapid decrease in the cerebral blood supply leads to hypoxia and lack of glucose. If severe hypoxia is sustained for more than a few minutes there is irreversible brain damage. The neurones are affected first, then the neuroglial cells and later the meninges and blood vessels. Conditions in which autoregulation breaks down include:

- cardiorespiratory arrest
- sudden severe hypotension
- carbon monoxide poisoning
- hypercapnia (excess blood carbon dioxide)
- drug overdosage with, e.g. narcotics, hypnotics, analgesics.

Changes in the cerebral circulation, leading to hypoxia, include:

- occlusion of a cerebral artery by, e.g. atheroma, thrombosis, rapidly expanding lesion, embolism
- arterial stenosis that occurs in arteritis, e.g. polyarteritis nodosa, tuberculous meningitis, syphilis, diabetes, degenerative changes in the elderly.

If the individual survives the initial ischaemia, there is infarction, necrosis and loss of function of the affected area of brain.

Stroke (cerebrovascular disease)

This condition is a common cause of death and disability, especially in the elderly. It occurs when a vascular disease suddenly interrupts flow of blood to the brain. The effects include paralysis of a limb or one side of the body and disturbances of speech and vision. The nature and extent of cerebral impairment depends on the size and location of the affected blood vessels. Predisposing factors include hypertension, cigarette smoking and diabetes mellitus. The main causes are listed below.

Cerebral infarction

This is caused by atheroma complicated by thrombosis (p. 117) or blockage of an artery by an embolus from, e.g. infective endocarditis. When complete recovery occurs within 24 hours, the event is called a *transient ischaemic attack* (TIA). Recurrence or complete stroke may follow.

Spontaneous intracranial haemorrhage

The haemorrage may be into the subarachnoid space or intracerebral (Fig. 7.50). It is commonly associated with an aneurysm or hypertension. In each case the escaped blood may cause arterial spasm, leading to ischaemia, infarction, fibrosis (gliosis) and hypoxic brain damage. A severe haemorrhage may be instantly fatal while repeated small haemorrhages have a cumula-

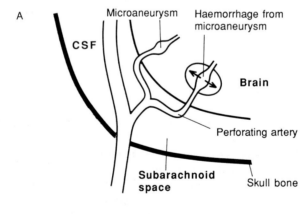

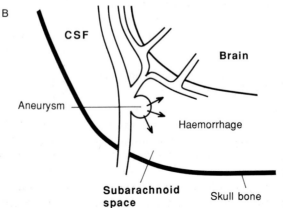

Figure 7.50
Types of haemorrhage causing stroke
A. Intracerebral
B. Subarachnoid.

tive effect in extending brain damage.

Intracerebral haemorrhage

Prolonged hypertension leads to the formation of multiple micro-aneurysms in the walls of very small arteries in the brain. Rupture of one or more of these, due to continuing rise in blood pressure, is usually the cause of intracerebral haemorrhage. The most common sites are branches of the middle cerebral artery in the region of the internal capsule and the basal nuclei (ganglia).

Severe haemorrhage. This causes compression and destruction of tissue, a sudden increase in ICP and distortion and herniation of the brain. Death follows when the vital centres in the medulla oblongata are damaged by haemorrhage or if there is coning due to increased ICP.

Less severe haemorrhage. This causes paralysis and loss of sensation of varying severity, affecting the side of the body opposite the haemorrhage. If the bleeding stops and does not recur an *apoplectic cyst* develops, i.e. the haematoma is walled off by gliosis, the blood clot is gradually absorbed and the cavity filled with tissue exudate. When the ICP returns to normal some functions may be restored, e.g. speech and movement of limbs.

Subarachnoid haemorrhage

This is mostly due to rupture of a berry aneurysm on one of the major cerebral arteries or bleeding from a congenitally malformed blood vessel. The blood may remain localised but usually spreads in the subarachnoid space round the brain and spinal cord, causing a general increase in ICP without distortion of the brain. The irritant effect of the blood may cause arterial spasm, leading to ischaemia, infarction, gliosis and the effects of localised

brain damage. It occurs most commonly in middle life, but occasionally in young people due to rupture of a malformed blood vessel.

Haemorrhage into tumours

Within the confined space of the skull, haemorrhage in a tumour exacerbates the increased ICP caused by the tumour.

Hypertension

Sustained hypertension causes brain damage when:

- microaneurysms rupture
- pulsation of hard tortuous arteries damages brain tissue in their immediate vicinity
- cerebral oedema in malignant hypertension leads to hypertensive encephalopathy.

Dementia

Alzheimer's disease

This condition was previously called pre-senile dementia and is the commonest cause of dementia. It is of unknown aetiology. Females are affected twice as often as males and it usually affects those over 60 years, the incidence increasing with age. Death usually occurs between 2 and 8 years after onset.

Huntington's disease (chorea)

This usually manifests itself between the ages of 30 and 50 years. It is caused by a genetic abnormality associated with deficient production of the neurotransmitter gamma

aminobutyric acid (GABA). The extrapyramidal changes are accompanied by cortical atrophy. There are uncoordinated involuntary movements especially of the facial muscles and, as the disease progresses, dementia develops.

Secondary dementias

Dementia may occur in association with other diseases:

- cerebrovascular disease—*multi-infarct dementia* is the result of the cumulative effect of several small cerebral infarcts leading to the gradually increasing impairment of mental function
- infections, e.g. encephalitis, neurosyphilis, human immunodeficiency virus (HIV), Creutzfeldt–Jakob disease
- cerebral trauma
- chronic abuse of alcohol and some drugs
- vitamin B deficiency
- effects of metabolic disorders, e.g. hypothyroidism, uraemia, liver failure.

Diseases of the extrapyramidal system

Parkinson's disease (paralysis agitans)

In this disease there is gradual destruction of the extrapyramidal neurones that produce dopamine, one of the chemical neurotransmitters. There is lack of control and coordination of muscle movement, resulting in:

- fixed muscle tone causing expressionless facial features, stiff shuffling gait and stooping posture
- muscle tremor, e.g. 'pill rolling' movement of the fingers.

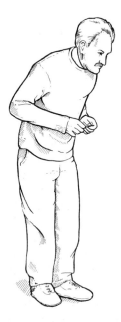

Figure 7.51 Shuffling gait of Parkinson's disease.

The cause is usually unknown but some cases are associated with:

- previous encephalitis lethargica (an epidemic virus disease in the 1920s that died out)
- repeated trauma as in, e.g. 'punch drunk' boxers
- tumours, causing midbrain compression
- drugs, e.g. phenothiazines
- heavy metal poisoning.

There is progressive physical disability but the intellect is not impaired (Fig. 7.51).

INFECTIONS OF THE CENTRAL NERVOUS SYSTEM

The brain and spinal cord are relatively well protected from microbial infection by the blood–brain barrier. When infection does occur microbes may be:

- blood-borne from infection elsewhere in the body, e.g. lung abscess

- introduced through a skull fracture, e.g. infection from the nose through the air sinuses of the frontal, sphenoid or ethmoid bone, from the middle ear through the temporal bone, the skin
- spread through the skull bones from, e.g. middle ear infection, mastoiditis, skull bone infection
- introduced during a surgical procedure, e.g. lumbar puncture.

The microbes usually involved are bacteria and viruses, occasionally protozoa and fungi. The infection may originate in the meninges (*meningitis*) or in the brain (*encephalitis*), then spread from one site to the other.

Pyogenic infection

Pyogenic meningitis

Pyogenic infection of the meninges may remain localised in the extradural or subdural space. If an abscess forms it may rupture into the subarachnoid space and spread to the brain, causing encephalitis and further abscess formation. Infection of the arachnoid mater tends to spread diffusely in the subarachnoid space round the brain and spinal cord.

Pyogenic encephalitis

This may involve single or multiple sites, usually with abscess formation. The microbes are either blood-borne or spread from adjacent meningeal infection. The effects include:

- inflammatory oedema and abscess formation lead to increased ICP, hypoxia and further brain damage.
- when meningitis follows encephalitis, healing takes place with the formation of fibrous adhesions which may interfere with CSF circulation and cause

hydrocephalus, or compress blood vessels, causing hypoxia.
- following encephalitis and brain abscess, healing is associated with gliosis and, as destroyed nerve cells are not replaced, loss of function depends on the site and extent of brain damage.

Virus infections

Virus infections of the nervous system are relatively rare even when caused by *neurotropic viruses*, i.e. those with an affinity for the nervous system. Viruses may cause meningitis, encephalitis or lesions of the neurones of spinal cord and peripheral nerves. Most viruses are blood-borne although a few travel along peripheral nerves, e.g. rabies virus and possibly polioviruses. They enter the body via:

- alimentary tract, e.g. poliomyelitis
- respiratory tract, e.g. shingles
- skin abrasions, e.g. rabies
- insect bites, e.g. encephalitis lethargica.

The effects of virus infections vary according to the site and the amount of tissue destroyed. Viruses are believed to damage nerve cells by:

- 'taking over' their metabolism
- stimulating an immune reaction which may explain why signs of some infections do not appear until there is a high antibody titre, 1 to 2 weeks after infection.

Viral meningitis

This is sometimes called 'aseptic' meningitis because cultures for bacteria are sterile. It is usually a relatively mild infection followed by complete recovery.

Viral encephalitis

Viral encephalitis may affect a wide variety of sites and, as nerve cells are not replaced, loss of function reflects the extent of damage. In severe infection neurones and neuroglia may be affected, followed by necrosis and gliosis. Early senility may develop or, if vital centres in the medulla oblongata are involved, death may ensue. In mild cases recovery is usually complete with little loss of function.

Herpes simplex encephalitis

This is an acute, often fatal, condition causing necrosis of areas of the cerebrum, usually the temporal lobes. If the patient survives the initial acute phase there may be residual dysfunction, e.g. behavioural disturbance and loss of memory.

Herpes zoster neuritis (shingles)

Herpes zoster viruses cause chickenpox (varicella) mainly in children and shingles (zoster) in adults. Susceptible children may contract chickenpox from a shingles sufferer. Adults infected with the viruses may show no immediate signs of disease. The viruses may remain dormant in posterior root ganglia of the spinal nerves then become active years later, causing shingles. The factors believed to reactivate them include:

■ local trauma involving the dermatome, i.e. the area supplied by the affected peripheral nerve
■ exposure of the dermatome to irradiation, e.g. sun, X-rays
■ depression of the immunological system, e.g. by drugs, old age, AIDS.

The posterior root ganglion becomes acutely inflamed. From there the *viruses* pass along the sensory nerve to the surface tissues supplied, e.g. skin, cornea. The tissues become inflamed and vesicles, containing serous fluid and viruses, develop along the course of the nerve. This is accompanied by persistent pain and hypersensitivity to touch (*hyperaesthesia*). Recovery is usually slow and there may be some loss of sensation, depending on the severity of the disease. The infection is usually unilateral and the most common sites are:

■ nerves supplying the trunk, sometimes two or three adjacent dermatomes (Fig. 7.39)
■ the ophthalmic division of the trigeminal nerve, causing *trigeminal neuralgia*, and, if vesicles form on the cornea, there may be ulceration, scarring and residual interference with vision.

Anterior poliomyelitis

This disease is usually caused by *polioviruses* and occasionally by other *enteroviruses*. The infection is spread by food contaminated by infected faecal matter and the initial virus multiplication occurs in the alimentary tract. The viruses are then blood-borne to the nervous system and invade anterior horn cells in the spinal cord. Usually there is a mild febrile illness with no indication of nerve cell damage. Paralytic disease is believed to be precipitated by muscular exercise during the early febrile stage. Irreversible damage to lower motor neurones causes muscle paralysis which, in the limbs, may lead to deformity because of the unopposed tonal contraction of antagonistic muscles. Death may occur due to paralysis of intercostal muscles or the diaphragm, or to destruction of the respiratory centre in the medulla oblongata.

Rabies

All warm-blooded animals are susceptible to the rabies virus, which is endemic in many countries but not in Britain. The main reservoirs of virus are wild animals, some of which may be carriers. These may infect domestic pets which then become the main source of human infection. The viruses multiply in the salivary glands and are present in large numbers in saliva. They enter the body through skin abrasions and are believed to travel to the brain along the nerves or lymph vessels adjacent to nerves. The incubation period varies from about 2 weeks to several months, possibly reflecting the distance viruses travel between the site of entry and the brain. Extensive damage to the basal nuclei, midbrain, medulla oblongata and the posterior root ganglia of the peripheral nerves causes meningeal irritation, extreme hyperaesthesia, muscle spasm and convulsions. *Hydrophobia* and overflow of saliva from the mouth are due to painful spasm of the throat muscles that inhibits swallowing. In the advanced stages muscle spasm may alternate with flaccid paralysis and death is usually due to respiratory muscle spasm or paralysis.

Not all people exposed to the virus contract rabies, but in those who do, the mortality rate is high.

Human immunodeficiency virus

The brain is often affected in indiviuals with AIDS resulting in, e.g.:

■ opportunistic infection
■ dementia.

Creutzfeldt–Jakob disease

This infective condition may be caused by a 'slow' virus the nature and transmission of which is poorly understood. It is a rapidly progressive form of dementia for which there is no known treatment so the condition is always fatal.

Myalgic encephalitis (ME)

This condition is also known as post-viral syndrome or chronic fatigue syndrome. It affects mostly teenagers and young adults and is believed to follow viral infection. The aetiology is unknown. The effects include malaise, severe fatigue, and myalgia. Recovery is usually spontaneous but sometimes results in chronic disability.

DEMYELINATING DISEASES

These diseases are caused either by injury to axons or by disorders of cells that secrete myelin, i.e. oligodendrocytes and Schwann cells.

Multiple (disseminated) sclerosis (MS)

In this disease there are areas of demyelinated white matter, called *plaques*, irregularly distributed throughout the brain and spinal cord. Nerve cells in the brain and spinal cord may also be affected because of the arrangement of satellite oligodendrocytes round cell bodies. In the early stages there may be little damage to axons. It usually develops between the ages of 20 and

40 years and there is an increased incidence of MS among siblings, especially twins, and parents of patients. It is not known whether this is due to genetic or environmental factors or a combination of both. The actual cause(s) of MS are not known but several factors have been suggested, more than one of which may be involved.

Environment before adolescence is suggested because the disease is most prevalent in people who spend their pre-adolescent years in temperate climates, and people who move to other climates after that age retain their susceptibility to MS. People moving into a temperate area during adolescence or later life appear not to be susceptible (Fig. 7.52).

Genetically abnormal myelin is present in many patients and may be antigenic, causing the development of autoimmunity.

Virus infection by slow-growing viruses has been suggested but so far none have been identified.

Effects of multiple sclerosis

Damage to grey matter leads to a variety of dysfunctions, depending on the sites and sizes of demyelinated plaques. Damage to white matter leads to muscle weakness, lack of coordination of movement and disturbed sensation, e.g. burning or pins and needles. The optic nerves are commonly involved early in the disease, leading to visual disturbances, especially blurring and double vision.

The disease pattern is usually one of relapses and remissions of widely varying duration. Each relapse causes further loss of nervous tissue and progressive dysfunction. In some cases there may be chronic progression without remission, or acute disease rapidly leading to death.

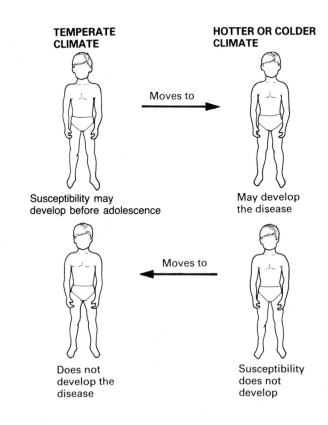

Figure 7.52 Climate and susceptibility to multiple sclerosis.

Acute disseminating encephalomyelitis

This is a rare but serious condition that may occur:

- during or very soon after a virus infection, e.g. measles, chickenpox, mumps, respiratory infection
- following primary immunisation against viral diseases, mainly in older children and adults.

The cause of the acute diffuse demyelination is not known. It has been suggested that autoimmunity to myelin is triggered either by viruses during a virus infection, such as measles or rubella, or by viruses present in vaccines. The effects vary considerably, according to the distribution and degree of demyelination. The early febrile state may progress to paralysis and coma. Most patients survive the initial phase and recover with no residual dysfunction or they may have severe impairment of a wide variety of neurological functions.

PHENYLKETONURIA

Some genetic abnormalities cause deficiency in the production of enzymes required at various stages in metabolic chains. This causes accumulation of the intermediate metabolite that the enzyme should catalyse, and high concentrations of some metabolites are toxic to the nervous system. Phenylketonuria is the most common disease of this type. When the gene necessary for the synthesis of the enzyme *phenylalanine hydroxylase* is absent, the amino acid *phenylalanine* is not converted to *tyrosine* in the liver. The phenylalanine accumulates in liver cells, then overflows into the blood and if not treated it impairs devel-

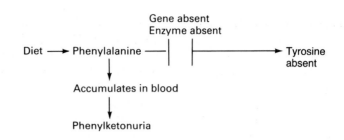

Figure 7.53   Phenylketonuria.

opment of the brain, causing severe mental retardation (Fig. 7.53).

EFFECTS OF POISONS ON THE CENTRAL NERVOUS SYSTEM

Many chemical substances encountered either as drugs or in the environment may damage the nervous system. Neurone metabolism may be disturbed directly or result from damage to other organs, e.g. liver, kidneys. The outcome depends on the toxicity of the substance, the dose and the duration of exposure, ranging from short-term neurological disturbance to encephalopathy which may cause coma and death.

DISEASES OF THE SPINAL CORD

Because space in the neural canal and intervertebral foramina is limited, any condition which distorts their shape or reduces the space may damage the spinal cord or peripheral nerve roots, or cause ischaemia by compressing blood vessels. Such conditions include:

- fracture and/or dislocation of vertebrae

- tumours of the meninges or vertebrae
- prolapsed intervertebral disc.

The effects of disease or injury depend on the severity of the damage, the type and position of the neurones involved, i.e. motor, sensory, proprioceptor, autonomic, connector neurones in reflex arcs in the spinal cord or in peripheral nerves.

Motor neurones

Upper motor neurone (UMN) lesions

Lesions of the UMNs above the level of the decussation of the pyramids affect the opposite side of the body, e.g. haemorrhage or infarction in the internal capsule of one hemisphere causes paralysis of the opposite side of the body. Lesions below the decussation level affect the same side of the body. The lower motor neurones are released from cortical control.

Lower motor neurone (LMN) lesions

The cell bodies of LMNs are in the spinal cord and the axons are part of peripheral nerves. Lesions of LMNs lead to weakness or paralysis of the muscles they supply.

Table 7.5 Summary of effects of damage to motor neurones

Upper motor neurone	Lower motor neurone
Muscle weakness and spastic paralysis	Muscle weakness and flaccid paralysis
Exaggerated tendon reflexes	Absence of tendon reflexes
Muscle twitching	Muscle wasting Contracture of muscles Impaired circulation

Table 7.5 gives a summary of the effects of damage to the motor neurones. The parts of the body affected depend on which neurones have been damaged and their site in the brain, spinal cord or peripheral nerve.

Motor neurone disease

This is a chronic progressive degeneration of motor neurones, occurring mainly in men between 60 and 70 years of age. The cause is not known. Motor neurones in the cerebral cortex, brain stem and anterior horns of the spinal cord are destroyed and replaced by gliosis. Early effects are usually weakness and twitching of the small muscles of the hand, and muscles of the arm and shoulder girdle. The legs are affected later. Death is usually due to the involvement of the respiratory centre in the medulla oblongata.

Sensory neurones

The sensory functions lost as a result of disease or injury depend on which neurones have been damaged and their position in the brain or spinal cord, or the peripheral nerve involved. In the brain, neurones connecting the thalamus and the cerebrum pass through the internal capsule. Damage in this area by, e.g. haemorrhage, usually from a berry aneurysm, may lead to loss of sensation but does not affect cerebellar function unless upper motor neurones have also been damaged. Spinal cord damage leads to loss of sensation and cerebellar function. Peripheral nerve damage leads to loss of reflex activity, loss of sensation and of cerebellar function.

Mixed motor and sensory conditions

Spinal cord

Subacute combined degeneration of the spinal cord

This condition most commonly occurs as a complication of pernicious anaemia. Vitamin B_{12} is associated with the formation and maintenance of myelin by Schwann cells and oligodendrocytes. Although degeneration of the spinal cord may be apparent before the anaemia it is arrested by treatment with vitamin B_{12}. This type of degeneration may occasionally complicate chronic conditions, such as diabetes mellitus, leukaemia, carcinoma.

The degeneration of nerve fibre myelin occurs in the posterior and lateral columns of white matter in the spinal cord, especially in the upper thoracic and lower cervical regions. Less frequently the changes occur in the posterior root ganglia and peripheral nerves. Demyelination of proprioceptor fibres leads to ataxia and involvement of upper motor neurones leads to increased muscle tone and spastic paralysis.

Compression of the spinal cord and nerve roots

The causes include:

- prolapsed intervertebral disc
- syringomyelia
- tumours: metastatic, meningeal or nerve sheath
- fractures with displacement of bone fragments.

Prolapsed intervertebral disc (Fig. 7.54)

This is the most common cause of compression of the spinal cord and/or nerve roots. The bodies of the vertebrae are separated by the intervertebral discs, each consisting of an outer rim of cartilage, the *annulus fibrosus*, and a central core of soft gelatinous material, the *nucleus pulposus*.

Prolapse of a disc is herniation of the nucleus pulposus, causing the annulus fibrosus and the posterior longitudinal ligament to protrude into the neural canal. It is most common in the lumbar region usually below the level of the spinal cord, i.e. below L2, so the injury is to nerve roots only. If it occurs in the cervical region, the cord may also be compressed. Herniation may occur suddenly or progressively due to one or more of the following factors: lifting weights using the back instead of the legs, bone disease, disc degeneration. The hernia may be:

- one-sided, causing pressure damage to a nerve root
- midline, compressing the spinal cord, the anterior spinal artery and possibly bilateral nerve roots.

The outcome depends upon the size of the hernia and the length of time the pressure is applied. Small herniations cause local pain due to pressure on the nerve endings in the posterior longitudinal ligament.

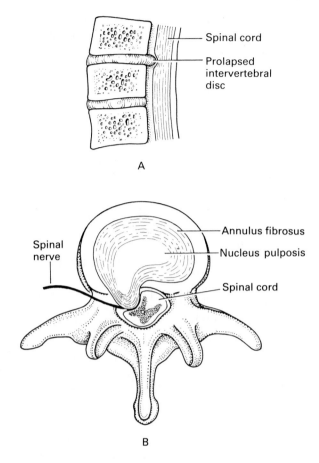

Figure 7.54 Prolapsed intervertebral disc. A. Viewed from the side. B. Viewed from above.

Large herniations may cause:

■ unilateral or bilateral paralysis
■ acute or chronic pain perceived to originate from the area supplied by the compressed sensory nerve, e.g. in the leg or foot
■ compression of the anterior spinal artery, causing ischaemia and possibly necrosis of the spinal cord
■ local muscle spasm due to pressure on motor nerves.

Syringomyelia

This dilatation of the central canal of the spinal cord occurs most commonly in the cervical region and is associated with congenital abnormality of the distal end of the fourth ventricle. As the central canal dilates, pressure causes progressive damage to sensory and motor neurones. Early effects include dissociated anaesthesia. i.e. insensibility to heat and pain, due to compression of the sensory fibres that cross the cord immediately they enter. In the long term there is destruction of motor and sensory tracts, leading to spastic paralysis and loss of sensation and reflexes.

Tumours and displaced fragments of fractured vertebrae

These may affect the spinal cord and nerve roots at any level. The pressure damage initially causes pain and later, if the pressure is not relieved, there may be loss of sensation and paralysis. The areas affected depend on the site of pressure.

DISEASES OF PERIPHERAL NERVES

Neuropathies

This is a group of diseases of peripheral nerves not associated with inflammation. They are classified as:

■ parenchymal, i.e. affecting neurones and/or myelin production and maintenance
■ interstitial, i.e. affecting blood vessels and/or connective tissue adjacent to nerves.

Parenchymal neuropathies

Polyneuropathy or damage to a number of neurones and their myelin sheaths occurs in, e.g.:

■ nutritional deficiencies, e.g. folic acid, vitamins B_1, B_2, B_6, B_{12}
■ metabolic disorders, e.g. diabetes mellitus
■ chronic diseases, e.g. renal failure, hepatic failure, carcinoma
■ toxic reactions to, e.g. lead, arsenic, mercury, carbon tetrachloride, aniline dyes and some drugs, such as phenytoin, chloroquine
■ infections, e.g. influenza, measles, typhoid fever, diphtheria, leprosy.

The long neurones are usually affected first, e.g. those supplying the feet and legs. The outcome depends upon the cause of the neuropathy and the extent of the damage.

Interstitial neuropathy

Usually only one neurone is damaged and the most common cause is ischaemia, due to:

- pressure applied to cranial nerves in cranial bone foramina due to distortion of the brain by increased ICP
- compression of a nerve in a confined space caused by surrounding inflammation and oedema, e.g. the median nerve in the carpal tunnel (see p. 404)
- external pressure on a nerve, e.g. an unconscious person lying with an arm hanging over the side of a bed or trolley
- compression of the axillary (circumflex) nerve by ill-fitting crutches
- trapping a nerve between the broken ends of a bone
- ischaemia due to thrombosis of blood vessels supplying a nerve.

The resultant dysfunction depends on the site and extent of the injury.

Neuritis

Acute idiopathic inflammatory polyneuropathy (Guillain–Barré syndrome)

This is a sudden, acute, progressive, bilateral ascending paralysis, beginning in the lower limbs and spreading to the arms, trunk and cranial nerves. It usually occurs 1 to 3 weeks after an upper respiratory tract infection. There is widespread inflammation accompanied by some demyelination of spinal, peripheral and cranial nerves and the spinal ganglia. Paralysis may affect all the limbs and the respiratory muscles. Patients who survive the acute phase usually recover completely in weeks or months.

Bell's palsy

Compression of a facial nerve in the temporal bone foramen causes paralysis of facial muscles on the affected side. The immediate cause is inflammation and oedema of the nerve but the underlying cause is unknown. The onset may be sudden or develop over several hours. Distortion of the features is due to muscle tone on the unaffected side, the affected side being expressionless. Recovery is usually complete within a few months.

DEVELOPMENTAL ABNORMALITIES OF THE NERVOUS SYSTEM

Spina bifida

This is a congenital malformation of the neural canal and spinal cord (Fig. 7.55). The neural arches of the vertebrae and dura mater are defective, most commonly in the lumbosacral region. The causes are not known. They may be of genetic origin or due to maternal upset, such as hypoxia, at a critical stage in development of the fetal vertebrae and spinal cord. The effects depend on the extent of the abnormality.

Occult spina bifida

The skin over the defect is intact and excessive growth of hair over the site may be the only sign of abnormality.

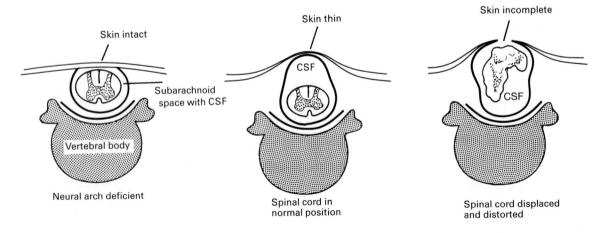

Figure 7.55 Spina bifida. A. Spina bifida occulta. B. Meningocele. C. Meningomyelocele.

Meningocele

The skin over the defect is very thin and there is dilatation of the subarachnoid space posteriorly. The spinal cord is correctly positioned.

Meningomyelocele

The subarachnoid space is dilated posteriorly, the spinal cord is displaced backwards and may be adherent to the posterior wall of the arachnoid dilatation. The skin is often deficient with leakage of CSF, and the meninges may become infected.

Hydrocephalus

(see p. 178)

TUMOURS OF THE NERVOUS SYSTEM

Most tumours of the nervous system are of neuroglial origin. Neurones are rarely involved because they do not normally multiply. Metastases of nervous tissue tumours are rare. Because of this, the rate of growth of a tumour is more important than the likelihood of spread outside the nervous system. In this context, 'benign' means slow-growing and 'malignant' rapid-growing. Signs of raised ICP appear after the limits of compensation have been reached.

Slow-growing tumours

These allow time for adjustment to compensate for increasing intracranial pressure, so the tumour may be quite large before its effects are evident. Compensation involves gradual reduction in the volume of cerebrospinal fluid and circulating blood.

Rapid-growing tumours

These do not allow time for adjustment to compensate for the rapidly increasing ICP, so the effects quickly become apparent. Complications include:

- neurological impairment, depending on tumour site and size
- effects of increased ICP (p. 177)
- necrosis of the tumour, causing haemorrhage and oedema.

Gliomas are usually astrocytomas, ranging from benign tumours to the highly malignant *glioblastoma multiforme*.

Meningiomas are usually benign, originating from arachnoid granulations.

Medulloblastomas are highly malignant neurone-cell tumours, occurring mainly in the cerebellum in children. They are believed to originate from primitive cells prior to differentiation into neurones and neuroglia.

Metastases in the brain

The most common primary sites are the breast, lungs and bone marrow (leukaemias). There are two forms:

- discrete multiple tumours, mainly in the cerebrum
- diffuse tumours in the arachnoid mater.

8
The special senses

The special senses of hearing, sight, smell and taste all have specialised nerve endings at the periphery, i.e. in the ears, eyes, nose and mouth, and in the brain. In the brain the incoming nerve impulses undergo complex processes of integration and coordination that result in perception and a variety of responses inside and outside the body. The ear is also involved in the maintenance of balance.

HEARING AND THE EAR

The ear is the organ of hearing. It is supplied by the eighth *cranial nerve*, i.e. the *cochlear part* of the *vestibulocochlear* nerve which is stimulated by vibrations caused by sound waves.

With the exception of the auricle (pinna), the structures that form the ear are encased within the petrous portion of the temporal bone.

Structure

The ear is divided into three distinct parts (Figs 8.1 and 8.7):

■ external ear
■ middle ear (tympanic cavity)
■ internal ear.

External ear

The external ear consists of the auricle (pinna) and the external acoustic meatus.

The auricle (pinna) (Fig. 8.2)
The auricle is the expanded portion projecting from the side of the head. It is composed of *fibroelastic cartilage* covered with skin. It is deeply grooved and ridged and the most prominent outer ridge is the *helix*.

The lobule is the soft pliable part at the lower extremity, composed of fibrous and adipose tissue richly supplied with blood capillaries.

External acoustic meatus (auditory canal)
This is a slightly 'S'-shaped tube about 2.5 cm long extending from the auricle to the *tympanic membrane* (ear drum). The lateral third is cartilaginous and the remainder is a canal in the temporal bone. The meatus is lined with hairy skin, continuous with that of the auricle. There are numerous *sebaceous* and *ceruminous*

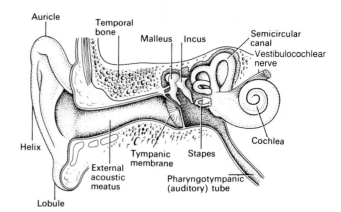

Figure 8.1 The parts of the ear.

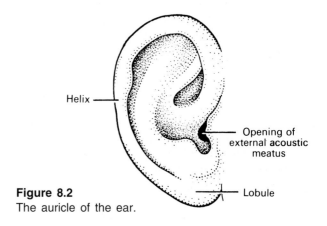

Figure 8.2
The auricle of the ear.

glands in the skin of the lateral third. Ceruminous glands are modified sweat glands that secrete *cerumen* (wax), a sticky material containing lysozyme and immunoglobulins. Foreign materials, e.g. dust, insects and microbes, are prevented from reaching the tympanic membrane by wax, hairs and the curvature of the meatus. Movements of the temporomandibular joint during chewing and speaking 'massage' the cartilaginous meatus, moving the wax towards the exterior.

The tympanic membrane (ear drum) (Fig. 8.3) completely separates the external acoustic meatus from the middle ear. It is oval-shaped with the slightly broader edge upwards and is formed by three types of tissue:

■ the outer covering of *hairless skin*
■ the middle layer of *fibrous tissue*
■ the inner lining of *mucous membrane* continuous with that of the middle ear.

Tympanic cavity or middle ear

This is an irregular-shaped cavity within the petrous portion of the temporal bone. The cavity, its contents

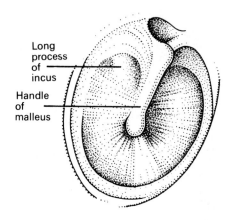

Figure 8.3 The tympanic membrane viewed through an auriscope showing the shadows cast by the malleus and the incus.

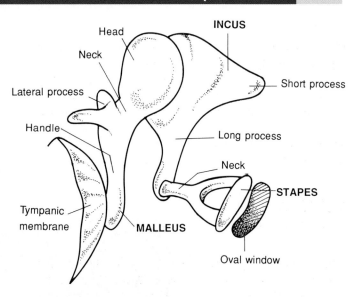

Figure 8.4 The auditory ossicles.

and the air sacs which open out of it are lined with either simple squamous or cuboidal epithelium. Air fills the cavity, reaching it through the *pharyngotympanic (auditory or Eustachian) tube* which extends from the nasopharynx. It is about 4 cm long and is lined with ciliated epithelium. The presence of air at atmospheric pressure on both sides of the tympanic membrane is maintained by the pharyngotympanic tube and enables the membrane to vibrate when sound waves strike it. The pharyngotympanic tube is normally closed but when there is unequal pressure across the tympanic membrane, e.g. at high altitude, it is opened by swallowing or yawning and the ears 'pop' equalising the pressure again.

The lateral wall of the middle ear is formed by the tympanic membrane.

The roof and floor are formed by the temporal bone.

The posterior wall is formed by the temporal bone with openings leading to the *mastoid antrum* through which air passes to the mastoid air cells.

The medial wall is a thin layer of temporal bone in which there are two openings:

■ oval window (fenestra vestibuli)
■ round window (fenestra cochleae).

The oval window is occluded by part of a small bone called the *stapes* and the round window, by a fine sheet of *fibrous tissue.*

Auditory ossicles (Fig. 8.4)

These are three very small bones that extend across the cavity from the tympanic membrane to the oval window (Fig. 8.1). They form a series of movable joints with each other and with the medial wall of the cavity at the oval window. They are: the *malleus, incus* and *stapes.*

The malleus is the lateral hammer-shaped bone. The handle is in contact with the tympanic membrane and the head forms a movable joint with the incus.

The incus is the middle anvil-shaped bone. Its body articulates with the malleus, the long process with the stapes, and it is stabilised by the short process, fixed by fibrous tissue to the posterior wall of the cavity.

The stapes is the medial stirrup-shaped bone. Its head articulates with the incus and its footplate fits into the oval window.

The three ossicles are held in position by fine ligaments.

Internal ear (Fig. 8.5)

The internal ear contains the organs of hearing and balance and is generally described in two parts, the *bony labyrinth* and the *membranous labyrinth.*

Bony labyrinth

This is a cavity within the temporal bone lined with periosteum. It is larger than, and encloses, the membranous labyrinth of the same shape which fits into it, like a tube within a tube. Between the bony and membranous labyrinths there is a layer of watery fluid called *perilymph* and within the membranous labyrinth there is a similarly watery *endolymph.*

The bony labyrinth consists of:

■ 1 vestibule
■ 1 cochlea
■ 3 semicircular canals.

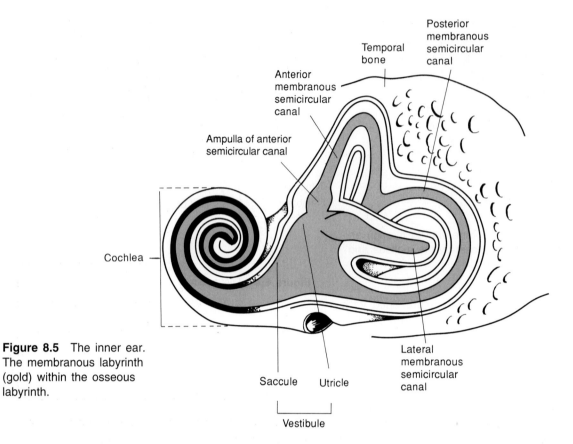

Figure 8.5 The inner ear. The membranous labyrinth (gold) within the osseous labyrinth.

Figure 8.6 A cross-section of the membranous cochlea showing the spiral organ (of Corti).

The vestibule is the expanded part nearest the middle ear. It contains the oval and round windows in its lateral wall.

The cochlea resembles a snail's shell. It has a broad base where it is continuous with the vestibule and a narrow apex, and it spirals round a central bony column.

The semicircular canals are three tubes arranged so that one is situated in each of the three planes of space. They are continuous with the vestibule.

Membranous labyrinth

The membranous labyrinth is the same shape as its bony counterpart and is separated from it by perilymph. It contains endolymph. It is divided into the same parts: the vestibule which contains the *utricle* and *saccule*, the cochlea and three semicircular canals (Fig. 8.5).

A cross-section (Fig. 8.6) shows the triangular shape of the membranous cochlea. Neuroepithelial cells and their nerve fibres lie on the *basilar membrane* or base of the triangle. Many of the neuroepithelial cells are long and narrow and are arranged side by side. These cell bodies and their nerve fibres form the the *spiral organ* (of Corti), the peripheral sensory organ that responds to vibration by initiating nerve impulses, eventually per-ceived as hearing by the brain. The nerve fibres combine to form the *auditory part of the vestibulocochlear nerve* (8th cranial nerve), which passes through a foramen in the temporal bone to reach the hearing area in the temporal lobe of the cerebrum.

Physiology of hearing

Every sound produces *sound waves* or vibrations in the air, which travel at about 332 metres (1088 feet) per second. The auricle, because of its shape, concentrates the waves and directs them along the auditory meatus causing the tympanic membrane to vibrate. Tympanic membrane vibrations are transmitted through the middle ear by movement of the ossicles (Fig. 8.7). At their medial end the footplate of the stapes rocks to and fro in the oval window, setting up fluid waves in the perilymph. These indent the membranous labyrinth, causing a wave motion in the endolymph, which stimulates the neuroepithelial cells of the spiral organ. The nerve impulses generated pass to the brain in the cochlear portion of the *vestibulocochlear nerve* (8th cranial nerve). The fluid wave is finally expended into the middle ear by vibration of the membrane of the round window. The vestibulocochlear nerve transmits the impulses to the hearing area in the cerebrum where sound is perceived and to various nuclei in the pons varolii and the midbrain.

Sound waves have properties of *pitch* and *volume*, or intensity (Fig. 8.8). Pitch is determined by the frequency of the sound waves and is measured in hertz (Hz). The volume depends on the amplitude of the sound waves and is measured in decibels (dB). Very loud noise is damaging to the ear.

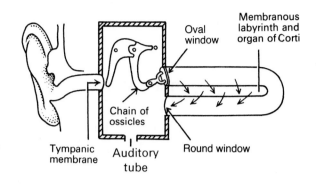

Figure 8.7A Diagram of the ear showing the passage of sound waves. The cochlea has been uncoiled.

EXTERNAL EAR	MIDDLE EAR	INNER EAR	
Sound waves in air	Mechanical movement of ossicles	Perilymph Fluid wave	Endolymph Fluid wave → Organ of corti → Fluid wave
Tympanic membrane	Oval window	Cochlear membrane	Round window

Figure 8.7B Summary of the transmission of sound through the ear.

Because of the structure of the basilar membrane sounds of different frequencies stimulate it at different places along its length allowing discrimination of pitch. Additionally, the greater the amplitude of the wave created in the endolymph, the greater the stimulation

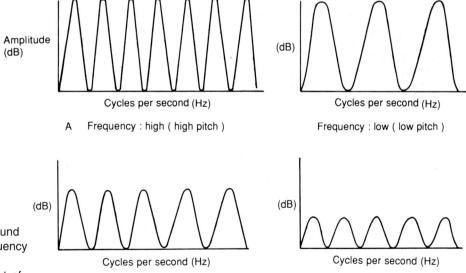

Figure 8.8 Behaviour of sound waves. A. Difference in frequency but of the same amplitude. B. Difference in amplitude but of the same frequency.

A   Frequency : high (high pitch)

Frequency : low (low pitch)

B   Amplitude : high (high volume)

Amplitude : low (low volume)

of the neuroepithelial cells in the spiral organ, enabling distinction of volume.

Semicircular canals and vestibule

The semicircular canals have no auditory function although they are closely associated with the cochlea. They provide information about the position of the head in space, contributing to maintenance of equilibrium and balance.

There are three semicircular canals, one lying in each of the three planes of space. They are situated above and behind the vestibule of the inner ear and open into it.

Structure (Fig. 8.9)

The semicircular canals, like the cochlea, are composed of an outer bony wall and inner membranous tubes or *ducts*. The membranous ducts contain endolymph and are separated from the bony wall by perilymph.

The utricle is a membranous sac which is part of the vestibule and the three membranous ducts open into it at their dilated ends, the *ampullae*. The *saccule* is a part of the vestibule and communicates with the utricle and the cochlea.

In the walls of the utricle, saccule and ampullae there are fine specialised epithelial cells with minute projections, called *hair cells*. Amongst the hair cells there

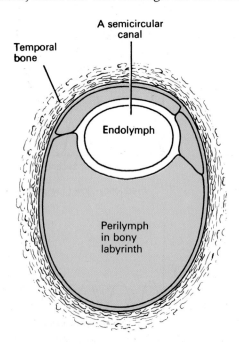

Figure 8.9 Transverse section of a semicircular canal.

are the minute nerve endings of the *vestibular part* of the vestibulocochlear nerve.

Physiology of balance

The semicircular canals, utricle and saccule are concerned with balance (Fig. 8.5). Any change of position of the head causes movement in the perilymph and endolymph which stimulates the nerve endings and the hair cells in the utricle, saccule and ampullae. The resultant nerve impulses are transmitted by the vestibular nerve which joins the cochlear nerve to form the *vestibulocochlear nerve*. The vestibular branch passes first to the *vestibular nucleus*, then to the *cerebellum*.

The cerebellum also receives nerve impulses from the eyes and the muscles and joints. Impulses from these three sources are coordinated and efferent nerve impulses pass to the cerebrum where position in space is perceived, and to skeletal muscles, maintaining posture and balance.

SIGHT AND THE EYE

The eye is the organ of the sense of sight situated in the orbital cavity and it is supplied by the *optic nerve* (2nd cranial nerve).

It is almost spherical in shape and is about 2.5 cm in diameter. The space between the eye and the orbital cavity is occupied by fatty tissue. The bony walls of the orbit and the fat help to protect the eye from injury.

Structurally the two eyes are separate but, unlike the ear, some of their activities are coordinated so that they function as a pair. It is possible to see with only one eye but three-dimensional vision is impaired when only one eye is used, especially in relation to the judgement of distance.

Structure (Fig. 8.10)

There are three layers of tissue in the walls of the eye. They are:

- the outer fibrous layer: sclera and cornea
- the middle vascular layer: choroid, ciliary body and iris
- the inner nervous tissue layer: retina.

Structures inside the eyeball are the lens, aqueous fluid (humour) and vitreous body.

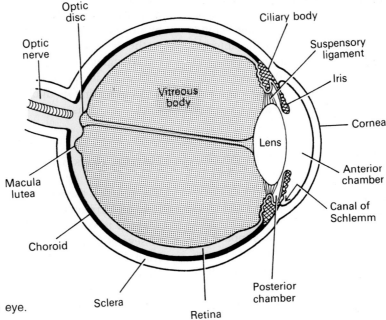

Figure 8.10 Section of the eye.

Sclera and cornea

The sclera, or white of the eye, forms the outermost layer of tissue of the posterior and lateral aspects of the eyeball and is continuous anteriorly with the transparent *cornea*. It consists of a firm fibrous membrane that maintains the shape of the eye and gives attachment to the *extraocular* or *extrinsic muscles* of the eye (p. 203).

Anteriorly the sclera continues as a clear transparent epithelial membrane, the *cornea*. Light rays pass through the cornea to reach the retina. The cornea is convex anteriorly and is involved in *refracting* or bending light rays to focus them on the retina.

Choroid (Figs 8.10 and 8.11)

The choroid lines the posterior five-sixths of the inner surface of the sclera. It is very rich in blood vessels and is a deep chocolate brown in colour. Light enters the eye through the pupil, stimulates the nerve endings in the retina then is absorbed by the choroid.

Ciliary body

The ciliary body is the anterior continuation of the choroid consisting of non-striated muscle fibres (*ciliary muscle*) and secretory epithelial cells. It gives attachment to the *suspensory ligament* which, at its other end, is attached to the capsule enclosing the lens. Contraction and relaxation of the ciliary muscle changes

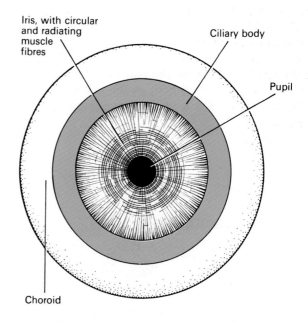

Figure 8.11 The choroid, ciliary body and iris. Viewed from the front.

the thickness of the lens which *bends*, or *refracts* light rays entering the eye to focus them on the retina. The epithelial cells secrete *aqueous fluid* into the anterior segment of the eye, i.e. the space between the lens and the cornea. The ciliary body is supplied by parasympathetic branches of the oculomotor nerve (3rd cranial nerve). Stimulation causes contraction of the muscle and accommodation of the eye (p. 202).

Iris

The iris is the visible coloured part of the eye and extends anteriorly from the ciliary body, lying behind the cornea in front of the lens. It divides the anterior segment of the eye into *anterior* and *posterior chambers* which contain *aqueous fluid* secreted by the ciliary body. It is a circular body composed of pigment cells and two layers of muscle fibres, one circular and the other radiating (Fig. 8.11). In the centre there is an aperture, the *pupil*.

The pupil varies in size depending upon the intensity of light. In bright light the circular muscle fibres of the iris contract and *constrict the pupil*. In dim light the radiating muscle fibres contract *dilating the pupil*.

The iris is supplied by parasympathetic and sympathetic nerves. Parasympathetic stimulation, supplied by the oculomotor nerve, constricts the pupil and sympathetic stimulation from the superior cervical ganglion dilates the pupil.

The colour of the iris is genetically determined and depends on the number of pigment cells present. Albinos have no pigment cells and people with blue eyes have fewer than those with brown eyes.

Lens (Fig. 8.12)

The lens is a *highly elastic* circular biconvex transparent body, lying immediately behind the pupil. It is suspended from the ciliary body by the *suspensory ligament* and enclosed within a transparent capsule. Its thickness is controlled by the ciliary muscle through the suspensory ligament. The lens bends light rays reflected by objects in front of the eye. It is the only structure in the eye that can vary its refractory power, achieved by changing its thickness. When the ciliary muscle contracts, it *moves forward*, releasing its pull on the lens, increasing its thickness. The nearer the object the thicker the lens.

Retina (Figs 8.13 and 8.14)

The retina is the innermost layer of the wall of the eye. It is an extremely delicate structure and is especially adapted to be stimulated by light rays. It is composed of several layers of nerve cell bodies and their fibres, lying on a pigmented layer of epithelial cells which attach it to the choroid. The layer highly sensitive to light is the *layer of rods and cones*.

The retina lines about three-quarters of the eyeball and is thickest at the back and thins out anteriorly to end just behind the ciliary body. Near the centre of the posterior part there is an area that appears yellow in colour, hence the name, *macula lutea*. In the centre of the area there is a little depression called the *fovea centralis*, consisting of only *cone-shaped cells*. Towards the anterior part of the retina there are fewer cone- than rod-shaped cells (Fig. 8.13).

The rods and cones contain photosensitive pigments involved in the conversion of light rays into nerve impulses. *Rhodopsin* (visual purple) is a pigment present in rods. It is degraded or *bleached* when exposed to light and its regeneration requires the presence of vitamin A. The time taken for the regeneration of rhodopsin, called *dark-adaptation*, is experienced when an individual moves from an area of bright light to one of darkness. Other pigments present in cones respond to different wavelengths of visible light and are responsible for colour vision. Rhodopsin is bleached by lower light intensity than the pigments in cones, e.g. as light intensity is reduced the shape of an object remains clear after its colour can no longer be seen.

About 0.5 cm to the nasal side of the macula lutea all the nerve fibres of the retina converge to form the *optic nerve* which passes through the sphenoid bone, eventually to reach the cerebral cortex in the occipital lobe of the cerebrum. The small area of retina where the optic nerve leaves the eye is the *optic disc* or *blind spot*. It has no light-sensitive cells.

Blood supply to the eye

The eye is supplied with arterial blood by the *ciliary arteries* and the *central retinal artery*. These are branches

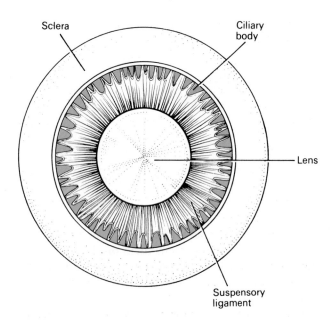

Figure 8.12 The lens and suspensory ligament viewed from the front. The iris has been removed.

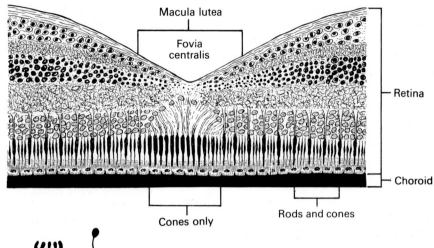

Figure 8.13A Magnified section of the retina.

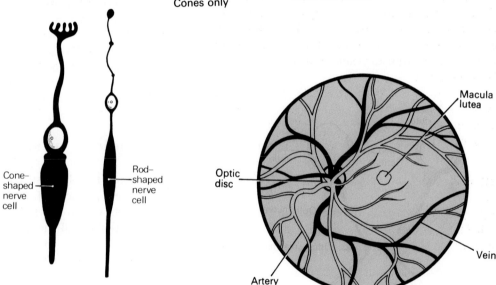

Figure 8.13B Cone- and rod-shaped cells in the retina.

Figure 8.14 The retina as seen through the pupil with an ophthalmoscope.

of the ophthalmic artery, one of the branches of the internal carotid artery.

Venous drainage is by a number of veins, including the *central retinal vein*, which eventually empty into the cavernous sinus.

The central retinal artery and vein are encased in the optic nerve, entering the eye at the optic disc.

Interior of the eyeball

The anterior segment of the eye, i.e. the space between the cornea and the lens, is incompletely divided into *anterior* and *posterior chambers* by the iris. Both chambers contain a clear *aqueous fluid (humour)* secreted into the posterior chamber by ciliary glands. It passes in front of the lens, through the pupil into the anterior chamber and returns to the venous circulation through the *canal of Schlemm* (scleral venous sinus) in the angle between the iris and cornea (Fig. 8.10). There is con-

tinuous production and drainage but the intraocular pressure remains fairly constant between 1.3 and 2.6 kPa (10 to 20 mmHg). An increase in the pressure causes *glaucoma* (p. 211). Aqueous fluid supplies nutrients and removes waste from the transparent structures in the front of the eye that have no blood supply, i.e. the cornea, lens and lens capsule.

Behind the lens and filling the cavity of the eyeball is the *vitreous body (humour)*. This is a soft, colourless, transparent, jelly-like substance composed of 99% water, some salts and mucoprotein. It maintains sufficient intraocular pressure to support the retina against the choroid and prevent the walls of the eyeball from collapsing.

The eye keeps its shape because of the intraocular pressure exerted by the vitreous body and the aqueous fluid. It remains fairly constant throughout life.

Optic nerves (second cranial nerves) (Fig. 8.15)

The fibres of the optic nerve originate in the retina of the eye. All the fibres converge to form the optic nerve about 0.5 cm to the nasal side of the macula lutea. The nerve pierces the choroid and sclera to pass backwards and medially through the orbital cavity. It then passes through the optic foramen of the sphenoid bone, backwards and medially to meet the nerve from the other eye at the *optic chiasma*.

Optic chiasma

This is situated immediately in front of and above the pituitary gland which is in the hypophyseal fossa of the sphenoid bone. In the optic chiasma the nerve fibres of the optic nerve from the *nasal side of each retina cross over* to the *opposite side*. The fibres from the *temporal side* do not cross but continue backwards on the same side.

Optic tracts

These are the pathways of the optic nerves, posterior to the optic chiasma. Each tract consists of the nasal fibres from the retina of one eye and the temporal fibres from the retina of the other. The optic tracts pass backwards through the cerebrum to synapse with nerve cells of the *lateral geniculate bodies* of the thalamus. From there the nerve fibres proceed backwards and medially as the *optic radiations* to terminate in the *visual area* of the cerebral cortex in the occipital lobes of the cerebrum. Other neurones originating in the lateral geniculate bodies convey impulses from the eyes to the *cerebellum* where, together with impulses from the semicircular canals of the ears and from the skeletal muscles and joints, they contribute to the maintenance of balance.

Physiology of sight

Light waves travel at a speed of 186 000 miles (300 000 kilometres) per second. Light is reflected into the eyes by objects within the field of vision. White light is a combination of all the colours of the visual spectrum (rainbow), i.e. red, orange, yellow, green, blue, indigo and violet. This can be demonstrated by passing white light through a glass prism which *refracts* or bends the rays of the different colours to a greater or lesser extent, depending on their wavelengths. Red light has the longest wavelength and violet the shortest (Fig. 8.16).

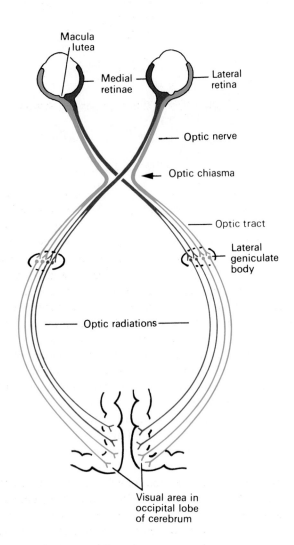

Figure 8.15 The optic nerves and their pathways.

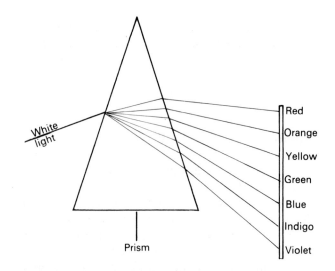

Figure 8.16 White light broken into the colours of the visible spectrum when passed through a prism.

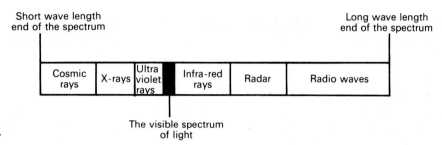

Figure 8.17 The spectrum of light.

This range of colour is the *spectrum of visible light*. In a rainbow, white light from the sun is broken up by raindrops which act as prisms and reflectors.

The spectrum of light

The spectrum of light is broad but only a small part is visible to the human eye (Fig. 8.17). Beyond the long end there are infrared (heat), radar and radio waves. Beyond the short end there are ultraviolet (UV), X-ray and gamma waves. UV light is not normally visible because it is absorbed by a yellow pigment in the lens. Following removal of the lens (cataract extraction), UV light is visible and it has been suggested that long-term exposure may damage the retina.

A specific colour is perceived when only one wavelength is *reflected* by the object and all the others are *absorbed*, e.g. an object appears red when only the red wavelength is reflected. Objects appear white when all wavelengths are reflected, and black when they are all absorbed.

In order to achieve clear vision, light reflected from objects within the visual field is focused on to the retina of both eyes. The processes involved in producing a clear image are *refraction of the light rays*, changing the *size of the pupils* and *accommodation of the eyes*.

Although these may be considered as separate processes, effective vision is dependent upon their coordination.

Refraction of the light rays

When light rays pass from a medium of one density to a medium of a different density they are refracted or bent (Fig. 8.18). This principle is used in the eye to focus light on the retina. Before reaching the retina light rays pass successively through the conjunctiva, cornea, aqueous fluid, lens and vitreous body. They are all more dense than air and, with the exception of the lens, they have a constant refractory power, similar to that of water. The conjunctiva plays a minor part in refraction.

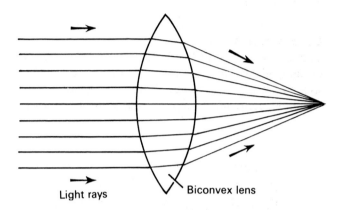

Figure 8.18 Refraction of light rays passing through media of different densities.

Lens

The lens is a biconvex elastic transparent body suspended behind the iris from the ciliary body by the suspensory ligament. It is the only structure in the eye that changes its refractive power. All light rays entering the eye need to be bent (refracted) to focus them on the retina. Light from distant objects needs least refraction and, as the object comes closer, the amount needed is increased. To increase the refractive power the ciliary muscle contracts, releasing its pull on the suspensory ligament and the anterior surface of the lens bulges forward, increasing its convexity. When the ciliary muscle relaxes it slips backwards, increasing its pull on the suspensory ligament, making the lens thinner (Fig. 8.19).

Size of the pupils

Pupil size influences accommodation by controlling the amount of light entering the eye. In a bright light the pupils are constricted. In a dim light they are dilated.

If the pupils were dilated in a bright light, too much light would enter the eye and damage the retina. In a dim light, if the pupils were constricted, insufficient light would enter the eye to activate the photosensitive pigments in the rods and cones which stimulate the nerve endings in the retina.

The iris consists of one layer of circular and one of radiating smooth muscle fibres. Contraction of the circular fibres constricts the pupil, and contraction of the radiating fibres dilates it. The size of the pupil is controlled by nerves of the autonomic nervous system. Sympathetic stimulation dilates the pupils and parasympathetic stimulation causes constriction.

Accommodation of the eyes to light
(Figs 8.19 and 8.20)

Close vision
In order to focus on near objects, i.e. within about 6 meters, the eye must make the following adjustments:

- constriction of the pupils
- convergence of the eyeballs
- changing the power of the lens.

Constriction of the pupils assists accommodation by reducing the width of the beam of light entering the eye so that it passes through the central curved part of the lens. Looking at near objects 'tires' the eyes more quickly, due to the continuous use of the ciliary muscle.

Convergence (movement of the eyeballs). Light rays from nearby objects enter the two eyes at different angles and for clear vision they must stimulate *corresponding areas* of the two retinae. Extraocular muscles move the eyes and to obtain a clear image they rotate the eyes so that they *converge* on the object viewed. This coordinated muscle activity is under autonomic control. When there is voluntary movement of the eyes both eyes move and convergence is maintained. The nearer an object is to the eyes the greater the eye rotation needed to achieve convergence, e.g. an individual focusing near the tip of his nose appears to be 'cross-eyed'. If convergence is not complete there is double vision, *diplopia*. After a period of time during which convergence is not possible the brain tends to ignore the impulses received from the divergent eye (squint p. 211).

Changing the power of the lens. Changes in the thickness of the lens are made to focus light on the retina. The amount of adjustment depends on the distance of the object from the eyes, i.e. the lens is thicker for near vision and at its thinnest when focusing on objects at more than 6 meters' distance (Fig. 8.19).

Distant vision. Objects more than 6 meters away from the eyes are focused on the retina without adjustment of the lens or convergence of the eyes.

Functions of the retina

The retina is the *photosensitive* part of the eye. The light-sensitive nerve cells are the *rods* and *cones*. Light rays cause chemical changes in photosensitive pigments in these cells and they emit nerve impulses which pass to the occipital lobes of the cerebrum via the optic nerves.

The rods are more sensitive than the cones. They are stimulated by *low-intensity or dim light*, e.g. by the dim light in the interior of a darkened room.

The cones are sensitive to *bright light and colour.* The different wavelengths of light stimulate photosensitive pigments in the cones, resulting in the perception of different colours. In a bright light the light rays are focused on the macula lutea.

The rods are more numerous towards the periphery of the retina. *Visual purple (rhodopsin)* is a photosensitive pigment present only in the rods. It is bleached by

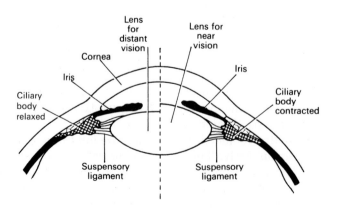

Figure 8.19   Diagram of the difference in the shape of the lens for near and distant vision.

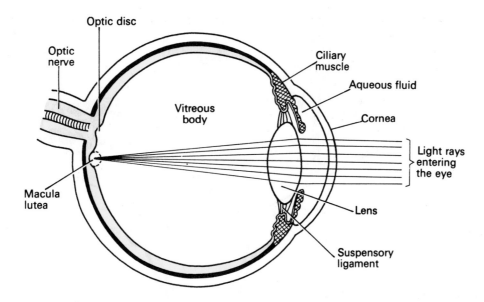

Figure 8.20 Section of the eye showing the focusing of light rays on the retina.

bright light and when this occurs the rods cannot be stimulated. Rhodopsin is quickly reconstituted when an adequate supply of vitamin A is available. When the individual moves from an area of bright light to one of dim light there is a variable period of time when it is difficult to see. The rate at which *dark adaptation* takes place is dependent upon the rate of reconstitution of rhodopsin. It is easier to see a dim star in the sky at night if the head is turned slightly away from it because light of low intensity is focused on the area of the retina where there is the greatest concentration of rods. If looked at directly the light intensity is not sufficient to stimulate the less sensitive cones in the area of the macula lutea. In dim evening light different colours cannot be distinguished because the light intensity is insufficient to stimulate colour-sensitive pigments in cones.

It is believed that the breakdown and reconstitution of the visual pigments in cones is similar to that of rods, but requires a stronger stimulus.

Binocular vision (Fig. 8.21)

Binocular or stereoscopic vision has certain advantages. Each eye 'sees' a scene slightly differently. There is an overlap in the middle but the left eye sees more on the left than can be seen by the other eye and vice versa. The images from the two eyes are fused in the cerebrum so that only one image is perceived.

Binocular vision provides a much more accurate assessment of one object relative to another, e.g. its distance, depth, height and width. Some people with monocular vision may find it difficult to judge the speed and distance of an approaching vehicle.

Extraocular muscles of the eye

The eyeballs are moved by six extrinsic muscles, attached at one end to the eyeball and at the other to the walls of the orbital cavity. There are four *straight* (rectus) muscles and two *oblique* muscles (Fig. 8.22). They are:

- medial rectus
- lateral rectus
- superior rectus
- inferior rectus
- superior oblique
- inferior oblique.

They consist of striated muscle fibres. Movement of the eyes to look in a particular direction is under voluntary control but coordination of movement, needed for convergence and accommodation to near or distant vision, is under autonomic control.

- *The medial rectus* rotates the eyeball inwards.
- *The lateral rectus* rotates the eyeball outwards.
- *The superior rectus* rotates the eyeball upwards.
- *The inferior rectus* rotates the eyeball downwards.
- *The superior oblique* rotates the eyeball so that the cornea turns in a downwards and outwards direction.
- *The inferior oblique* rotates the eyeball so that the cornea turns upwards and outwards.

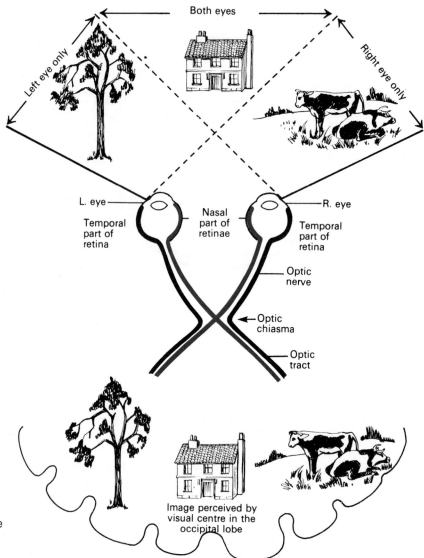

Figure 8.21 Diagram of the parts of the visual field—monocular and binocular.

Nerve supply to the muscles of the eye

The oculomotor (3rd cranial) nerve supplies the:

- superior rectus
- inferior rectus
- medial rectus } extrinsic muscles
- inferior oblique
- iris
- ciliary muscle } intrinsic muscles.

The trochlear (4th cranial) nerve supplies the superior oblique.

The abducent (6th cranial) nerve supplies the lateral rectus.

Accessory organs of the eye

The eye is a delicate organ which is protected by several structures (Figs 8.23 and 8.24):

- eyebrows
- eyelids and eyelashes
- lacrimal apparatus.

Eyebrows

These are two arched ridges of the supraorbital margins of the frontal bone. Numerous hairs (eyebrows) project obliquely from the surface of the skin. They protect the anterior aspect of the eyeball from sweat, dust and other foreign bodies.

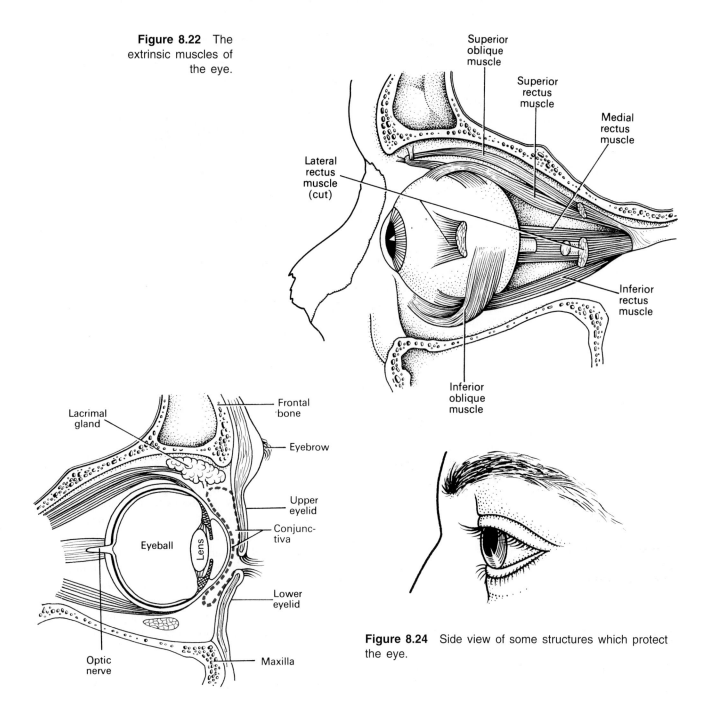

Figure 8.22 The extrinsic muscles of the eye.

Figure 8.23 Section of the eye and its accessory structures.

Figure 8.24 Side view of some structures which protect the eye.

Eyelids (palpebrae)

The eyelids are two movable folds of tissue situated above and below the front of each eye. On their free edges there are short curved hairs, the eyelashes. The layers of tissue which form the eyelids are:

■ a thin covering of skin
■ a thin sheet of areolar tissue

■ two muscles—the *orbicularis oculi* and *levator palpebrae superioris*
■ a thin sheet of dense connective tissue, the *tarsal plate*, larger in the upper than in the lower eyelid, which supports the other structures
■ a lining of *conjunctiva*.

Conjunctiva

This is a fine transparent membrane which lines the eyelids and is reflected on to the front of the eyeball. Where it lines the eyelids it consists of highly vascular columnar epithelium. Corneal conjunctiva consists of less-vascular stratified epithelium. When the eyelids are closed the conjunctiva becomes a closed sac (Fig. 8.23). It protects the delicate cornea and the front of the eye. When drops of a drug are put into the eye they are placed in the lower conjunctival sac. The medial and lateral angles of the eye where the upper and lower lids come together are called respectively the *medial canthus* and the *lateral canthus*.

Eyelid margins

Along the edges of the lids there are numerous *sebaceous glands*, some with ducts opening into the hair follicles of the *eyelashes* and some on to the eyelid margins between the hairs. *Meibomian glands* (tarsal glands) are modified sebaceous glands embedded in the tarsal plates with ducts that open on to the inside of the free margins of the eyelids. They secrete an oily material that is spread over the conjunctiva by blinking which delays evaporation of tears.

Functions

The eyelids and *eyelashes* protect the eye from injury:

- reflex closure of the lids occurs when the conjunctiva or eyelashes are touched, when an object comes close to the eye or when a bright light shines into the eye—this is called the *conjunctival* or *corneal reflex*
- blinking at about 3- to 7-second intervals spreads tears and Meibomian secretions over the cornea, preventing drying.

When the *orbicularis oculi* contracts the eyes close. When the *levator palpebrae* contract the eyelids open.

Lacrimal apparatus (Fig. 8.25)

For each eye this consists of:

- 1 lacrimal gland and its ducts
- 2 lacrimal canaliculi
- 1 lacrimal sac
- 1 nasolacrimal duct.

The lacrimal glands are situated in recesses in the frontal bones on the lateral aspect of each eye just behind the supraorbital margin. Each gland is approximately the size and shape of an almond, and is composed of *secretory epithelial cells*. The glands secrete *tears* composed of water, mineral salts, antibodies, and *lysozyme*, a bactericidal enzyme.

The tears leave the lacrimal gland by several small

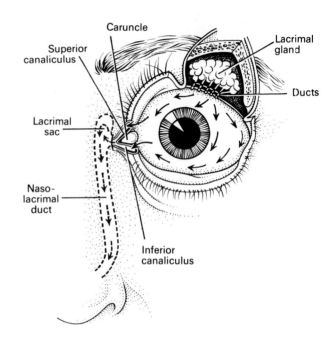

Figure 8.25 The lacrimal apparatus. Arrows show the direction of the flow of tears.

ducts and pass over the front of the eye under the lids towards the medial canthus where they drain into the *two lacrimal canaliculi*; the opening of each is called the *punctum*. The two canaliculi lie one above the other, separated by a small red body, the *caruncle*. The tears then drain into the *lacrimal sac* which is the upper expanded end of the *nasolacrimal duct*. This is a membranous canal approximately 2 cm long, extending from the lower part of the lacrimal sac to the nasal cavity, opening at the level of the inferior concha. Normally the rate of secretion of tears keeps pace with the rate of drainage. When a foreign body or other irritant enters the eye the secretion of tears is greatly increased and the conjunctival blood vessels dilate. Secretion of tears is also increased in emotional states.

Functions

The fluid that fills the conjunctival sac consists of tears and the secretion of Meibomian glands and is spread over the cornea by blinking. The functions of this mixture of fluids include:

- washing away irritating materials, e.g. dust, grit
- the bacteriocidal enzyme lysozyme prevents microbial infection
- its oiliness delays evaporation and prevents drying of the conjunctiva
- nourishment of the cornea.

SENSE OF SMELL

The nose has a dual function: respiration (Ch. 10) and sense of smell (Fig. 8.26).

Olfactory nerves (first cranial nerves)

These are the sensory nerves of smell. They have their origins in special chemoreceptor nerve cells in the mucous membrane of the roof of the nose above the superior nasal conchae. On each side of the nasal septum nerve fibres from the cell bodies pass through the *cribriform plate of the ethmoid bone* to the *olfactory bulb* where interconnections and synapses occur. From the bulb, bundles of nerve fibres form the *olfactory tract* which passes backwards to the olfactory area in the *temporal lobe* of the cerebral cortex in each hemisphere where the impulses are interpreted and odour perceived. (Fig. 8.27).

Physiology of smell

The sense of smell in human beings is generally less acute than in other animals. All odorous materials give off chemical particles which are carried into the nose with the inhaled air and stimulate the nerve cells of the olfactory region when dissolved in mucus.

The air entering the nose is heated and convection currents carry eddies of inspired air from the main stream to the roof of the nose. 'Sniffing' concentrates more particles more quickly in the roof of the nose. This increases the number of olfactory receptor cells stimulated and thus the perception of the smell. The sense of smell may affect the appetite. If the odours are pleasant the appetite may improve and vice versa. The sense of smell may create long-lasting memories, especially to distinctive odours, e.g. hospital smells, favourite or least-liked foods.

Adaptation. When an individual is continuously exposed to an odour, perception of the odour quickly decreases and eventually ceases. This loss of perception only affects that specific odour and adaptation probably

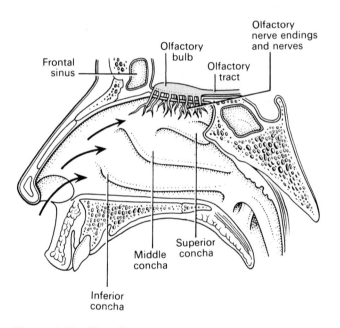

Figure 8.26 The olfactory structures.

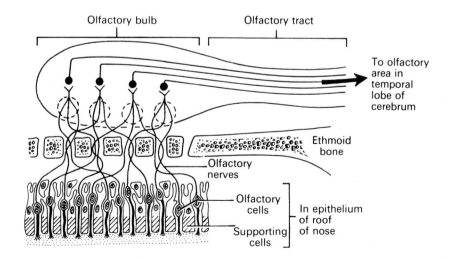

Figure 8.27 An enlarged section of the olfactory apparatus in the nose and on the inferior surface of the cerebrum.

occurs both in the cerebrum and in the nerve endings in the nose.

Inflammation of the nasal mucosa prevents odorous substances from reaching the olfactory area of the nose, causing loss of the sense of smell. The usual cause is the common cold.

SENSE OF TASTE

Taste buds are found in the papillae of the tongue and widely distributed in the epithelium of the tongue, soft palate, pharynx and epiglottis. They consist of small bundles of cell bodies and nerve endings of the glosso-pharyngeal, facial and vagus nerves (cranial nerves VII, IX and X). Some of the cells have hair-like microvilli on their free border, projecting towards tiny pores in the epithelium (Fig. 8.28). The nerve cells are stimu-lated by chemical substances in solution that enter the pores. Nerve impulses are generated and transmitted to the thalamus then to the *taste area* in the cerebral cortex, one in each hemisphere, where taste is perceived.

Physiology of taste

Four fundamental sensations of taste have been de-scribed—sweet, sour, bitter and salt. This is probably an oversimplification because perception varies widely and many 'tastes' cannot be easily classified. However, some tastes consistently stimulate taste buds in specific parts of the tongue (Fig. 12.11):

- sweet and salty, mainly at the tip
- sour, at the sides
- bitter, at the back.

The sense of taste is impaired when the mouth is dry and there is insufficient saliva water to dissolve stimu-lating chemicals in food.

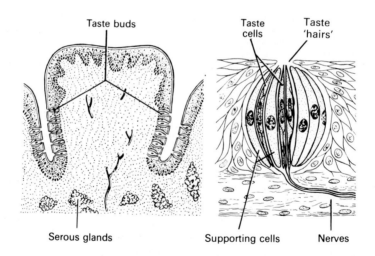

Figure 8.28 *Left*: A section of the vallate papilla.   *Right*: A section of a taste bud—greatly magnified.

DISEASES OF THE EAR

External otitis

Infection by *Staphylococcus aureus* is the usual cause of localised inflammation (boils) in the external auditory meatus. When more generalised, the inflammation may be caused by bacteria or fungi or by an allergic reaction to, e.g. dandruff, soaps, hair sprays, hair dyes.

Acute otitis media

This is inflammation of the middle ear and may be due to spread of microbes from the:

- upper respiratory tract through the auditory (Eustachian) tube
- outer ear through a perforation in the tympanic membrane.

Microbial infection leads to the accumulation of pus and the outward bulging of the tympanic membrane. Sometimes there is rupture of the tympanic membrane and purulent discharge from the ear. The spread of infection may cause mastoiditis and labyrinthitis. As the petrous portion of the temporal bone is very thin the infection may spread through the bone and cause meningitis, encephalitis and brain abscess.

Serous otitis media

Effusion of fluid in the middle ear follows obstruction of the auditory tube by, e.g. pharyngeal inflammation or a tumour. Air already present in the middle ear is absorbed and a negative pressure develops. At first there is retraction of the tympanic membrane, then fluid is drawn into the low-pressure cavity from surrounding blood vessels. There may or may not be secondary infection.

Chronic otitis media

In this condition there is permanent perforation of the tympanic membrane following acute otitis media, mechanical or blast injuries. A serious complication occurs when the membrane has been ruptured for some time and squamous epithelial cells from the external ear grow into the middle ear, forming a *cholesteatoma*. This consists of desquamated epithelial cells and purulent material. Continued development of cholesteatoma may lead to:

- destruction of the ossicles and conduction deafness
- erosion of the roof of the middle ear and meningitis
- spread of infection to the inner ear that may cause labyrinthitis.

Menière's disease

In this condition there is excessive endolymph causing generalised dilatation and increased pressure within the membranous labyrinth with destruction of the sensory cells in the ampulla and cochlea. It is usually unilateral at first but both ears may be affected later. The cause is not known. Menière's disease is associated with recurrent episodes of incapacitating dizziness (vertigo), nausea and vomiting, lasting for several hours. Periods of remission vary from days to months. During and between attacks there may be continuous ringing in the affected ear (tinnitus). Loss of hearing is experienced during episodes, and permanent deafness gradually develops over a period of years as the spiral organ (of Corti) is destroyed.

Labyrinthitis

This may be caused by spread of infection from the middle ear. In some generalised viral diseases the spiral organ of Corti is destroyed, causing sudden total nerve deafness in the affected ear. The virus infections include mumps, rubella, chickenpox and influenza.

Motion sickness

Repetitive motion causes excessive stimulation of the semicircular canals and vestibular apparatus and results in nausea and vomiting in some people.

Deafness in young children

This is usually sensorineural (perceptive) deafness and may be due to:

- genetic abnormality
- rubella in the mother in the first 3 months of pregnancy
- acute hypoxia at birth, or soon after.

Deafness in older children and adults

Conductive deafness
This is due to impaired transmission of sound waves from the outside to the oval window. It may be caused by:

- wax in the external auditory meatus
- acute or chronic otitis media
- *otosclerosis*, a common age-related condition, in which the footplate of the stapes becomes fused to the oval window by connective tissue
- traumatic rupture of the tympanic membrane and dislocation of the ossicles by, e.g. excessive force used when syringeing an ear, attempting to remove a foreign body, a severe blow to the head, an explosion

- haemorrhage into the middle ear, e.g. following a skull fracture.

Sensorineural (perceptive) deafness

This is the result of disease of the cochlea, the cochlear branch of the vestibulocochlear nerve or hearing area of the brain. The individual usually hears noise but cannot discriminate between sounds, i.e. hears but cannot understand. Causes include:

- presbycusis (the deafness of old age) due to degeneration of the sensory cells of the organ of Corti—perception of high-frequency sounds is impaired first and later, low-frequency sounds may also be affected
- Ménière's disease, progressive destruction of the organ of Corti
- trauma caused by:
  —exposure to high-pitched loud noise for a prolonged period
  —fracture of the base of the skull, involving the petrous portion of the temporal bone
- vascular changes in which the blood supply to the inner ear is interrupted
- labyrinthitis due to general virus diseases or to infection spread from the middle ear
- disease of, or injury to, the vestibulocochlear nerve
- aminoglycoside drugs, e.g. streptomycin.

DISEASES OF THE EYE

Inflammation

Stye (hordeolum)

This is an acute and painful pyogenic infection of sebaceous or Meibomian glands of the eyelid margin. A 'crop' of styes may occur due to localised spread to adjacent glands. Infection of Meibomian (tarsal) glands may block their ducts, leading to cyst formation (*chalazion*) which may damage the cornea. The most common infecting organism is *Staphylococcus aureus*.

Blepharitis

This is microbial or allergic inflammation of the eyelid margins. The most common causes are staphylococcal infection, seborrhoea (excessive sebaceous gland secretion) or allergy to dandruff. If ulceration occurs, healing by fibrosis may distort the eyelid margins, preventing complete closure of the eye. This may lead to drying of the eye, conjunctivitis and possibly corneal ulceration.

Conjunctivitis

Inflammation of the conjunctiva may be caused by irritants, such as smoke, dust, wind, cold or dry air, microbial infection or allergic reactions. Microbial infection is usually by staphylococci, streptococci, pneumococci, herpes zoster (shingles), herpes simplex or measles viruses. Gonococcal infection may be acquired by the baby at birth if the mother is infected. Infection may spread to the cornea, causing ulceration and patches of opacity when the ulcers heal. Allergic conjunctivitis may be a complication of other autoimmune diseases or be caused by a wide variety of antigens encountered in the environment, e.g. dust, pollen, fungus spores, animal dander, cosmetics, hair sprays, soaps. The condition sometimes becomes chronic.

Trachoma

This is a chronic inflammatory condition caused by *Chlamydia trachomatis* in which fibrous tissue forms in the conjunctiva and cornea, leading to eyelid deformity and possibly blindness. It occurs mostly where there is poor hygiene, especially in the Middle East, Africa and Southeast Asia. The microbes are usually spread by flies, communal use of contaminated washing water, cross-infection between mother and child, contaminated towels and clothing.

A different type of *Chlamydia trachomatis* infects the genital tract and, if transferred to the eyes, causes chlamidial ophthalmia in adults. Neonatal conjunctivitis occurs when the microbes contaminate the baby's eyes during delivery.

Corneal ulcer

This is local necrosis of corneal tissue, usually associated with corneal infection (*keratitis*) following trauma, or infection spread from the conjunctiva or eyelids. The most common infecting microbes are staphylococci, streptococci, pneumococci and herpes simplex viruses. Acute pain, photophobia and lacrimation interfere with sight during the acute phase. Extensive ulceration and healing by fibrosis cause opacity of the cornea and irreversible loss of sight.

Inflammation of the uveal tract (iris, ciliary body, choroid)

Anterior uveitis (iritis, iridocyclitis). Iridocyclitis (inflammation of iris and ciliary body) is the more common and it may be acute or chronic. The infection may have spread from the outer eye but in most cases the cause is unknown. There is usually moderate to severe pain, redness, lacrimation and photophobia. In severe cases adhesions form between the iris and lens capsule, preventing the circulation of aqueous fluid in the posterior and anterior chambers. This may cause the lens to bulge and occlude the scleral venous sinus (canal of Schlemm), raising intraocular pressure, i.e. a form of *glaucoma*. Acute infection usually resolves in several days or weeks while the chronic form may last for months or years.

Posterior uveitis (choroiditis, chorioretinitis) Chorioretinitis is the more common condition. It may be caused by spread of infection from the front of the eye or be secondary to a wide variety of systemic conditions, including rheumatoid arthritis, Reiter's syndrome, ulcerative colitis, brucellosis. Complications that may occur include retinal detachment due to accumulation of inflammatory exudate, secondary glaucoma, cataract.

Glaucoma

This is a group of conditions in which there is increased intraocular pressure due to defective drainage of aqueous fluid through the scleral venous sinus (canal of Schlemm) in the angle between the iris and cornea in the anterior chamber. The extent of visual impairment varies from minor to complete blindness.

Primary glaucomas

Chronic open-angle glaucoma. There is a gradual painless rise in intraocular pressure with progressive loss of vision. Peripheral vision is lost first but may not be noticed until only central (*tunnel*) vision remains. As the condition progresses, atrophy of the optic disc occurs leading to irreversible blindness. It is commonly bilateral and occurs mostly in people over 40 years of age. The cause is not known but there is a familial tendency.

Acute closed-angle glaucoma. This is most common in people over 60 years of age and usually affects one eye. During life the crystalline lens gradually increases in size, pushing the iris forward. In dim light when the pupil dilates the lax iris bulges still further forward, and may come into contact with the cornea and close the scleral venous sinus (canal of Schlemm), raising the intraocular pressure. An acute attack may abort if the iris responds to bright light, constricting the pupil and releasing the pressure on the scleral venous sinus. After repeated attacks spontaneous recovery may be incomplete, leading to further increase in intraocular pressure accompanied by severe pain, headache, nausea and vomiting. The cornea becomes oedematous and opaque and vision is progressively impaired following each attack.

Chronic closed-angle glaucoma. Following repeated moderately severe attacks of acute glaucoma the angle between the iris and cornea is gradually reduced and the scleral venous sinus obstructed by adhesions. Although the intraocular pressure rises there is usually little pain. Peripheral vision deteriorates first followed by atrophy of the optic disc and blindness.

Congenital glaucoma. This abnormal development of the anterior chamber is often familial or due to maternal infection with rubella in early pregnancy.

Secondary glaucoma

The most common primary disorder is uveitis with the formation of adhesions between the iris and lens capsule that obstruct the flow of aqueous fluid from the posterior to the anterior chamber. Other primary conditions include intraocular tumours, enlarged cataracts, central retinal vein occlusion, intraocular haemorrhage, trauma to the eye.

Strabismus (squint, cross-eye)

This is the inability of the eyes to move so that the same image falls on the corresponding parts of the retina in both eyes. It is caused by extraocular muscle weakness or defective nerve supply to the muscle, i.e. defective cranial nerves III, IV or VI. In most cases the image falling on the squinting eye is suppressed by the brain, otherwise there is double vision (diplopia).

Cataract

This is opacity of the lens which may be degenerative or congenital, bilateral or unilateral. In *degenerative cataract* there is gradual development of lens opacity that may be due to senile degeneration, X-rays, infrared rays (heat), trauma, diabetes mellitus, uveitis and some drugs, e.g. long-term use of corticosteroids. Senile cataract usually develops in older age groups. Other degenerative forms may develop at an earlier age depending on the primary cause. *Congenital cataract* may be due to genetic abnormality, e.g. Down's syndrome, or maternal infection in early pregnancy, e.g. rubella.

The extent of visual impairment depends on the location and extent of the opacity.

Retinopathies

Vascular retinopathies

Occlusion of the central retinal artery or vein causes sudden painless unilateral loss of vision. *Arterial occlusion* is usually due to embolism from, e.g. atheromatous plaques, endocarditis, retinal artery sclerosis. *Venous occlusion* is usually associated with arteriosclerosis in the elderly or with venous thrombosis elsewhere in the body. The retinal veins become distended and retinal haemorrhages occur. Predisposing factors include glaucoma, diabetes mellitus, hypertension, increased blood viscosity.

Diabetic retinopathy

This occurs in Type I and Type II diabetes mellitus (p. 233) and changes in retinal blood vessels are associated more with the duration of diabetes than with its severity. Capillary microaneurysms develop and later there may be proliferation of blood vessels. Haemorrhages, fibrosis and secondary retinal detachment may occur, leading to retinal degeneration and loss of vision.

Retinal detachment

This painless condition occurs when a tear or hole in the retina allows fluid to accumulate between the layers of retinal cells or between the retina and choroid. It is usually localised at first but as fluid collects the detachment spreads. There are spots before the eyes, flashing lights due to abnormal stimulation of sensory cells, and progressive loss of vision. In many cases the cause is unknown but it may be associated with trauma to the eye or head, tumours, haemorrhage, cataract surgery when the pressure in the eye is reduced or diabetic retinopathy.

Retrolental fibroplasia

This condition may occur in premature babies who receive oxygen therapy at high concentrations for long periods of time. The high oxygen tension in the blood may cause constriction of immature retinal arterioles. After oxygen therapy ceases there is disordered development of retinal blood vessels and the formation of fibrovascular tissue in the vitreous body causing varying degrees of interference with light transmission. Blindness may be caused by haemorrhage in the vitreous body, detachment of the retina or in very severe cases, by formation of an opaque membrane behind the lens.

Retrolental fibroplasia of unknown cause occasionally occurs in infants who have not received oxygen therapy.

Retinitis pigmentosa

This is an hereditary disease in which there is degeneration of the retina, mainly affecting the rods. Defective vision in dim light usually becomes apparent in early childhood, leading to tunnel vision and eventually, blindness.

Keratomalacia

In this condition there is corneal ulceration, usually with secondary infection. The lacrimal glands and conjunctiva may be involved. It is caused by chronic vitamin A and protein deficiency in the diet. There may be softening or even perforation of the cornea. Night blindness (defective adaptation to dim light) is usually an early sign of deficiency of vitamin A which is required for the reconstitution of rhodopsin (visual purple) after it has been exposed to light.

Tumours

Choroidal malignant melanoma

This is the most common ocular malignancy and it occurs mostly in older people. Vision is not usually affected until the tumour causes retinal detachment, usually when well advanced. The tumour spreads locally in the choroid, and blood-borne metastases develop mainly in the liver, bones, lungs and brain.

Retinoblastoma

This is a malignant tumour derived from embryonic retinal cells. It is usually evident before the age of 4 years and may be bilateral. It spreads locally to the vitreous body and may grow along the optic nerve, invading the brain.

Disorders of the lacrimal apparatus

Acute dacryoadenitis

This is inflammation of the lacrimal gland, usually unilateral. It may be due to spread of infection from the eyelids or surrounding structures, or be associated with measles, mumps or influenza. The infection usually resolves but occasionally an abscess forms.

Dacryocystitis

This inflammation of the lacrimal sac is usually associated with partial or complete obstruction of the lacrimal duct. In infants there may be congenital stenosis of the duct. In adults the blockage may be due to nasal trauma, deviated nasal septum, nasal polyp or acute inflammatory nasal congestion.

REFRACTIVE ERRORS OF THE EYE

In the *emetropic*, or normal, eye light from near and distant objects is focused on the retina (Fig. 8.29A).

In *hypermetropia*, or farsightedness, a near image is focused behind the retina because the eyeball is too short (Fig. 8.29B). A convex lens corrects this (Fig. 8.29C). Distant objects are focused normally.

In *myopia*, or nearsightedness, the eyeball is too long and distant objects are focused in front of the retina (Fig. 8.29D). Correction is achieved using a concave lens (Fig. 8.29E). Near objects are seen in focus as the eye can accommodate normally.

Astigmatism results in blurred vision when there is abnormal curvature of part of the cornea or lens that prevents focusing on the retina. Correction requires cylindrical lenses.

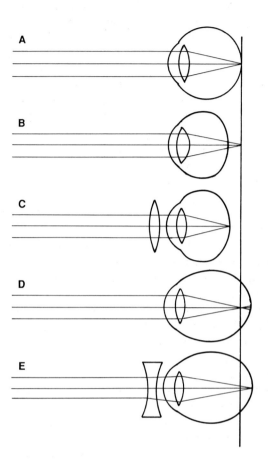

Figure 8.29 Common refractive errors of the eye and corrective lenses.
A. Normal eye.
B. and C. Farsightedness.
D. and E. Nearsightedness.

9

The endocrine system

The endocrine system consists of glands widely separated from each other with no direct anatomical links (Fig. 9.1). They are commonly referred to as the *ductless glands* because the *hormones* they secrete pass *directly* into the bloodstream.

A *hormone* is a chemical messenger which, having been formed in one organ or gland, is carried in the blood to another organ (*target organ* or *tissue*), probably quite distant, where it influences activity, growth, nutrition.

Homeostasis, i.e. equilibrium, of the internal environment of the body is maintained partly by the autonomic nervous system and partly by the endocrine system. The autonomic nervous system is concerned with rapid changes, while hormones of the endocrine system are mainly involved in slower and more precise adjustments.

The endocrine system consists of a number of distinct glands and some tissues in other organs. Although the hypothalamus is classified as a part of the brain and not as an endocrine gland it has a direct controlling effect on the pituitary gland and an indirect effect on many others. The endocrine glands are:

- 1 pituitary gland
- 1 thyroid gland
- 4 parathyroid glands
- 2 adrenal (suprarenal) glands
- the pancreatic islets (islets of Langerhans)
- 1 pineal gland or body
- 1 thymus gland
- 2 ovaries in the female
- 2 testes in the male.

The ovaries and the testes secrete hormones associated with the reproductive system. Their functions are described in Chapter 18.

PITUITARY GLAND AND HYPOTHALAMUS (FIGS 9.2 and 9.3)

The pituitary gland and the hypothalamus act as a unit, regulating the activity of most of the other endocrine glands. The pituitary gland lies in the hypophyseal fossa of the sphenoid bone below the hypothalamus, to which it is attached by a *stalk*. It is the size of a pea, weighs about 4 g and consists of three distinct parts that originate from different types of cells. The *adenohypophysis* (anterior lobe) is an upgrowth of glandular tissue from the pharynx and the *neurohypophysis* (posterior lobe) is a downgrowth of nervous tissue from the brain. There is a network of nerve fibres between

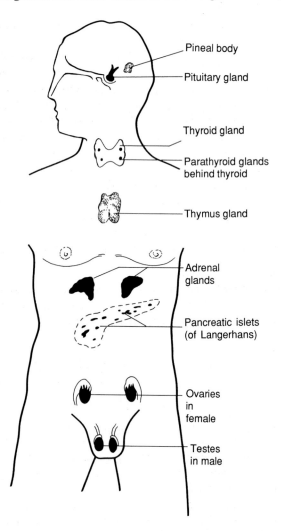

Figure 9.1 Diagram of the positions in the body of the endocrine glands.

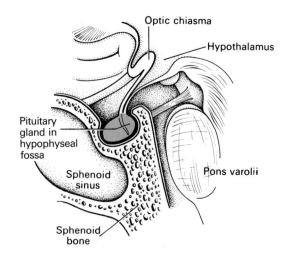

Figure 9.2 The position of the pituitary gland and its associated structures.

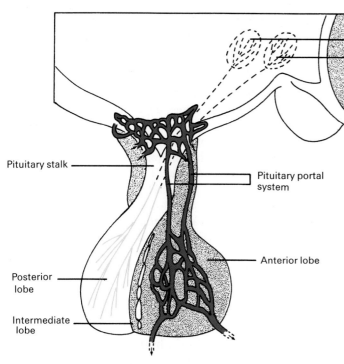

Paraventricular nucleus
Supraoptic nucleus
Pituitary stalk
Pituitary portal system
Anterior lobe
Posterior lobe
Intermediate lobe

Figure 9.3 The parts of the pituitary gland and its relation to the hypothalamus.

the hypothalamus and the neurohypophysis and the adenohypophysis. Between these lobes there is a thin strip of tissue called the *intermediate lobe*. Hormones are found in this part only during fetal life and in pregnancy but their functions are not known.

Blood supply

Arterial blood is supplied by branches from the internal carotid artery.

The *anterior lobe* of the pituitary gland is supplied indirectly by blood that has already passed through a capillary bed in the hypothalamus. This network of blood vessels, *the pituitary portal system*, conveys blood from the hypothalamus to the anterior lobe where it enters thin-walled vascular sinusoids and is in very close contact with the cells. The blood pressure in the sinusoids is lower than in the portal system. As well as providing oxygen and nutrition this blood conveys the *releasing* and *inhibiting hormones* secreted by the *hypothalamus* that influence the secretion and release of hormones formed in the anterior lobe.

The *posterior lobe* is supplied directly by a branch from the carotid artery.

Venous blood from both lobes, containing hormones, leaves the gland in short veins that enter the venous sinuses between the layers of dura mater.

Adenohypophysis (anterior lobe)

Some of the hormones secreted by the anterior lobe stimulate or inhibit secretion by other endocrine glands (target glands) while others have a direct effect on target tissues. Table 9.1 shows the main relationship between the hypothalamus, the adenohypophysis and the target glands or tissues.

The release of anterior pituitary hormones follows stimulation of the gland by *releasing hormones* produced by the hypothalamus and conveyed to the gland through the pituitary portal system of blood vessels. The whole

Table 9.1 Hormones of the hypothalamus and adenohypophysis

Hypothalamus	Adenohypophysis	Target gland or tissue
GHRH	GH	Many glands
		All tissues
GHRIH	GH inhibition	Thyroid gland
		Islets of Langerhans
		All tissues
TRH	TSH	Thyroid gland
CRH	ACTH	Adrenal cortex
None	PRL	Breast
PIF	PRL inhibition	Breast
LHRH or	FSH	Ovaries and testes
GnRH	LH	Ovaries and testes

GHRH = growth hormone releasing hormone
GH = growth hormone (somatotrophin)
GHRIH = growth hormone release inhibiting hormone (somatostatin)
TRH = thyroid releasing hormone
TSH = thyroid stimulating hormone
CRH = corticotrophin releasing hormone
ACTH = adrenocorticotrophic hormone
PRL = prolactin (lactogenic hormone)
PIF = prolactin inhibiting factor (dopamine)
LHRH = luteinising hormone releasing hormone
GnRH = gonadotrophin releasing hormone
FSH = follicle stimulating hormone
LH = luteinising hormone

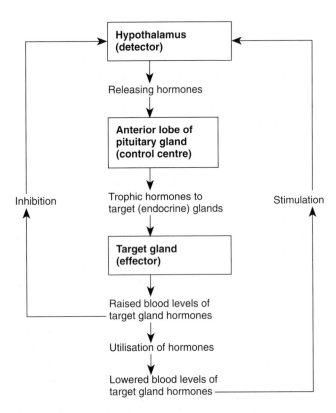

Figure 9.4 Negative feedback regulation of secretion of hormones by the anterior lobe of the pituitary gland.

system is controlled by a *negative feedback mechanism*. That is, when there is a low level of a hormone in the blood supplying the hypothalamus it produces the appropriate releasing hormone which stimulates release of hormone by the anterior pituitary and this in turn stimulates the target gland to produce and release its hormone. As a result the blood level of that hormone rises and inhibits the secretion of releasing factor by the hypothalamus (Fig. 9.4).

There are several hormones secreted by the adeno-hypophysis (Table 9.1).

Growth hormone

Growth hormone (GH) is synthesised by the adeno-hypophysis. Its release is stimulated by GHRH and inhibited by GHRIH (*somatostatin*), both secreted by the hypothalamus. GH promotes growth of the skeleton, muscles, connective tissue and organs such as kidneys, liver, intestines, pancreas, adrenal glands. Somatostatin inhibits secretion of GH, TSH, ACTH, gastrin, cholecystokinin (CCK), glucagon, insulin, renin. It also inhibits secretion of gastric juice, emptying of the stomach, and platelet aggregation, and it diminishes

the production and transmission of nerve impulses. Increased secretion is stimulated by exercise, anxiety, sleep and hypoglycaemia.

Thyroid stimulating hormone (TSH)

This hormone is synthesised by the adenohypophysis and its release is stimulated by TRH from the hypothalamus. It stimulates growth and activity of the thyroid gland which secretes the hormones *thyroxine* (T_4) and *triiodothyronine* (T_3). There is a circadian rhythmical release of TSH. It is highest between 9 p.m. and 6 a.m. and lowest between 4 p.m. and 7 p.m. Secretion is also regulated by a negative feedback mechanism (Fig. 9.4). When the blood level of thyroid hormones is high, secretion of TSH is reduced, and vice versa.

Adrenocorticotrophic hormone (corticotrophin, ACTH)

Corticotrophin releasing hormone (CRH) from the hypothalamus promotes the synthesis and release of ACTH by the adenohypophysis. This stimulates the flow of blood to the adrenal cortex, increases the concentration of cholesterol and steroids within the gland and increases the output of steroid hormones, especially *cortisol*. Production of CRH is believed to be influenced by:

- nerve impulses from the higher centres
- a low blood level of cortisol
- physical stress, especially exercise
- emotional stress
- hypoglycaemia
- negative feedback mechanisms stimulated by increased blood ACTH and cortisol.

ACTH levels are highest at about 8 a.m. and fall to their lowest about midnight, although high levels sometimes occur at midday and 6 p.m. This circadian rhythm is maintained throughout life. It is associated with the sleep pattern and adjustment to changes takes several days, following, e.g. shift work changes, travel to a different time zone (jet lag).

Prolactin

This hormone stimulates *lactation* (milk production) and has a direct effect on the breasts immediately after parturition. The blood level of prolactin is not dependent on a hypothalamic releasing factor but it is lowered by the inhibiting factor, *dopamine*, and by an increased blood level of prolactin. Suckling stimulates prolactin secretion and the resultant high blood level is a factor in reducing the incidence of conception during lactation.

Prolactin together with oestrogens, corticosteroids, insulin and thyroxine is involved in initiating and maintaining lactation. The circadian rhythm of prolactin secretion is related to sleep, i.e. it is raised during any period of sleep, night and day. Emotional stress increases production.

Gonadotrophic hormones

These are released in response to luteinising hormone releasing hormone (LHRH), also known as gonadotrophin releasing hormone (GnRH), from the hypothalamus. After puberty the anterior lobe secretes *two gonadotrophic* or *sex hormones* in females and males:

- follicle stimulating hormone (FSH)
- luteinising hormone (LH).

Female gonadotrophic hormones. The *follicle stimulating hormone* stimulates the development and ripening of the ovarian follicle (Ch. 18). During its development the ovarian follicle secretes its own hormone, *oestrogen*. As the level of oestrogen increases in the blood so FSH secretion is reduced.

The *luteinising hormone* promotes the final maturation of the ovarian follicle and ovulation (discharge of the mature ovum). Its main function is to promote the formation of the *corpus luteum* which secretes the second ovarian hormone, *progesterone*. As the level of progesterone in the blood increases there is a gradual reduction in the production of the luteinising hormone.

Male gonadotrophic hormones. The *follicle stimulating hormone* stimulates the epithelial tissue of the *seminiferous tubules* in the testes to produce *spermatozoa* (male germ cells or gametes).

The *luteinising hormone*, also called *interstitial cell stimulating hormone* (ICSH) in males, stimulates the *interstitial cells* in the testes to secrete the hormone *testosterone*.

Neurohypophysis (posterior lobe)

The posterior lobe of the pituitary gland is composed of secretory cells called *pituicytes* and nerve fibres which arise from cells in the hypothalamus, the *supraoptic nucleus* and the *paraventricular nucleus*.

The hormones released by the neurohypophysis, *oxytocin* and *antidiuretic hormone* (ADH or *vasopressin*), are synthesised by the cells of the hypothalamus and migrate along nerve fibres to the posterior pituitary where they are stored in the nerve endings. Each hormone is released in response to a different stimulus (Fig. 9.5A and B).

Oxytocin

Oxytocin promotes contraction of uterine muscle and contraction of myoepithelial cells of the lactating breast, squeezing milk into the large ducts behind the nipple. In late pregnancy the uterus becomes very sensitive to oxytocin. The amount secreted is increased just before and during labour and by the suckling baby.

Antidiuretic hormone (ADH) or vasopressin

This hormone has two main functions:

1. *Antidiuretic effect.* It increases the permeability to water of the distal convoluted and collecting tubules of the nephrons of the kidneys (Ch. 13). As a result the reabsorption of water from the glomerular filtrate is increased. The amount of ADH secreted is influenced by the osmotic pressure of the blood circulating to the osmoreceptors in the hypothalamus. As the osmotic pressure rises the secretion of ADH increases and more water is reabsorbed. Conversely, when the osmotic pressure of the blood is low, the secretion of ADH is reduced, less water is reabsorbed and more urine is produced (Fig. 13. 10). The blood level is increased in dehydration and following haemorrhage.

2. *Pressor effect.* In pharmacological doses, ADH stimulates contraction of smooth muscle, especially in blood vessel walls of the skin and abdominal organs, raising the blood pressure. It is not clear whether physiological amounts have a significant pressor effect.

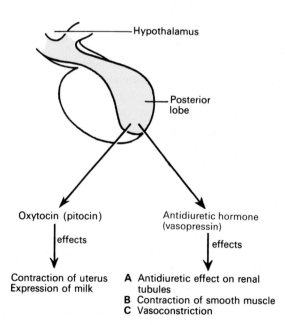

Figure 9.5A The hormones secreted by the posterior lobe of the pituitary gland (neurohypophysis) and their main functions.

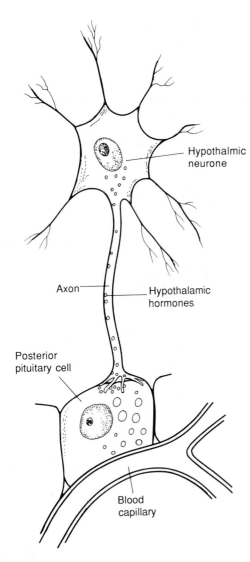

Figure 9.5B Relationship between hypothalamus and posterior pituitary cells in the secretion and storage of oxytocin and ADH.

THYROID GLAND (FIG. 9.6)

The thyroid gland is situated in the neck in front of the larynx and trachea at the level of the 5th, 6th and 7th cervical and 1st thoracic vertebrae. It is a highly vascular gland surrounded by a fibrous capsule. It consists of *two lobes*, one on either side of the thyroid cartilage and upper cartilaginous rings of the trachea. The lobes are joined by a narrow *isthmus*, lying in front of the trachea.

The lobes are roughly cone-shaped, about 5 cm long and 3 cm wide.

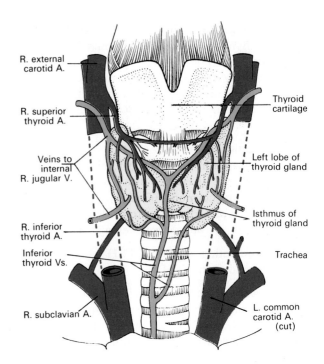

Figure 9.6 The position of the thyroid gland and its associated structures.

The *arterial blood supply* to the gland is through the superior and inferior thyroid arteries. The superior thyroid artery is a branch of the external carotid artery and the inferior thyroid artery is a branch of the subclavian artery.

The *venous return* is by the thyroid veins which drain into the internal jugular veins.

Two parathyroid glands lie against the posterior surface of each lobe and are sometimes embedded in thyroid tissue. The recurrent laryngeal nerve passes upwards close to the lobes of the gland and on the right side it lies near the inferior thyroid artery (Fig. 9.9).

The gland is composed of cubical epithelial cells which form closed spherical follicles (Fig. 9.7), containing a thick, sticky, semifluid, structureless protein called *colloid* in conjunction with which thyroid hormones are stored. Between the follicles there are parafollicular cells, also called C-cells, which secrete the hormone *calcitonin*.

Functions (Fig. 9.8)

Thyroxine (T$_4$) and triiodothyronine (T$_3$)

Iodine is essential for the formation of the thyroid gland hormones, T$_3$ and T$_4$. It is ingested in food and most of it is taken up by the gland and used in hormone for-

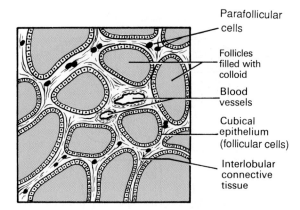

Figure 9.7 The microscopic structure of the thyroid gland.

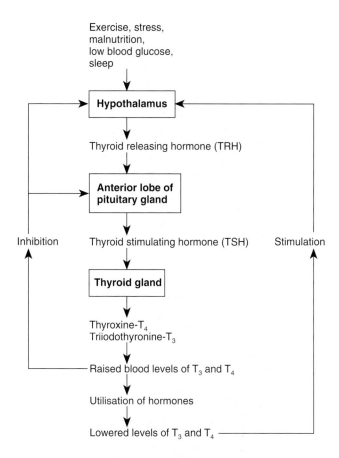

Figure 9.8 Regulation of the secretion of thyroxine and triiodothyronine.

mation. After secretion, thyroid hormones combine with colloid and are stored in the follicles as *thyroglobulin*. Their release into the blood is regulated by *thyroid stimulating hormone* (TSH) from the adenohypophysis. Secretion of TSH is stimulated by the *thyroid releasing hormone* (TRH) from the hypothalamus and secretion of TRH is stimulated by exercise, stress, malnutrition, low plasma glucose, sleep. The level of secretion of TSH depends on the plasma levels of T_3 and T_4 because these hormones affect the sensitivity of the adenohypophysis to TRH. Increased levels of T_3 and T_4 decrease TSH secretion and vice versa (Fig. 9.8). When the supply of iodine is deficient, excess TSH is secreted and there is proliferation of thyroid gland cells and enlargement of the gland. Secretion of T_3 and T_4 begins about the third month of fetal life and is increased at puberty and in women during the reproductive years, especially during pregnancy. Otherwise, it remains fairly constant throughout life.

The method of action of T_3 and T_4 is not known. They may act indirectly through cell enzymes and by enhancing the effects of other hormones, e.g. the catecholamines: adrenaline and noradrenaline. T_3 and T_4 are essential for physical growth and mental development and they have an important function in metabolism. Effects include the regulation of:

- basal metabolic rate (BMR)—the rate at which cells utilise oxygen when the body is at rest (p. 311)
- carbohydrate, protein and lipid metabolism
- normal functioning of the nervous and cardiovascular systems
- motility of the gastrointestinal tract (peristalsis)
- the female reproductive cycle and lactation (Ch. 18).

Calcitonin

This is secreted by the C-cells in the thyroid gland. It acts on bone and the kidneys to reduce the blood calcium level. It reduces the reabsorption of calcium from bones and inhibits reabsorption of calcium by the renal tubules. Its effect is opposite to that of parathormone (parathyrin, PTH), the hormone secreted by the parathyroid glands. Release of calcitonin is stimulated by an increase in ionised calcium in the blood.

PARATHYROID GLANDS
(FIG. 9.9)

There are four small parathyroid glands, two embedded in the posterior surface of each lobe of the thyroid gland. They are surrounded by fine connective tissue capsules. The cells forming the glands are spherical in shape and are arranged in columns with channels containing blood between them.

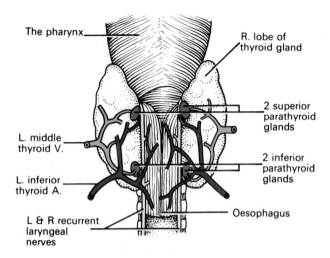

Figure 9.9 The positions of the parathyroid glands and their related structures, viewed from behind.

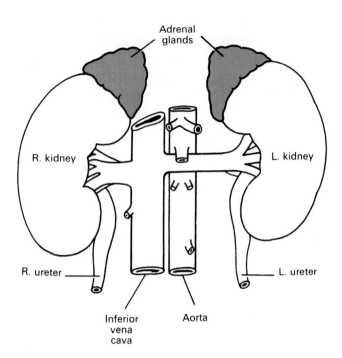

Figure 9.10 The positions of the adrenal glands and some of their associated structures.

Function

The function of the parathyroid glands is to secrete the hormone *parathormone* (parathyrin, PTH). Secretion is regulated by the blood level of *ionised calcium*. When this falls, secretion of PTH is increased and vice versa.

The main function of PTH is to maintain the blood concentration of calcium within normal limits. This is achieved by influencing the amount of calcium absorbed from the small intestine and reabsorbed from the renal tubules. If these sources provide inadequate supplies PTH stimulates osteoblasts and osteocytes to resorb calcium from bones.

Parathormone and calcitonin from the thyroid gland act together to maintain homeostasis of ionised calcium levels in the blood, i.e. within normal limits. This is needed for:

- muscle contraction
- blood clotting
- nerve impulse transmission.

ADRENAL OR SUPRARENAL GLANDS (FIG. 9.10)

There are two adrenal glands, one situated on the upper pole of each kidney enclosed within the renal fascia. They are about 4 cm long and 3 cm thick.

The *arterial blood supply* to the glands is by branches from the abdominal aorta and renal arteries.

The *venous return* is by suprarenal veins. The right gland drains into the inferior vena cava and the left into the left renal vein.

The glands are composed of two parts which differ both anatomically and physiologically. The outer part is the *cortex* and the inner part, the *medulla*. The cortex is essential to life but the medulla is not.

Adrenal cortex

The adrenal cortex produces three groups of hormones from cholesterol. They are collectively called *adrenocorticocoids* (corticosteroids, corticoids). They are:

- glucocorticoids
- mineralocorticoids
- androgens (sex hormones).

The hormones in each group have different characteristic actions but due to their structural similarity their actions may overlap.

Glucocorticoids

Cortisol (hydrocortisone) and *corticosterone* are the main glucocorticoids. They are essential for life. Secretion is stimulated by ACTH from the anterior pituitary and

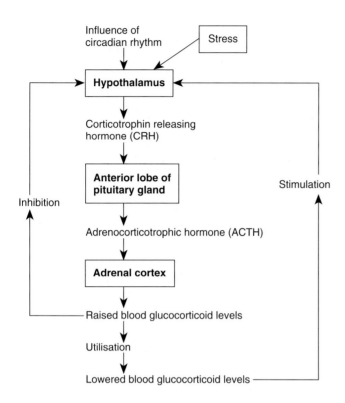

Figure 9.11 Regulation of glucocorticoid secretion.

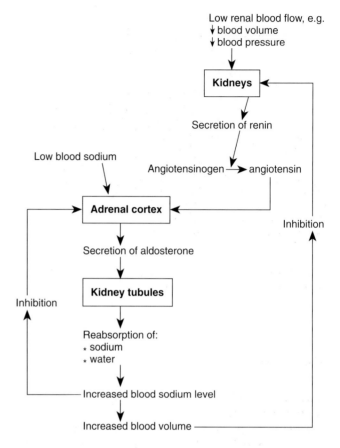

Figure 9.12 Regulation of aldosterone secretion.

by stress (Fig. 9.11). In non-stressful conditions secretion has marked circadian variations. The highest level of hormones occurs between 4 a.m. and 8 a.m. and the lowest, between midnight and 3 a.m. When the sleeping and waking pattern is changed it takes several days for adjustment of the ACTH/cortisol secretion to take place. This may be a factor in jet lag and in the difficulties experienced by some people when they change from day- to night-shift work and vice versa.

Glucocorticoids have widespread effects on body systems. The main functions include:

- regulation of carbohydrate metabolism
- promotion of the formation and storage of glycogen
- *gluconeogenesis* (formation of new glucose, p. 312) from, e.g. protein, raising the blood glucose level
- promotion of sodium and water reabsorption from the renal tubules.

In pathological and pharmacological quantities glucocorticoids:

- have an anti-inflammatory action
- suppress the immune response
- suppress the response of tissues to injury
- delay wound healing.

Mineralocorticoids (aldosterone)

Aldosterone is the main mineralocorticoid. Its functions are associated with the maintenance of the electrolyte balance in the body. It stimulates the reabsorption of sodium by the renal tubules and when the amount of *sodium reabsorbed* is increased the amount of *potassium excreted* is increased. Indirectly this affects water excretion as water and electrolyte excretion are related.

The amount of aldosterone produced is influenced by the sodium level in the blood. If there is a fall in the sodium blood level, more aldosterone is secreted and more sodium reabsorbed (Fig. 9.12).

Renin–angiotensin–aldosterone system. When renal blood flow is reduced the enzyme *renin* is secreted by kidney cells. This promotes the conversion of *angiotensinogen*, produced by the liver, to *angiotensin* which stimulates the production of aldosterone by the adrenal cortex. Aldosterone increases the reabsorption of sodium and water and the excretion of potassium by the kidneys. This raises the blood volume and the flow of blood through the kidneys, suppressing renin production and reducing aldosterone secretion (p. 344).

Androgens (sex hormones)

Sex hormones produced by the adrenal cortex are believed to have little significance compared to those produced by other glands, especially in females. They are associated with deposition of protein in muscles and retention of nitrogen, especially in males.

Adrenal medulla

The medulla is completely surrounded by the cortex. It is an outgrowth of tissue from the same source as the nervous system and its functions are closely allied to those of the sympathetic part of the autonomic nervous system. It is stimulated by its extensive sympathetic nerve supply to produce the *catecholamines, adrenaline* and *noradrenaline* in the ratio 1:4.

Noradrenaline

This is the postganglionic chemical transmitter of the sympathetic nervous system. The adrenal medulla is not essential to life but its hormones greatly assist the body in its response to adverse environmental conditions. The main function of noradrenaline is maintenance of blood pressure by causing general vasoconstriction, except of the coronary arteries.

Adrenaline

Adrenaline is associated with potentiating the conditions needed for 'fight or flight' after the initial sympathetic stimulation, by, e.g.:

- constricting skin blood vessels
- dilating blood vessels of muscles, heart and brain
- converting glycogen to glucose
- increasing the metabolic rate
- dilating the pupils
- dilating the bronchioles, allowing an increase in air intake.

Adrenaline and noradrenaline are released in response to stimulation of the sympathetic nervous system (p. 171) and by stressors.

Response to stress

When the body is under stress homeostasis is disturbed. To restore it and, in some cases, to maintain life there are immediate and, if necessary, longer-term responses.

The *immediate response* is sometimes described as preparing for 'fight or flight'. This is mediated by the sympathetic part of the autonomic nervous system and the principal effects are listed in Figure 9.13.

In the *longer term*, ACTH from the anterior lobe of the pituitary gland stimulates the release of glucocorticoids and mineralocorticoids from the adrenal cortex. The effects of these hormones in the long term increase or decrease the response to stress.

PANCREATIC ISLETS

The cells which make up the pancreatic islets (islets of Langerhans) are found in clusters irregularly distributed throughout the substance of the pancreas. Unlike the pancreatic tissue which produces a digestive juice there are no ducts leading from the clusters of islet cells. Their secretion passes directly into the pancreatic veins and circulates throughout the body.

There are three main types of cells in the pancreatic islets:

- α cells that secrete *glucagon*
- β cells that secrete *insulin*
- δ cells that secrete several substances including *somatostatin* (GHRIH, p. 217).

The normal blood glucose level is between 2.5 and 5.3 mmol/litre (45 to 95 mg/100 ml). Homeostasis of blood glucose levels is maintained mainly by the actions of insulin and glucagon. These hormones act in a complementary manner:

- glucagon increases blood glucose levels
- insulin reduces blood glucose levels.

Insulin

The main function of insulin is to participate in maintaining homeostasis of blood glucose and to promote other metabolic activities that are anabolic. When absorbed nutrients, especially glucose, are in excess of immediate needs insulin promotes storage. It reduces high blood nutrient levels by:

- acting on cell membranes and stimulating uptake and utilisation of glucose by muscle and connective tissue cells
- increasing conversion of glucose to glycogen, especially in the liver and skeletal muscles
- accelerating uptake of amino acids by cells, and the synthesis of protein
- promoting synthesis of fatty acids and storage of fat in adipose tissue

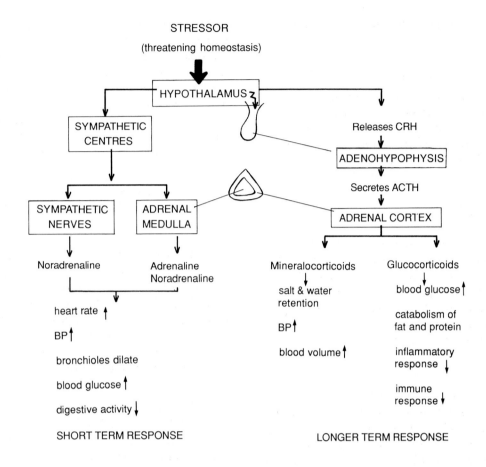

Figure 9.13 Responses to stressors that threaten homeostasis.
CRH = corticotrophin releasing hormone.
ACTH = adrenocorticotrophic hormone.

■ preventing the breakdown of protein and fat, and *gluconeogenesis* (formation of new sugar from, e.g. protein).

Secretion of insulin is stimulated by increased blood glucose and amino acid levels, and gastrointestinal hormones, e.g. gastrin, secretin and cholecystokinin. Secretion is decreased by sympathetic stimulation, adrenaline, cortisol and somatostatin (GHRIH) secreted by cells of the pancreatic islets.

Insulin is a polypeptide consisting of about 50 amino acids. Amounts are expressed in international units (IU) and 1 unit is about 40 μg.

Glucagon
The effects of glucagon increase blood glucose levels by stimulating, e.g.:

■ conversion of glycogen to glucose (in the liver and skeletal muscles)
■ gluconeogenesis.

Somatostatin (GHRIH)
The effect of this hormone, also produced by the hypothalamus, is to inhibit the secretion of both insulin and glucagon.

PINEAL GLAND OR BODY

The pineal gland is a small body situated under the brain behind the third ventricle. It is connected to the brain by a short stalk containing nerves, many of which terminate in the hypothalamus. It is about 10 mm long, is reddish brown in colour and is surrounded by a capsule.

Melatonin
This is the hormone secreted by the pineal gland. Secretion is influenced by the amount of light entering

the eye and levels fluctuate during each 24-hour period, being highest at night and lowest around midday. Although its functions are not fully understood, it is believed to be associated with:

■ coordination of the circadian and diurnal rhythms of many tissues, possibly by influencing the hypothalamus
■ inhibition of growth and development of the sex organs before puberty, possibly by preventing synthesis or release of gonadotrophins.

The gland tends to atrophy after puberty and may become calcified in later life.

THYMUS GLAND

The location and structure of the thymus gland are described on p. 138.

Thymosin
This is the hormone secreted by the thymus gland and is required for the development of T-lymphocytes for cell-mediated immunity (Ch. 4).

LOCAL HORMONES

A number of hormones are secreted by cells not in glands and widely dispersed in the body.

Histamine
This hormone is synthesised by mast cells in the tissues and basophils in blood. It is released as part of the inflammatory process, increasing capillary permeability and dilatation. It also causes contraction of smooth muscle of the bronchi and alimentary tract and stimulates the secretion of gastric juice.

Serotonin (5-hydroxytryptamine)
This is present in platelets, in the brain and in the intestinal wall. It causes intestinal secretion and contraction of smooth muscle. Serum obtained from clotted blood may cause vasoconstriction due to the presence of serotonin released from damaged platelets.

Prostaglandins
This is a group of substances produced from fatty acids by cells in most tissues. The members of the group have wide and varied effects and are believed to act inside cells, probably by modifying cellular responses to other stimuli.

Leukotrienes, released from mast cells, may assist in promoting allergic responses and inflammatory reactions. They cause bronchoconstriction, vasoconstriction, increase small blood vessel permeability and attract neutrophils and eosinophils to sites of inflammation. They are present in high concentrations in joints in rheumatoid arthritis.

Thromboxanes are synthesised by platelets and when released they cause vasoconstriction and platelet aggregation, thus contributing to the process of blood coagulation.

Prostacyclin is synthesised by endothelial and smooth muscle cells in the walls of blood vessels, causing vasodilatation and inhibition of platelet aggregation.

In addition the *prostaglandins* act as local hormones and have wide-ranging effects. They are believed to influence:

■ the response of the pituitary gland to hypothalamic hormones
■ the regulation of the female reproductive cycle
■ body temperature in some inflammatory conditions
■ the effects of neurotransmitters
■ the production of renin by the kidneys
■ the intensity of pain
■ platelet aggregation.

Gastrointestinal hormones
Several local hormones that influence the secretion of digestive juices are described in Chapter 11.

DISORDERS OF THE ADENOHYPOPHYSIS

These disorders result in hypersecretion or hyposecretion of one or more *hormones*. The abnormalities described here are those in which there is a general effect but no specific target gland. The abnormalities of *stimulating hormones* are included with the descriptions of their target glands.

Hypersecretion of adenohypophyseal hormones

Gigantism and acromegaly

The most common cause is prolonged hypersecretion of growth hormone (GH), usually by a hormone-secreting tumour. The conditions are only occasionally due to excess growth hormone releasing hormone (GHRH) secreted by the hypothalamus. As the tumour increases in size the pressure in the gland and surrounding tissues leads to:

- hyposecretion of other hormones of both the anterior and posterior lobes
- hyposecretion of hormone-releasing factors by the hypothalamus
- damage to the optic nerves, causing visual disturbances.

Effects of excess GH
These include:

- excessive growth of bones
- enlargement of internal organs
- growth of excess connective tissue
- enlargement of the heart and a rise in blood pressure

- reduced glucose tolerance and a predisposition to diabetes mellitus.

Gigantism occurs when there is excess GH while epiphyseal cartilages of long bones are still growing, i.e. before ossification of bones is complete. It is evident mainly in the bones of the limbs and affected

individuals may grow to heights of 7 to 8 feet (Fig. 9.14).

Acromegaly occurs when there is excess GH after ossification is complete. The bones become abnormally thick due to ossification of periosteum and there is thickening of the soft tissues. These changes are most noticeable as coarse facial features and excessively large hands and feet (Fig. 9.15).

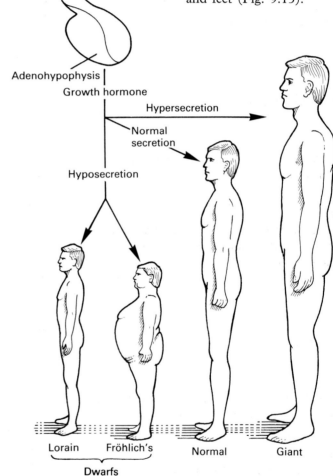

Figure 9.14 Effects of normal and abnormal growth hormone secretion.

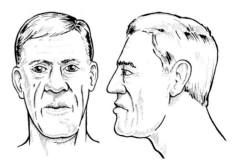

Figure 9.15 Facial features in acromegaly.

Hyperprolactinaemia

This is caused by a hormone-secreting tumour. It causes sterility and amenorrhoea in women and impotence in men.

Hyposecretion of adenohypophyseal hormones

The number of hormones and the extent of hyposecretion varies. Panhypopituitarism is absence of all hormones. Causes of hyposecretion include:

- non-secretory pituitary tumours
- trauma, usually caused by fractured base of skull or surgery
- pressure caused by a tumour adjacent to the gland, e.g. glioma, meningioma
- ischaemic necrosis, e.g. hypotension, following antepartum or postpartum haemorrhage
- ionising radiation or cytoxic drugs.

Simmonds' disease (Sheehan's syndrome)

This is panhypopituitarism in adults. One cause is *Sheehan's syndrome*, which sometimes affects women following a difficult labour, especially if there has been haemorrhage and a substantial fall in blood pressure. Because of the arrangement of the blood supply, the gland is unusually susceptible to a fall in systemic blood pressure and becomes necrosed. The immediate effect may be failure of lactation and, later, deficient stimulation of target glands, resulting in hyposecretion of hormones by the thyroid, adrenal cortex and the sex glands. The outcome depends on the extent of pituitary necrosis and

hormone deficiency. In severe cases death may occur due to hypothyroidism and glucocorticoid deficiency.

Pituitary dwarfism (Lorain–Lévi syndrome)

This is caused by severe deficiency of GH, and possibly of other hormones, in childhood. The individual is of small stature but is well proportioned and mental development is not affected. Puberty is delayed and there may be episodes of hypoglycaemia. The condition may be due to genetic abnormality or to pressure caused by a tumour but in the majority of cases the cause is unknown.

Fröhlich's syndrome

In this condition there is panhypopituitarism but the main features are associated with deficiency of GH, FSH and LH. In children the effects are diminished growth, lack of sexual development, obesity with female distribution of fat and retarded mental development. In a similar condition in adults, obesity and sterility are the main features. The hypothalamus may also be involved. It may be caused by a tumour but in most cases the cause is unknown.

DISORDERS OF THE NEUROHYPOPHYSIS

Diabetes insipidus

This is a relatively rare condition caused by hyposecretion of ADH due to damage to the hypothalamus by, e.g. trauma, tumour, encephalitis. Water reabsorption by the kidneys is deficient, leading to

excretion of excessive amounts of dilute urine, often more than 10 litres daily, causing dehydration, extreme thirst and polydipsia. Water balance is disturbed unless fluid intake is greatly increased to compensate for excess losses.

DISORDERS OF THE THYROID GLAND

These fall into three main categories:

- abnormal secretion of thyroid hormones (T_3 and T_4) —hyperthyroidism —hypothyroidism
- enlargement of the thyroid gland (*goitre*)
- solitary masses (*tumours*).

The disorders may occur in the hypothalamus, anterior pituitary or thyroid gland, or be due to insufficient intake of iodine in the diet. The main effects are caused by an abnormally high or low metabolic rate (MR).

Abnormal secretion of thyroid hormones

Hyperthyroidism (thyrotoxicosis)

This syndrome arises as the body tissues are exposed to excessive levels of T_3 and T_4. The main effects are due to increased MR. A temporary increase may be tolerated but sustained increase causes:

- cardiac arrhythmias, because the heart becomes overstressed as it tries to supply extra oxygen and nutrition to the hyperactive body cells
- increased gluconeogenesis from body protein to provide extra

energy, causing loss of weight, muscle wasting and weakness

■ diminished glucose tolerance and glycosuria

■ excess heat production as a by-product of the raised MR

■ physical restlessness and mental excitability due to neurone hyperactivity.

The gland enlarges and may develop single or multiple hormone-secreting nodules or diffuse hyperplasia of secretory cells in *Graves' disease* and in *toxic nodular goitre*.

Graves' disease (exophthalmic goitre)

This is the most common cause of thyrotoxicosis. There is diffuse hyperplasia of the thyroid gland with excess secretion of T_3 and T_4. It affects women more commonly than men. It is caused by an autoimmune reaction to thyroid tissue and thyroglobulin resulting in the development of autoantibodies that mimic the action of TSH. High levels of T_3 and T_4 are then secreted which are not subject to the normal negative feedback control mecha-

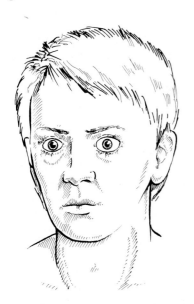

Figure 9.16 Features of Graves' disease.

nism but do depress secretion of TRH from the hypothalamus and TSH from the anterior pituitary.

Exophthalmos (protrusion of the eyeballs), due to the deposition of excess fat and fibrous tissue behind the eyes, is often present in Graves' disease (Fig. 9.16). It may be caused by autoimmunity different from that associated with hyperplasia of the gland. Effective treatment of thyrotoxicosis does not reduce the exophthalmos. In severe cases the eyelids may not completely cover the eyes during blinking and sleep, leading to drying of the conjunctiva and predisposing to infection. It does not occur in other forms of thyrotoxicosis.

Toxic nodular goitre

In this type of hyperthyroidism excess secretion of T_3 and T_4 produces the general effects of increased MR described above. Exophthalmos is absent. Cardiac arrhythmia may be severe and death may occur due to cardiac failure.

Hypothyroidism

Insufficient secretion of T_3 and T_4 causes cretinism in children and myxoedema in adults.

Cretinism (Fig. 9.17)

The retarded mental and physical development is associated with hyposecretion of T_3 and T_4. In late intrauterine life and for the first few months after birth these hormones are essential for development of the brain and bones. The child received hormones from the mother before birth so appears normal at first but within a few weeks or months it becomes evident that physical and mental development are retarded, usually first noticed by the mother.

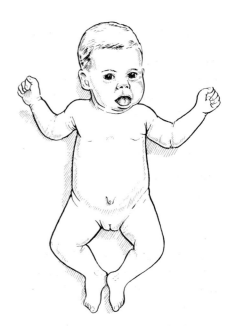

Figure 9.17 Features of cretinism.

Unless treatment begins early in life the individual remains severely mentally retarded, has disproportionately short limbs, a large protruding tongue, coarse dry skin, poor abdominal muscle tone and an umbilical hernia.

Endemic cretinism occurs in mountainous areas and areas far from the sea where soil and plant iodine content is very low. There is usually a family history of goitre extending over two or three generations. Iodine deficiency in the fetus causes developmental errors in early intrauterine life.

Sporadic cretinism is due to congenital underdevelopment in complete absence of the thyroid gland. The cause is unknown.

Myxoedema (Fig. 9.18)

This condition is common in the elderly and is five times more common in females than males.

Deficiency of T_3 and T_4, occurring after normal mental and physical development is complete, results in an abnormally low MR and lack

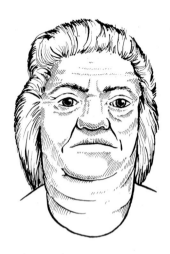

Figure 9.18 Features of myxoedema.

of response to demand for increased energy, e.g. by muscles during exercise. Mental and physical processes become slower and there is reduced heat production with persistent feeling of cold even when the environmental temperature is high. The features become coarse, the hair lacks lustre, becomes brittle and tends to fall out. Causes of myxoedema include:

- autoimmune thyroiditis, i.e. atrophy of the gland due to autoimmunity in which T_3, T_4 and thyroid gland tissue are the antigens
- severe and prolonged iodine deficiency
- deficiency of TRH and/or TSH
- surgical removal of excess thyroid tissue
- administration of excess antithyroid drugs.

Autoimmune thyroiditis

The variants of this disease are Hashimoto's disease, primary myxoedema and focal thyroiditis. In all types there is autoimmunity to T_3, T_4, thyroglobulin and thyroid gland cells. The antibodies prevent syn-

thesis and release of the hormones, causing myxoedema. The gland becomes swollen due to accumulation of lymphocytes and plasma cells. The causes are not known.

Simple goitre

In this condition there is enlargement of the thyroid gland and deficient secretion of T_3 and T_4 in spite of excess TRH and TSH. There is diffuse or nodular hyperplasia of the gland (Fig. 9.19). Sometimes the extra thyroid tissue is able to maintain normal hormone levels but if not, myxoedema develops. Underlying causes include:

- persistent iodine deficiency
- genetic abnormality
- chemicals that interfere with hormone synthesis, e.g. some drugs, including antithyrotoxicosis drugs, resorcinol, para-aminosalicylic acid, sulphonylureas.

The enlarged gland may cause pressure damage to adjacent tissues, especially if it lies in an abnormally low position, i.e. behind the ster-

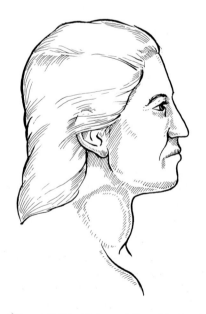

Figure 9.19 Enlarged thyroid gland in simple goitre.

num. The structures most commonly affected are the oesophagus, causing dysphagia; trachea, causing dyspnoea; recurrent laryngeal nerve, causing hoarseness of voice.

Tumours of the thyroid gland

Benign tumours

Single and multiple adenomas are fairly common and many solitary nodules become cystic. If the adenoma secretes hormones, thyrotoxicosis may develop. The tumours have a tendency to become malignant especially in the elderly.

Malignant tumours

These are relatively rare and the type of cell varies from well differentiated to anaplastic. The most common mode of spread is infiltration of the surrounding tissues, especially the trachea and recurrent laryngeal nerve, although blood spread to the lungs and bones may occur.

DISORDERS OF THE PARATHYROID GLANDS

Hyperparathyroidism

Excess secretion of parathormone (PTH), usually by benign tumours of the gland, causes reabsorption of calcium from bones, raising the blood calcium level. The effects may be:

- formation of renal calculi complicated by pyelonephritis and renal failure

- muscle weakness
- general fatigue
- calcification of soft tissue.

Hypoparathyroidism

Parathormone (PTH) deficiency causes an abnormally low level of ionised calcium in the blood. This reduces absorption of calcium from the small intestine and reabsorption from bones and glomerular filtrate. Low blood calcium causes:

- increased skeletal muscle tone and, in severe cases, *tetany* (Fig. 9.20)
- development of cataract (opacity of the lens) and brittle nails
- behavioural disturbances and, in extreme cases, dementia
- paraesthesia
- convulsions.

The causes of hypoparathyroidism include:

- damage to or removal of the glands during thyroidectomy
- ionising radiation, usually from radioactive iodine used to treat hyperthyroidism
- development of autoimmunity to parathyroid gland cells and PTH

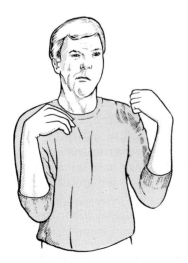

Figure 9.20 Characteristic positions adopted during tetanic spasms.

- congenital abnormality of the glands.

Tetany (carpopedal spasm)

This is caused by low blood levels of ionised calcium. There are very strong painful spasms of skeletal muscles, causing characteristic bending inwards of the hands, forearms and feet (Fig. 9.20). In children there may be laryngeal spasm and convulsions. It is associated with:

- hypoparathyroidism
- defective absorption from the intestine or dietary deficiency of calcium
- excretion of excess calcium in the urine in chronic renal failure
- alkalosis, due to persistent vomiting, ingestion of excess alkali to alleviate gastric disturbances or hyperventilation, which cause a fall in ionised calcium although the total calcium level is unchanged.

DISORDERS OF THE ADRENAL CORTEX

Hypersecretion of glucocorticoids (Cushing's syndrome)

Cortisol is the main glucocorticoid hormone secreted by the adrenal cortex. Causes of hypersecretion include:

- hormone-secreting adrenal tumours, benign or malignant
- hypersecretion of adrenocorticotrophic hormone (ACTH) by the pituitary
- abnormal secretion of ACTH by a non-pituitary tumour, e.g.

bronchial carcinoma, pancreatic tumour, carcinoid tumours
- prolonged therapeutic use of ACTH or glucocorticoids in high doses.

Hypersecretion of cortisol has a wide variety of effects but they may not all be present (Fig. 9.21). They include:

- painful adiposity of the face (*moon face*), neck and trunk
- excess protein catabolism, causing thinning of subcutaneous tissue and muscle wasting, especially of the limbs
- diminished protein synthesis
- suppression of growth hormone, causing arrest of growth in children
- osteoporosis and kyphosis if vertebral bodies are involved
- pathological fractures
- excessive gluconeogenesis with hyperglycaemia and glycosuria
- atrophy of lymphoid tissue and depressed immune response
- susceptibility to infection due to reduced febrile response, depressed immune response and phagocytosis, impaired migration of phagocytes
- insomnia, excitability, euphoria, psychotic depression
- hypertension
- menstrual disturbances
- formation of renal calculi
- peptic ulceration.

Hyposecretion of glucocorticoids

Inadequate secretion of cortisol causes diminished gluconeogenesis, low blood glucose, muscle weakness and pallor. It may be primary, i.e. due to adrenal cortex disease, or secondary due to deficiency of ACTH from the anterior pituitary. In primary deficiency there is also hyposecretion of aldosterone but in secondary deficiency, aldosterone secretion is not usually affected.

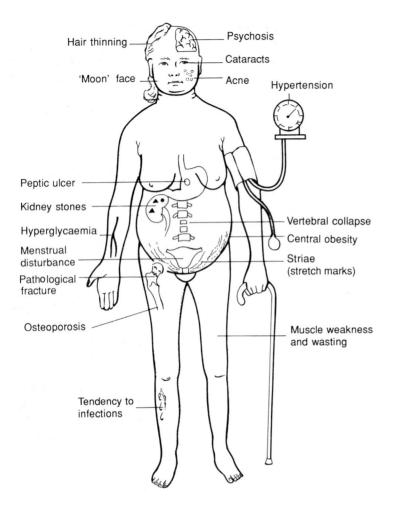

Hair thinning

'Moon' face

Psychosis

Cataracts

Acne

Hypertension

Peptic ulcer

Kidney stones

Hyperglycaemia

Menstrual disturbance

Pathological fracture

Osteoporosis

Vertebral collapse

Central obesity

Striae (stretch marks)

Muscle weakness and wasting

Tendency to infections

Figure 9.21 The systemic features of Cushing's syndrome.

Hypersecretion of mineralocorticoids

Excess aldosterone affects kidney function, causing:

- excessive reabsorption of sodium chloride and water, causing hypertension
- excessive excretion of potassium, causing hypokalaemia which leads to cardiac arrhythmia, alkalosis, syncope and muscle weakness.

Primary aldosteronism (Conn's syndrome)

This is due to an excessive secretion of mineralocorticoids, independent of renin/angiotensin secretion. It may be caused by a tumour, usually affecting only one adrenal gland, or there may be bilateral hyperplasia of unknown origin.

Secondary aldosteronism

This is caused by overstimulation of normal glands by the excessively high blood levels of renin and angiotensin that result from low renal perfusion or low blood sodium chloride.

Hyposecretion of mineralocorticoids

Hypoaldosteronism results in failure of the kidneys to regulate sodium, potassium and water excretion, leading to:

- blood sodium deficiency and potassium excess
- dehydration, low blood volume and low blood pressure, especially if arteriolar constriction is defective due to deficiency of noradrenaline.

There is usually hyposecretion of other cortical hormones, as in Addison's disease.

Chronic adrenal cortex insufficiency (Addison's disease)

This is due to hyposecretion of all adrenal cortex hormones. The most common causes are autoimmunity to cortical cells, metastatic tumours and infections. Autoimmune disease of some other glands is associated with Addison's disease, e.g. thyroiditis, thyrotoxicosis, hypoparathyroidism. The outstanding effects are:

- muscle weakness and wasting
- gastrointestinal disturbances, e.g. vomiting, diarrhoea, anorexia
- increased pigmentation of the skin, especially of exposed areas, due to excess ACTH and the related melanin-stimulating hormone secreted by the adenohypophysis
- listlessness and tiredness
- hypoglycaemia
- mental confusion
- menstrual disturbances and loss of body hair in women
- electrolyte imbalance, including low blood sodium and chloride and high potassium levels
- chronic dehydration, low blood volume and hypotension.

The adrenal glands have a considerable reserve of tissue and Addison's disease is not usually severely debilitating unless more than 90% of cortical tissue is destroyed.

Acute adrenal cortical insufficiency (Addisonian crisis)

This is characterised by sudden severe vomiting, fluid loss, electrolyte imbalance and, in severe cases, circulatory collapse. It arises when an individual with chronic adrenal cortex insufficiency is subject to stress, e.g. an acute infection.

DISORDERS OF THE ADRENAL MEDULLA

Tumours

Hormone-secreting tumours are the main abnormality. The effects of excess adrenaline and noradrenaline include:

- hypertension, often associated with arteriosclerosis and cerebral haemorrhage
- raised blood glucose and glycosuria
- excessive sweating and alternate flushing and blanching
- raised metabolic rate.

Phaeochromocytoma

This is a *benign tumour*, occurring in one or both glands. The secretion of hormones may be at a steady high level or in intermittent bursts, usually triggered by injury in the region of the tumour.

Neuroblastoma

This is a *malignant tumour*, occurring in infants and children under 15 years of age. Tumours that develop early tend to be highly malignant but there may be sponta-

neous regression. Haemorrhagic necrosis and calcification may destroy the gland. The tumour spreads rapidly to the thoracic lymph nodes, liver and bones.

DISORDERS OF THE PANCREATIC ISLETS

Diabetes mellitus

This is due to deficiency or absence of insulin or to interference with insulin activity causing varying degrees of disruption of carbohydrate and fat metabolism and storage, excessive gluconeogenesis from protein catabolism and water and electrolyte imbalance.

Type I insulin-dependent diabetes mellitus (IDDM)

This occurs mainly in children and young adults and the onset is usually sudden. The deficiency or absence of insulin is due to the destruction of islet cells. The causes are unknown but there is a familial tendency, suggesting genetic involvement. In many cases an autoimmune reaction has occurred in which antibodies to islet cells are present. The antigen is probably cells previously damaged by infection.

Type II non-insulin-dependent diabetes mellitus (NIDDM)

This is the most common form of diabetes. Most patients are obese and it tends to develop in women over 75 years and men over 65 years. The cause is unknown. Insulin secretion may be below or above

normal. Deficiency of glucose inside body cells may occur when there is hyperglycaemia and a high insulin level. This may be due to changes in cell walls which block the insulin-assisted movement of glucose into cells.

Secondary diabetes

This may develop as a complication of:

- other autoimmune endocrine diseases, e.g. acromegaly, thyrotoxicosis
- acute and chronic pancreatitis
- some drugs, especially when used to treat genetically susceptible people, e.g. corticosteroids, ACTH, thiazide diuretics
- secondary to other hormonal disturbances involving, e.g. growth hormone, thyroid hormones, cortisol, adrenaline.

Effects of diabetes mellitus

Raised blood glucose level
After the intake of a carbohydrate meal the blood glucose level remains high because:

- glucose metabolism by body cells is defective
- conversion of glucose to glycogen in the liver and muscles is diminished
- there is gluconeogenesis from protein in response to the deficient intracellular glucose.

Glycosuria and polyuria
The concentration of glucose in the glomerular filtrate is the same as in the blood and, although diabetes raises the renal threshold for glucose, it is not all reabsorbed by the tubules (p. 342). The remaining glucose in the filtrate raises the

osmotic pressure, water reabsorption is reduced and the volume of urine produced is increased. This causes electrolyte imbalance and excretion of urine of high specific gravity. Polyuria leads to hypovolaemia, extreme thirst and polydipsia.

Weight loss

In diabetes, cells fail to metabolise glucose, resulting in weight loss due to:

- gluconeogenesis from amino acids and body protein, causing tissue wasting and further increase in blood glucose
- catabolism of excess body fat, releasing some of its energy and excess production of ketoacids.

Ketoacidosis

This is due to the accumulation of the intermediate fat metabolite, acetyl coenzyme A, because it cannot enter the citric acid cycle without acetoacetic acid, a glucose intermediate metabolite (Fig. 12.50). In diabetes the amount of available oxaloacetic acid is reduced because glucose metabolism is reduced. As a result excess acetyl coenzyme A is converted to ketoacid which lowers the pH of the body fluids, causing acidosis. The effects are:

- hyperventilation and the excretion of excess bicarbonate
- acidification of urine and high filtrate osmotic pressure which leads to excessive loss of ammonia, sodium, potassium and water
- coma due to a combination of low blood pH (acidosis), high plasma osmotic pressure and electrolyte imbalance.

Complications of diabetes mellitus

Diabetic ketoacidosis (diabetic coma, hyperglycaemic coma)

Ketoacidosis develops due to increased insulin requirement or increased resistance to insulin due to some added stress, such as pregnancy, microbial infection, infarction, cerebrovascular accident. The inadequate supply of insulin may also be due to failure by the patient to administer the prescribed dose or inadequate adjustment of the prescribed dose to meet the patient's increased needs. In some cases severe and dangerous ketoacidosis may occur without loss of consciousness.

The factors that predispose to the development of hyperglycaemic coma in either type of diabetes include:

- hypovolaemia with severe dehydration due to persistent polyuria
- high blood osmotic pressure due to excess blood glucose, leading to electrolyte imbalance
- dehydration due to polyuria
- acidosis due to accumulation of ketoacids
- excretion of acetone in urine and breath.

Hypoglycaemic coma

This occurs in insulin-dependent diabetics when the insulin administered is in excess of that needed to balance the food intake and expenditure of energy. Because neurones are more dependent on glucose for their energy needs than are other cells,

glucose deprivation causes disturbed neural function, leading to coma and, if prolonged, irreversible damage. Hypoglycaemia may be the result of:

- accidental overdose of insulin
- delay in taking food after insulin administration
- gastrointestinal disturbances in which carbohydrate absorption is diminished, e.g. vomiting, diarrhoea
- increased metabolic rate in, e.g. unexpected exercise, acute febrile illness
- an insulin-secreting tumour, especially if it produces irregular bursts of secretion.

Cardiovascular disturbances

Changes in blood vessels occur even when the disease is well controlled by diet and insulin.

Diabetic macroangiopathy

The most common lesions are atheroma and calcification of the tunica media of the large muscular arteries. In insulin-dependent diabetics these changes may occur at a relatively early age. The most common sequelae are peripheral vascular disease, myocardial infarction, cerebral ischaemia and infarction.

Diabetic microangiopathy

There is thickening of the epithelial basement membrane of arterioles, capillaries and sometimes of venules. These changes may lead to:

- peripheral vascular disease, progressing to gangrene
- retinopathy, in which microaneurysms and small

haemorrhages cause numerous small necrotic points in the retina, leading to loss of sight
- glomerulosclerosis, leading to nephrotic syndrome and renal failure
- peripheral neuropathy, especially when myelination is defective.

Infection

Diabetics are highly susceptible to infection, especially by bacteria and fungi, possibly because phagocyte activity is depressed by insufficient intracellular glucose. Infection may cause:

- complications in areas affected by peripheral neuropathy and changes in blood vessels, e.g. in the feet when sensation and blood supply are impaired
- boils and carbuncles
- vaginal candidiasis (thrush)
- pyelonephritis.

Renal failure

This is due to vascular changes and infection, and is a common cause of death in diabetics.

Section 3
Intake of raw materials and elimination of waste

10
The respiratory system

The cells of the body need energy for their chemical activity that maintains homeostasis. Most of this energy is derived from chemical reactions which can only take place in the presence of oxygen (O_2). The main waste product of these reactions is carbon dioxide (CO_2). The respiratory system provides the route by which the supply of oxygen present in the atmospheric air gains entry to the body and it provides the route of excretion of carbon dioxide.

The condition of the atmospheric air entering the body varies considerably according to the external environment, e.g. it may be dry, cold and contain dust particles or it may be moist and hot. As the air breathed in moves through the air passages to reach the lungs, it is warmed or cooled to body temperature, moistened to become saturated with water vapour and 'cleaned' as particles of dust stick to the mucus which coats the lining membrane. Blood provides the transport system for these gases between the lungs and the cells of the body. Exchange of gases between the blood and the lungs is called *external respiration* and that between the blood and the cells *internal respiration*. The organs of the respiratory system are:

- nose
- pharynx
- larynx
- trachea
- two bronchi (one bronchus to each lung)
- bronchioles and smaller air passages
- two lungs and their coverings—the pleura
- muscles of respiration—the intercostal muscles and the diaphragm.

A general view of the organs of the respiratory system is given in Figure 10.1.

NOSE AND NASAL CAVITY

Position and structure

The nasal cavity is the first of the respiratory organs and consists of a large irregular cavity divided into two equal passages by a *septum*. The posterior bony part of the septum is formed by the perpendicular plate of the ethmoid bone and the vomer. Anteriorly it consists of hyaline cartilage (Fig. 10.2).

The roof is formed by the cribriform plate of the ethmoid bone, and the sphenoid bone, frontal bone and nasal bones.

The floor is formed by the roof of the mouth and consists of the hard palate in front and the soft palate behind. The hard palate is composed of the maxilla

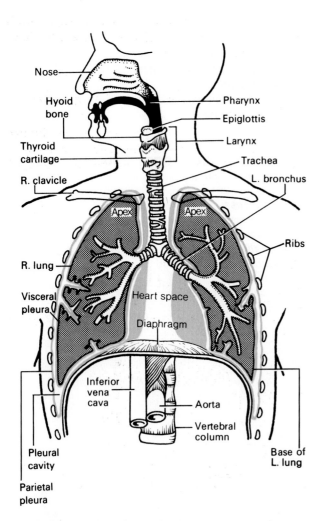

Figure 10.1 The organs of respiration. Pleura in gold.

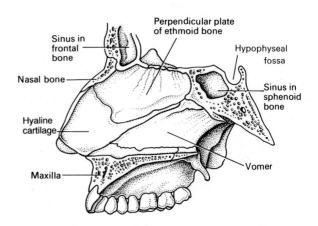

Figure 10.2 Structures forming the nasal septum.

and palatine bones and the soft palate consists of involuntary muscle.

The medial wall is formed by the *septum.*

The lateral walls are formed by the maxilla, the ethmoid bone and the inferior conchae (Fig. 10.3).

The posterior wall is formed by the posterior wall of the pharynx.

Lining of the nose

The nose is lined with very vascular *ciliated columnar epithelium* (ciliated mucous membrane) which contains mucus-secreting goblet cells (Figs 10.4 and 10.5). At the anterior nares this blends with the skin and posteriorly it extends into the nasal part of the pharynx.

Openings into the nasal cavity

The anterior nares, or nostrils, are the openings from the exterior into the nasal cavity. Hairs are present in this area.

The posterior nares are the openings from the nasal cavity into the pharynx.

The paranasal sinuses are cavities in the bones of the face and the cranium which contain air. There are tiny openings between the paranasal sinuses and the nasal cavity. They are lined with mucous membrane, continuous with that of the nasal cavity. The main sinuses are:

- maxillary sinuses in the lateral walls (Fig. 10.5)

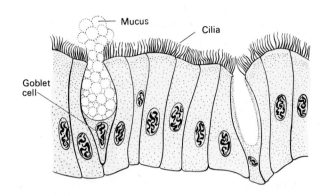

Figure 10.4   Ciliated columnar epithelium with goblet cells.

- frontal and sphenoidal sinuses in the roof (Fig. 10.3)
- ethmoidal sinuses in the upper part of the lateral walls (Fig. 10.3).

The nasolacrimal ducts extend from the lateral walls of the nose to the conjunctival sacs of the eye (p. 206). They drain tears from the eyes.

Respiratory function of the nose

The nose is the first of the respiratory passages through which the inspired air passes. The function of the nose is to begin the process by which the air is *warmed, moistened and 'filtered'.*

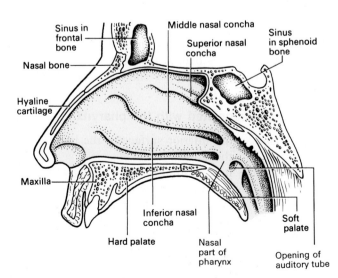

Figure 10.3   Lateral wall of right nasal cavity. Epithelium in yellow.

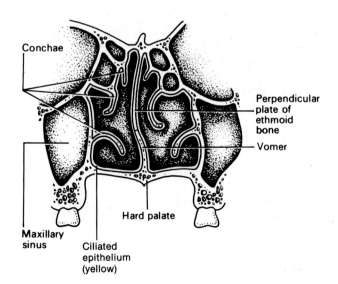

Figure 10.5   Interior of the nose viewed from the front.

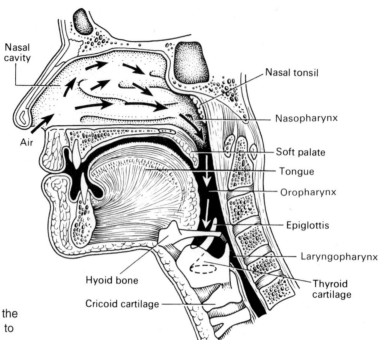

Figure 10.6 Arrows showing the pathways of air from the nose to the larynx.

The projecting *conchae* (Figs 10.3 and 10.6) increase the surface area and cause turbulence, spreading inspired air over the whole nasal surface. The large surface area maximises warming, humidification and filtering.

Warming is due to the immense vascularity of the mucosa. This explains the large blood loss when a nosebleed (epistaxis) occurs.

Filtering and cleaning of air occurs as hairs at the anterior nares trap larger particles. Smaller particles such as dust and microbes settle and adhere to the mucus. Mucus protects the underlying epithelium from irritation and prevents drying. Synchronous beating of the cilia wafts the mucus towards the throat where it is swallowed or expectorated.

Humidification occurs as air travels over the moist mucosa and becomes saturated with water vapour. Irritation of the nasal mucosa results in *sneezing*, a reflex action that forcibly expels an irritant.

Olfactory function of the nose

The nose is the organ of the sense of smell. There are nerve endings that detect smell, located in the roof of the nose in the area of the cribriform plate of the ethmoid bones and the superior conchae. These nerve endings are stimulated by chemical substances given

off by odorous materials. The resultant nerve impulses are conveyed by the *olfactory nerves* to the brain where the sensation of smell is perceived (p. 207).

PHARYNX

Position

The pharynx is a tube 12 to 14 cm long that extends from the base of the skull to the level of the 6th cervical vertebra. It lies behind the nose, mouth and larynx and is wider at its upper end.

Structures associated with the pharynx

Superiorly — the inferior surface of the base of the skull

Inferiorly — it is continuous with the oesophagus

Anteriorly — the wall is incomplete because of the openings into the nose, mouth and larynx

Posteriorly — areolar tissue, involuntary muscle and the bodies of the first six cervical vertebrae

For descriptive purposes the pharynx is divided into three parts: *nasopharynx, oropharynx* and *laryngopharynx*.

The **nasopharynx**, or nasal part of the pharynx, lies behind the nose above the level of the soft palate. On its lateral walls are the two openings of the *auditory tubes*, one leading to each middle ear. On the posterior wall there are the *pharyngeal tonsils* (adenoids), consisting of lymphoid tissue. They are most prominent in children up to approximately 7 years of age. Thereafter they gradually atrophy.

The **oropharynx**, or oral part of the pharynx, lies behind the mouth, extending from below the level of the soft palate to the level of the upper part of the body of the 3rd cervical vertebra. The lateral walls of the pharynx blend with the soft palate to form two folds on each side. Between each pair of folds there is a collection of lymphoid tissue called the *palatine tonsil*.

During swallowing, the nasal and oral parts are separated by the soft palate and the *uvula*.

The **laryngopharynx**, or laryngeal part of the pharynx, extends from the oropharynx above and continues as the oesophagus below, i.e. from the level of the 3rd to the 6th cervical vertebrae.

Structure

The pharynx is composed of three layers of tissue:

1. *Mucous membrane lining*. The mucosa varies slightly in the different parts. In the nasopharynx it is continuous with the lining of the nose and consists of *ciliated columnar epithelium*; in the oropharynx and laryngopharynx it is formed by tougher *stratified squamous epithelium* which is continuous with the lining of the mouth and oesophagus.
2. *Fibrous tissue*. This forms the intermediate layer. It is thicker in the nasopharynx, where there is little muscle, and becomes thinner towards the lower end, where the muscle layer is thicker.
3. *Muscle tissue* consists of several involuntary *constrictor muscles* that play an important part in the mechanism of swallowing (deglutition) which, in the pharynx, is not under voluntary control. The upper end of the oesophagus is closed by the lower constrictor muscle, except during swallowing.

Blood and nerve supply

Blood is supplied to the pharynx by several branches of the facial artery. The venous return is into the facial and internal jugular veins.

The nerve supply is from the pharyngeal plexus, formed by parasympathetic and sympathetic nerves.

Parasympathetic supply is by the *vagus* and *glossopharyngeal* nerves. Sympathetic supply is by nerves from the *superior cervical ganglia* (p. 171).

Functions

Passageway for air and food. The pharynx is an organ involved in both the respiratory and the digestive systems: air passes through the nasal and oral parts, and food through the oral and laryngeal parts.

Warming and humidifying. By the same methods as in the nose, the air is further warmed and moistened as it passes through the pharynx.

Taste. There are olfactory nerve endings of the sense of taste in the epithelium of the oral and pharyngeal parts.

Hearing. The auditory tube, extending from the nasal part to each middle ear, allows air to enter the middle ear. Satisfactory hearing depends on the presence of air at atmospheric pressure on each side of the *tympanic membrane* (ear drum) (p. 193).

Protection. The lymphatic tissue of the pharyngeal and laryngeal tonsils produces antibodies in response to antigens, e.g. microbes (Ch. 4). The tonsils are larger in children and tend to atrophy in adults.

LARYNX

Position

The larynx or 'voice box' extends from the root of the tongue and the hyoid bone to the trachea. It lies in front of the laryngopharynx at the level of the 3rd, 4th, 5th and 6th cervical vertebrae. Until puberty there is little difference in the size of the larynx between the sexes. Thereafter it grows larger in the male, which explains the prominence of the 'Adam's apple' and the generally deeper voice.

Structures associated with the larynx

Superiorly — the hyoid bone and the root of the tongue
Inferiorly — it is continuous with the trachea
Anteriorly — the muscles attached to the hyoid bone and the muscles of the neck
Posteriorly — the laryngopharynx and 3rd to 6th cervical vertebrae
Laterally — the lobes of the thyroid gland

Structure

Cartilages
The larynx is composed of several irregularly shaped cartilages attached to each other by ligaments and membranes. The main cartilages are:

- 1 thyroid cartilage ⎫
- 1 cricoid cartilage ⎬ hyaline cartilage
- 2 arytenoid cartilages ⎭
- 1 epiglottis   — elastic fibrocartilage.

The thyroid cartilage is the most prominent and consists of two flat pieces of hyaline cartilage, or *laminae*, fused anteriorly, forming the *laryngeal prominence* (Adam's apple). Immediately above the laryngeal prominence the laminae are separated, forming a V-shaped notch known as the *thyroid notch*. The thyroid cartilage is incomplete posteriorly and the posterior border of each lamina is extended to form two processes called the *superior* and *inferior cornu* (Fig. 10.7).

The upper part of the thyroid cartilage is lined with stratified squamous epithelium like the larynx, and the lower part with ciliated columnar epithelium like the trachea. There are many muscles attached to its outer surface.

The cricoid cartilage lies below the thyroid cartilage and is also composed of hyaline cartilage. It is shaped like a signet ring, completely encircling the larynx with the narrow part anteriorly and the broad part posteriorly. The broad posterior part articulates with the arytenoid cartilages above and with the inferior cornu of the thyroid cartilage below. It is lined with ciliated columnar epithelium and there are muscles and ligaments attached to its outer surface (Fig. 10.8). The lower border of the cricoid cartilage marks the end of the upper respiratory tract.

The arytenoid cartilages are two roughly pyramid-shaped hyaline cartilages situated on top of the broad part of the cricoid cartilage forming part of the posterior wall of the larynx. They give attachment to the vocal cords and to muscles and are lined with ciliated columnar epithelium.

The epiglottis is a leaf-shaped fibroelastic cartilage attached to the inner surface of the anterior wall of the thyroid cartilage immediately below the thyroid notch. It rises obliquely upwards behind the tongue and the body of the hyoid bone. It is covered with stratified squamous epithelium.

Ligaments and membranes
There are several ligaments that attach the cartilages to each other and to the hyoid bone (Figs 10.9, 10.10 and 10.11).

Blood and nerve supply

Blood is supplied to the larynx by the superior and inferior laryngeal arteries and drained by the thyroid veins, which join the internal jugular vein.

The parasympathetic nerve supply is from the superior laryngeal and recurrent laryngeal nerves, which are branches of the vagus nerves, and the sympathetic nerves are from the superior cervical ganglia, one on each side. These provide the motor nerve supply to the muscles of the larynx and sensory fibres to the lining membrane.

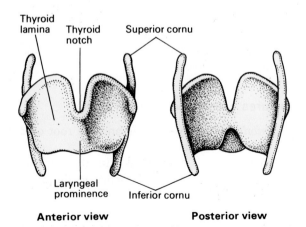

Figure 10.7 Thyroid cartilage.

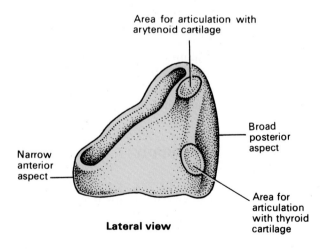

Figure 10.8 Cricoid cartilage.

Interior of the larynx

The *vocal cords* are two pale folds of mucous membrane with cord-like free edges which extend from the inner wall of the thyroid prominence anteriorly to the arytenoid cartilages posteriorly.

Contraction of the lateral cricoarytenoid muscles rotate the arytenoid cartilages medially, pulling the vocal cords together and narrowing the gap between them, thus forming the *chink of glottis* (Fig. 10.12). If air is forced through this chink it causes vibration of the cords and sound is produced. Contraction of the posterior cricoarytenoid muscles rotates the cartilages laterally, abducting the vocal cords. No sound is produced but a greater volume of air can be taken into and out of the lungs.

Functions of the larynx

Production of sound. Sound has the properties of *pitch*, *volume* and *resonance*.

- Pitch of the voice depends upon the *length* and *tightness* of the cords. At puberty, the male vocal cords begin to grow longer, hence the lower pitch of the adult male voice.
- Volume, or loudness, of the voice depends upon the *force* with which the cords vibrate. The greater the force of expired air the more the cords vibrate and the louder the sound emitted.
- Resonance, or tone, is dependent upon the shape of the mouth, the position of the tongue and the lips, the facial muscles and the air in the paranasal sinuses.

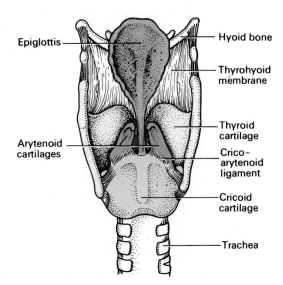

Figure 10.9 Larynx—viewed from behind.

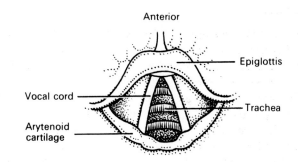

Figure 10.11 Interior of the larynx viewed from above.

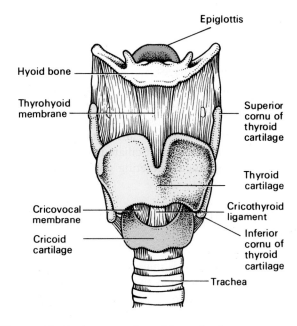

Figure 10.10 Larynx—viewed from the front.

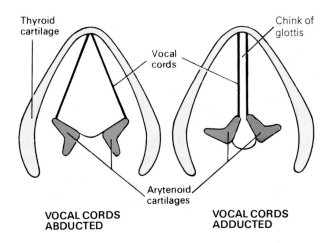

Figure 10.12 Diagram of the extreme positions of the vocal cords.

Speech occurs during expiration when the sounds produced by the vocal cords are manipulated by the tongue, cheeks and lips.

Protection of the lower respiratory tract. During swallowing (deglutition) the larynx moves upwards, occluding the opening into it from the pharynx. This ensures that food passes into the oesophagus and not into the lower respiratory passages (p. 243).

Passageway for air between the pharynx and trachea.

Humidifying, filtering and warming continue as inspired air travels through the larynx.

TRACHEA

Position

The trachea or windpipe is a continuation of the larynx and extends downwards to about the level of the 5th thoracic vertebra where it divides (bifurcates) at the *carina* into the right and left bronchi, one bronchus going to each lung. It is approximately 10 to 11 cm long and lies mainly in the median plane in front of the oesophagus.

Structures associated with the trachea (Fig. 10.13)

Superiorly — the larynx
Inferiorly — the right and left bronchi
Anteriorly — upper part: the isthmus of the thyroid gland
lower part: the arch of the aorta and the sternum
Posteriorly — the oesophagus separates the trachea from the vertebral column
Laterally — the lungs and the lobes of the thyroid gland.

Structure

The trachea is composed of from 16 to 20 incomplete (C-shaped) rings of hyaline cartilages situated one above the other. The cartilages are incomplete posteriorly. Connective tissue and involuntary muscle join the cartilages and form the posterior wall where they are incomplete. The soft tissue posterior wall is in contact with the oesophagus.

There are three layers of tissue which 'clothe' the cartilages of the trachea.

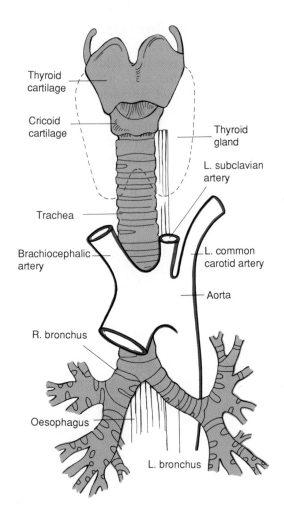

Figure 10.13   The trachea and some of its associated structures.

The outer layer consists of fibrous and elastic tissue and encloses the cartilages.

The middle layer consists of cartilages and bands of smooth muscle that wind round the trachea in a helical arrangement. There is some areolar tissue, containing blood and lymph vessels and autonomic nerves.

The inner lining consists of ciliated columnar epithelium, containing mucus-secreting goblet cells.

Blood and nerve supply, lymph drainage

The arterial blood supply is mainly by the inferior thyroid and bronchial arteries and the *venous return* is by the inferior thyroid veins into the brachiocephalic veins.

The *nerve supply* is by parasympathetic and sympathetic fibres. Parasympathetic supply is by the recurrent laryngeal nerves and other branches of the vagi. Sympathetic supply is by nerves from the sympathetic ganglia.

Lymph from the respiratory passages passes through lymph nodes situated round the trachea and in the carina, the area where it divides into two bronchi.

Functions

Support and patency

The arrangement of cartilage and elastic tissue prevents kinking and obstruction of the airway as the head and neck move. The absence of cartilage posteriorly allows the trachea to dilate and constrict in response to nerve stimulation, and for indentation as the oesophagus distends during swallowing. The cartilages prevent collapse of the tube when the internal pressure is less than intrathoracic pressure, i.e. at the end of forced expiration.

Mucociliary escalator

This is the synchronous and regular beating of the cilia of the mucous membrane lining that wafts mucus with adherent particles upwards towards the larynx where it is swallowed or expectorated (Fig. 10.14).

Cough reflex

Nerve endings in the larynx, trachea and bronchi are sensitive to irritation that generates nerve impulses which are conducted by the vagus nerves to the respiratory centre in the brain stem (p. 256). The reflex motor response is deep inspiration followed by closure of the glottis. The abdominal and respiratory muscles then contract and suddenly the air is released under pressure expelling mucus and/or foreign material from the mouth.

Warming, humidifying and filtering of air continue as in the nose, although air is normally saturated and at body temperature when it reaches the trachea.

BRONCHI AND SMALLER AIR PASSAGES

The two bronchi are formed when the trachea divides, i.e. about the level of the 5th thoracic vertebra (Fig. 10.15).

The right bronchus is a wider, shorter tube than the left bronchus and it lies in a more vertical position. It

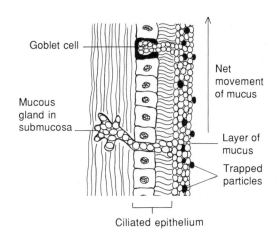

Figure 10.14 Diagram of microscopic view of ciliated mucous membrane.

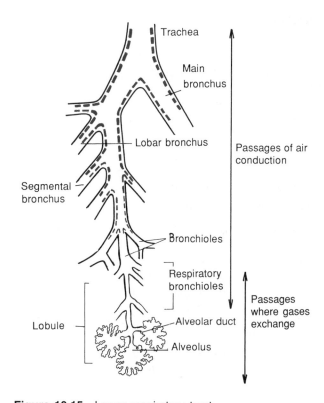

Figure 10.15 Lower respiratory tract.

is approximately 2.5 cm long. After entering the right lung at the hilum it divides into three branches, one of which passes to each lobe. Each branch then subdivides into numerous smaller branches.

The left bronchus is about 5 cm long and is narrower than the right. After entering the lung at the hilum it divides into two branches, one of which goes to each lobe. Each branch then subdivides into progressively smaller tubes within the lung substance.

Bronchi and bronchioles

Structure

The bronchi are composed of the same tissues as the trachea. They are lined with ciliated columnar epithelium. The bronchi progressively subdivide into *bronchioles* (Fig. 10.15), *terminal bronchioles, respiratory bronchioles, alveolar ducts* and finally, *alveoli*. Towards the distal end of the bronchi the cartilages become irregular in shape and are absent at the bronchiole level. In the absence of cartilage the smooth muscle in the walls of the bronchioles becomes thicker and is responsive to autonomic nerve stimulation and irritation. Ciliated mucous membrane changes gradually to cuboidal-shaped cells in the distal bronchioles.

Blood and nerve supply, lymph drainage

The arterial blood supply to the walls of the bronchi and smaller air passages is through branches of the *right and left bronchial arteries* and the *venous return* is mainly through the bronchial veins. On the right side they empty into the azygos vein and on the left into the superior intercostal vein (Figs 5.40 and 5.41)

The nerve supply is by parasympathetic and sympathetic nerves. The vagus nerves (parasympathetic) stimulate contraction of smooth muscle in the bronchial tree, causing bronchoconstriction, and sympathetic stimulation causes bronchodilatation (Ch. 7).

The lymphatic vessels and lymph nodes. Lymph is drained from the walls of the air passages in a network of lymph vessels. It passes through lymph nodes situated around the trachea and bronchial tree then into the thoracic duct on the left side and the right lymphatic duct on the other.

Functions of air passages not involved in gaseous exchange

Control of air entry
The diameter of the respiratory passages may be altered by contraction or relaxation of the involuntary muscles in their walls, thus regulating the volume of air entering the lungs. These changes are controlled by the autonomic nerve supply: parasympathetic stimulation causes constriction and sympathetic stimulation causes dilatation (p. 174).

The following functions continue as in the upper airways:

- warming and humidifying
- support and patency
- removal of particulate matter
- cough reflex.

Respiratory bronchioles and alveoli

Structure

Lobules are the blind ends of the respiratory tract distal to the terminal bronchioles, consisting of: *respiratory bronchioles, alveolar ducts* and *alveoli* (tiny air sacs) (Fig. 10.15). The walls gradually become thinner until muscle and connective tissue fade out leaving a single layer of simple squamous epithelial cells in the alveolar ducts and alveoli. These distal respiratory passages are supported by a loose network of elastic connective tissue in which macrophages, fibroblasts, nerves and blood and lymph vessels are embedded. The alveoli are surrounded by a network of capillaries. The exchange of gases during respiration takes place across two membranes, the alveolar and capillary membranes.

Interspersed between the squamous cells are other cells that secrete *surfactant*, a phospholipid fluid which prevents the alveoli from drying out. In addition, surfactant reduces surface tension and prevents alveolar walls collapsing during expiration. Secretion of surfactant into the distal air passages and alveoli begins about the 35th week of fetal life. Its presence in newborn babies facilitates expansion of the lungs and the establishment of respiration. It may not be present in sufficient amounts in the immature lungs of premature babies, causing difficulty in establishing respiration.

Functions of respiratory bronchioles and alveoli

External respiration (p. 255)

Defence against microbes—cells in connective tissue protect against infection and inhaled foreign particles not trapped by mucus. Lymphocytes and plasma cells produce antibodies in the presence of antigens, and macrophages and polymorphonuclear lymphocytes are phagocytic. These cells are most active in the distal air passages where ciliated epithelium has been replaced by flattened cells.

Warming and humidifying continue as in the upper airways. Inhalation of dry or inadequately humidified air over a period of time causes irritation of the mucosa and facilitates the establishment of pathogenic microbes.

LUNGS

Position and associated structures
(Fig. 10.16)

There are two lungs, one lying on each side of the midline in the thoracic cavity. They are cone-shaped and are described as having an *apex*, a *base, costal surface* and *medial surface.*

The apex is rounded and rises into the root of the neck, about 25 mm (1 inch) above the level of the middle third of the clavicle. The structures associated with it are the first rib and the blood vessels and nerves in the root of the neck.

The base is concave and semilunar in shape and is closely associated with the thoracic surface of the diaphragm.

The costal surface is convex and is closely associated with the costal cartilages, the ribs and the intercostal muscles.

The medial surface is concave and has a roughly triangular-shaped area, called the *hilum*, at the level of the 5th, 6th and 7th thoracic vertebrae. Structures which form the *root of the lung* enter and leave at the hilum. These include (Fig. 10.17):

- 1 bronchus
- 1 pulmonary artery
- 2 pulmonary veins
- 1 bronchial artery
- bronchial veins
- lymph vessels
- parasympathetic and sympathetic nerves.

The area between the lungs is the *mediastinum*. It is occupied by the heart, great vessels, trachea, right and left bronchi, oesophagus, lymph nodes, lymph vessels and nerves.

Organisation of the lungs

The *right lung* is divided into three distinct lobes: superior, middle and inferior.

The *left lung* is smaller as the heart is situated left of the midline. It is divided into only two lobes: superior and inferior.

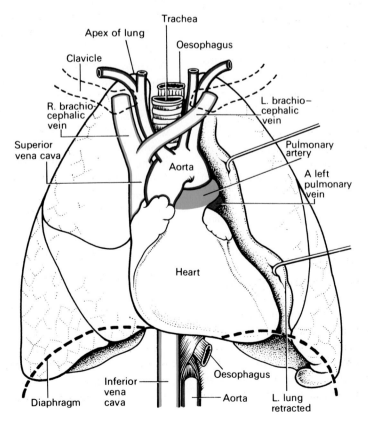

Figure 10.16 Organs associated with the lungs.

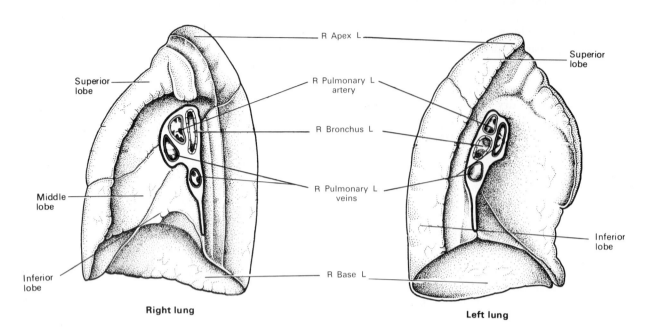

Superior lobe
Middle lobe
Inferior lobe

R Apex L
R Pulmonary L artery
R Bronchus L
R Pulmonary L veins
R Base L

Superior lobe
Inferior lobe

Right lung

Left lung

Figure 10.17 The parts of the lungs and some structures entering at the hilum.

Pleura and pleural cavity

The pleura consists of a closed sac of serous membrane (one for each lung) which contains a small amount of serous fluid. The lung is invaginated into this sac so that it forms two layers: one adheres to the lung and the other to the wall of the thoracic cavity (Figs 10.1 and 10.18).

The visceral pleura is adherent to the lung covering each lobe and passing into the fissures which separate them.

The parietal pleura is adherent to the inside of the chest wall and the thoracic surface of the diaphragm. It remains detached from the adjacent structures in the mediastinum and is continuous with the visceral pleura round the edges of the hilum.

The *pleural cavity* is only a potential space in health. The two layers of pleura are separated by only a thin film of serous fluid which allows them to glide over each other, preventing friction between them during breathing. The serous fluid is secreted by the epithelial cells of the membrane.

The two layers of pleura, with serous fluid between them, behave in the same way as two pieces of glass separated by a thin film of water. They glide over each other easily but can only be pulled apart with difficulty, because of the surface tension between the membranes and the fluid. If either layer of pleura is punctured, the underlying lung collapses due to its inherent property of elastic recoil.

Interior of the lungs

The lungs are composed of the bronchi and smaller air passages, alveoli, connective tissue, blood vessels, lymph vessels and nerves. The left lung is divided into two lobes and the right, into three (Fig. 10.17). Each lobe is made up of a large number of lobules (Fig. 10.19).

Pulmonary blood supply (Fig. 10.20)

The *pulmonary artery* divides into two, one branch conveying *deoxygenated blood* to each lung. Within the lungs each pulmonary artery divides into many branches which eventually end in a dense capillary network around the walls of the alveoli (Fig. 10.21). The walls of the alveoli and those of the capillaries each consist of only one layer of flattened epithelial cells. The exchange of gases between air in the alveoli and blood in the capillaries takes place across these two very fine membranes. The pulmonary capillaries join up, eventually becoming *two pulmonary veins* in each lung. They leave the lungs at the hilum and convey *oxygenated blood* to the left atrium of the heart. The innumerable blood capillaries and blood vessels in the lungs are supported by connective tissue.

The blood supply to the respiratory passages, lymphatic drainage and nerve supply has already been described (p. 248).

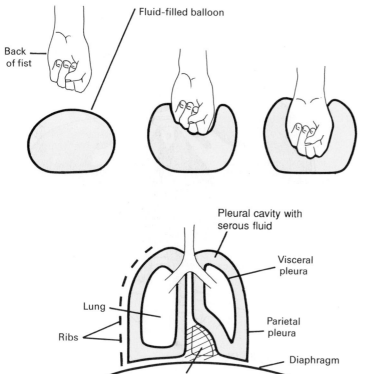

Figure 10.18 Diagram of the relationship of the pleura and the lungs. Hatched area is the mediastinum.

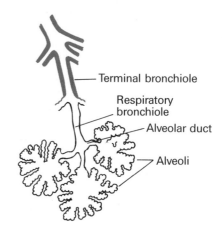

Figure 10.19 Diagram of a lung lobule.

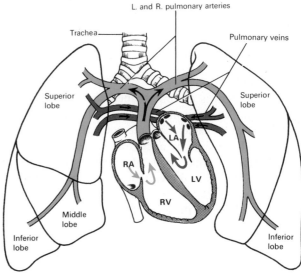

Figure 10.20 Diagram of the flow of blood between the heart and lungs.

RESPIRATION

Inflation and deflation of the lungs ensures that regular exchange of gases takes place between the alveoli and the external air. This is dependent upon the arrangement of the pleura, the contraction and relaxation of the muscles of respiration and the elastic connective tissue.

Muscles of respiration

The expansion of the chest during inspiration occurs as a result of muscular activity, partly voluntary and partly involuntary. The main muscles of respiration in normal quiet breathing are the *intercostal muscles* and the *diaphragm*. During difficult or deep breathing they are assisted by the muscles of the neck, shoulders and abdomen.

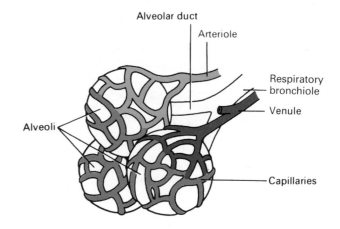

Figure 10.21 Diagram of the capillary network surrounding the alveoli.

Intercostal muscles

There are 11 pairs of intercostal muscles that occupy the spaces between the 12 pairs of ribs. They are arranged in two layers, the external and internal intercostal muscles (Fig. 10.22).

The external intercostal muscle fibres extend in a downwards and forwards direction from the lower border of the rib above to the upper border of the rib below.

The internal intercostal muscle fibres extend in a downwards and backwards direction from the lower border of the rib above to the upper border of the rib below, crossing the external intercostal muscle fibres at right angles.

The first rib is fixed. Therefore, when the intercostal muscles contract they pull all the other ribs towards the first rib. Because of the shape of the ribs they move outwards when pulled upwards. In this way the thoracic cavity is enlarged anteroposteriorly and laterally. The intercostal muscles are stimulated to contract by the *intercostal nerves*.

Diaphragm

The diaphragm is a dome-shaped structure separating the thoracic and abdominal cavities. It forms the floor of the thoracic cavity and the roof of the abdominal cavity and consists of a central tendon from which muscle fibres radiate to be attached to the lower ribs and sternum and to the vertebral column by two crura. When the muscle of the diaphragm is relaxed, the central tendon is at the level of the 8th thoracic vertebra

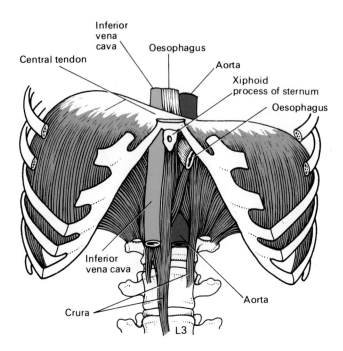

Figure 10.23   Diaphragm.

(Fig. 10.23). When it contracts, its muscle fibres shorten and the central tendon is pulled downwards, enlarging the thoracic cavity in length. This decreases pressure in the thoracic cavity and increases it in the abdominal and pelvic cavities. The diaphragm is supplied by the *phrenic nerves*.

The intercostal muscles and the diaphragm contract *simultaneously* ensuring the enlargement of the thoracic cavity in all directions, that is from back to front, side to side and top to bottom (Fig. 10.24).

Cycle of respiration

This occurs 12 to 15 times per minute and consists of three phases:

- inspiration
- expiration
- pause.

As described previously, the visceral pleura is adherent to the lungs and the parietal pleura to the inner wall of the thorax and to the diaphragm. Between them there is a thin film of serous fluid (p. 250).

Inspiration

When the capacity of the thoracic cavity is increased by simultaneous contraction of the intercostal muscles

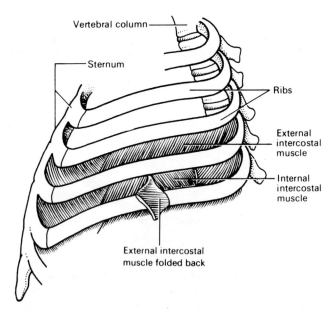

Figure 10.22   The intercostal muscles and the bones of the thorax.

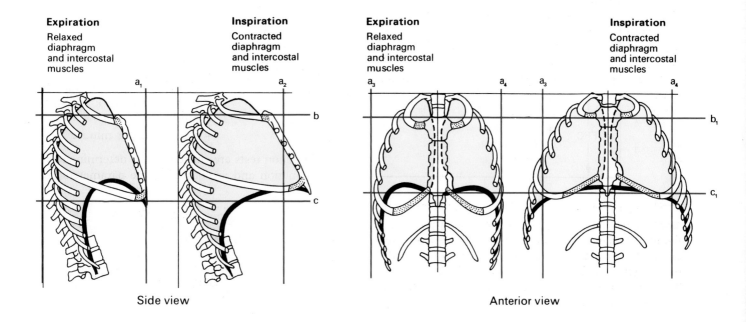

Expiration
Relaxed diaphragm and intercostal muscles

Inspiration
Contracted diaphragm and intercostal muscles

Expiration
Relaxed diaphragm and intercostal muscles

Inspiration
Contracted diaphragm and intercostal muscles

Side view

Anterior view

Figure 10.24 Diagram of the changes in capacity of the thoracic cavity (and the lungs) during breathing.

and the diaphragm, the parietal pleura moves with the walls of the thorax and the diaphragm. This reduces the pressure in the pleural cavity to a level considerably lower than atmospheric pressure. The visceral pleura follows the parietal pleura. During this process the lungs are stretched and the pressure within the alveoli and in the air passages is reduced, drawing air into the lungs in an attempt to equalise the atmospheric and alveolar air pressures.

The process of inspiration is *active*, as it requires expenditure of energy for muscle contraction. The negative pressure created in the thoracic cavity aids venous return to the heart and is known as the *respiratory pump*.

Expiration

Relaxation of the intercostal muscles and the diaphragm results in downward and inward movement of the rib cage (Fig. 10.24) and elastic recoil of the lungs. As this occurs, the pressure of gases inside the thorax exceeds that in the atmosphere and therefore air is expelled from the respiratory tract. The lungs still contain some air and are prevented from complete collapse by the intact pleura. This process is *passive* as it does not require the expenditure of energy.

After expiration, there is a *pause* before the next cycle begins.

Physiological variables affecting respiration

Elasticity. Loss of elasticity of the connective tissue in the lungs necessitates forced expiration and increased effort on inspiration.

Compliance. This is a measure of the distensibility of the lungs, i.e. the effort required to inflate the alveoli. When compliance is low the effort needed to inflate the lungs is greater than normal, e.g. in some diseases where elasticity is reduced or when insufficient surfactant is present.

Airflow resistance. When this is increased, e.g. in bronchoconstriction, more respiratory effort is required to inflate the lungs.

Lung volumes and capacities
(Fig. 10.25)

In normal quiet breathing there are about 15 complete respiratory cycles per minute. The lungs and the air passages are never empty and, as the exchange of gases takes place only across the walls of the alveolar ducts and alveoli, the remaining capacity of the respiratory

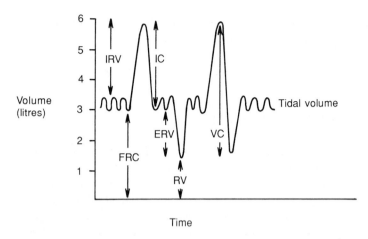

Figure 10.25 Lung volumes and capacities: IRV = inspiratory reserve volume; IC = inspiratory capacity; FRC = functional reserve capacity; ERV = expiratory reserve volume; RV = residual volume; VC = vital capacity.

passages is called the *anatomical dead space* (about 150 ml).

Tidal volume (TV): is the amount of air which passes into and out of the lungs during each cycle of quiet breathing (about 500 ml).

Inspiratory reserve volume (IRV): is the extra volume of air that can be inhaled into the lungs during maximal inspiration.

Inspiratory capacity (IC): is the amount of air that can be inspired with the maximum effort. It consists of the tidal volume (500 ml) plus the *inspiratory reserve volume*.

Functional residual capacity (FRC): is the amount of air remaining in the air passages and alveoli at the end of quiet expiration. Tidal air mixes with this air, causing relatively small changes in the composition of alveolar air. As blood flows continuously through the pulmonary capillaries this means that the interchange of gases is not interrupted between breaths, preventing marked changes in the concentration of blood gases. The functional residual volume also prevents collapse of the alveoli on expiration.

Expiratory reserve volume (ERV): is the largest volume of air which can be expelled from the lungs during maximal expiration.

Residual volume (RV): cannot be directly measured but is the volume of air remaining in the lungs after forced expiration.

Vital capacity (VC): is the maximum volume of air which can be moved into and out of the lungs:

VC = Tidal volume + IRV + ERV

Alveolar ventilation. This is the volume of air that moves into and out of the alveoli per minute. It is equal to the tidal volume minus the anatomical dead space, multiplied by the respiratory rate:

Alveolar ventilation = (TV – anatomical dead space) × respiratory rate
= (500 – 150) ml × 15 per minute
= 5.25 litres per minute

Lung function tests are carried out to determine respiratory function and are based on the parameters outlined above.

Composition of air

Atmospheric pressure at sea level is 101.3 kilopascals (kPa)* or 760 mmHg. With the increase in height above sea level, atmospheric pressure is progressively reduced and at 5500 m (18 000 ft) it is about half that at sea level. Under water, pressure increases by approximately 1 atmosphere per 10 m below sea level.

Air is a mixture of gases: nitrogen, oxygen, carbon dioxide, water vapour and small quantities of inert gases. The percentage of each is listed in Table 10.1. Each gas in the mixture exerts a part of the total pressure proportional to its concentration, i.e. the *partial pressure* (Table 10.2). This is denoted as, e.g. PO_2, PCO_2.

Alveolar air

The composition of alveolar air remains fairly constant and is different from atmospheric air. It is saturated with water vapour and contains more carbon dioxide, and less oxygen. Saturation with water vapour provides 6.3 kPa (47 mmHg) thus reducing the partial pressure of all the other gases present. Gaseous exchange be-

Table 10.1 The composition of inspired and expired air

	Inspired air %	Expired air %
Oxygen	21	16
Carbon dioxide	0.04	4
Nitrogen and rare gases	78	78
Water vapour	Variable	Saturated

---

* 1 mmHg = 133.3 Pa = 0.133 kPa
   1 kPa = 7.5 mmHg

Gas	Alveolar air kPa mmHg		Deoxygenated blood kPa mmHg		Oxygenated blood kPa mmHg	
Oxygen	13.3	100	5.3	40	13.3	100
Carbon dioxide	5.3	40	5.8	44	5.3	40
Nitrogen and other inert gases	76.4	573	76.4	573	76.4	573
Water vapour	6.3	47				
	101.3	760				

Table 10.2 Partial pressures of gases

tween the alveoli and the bloodstream (*external respiration*) is a continuous process, as the alveoli are never empty, so it is independent of the respiratory cycle. During each inspiration only some of the alveolar gases are exchanged.

Expired air
This is a mixture of alveolar air and atmospheric air in the dead space. Its composition is shown in Table 10.2.

Diffusion of gases

Exchange of gases occurs when a difference in partial pressure exists across semipermeable membranes. Gases move by diffusion from the higher concentration to the lower until equilibrium is established. Atmospheric nitrogen is not used by the body so its partial pressure remains unchanged and is the same in inspired and expired air, alveolar air and in the blood.

External respiration

This is exchange of gases by diffusion between the alveoli and the blood. Each alveolar wall is one cell thick and is surrounded by a network of tiny capillaries. The total area for gas exchange in the lungs is 70 to 80 square metres. Carbon dioxide diffuses from venous blood along its concentration gradient into the alveoli until equilibrium with alveolar air is reached. By the same process, oxygen diffuses from the alveoli into the blood. The slow flow of blood through the capillaries increases the time available for diffusion to occur. When blood leaves the alveolar capillaries, the oxygen and carbon dioxide concentrations are in equilibrium with those of alveolar air (Fig. 10.26).

Internal respiration

This is exchange of gases between blood in the capillaries and the body cells. When there is a difference in partial pressures, oxygen diffuses outwards from the arterial end of capillaries into the surrounding extracellular fluid, then through cell walls. The process involved is that of diffusion from a higher concentration of oxygen in the blood to a lower concentration in the

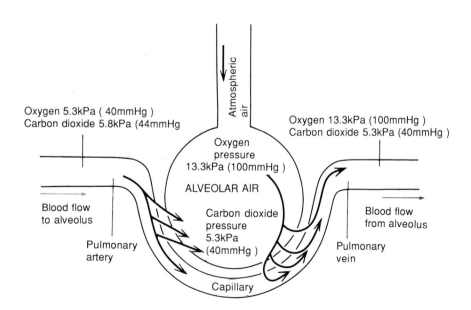

Figure 10.26 External respiration: the interchange of gases between air in the alveoli and the blood capillaries.

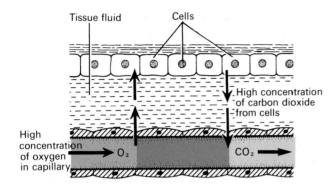

Figure 10.27 Internal respiration: the interchange of gases between capillaries and the tissues.

cells, i.e. down the concentration gradient (Fig. 10.27). Carbon dioxide diffuses from the cells into the extracellular fluid then into the bloodstream towards the venous end of the capillary.

Transport of gases in the bloodstream

Transport of blood oxygen and carbon dioxide is essential for internal respiration to occur.

Oxygen
Oxygen is carried in the blood:

- in chemical combination with haemoglobin as *oxyhaemoglobin*
- in solution in plasma water.

Oxyhaemoglobin is an unstable compound that under certain conditions readily dissociates releasing oxygen. Factors that increase dissociation include raised carbon dioxide content of tissue fluid, raised temperature and 2,3-diphosphoglycerate (2,3-DPG is a substance present in red blood cells). In active tissues there is increased production of carbon dioxide and heat which leads to increased release of oxygen. In this way oxygen is available to tissues in greatest need. When oxygen leaves the erythrocyte, the deoxygenated haemoglobin turns purplish in colour.

Carbon dioxide
Carbon dioxide is one of the waste products of metabolism. It is excreted by the lungs and is transported by three mechanisms:

- most of it is in the form of bicarbonate ions (HCO_3^-) in the plasma

- some is dissolved in the plasma
- some is carried in erythrocytes, loosely combined with haemoglobin as *carbaminohaemoglobin*.

Control of respiration

Control of respiration is normally involuntary. Voluntary control is exerted during activities such as speaking and singing but is overridden if homeostasis of arterial PO_2 or PCO_2 is threatened, i.e. if there is high arterial PCO_2 (*hypercapnia*) or low arterial PO_2 (*hypoxia*).

The respiratory centre
This is formed by groups of nerve cells that control the rate and depth of respiration. They are situated in the brain stem, in the *medulla oblongata* and the *pons varolii*. The interrelationship between these groups of cells is complex. In the medulla there are *inspiratory neurones* and *expiratory neurones*. Neurones in the *pneumotaxic* and *apneustic centres*, situated in the pons, influence the inspiratory and expiratory neurones of the medulla.

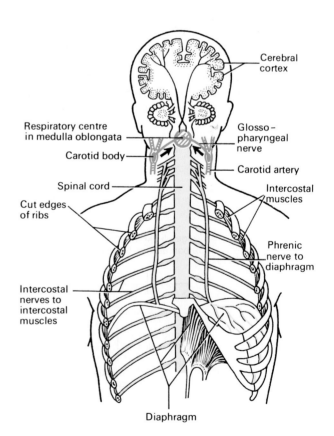

Figure 10.28 Diagram of some of the nerves involved in the control of respiration.

Motor impulses leaving the respiratory centre pass in the *phrenic* and *intercostal nerves* to the diaphragm and intercostal muscles respectively (Fig. 10.28).

Chemoreceptors

These are receptors that respond to changes in the partial pressures of oxygen and carbon dioxide in the blood and cerebrospinal fluid. They are located centrally and peripherally.

Central chemoreceptors are on the surface of the medulla oblongata and are bathed in cerebrospinal fluid. When the arterial PCO_2 rises even slightly, the central chemoreceptors respond by stimulating the respiratory centre, increasing ventilation of the lungs and reducing arterial PCO_2. The sensitivity of the central chemoreceptors to raised arterial PCO_2 is the most important factor in maintaining homeostasis of blood gases in health. A small reduction in PO_2 has the same, but less pronounced effect, but a substantial reduction has a depressing effect.

Peripheral chemoreceptors are situated in the arch of the aorta and in the carotid bodies (Fig. 10.28). They are more sensitive to small rises in arterial PCO_2 than to similarly low arterial PO_2 levels. Nerve impulses, generated in the peripheral chemoreceptors, are conveyed by the *glossopharyngeal* and *vagus nerves* to the medulla and stimulate the respiratory centre. The rate and depth of breathing are then increased. An increase in blood acidity (decreased pH or raised [H+]) stimulates the peripheral chemoreceptors, resulting in increased ventilation, increased CO_2 excretion and reduced blood pH.

Other factors that influence respiration

Breathing may be modified by the higher centres in the brain by:

- speech, singing
- emotional displays, e.g. crying, laughing, fear
- drugs, e.g. sedatives, alcohol
- sleep.

Temperature influences breathing. In fever respiration is increased due to increased metabolic rate while in hypothermia it is depressed, as is metabolism. Temporary changes in respiration occur in swallowing, sneezing and coughing.

The *Hering–Breuer reflex* prevents over-inflation of the lungs. Stretch receptors situated in the thoracic wall generate nerve inhibitory impulses when the lungs have inflated. They travel via the vagus nerves to the respiratory centre.

Normally, quiet breathing is adequate to maintain arterial PO_2 and PCO_2 levels; however, on strenuous exercise, both the rate and depth of breathing increase, increasing oxygen uptake and carbon dioxide excretion in order to meet increased needs and so maintain homeostasis. When intense respiratory effort is required, the *accessory muscles of respiration* are used. The most important is the *sternocleidomastoid* (Fig. 17.1). Contraction of these muscles in addition to the diaphragm and intercostal muscles ensures the maximum increase in the capacity of the thoracic cavity.

Effective control of respiration enables the body to maintain homeostasis of blood gases over a wide range of physiological, environmental and pathological conditions.

DISORDERS OF THE UPPER RESPIRATORY TRACT

Inflammation

Upper respiratory tract infections are usually caused by viruses which lower the resistance of the mucous membrane and allow bacteria dormant in the tract to invade the tissues. Such infections are not usually a threat to life unless:

- they spread to the lungs or other organs
- inflammatory swelling and exudate block the airway.

Acute inflammation

Microbes are usually spread by droplet infection, in dust or by contaminated equipment and dressings. If not completely resolved, acute infection may become chronic.

Viral infections

Viruses are the initial cause of most upper respiratory tract infections and are small enough to pass through cell walls. They multiply inside the cells and cannot be killed by most antibacterial or antifungal agents that are unable to penetrate cell walls. Antimicrobial agents that can enter cells tend to damage host cells so their use is limited. Interferons secreted by lymphocytes provide some degree of protection against viruses by limiting their ability to replicate (p. 69).

Viral infections cause acute inflammation of mucous membrane, leading to tissue congestion and profuse exudate of watery fluid. Secondary infection by bacteria usually results in purulent discharge. Viral upper respiratory tract infections include:

- common cold
- pharyngitis
- tracheitis
- tonsillitis
- influenza
- laryngotracheobronchitis (croup in young children)
- laryngitis.

Viral infections commonly cause severe illness and sometimes death in infants and young children. In adults influenza is an incapacitating condition but is rarely fatal unless infection spreads to the lungs.

Hay fever

In this condition, *atopic* ('immediate') hypersensitivity develops to foreign proteins (antigens), e.g. pollen, mites in pillow feathers, animal dander. The acute non-microbial inflammation of nasal mucosa and conjunctiva causes *rhinorrhoea* (excessive watery exudate from the nose), redness of the eyes and excessive secretion of tears. The first time the antigen is encountered and absorbed, IgE antibodies are produced by B-lymphocytes which adhere to the surface of mast cells and basophils in the mucosa. Subsequent contact with the same antigen causes an immediate antigen/antibody reaction, stimulating the release of histamine and related substances from the granules of mast cells and basophils. These substances cause vasodilatation, increased permeability of capillary walls, hypersecretion by glands and swelling of tissues (see Fig. 4.16). Atopic hypersensitivity tends to run in families, but no genetic factor has yet been identified. Other forms of atopic hypersensitivity include:

- extrinsic asthma (p. 260)
- eczema in infants and young children
- food allergies.

Acute sinusitis

This is usually caused by spread of microbes from the nose and pharynx to the mucous membrane lining the paranasal sinuses in maxillary, sphenoidal, ethmoidal and frontal bones. The primary virus infection is usually followed by bacterial infection, e.g. *Streptococcus pyogenes, Streptococcus pneumoniae, Staphylococcus aureus*. The congested mucosa may block the openings between the nose and the sinuses, preventing drainage of mucopurulent discharge. If there are repeated attacks or if recovery is not complete, the infection may become chronic.

Acute pharyngitis

This usually accompanies common colds and tonsillitis. Viruses, with superimposed bacterial infection, cause acute inflammation of the mucous membrane of the pharynx, nose and sinuses.

Acute laryngitis and tracheitis

The larynx and trachea are subject to the same viral and bacterial infections as the nose and pharynx. The infection may become chronic, expecially in tobacco smokers and people who live or work in a polluted atmosphere. Acute inflammation may follow damage caused by an endotracheal tube, especially if it is used for long periods or has an inflated cuff.

Nasal polyps

These are small pear-shaped masses, covered with mucous membrane, that protrude into the nasal cavity. They consist of oedematous connective tissue, lymphocytes and plasma cells. Each polyp is suspended by a mucous membrane pedicle, usually from the lateral wall of the cavity. Chronic inflammation of the nasal mucous membrane is the main predisposing factor.

Enlarged pharyngeal tonsils (adenoids)

Adenoids consist of lymphoid tissue that reacts to foreign material and produces appropriate specific antibodies. Temporary enlargement is a protective reaction to infection of nasal and pharyngeal mucosa. After repeated inflammatory episodes the adenoids may remain enlarged due to fibrosis, causing partial or complete obstruction of the airway and preventing nasal breathing, especially in children.

Tonsillitis

Viruses and *Streptococcus pyogenes* are common causes of inflammation of the palatine tonsils, palatine arches and walls of the pharynx. Severe infection may lead to suppuration and abscess formation (*quinsy*). Occasionally the infection spreads into the neck causing cellulitis. Following acute tonsillitis, swelling subsides and the tonsil returns to normal but repeated infection may lead to chronic inflammation, fibrosis and permanent enlargement. Endotoxins from tonsillitis caused by *Streptococcus pyogenes* are associated with the development of rheumatic fever and glomerulonephritis.

Diphtheria

This is an infection of the pharynx, caused by *Corynebacterium diphtheriae*, that may extend to the nasopharynx and trachea. A thick fibrous membrane forms over the area and may obstruct the airway. Powerful exotoxins may severely damage cardiac and skeletal muscle, the liver, kidneys and adrenal glands. Where immunisation is widespread diphtheria is comparatively rare.

Tumours

Benign (haemangiomata)

These occur in the nasal septum. They consist of abnormal proliferations of blood vessels interspersed with collagen fibres of irregular size and arrangement. The blood vessels tend to rupture and cause persistent bleeding (epistaxis).

Malignant

Carcinoma of the nose, sinuses, nasopharynx and larynx is relatively rare.

DISEASES OF THE BRONCHI

Acute bronchitis

This is usually a secondary bacterial infection of the bronchi. It is usually preceded by a common cold or influenza and it may also complicate measles and whooping cough in children. The viruses depress normal defence mechanisms, allowing bacteria already present in the respiratory tract to multiply, e.g. *Streptococcus pneumoniae, Haemophilus influenzae, Streptococcus pyogenes, Staphylococcus aureus*. Downward spread of infection may lead to bronchiolitis, and bronchopneumonia may develop, especially in children and in debilitated, often elderly, adults.

Chronic bronchitis

Chronic bronchitis is defined clinically when an individual has had a cough with sputum for 3 months in 2 successive years. It is a progressive inflammatory disease resulting from prolonged irritation of the bronchial epithelium. One or more of the following predisposing factors are usually present:

- acute bronchitis commonly caused by *Haemophilus influenzae* or *Streptococcus pneumoniae*
- cigarette smoking
- atmospheric pollutants, e.g. motor vehicle exhaust fumes, industrial chemicals, sulphur dioxide, urban fog
- previous episodes of acute bronchitis.

It develops mostly in middle-aged men who are chronic heavy smokers and may have a familial predisposition. The changes occurring in the mucous membrane of the bronchi include:

- thickening
- increase in the number and size of mucous glands
- oedema
- reduction in the number of ciliated cells
- narrowing of bronchioles due to fibrosis following repeated inflammatory episodes.

Reduced ciliary activity causes stagnation in the bronchi of the excessive amount of mucus secreted. If the mucus and bronchial lining are colonised by bacteria, pus is formed. Stagnant mucus may partially or completely obstruct small bronchioles. The severe difficulty in breathing (*dyspnoea*) with active expiratory effort raises the air pressure in the alveoli and may rupture the alveolar walls, causing *emphysema* (p. 260). Damp cold conditions tend to exacerbate the disease, and spread of infected mucus to the alveoli may cause pneumonia. As the disease progresses inflamed tissue of the bronchi is progressively replaced by fibrous tissue. Ventilation of the lungs is severely impaired, causing breathlessness, leading to hypoxia, pulmonary hypertension and right-sided heart failure. As respiratory failure develops, arterial blood PO_2 is reduced (*hypoxia*) and is accompanied by a rise in arterial blood PCO_2 (*hypercapnia*). When the condition becomes more severe, the respiratory centre in the medulla responds to hypoxia rather than to hypercapnia.

Bronchial asthma

There are two types of bronchial asthma, *extrinsic* and *intrinsic*. In both types the mucous membrane and muscle layers of the bronchi become thickened and the mucous glands enlarge reducing airflow in the lower respiratory tract. During an asthmatic attack spasmodic contraction of bronchial muscle (*bronchospasm*) constricts the airway and there is excessive secretion of thick sticky mucus which further reduces the airway. Inspiration is normal but only partial expiration is achieved. The lungs become hyperinflated and there is severe dyspnoea and wheezing. The duration of attacks usually varies from a few minutes to hours, and very occasionally, days (*status asthmaticus*). In severe acute attacks the bronchi may be obstructed by mucus plugs, leading to acute respiratory failure, hypoxia and possibly death.

Non-specific factors that may precipitate asthma attacks include:

■ cold air
■ cigarette smoking
■ air pollution
■ upper respiratory tract infection
■ emotional stress
■ strenuous exercise.

Extrinsic asthma (allergic, atopic)

This type occurs in children and young adults who have atopic (Type 1) hypersensitivity to foreign protein, e.g. pollen, dust containing mites from carpets, feather pillows, animal dander, fungi. A history of infantile eczema or food allergies is common.

The same disease process occurs as in hay fever. Antigens (allergens) are inhaled and absorbed by the bronchial mucosa. This stimulates the production of IgE antibodies that bind to the surface of mast cells and basophils round the bronchial blood vessels. When the allergen is encountered again, the antigen/antibody reaction results in the release of histamine and other related substances that stimulate mucus secretion and muscle contraction. Attacks tend to become less frequent and less severe with age (Fig. 4.16).

Intrinsic (chronic) asthma

This type occurs later in adult life and there is no history of childhood allergic reactions. It is associated with chronic inflammation of the upper respiratory tract, e.g. chronic bronchitis, nasal polyps. Antigens are rarely identified but drug hypersensitivity may develop later, especially to aspirin and penicillin. Attacks tend to increase in severity and there may be irreversible damage to the lungs. Eventually, impaired lung ventilation leads to hypoxia, pulmonary hypertension and right-sided heart failure.

Bronchiectasis

This is permanent abnormal dilatation of bronchi and bronchioles. It is associated with chronic bacterial infection and in some cases there is a history of childhood bronchiolitis and bronchopneumonia, cystic fibrosis, or bronchial tumour. The bronchi become obstructed by mucus, pus and inflammatory exudate and the alveoli *distal* to the blockage collapse as trapped air is absorbed. Interstitial elastic tissue degenerates and is replaced by fibrous adhesions that attach the bronchi to the parietal pleura. The pressure of inspired air in these damaged bronchi leads to dilatation *proximal* to the blockage. The persistent severe coughing to remove copious purulent sputum causes intermittent increases in pressure in the blocked bronchi, leading to further dilatation.

The lower lobe of the lung is usually affected. Suppuration is common. If a blood vessel is eroded, haemoptysis may occur or pyaemia, leading to abscess formation elsewhere in the body, commonly the brain. Progressive fibrosis of the lung leads to hypoxia, pulmonary hypertension and right-sided heart failure.

DISORDERS OF THE LUNGS

Emphysema (Fig. 10.29)

Pulmonary emphysema

In this form of the disease there is irreversible distension of the respiratory bronchioles, alveolar ducts and alveoli reducing the surface area for the exchange of gases. There are two main types and both are usually present.

Panacinar emphysema
The walls between *adjacent alveoli* break down, the *alveolar ducts* dilate and there is loss of interstitial elastic tissue. The lungs become distended and their capacity is increased. Because the volume of air

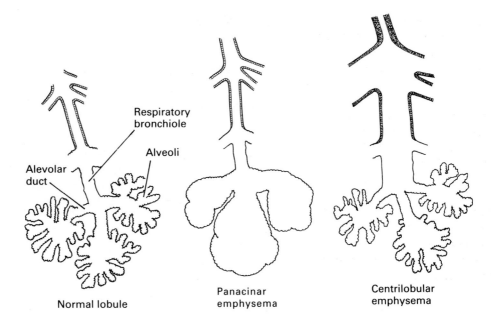

Figure 10.29 Emphysema.

Respiratory bronchiole

Alveoli

Alevolar duct

Normal lobule

Panacinar emphysema

Centrilobular emphysema

in each breath remains unchanged it constitutes a smaller proportion of the total volume of air in the distended alveoli, reducing the partial pressure of oxygen. The merging of alveoli reduces the surface area for diffusion of gases. Homeostasis of arterial blood O_2 and CO_2 levels is maintained at rest by hyperventilation. As the disease progresses the combined effect of these changes may lead to hypoxia, pulmonary hypertension and eventually right-sided heart failure. Predisposing factors include:

- cigarette smoking, believed to promote the release of proteolytic enzymes from mast cells and basophils in the lungs
- acute inflammation of bronchi and lungs
- increased pressure caused by coughing which stretches the already damaged structures
- congenital deficiency of an antiproteolytic enzyme, α_1-antitrypsin, which causes deficiency of supporting elastic tissue in the lungs.

Centrilobular emphysema
In this form there is irreversible dila-

tation of the *respiratory bronchioles* in the centre of lobules. When inspired air reaches the dilated area the pressure falls, leading to a reduction in alveolar air pressure, reduced ventilation efficiency and reduced partial pressure of oxygen. As the disease progresses the resultant hypoxia leads to pulmonary hypertension and right-sided heart failure. Predisposing conditions, exacerbated by persistent severe coughing, include recurrent bronchiolitis, pneumoconiosis, chronic bronchitis and cigarette smoking.

Interstitial emphysema

Air may gain access to thoracic interstitial tissues when a lung is ruptured in one of the following ways:

- from the outside by injury, e.g. fractured rib, stab wound
- from the inside when an alveolus ruptures through the pleura, e.g. during an asthmatic attack, in bronchiolitis, coughing as in whooping cough.

The air in the tissues usually tracks upwards to the soft tissues of the

neck where it is gradually absorbed, causing no damage. A large quantity in the mediastinum may limit heart movement.

Pneumonia (Fig. 10.30)

This occurs when protective processes fail to prevent inhaled or blood-borne microbes reaching and *colonising* the lungs. The following are some predisposing factors.

Impaired coughing. The effectiveness of coughing as an aid to the removal of infected mucus may be reduced when the individual is unconscious or by damage to:

- sensory nerve endings in the walls of the respiratory passages
- the cough reflex centre in the medulla oblongata
- nerves to the respiratory passages, lungs and muscles of respiration
- the diaphragm and intercostal muscles.

Voluntary inhibition may occur if coughing causes pain, e.g. following abdominal surgery.

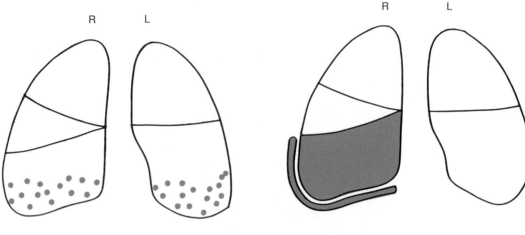

Figure 10.30 The distribution of lesions in broncho- and lobar pneumonia. A. Bronchopneumonia: focal inflammation centred on the airways and often bilateral. B. Lobar pneumonia: diffuse inflammation affecting the entire lobe. Pleural exudate is common.

Damage to the epithelial lining of the tract. Ciliary action may be impaired or the epithelium destroyed by, e.g. tobacco smoking, inhaling noxious gases, infection.

Defective alveolar phagocytosis. Depressed macrophage activity may be caused by tobacco smoking, alcohol, anoxia, oxygen toxicity.

Pulmonary oedema and congestion. Bronchopneumonia frequently occurs in patients with hypostatic pulmonary oedema and congestive heart failure. The relationship is not clear.

General lowering of resistance to infection. Factors involved include:

- leukopenia
- chronic diseases
- impaired immune response caused by, e.g. ionising radiation, corticosteroid drugs
- unusually virulent infections
- hypothermia.

Lobar pneumonia

This is infection of one or more lobes by *Streptococcus pneumoniae*, mainly Type 1, 2 and 3. The infection leads to production of watery inflammatory exudate in the alveoli. This accumulates and fills the lobule then overflows into adjacent lobules, spreading the microbes. It is of sudden onset and pleuritic pain accompanies inflammation of the visceral pleura. If not treated by antibacterial drugs the disease goes through a series of stages followed by resolution and reinflation of the lobes in 2 to 3 weeks.

Complications of lobar pneumonia

Incomplete resolution. If the fibrous exudate, formed as the infection subsides, is not completely cleared it may become permanently solid, tough, leathery and airless, reducing the surface area for gaseous exchange.

Pleural effusion and empyema. When infection spreads to the pleura, inflammatory exudate accumulates (*effusion*) in the pleural cavity and pus is formed (*empyema*). Healing may lead to formation of fibrous adhesions which prevent normal expansion of the lung.

Spread of infection may be to local tissues or cause:

- pericarditis
- acute endocarditis
- meningitis
- acute otitis media
- arthritis.

Lung abscess may develop but only rarely when antimicrobial drugs are available.

Cardiac complications include endocarditis or toxic myocarditis that may lead to heart failure, especially in elderly people.

Bronchopneumonia

Infection is spread from the bronchi to terminal bronchioles and alveoli. As these become inflamed, fibrous exudate accumulates and there is an influx of leukocytes. Small foci of consolidation develop. There is frequently incomplete resolution with fibrosis. Bronchiectasis is a common complication leading to further acute attacks, lung fibrosis and progressive destruction of lung substance. Bronchopneumonia occurs most commonly in infancy and old age, and death is fairly common, especially when the condition complicates debilitating diseases. Predisposing factors include:

- debility due to, e.g., cancer, uraemia, cerebral haemorrhage, congestive heart failure, malnutrition, hypothermia
- chronic bronchitis
- bronchiectasis
- cystic fibrosis
- general anaesthetics which depress respiratory and ciliary activity
- acute viral infections
- inhalation of gastric contents in, e.g. unconsciousness, very deep sleep, following excessive alcohol consumption, drug overdose
- inhalation of infected material from the paranasal sinuses or upper respiratory tract.

Microbes causing bronchopneumonia

Staphylococcus aureus. Infection is usually preceded by influenza, measles, whooping cough or chronic lung disease. Incomplete resolution may cause abscess formation, with rupture into the pleural cavity, empyema and possibly pneumothorax. Pleural adhesions may form during healing and limit lung expansion.

Friedländer's bacillus (Klebsiella pneumoniae). This commensal is sometimes present in the upper respiratory tract, especially where there is advanced dental caries. It commonly causes pneumonia in men over 50 years and is often associated with diabetes mellitus and alcoholism.

Legionella pneumonophila. These microbes are widely distributed in water tanks, shower heads and air conditioning systems, and are therefore commonly found in institutions such as hospitals and hotels. They may cause a severe form of pneumonia (*Legionnaires' disease*),

complicated by gastrointestinal disturbances, headache, mental confusion and renal failure.

Streptococcus pyogenes. Infection is usually preceded by influenza or measles. In very severe cases death may occur within a few days.

Pseudomonas pyocyanea. This is a commensal in the bowel that may cause a type of pneumonia acquired by cross-infection in hospitals, especially in patients with mechanically assisted ventilation or tracheostomy. It is resistant to many antibacterial agents and multiplies at room temperature in, e.g., water, soap solution, eye drops, ointments, weak antiseptics.

Streptococcus pneumoniae (pneumococcus). This is a commensal in the respiratory tract which may cause lobar pneumonia or bronchopneumonia, usually preceded by virus infection. It affects mainly debilitated bed-ridden patients when there is stagnation of mucus in the respiratory passages.

Other organisms. Some viruses, protozoa and fungi may cause pneumonia in people whose general resistance is lowered or whose immune systems are depressed by, e.g. drugs.

Lung abscess

Local suppuration and necrosis within the lung substance is most commonly caused by: *Streptococcus viridans, Streptococcus pyogenes, Streptococcus pneumoniae, Staphylococcus aureus.*

Sources of infection

Inhalation. Infected matter from the paranasal sinuses, gums and the upper respiratory passages may be inhaled. An important predisposing factor is inhalation of regurgitated

gastric contents that may occur during coma, emergency anaesthesia, very deep sleep, following alcohol consumption, drug overdose, sniffing volatile gases from, e.g. glue (*aspiration pneumonia*). The hydrochloric acid and food particles cause severe irritation of the upper respiratory tract, allowing bacteria already present to invade the tissues and spread to the lungs.

Pneumonia. Lung abscess may complicate pneumonia, especially when the latter is caused by *Staphylococcus aureus, Streptococcus pneumoniae* or Friedländer's bacillus.

Septic embolism. Thrombophlebitis and right-sided endocarditis are the main sources of septic emboli that cause lung abscess.

Traumatic penetration of the lung. Pathogenic microbes may enter the lung when both skin and lung are penetrated, e.g. in compound fracture of rib, stab wound, gunshot wound, during surgery.

Local spread of infection. Microbes may spread from the pleural cavity, oesophagus, spine or a subphrenic abscess. Recovery from lung abscess may be complete or lead to complications, e.g.:

- chronic suppuration
- septic emboli may spread to other parts of the body, e.g. the brain, causing cerebral abscess or meningitis
- subpleural abscesses may spread and cause empyema and possibly bronchopleural fistula formation
- erosion of a pulmonary blood vessel, leading to haemorrhage.

Tuberculosis

This infection is caused by one of two forms of mycobacteria.

Mycobacterium tuberculosis. Man is the main host. The microbes cause pulmonary tuberculosis and are spread either by droplet infection from an individual with active tuberculosis, or in dust contaminated by infected sputum.

Mycobacterium bovis. Animals are the main host. The microbes are usually spread to man by untreated milk from infected cows, causing infection of the alimentary tract. In Britain the incidence has been greatly reduced by the elimination of bovine tuberculosis and the pasteurisation of milk. It is still a significant infection in many countries.

Phases of pulmonary tuberculosis

Primary tuberculosis

When microbes are inhaled they colonise a lung bronchiole, usually towards the apex of the lung. There may be no evidence of clinical disease during the initial stage of non-specific inflammation. Later, cell-mediated T-lymphocytes respond to the microbes (antigens) and the individual becomes *sensitised*. Macrophages surround the microbes at the site of infection, forming *Ghon foci* (tubercles). Some macrophages containing live microbes are spread in lymph and infect hilar lymph nodes. *Primary complexes* are formed, consisting of Ghon foci plus infected hilar lymph nodes. Necrosis (caseation) may reduce the core of foci to a cheese-like substance consisting of dead macrophages, dead lung tissue and live and dead microbes. Primary tuberculosis is usually asymptomatic. There are various outcomes:

■ the disease may be permanently arrested, the foci becoming fibrosed and calcified
■ microbes may survive in the foci and become the source of *postprimary infection* months or years later

■ the disease may spread:
—throughout the lung, forming multiple small foci; to the respiratory passages, causing bronchopneumonia or bronchiectasis; to the pleura causing pleurisy, with or without effusion
—to other parts of the body via lymph and blood leading to wide spread of the infection and the development of numerous small foci throughout the body (*miliary tuberculosis*).

Weight loss and malaise develop insidiously, and night sweats are common.

Secondary (postprimary) tuberculosis

This phase occurs only in people *previously sensitised* by a primary lesion, usually situated in the apex of one or both lungs. It may be caused by a new infection or by reactivation of infection by microbes surviving in Ghon foci. As sensitisation has already occurred, T-lymphocytes stimulate an immediate immune reaction, followed by phagocytosis. The subsequent course of the disease is variable, e.g.:

■ it may be arrested, healing occurring with fibrosis and calcification of the foci
■ foci, containing live microbes, may be walled off by fibrous tissue, becoming a potential source of future infection
■ live microbes in foci may break out through the fibrous walls and cause further infection
■ pleurisy with or without effusion or empyema may develop
■ haemoptysis (expectoration of blood-stained sputum) may occur if a small blood vessel is eroded and bleeds into the respiratory tract
■ caseous material containing live microbes may be expectorated,

leaving cavities in the lung, and become a source of infection of:
—the other lung, bronchi, trachea and larynx
—the alimentary tract when microbes are swallowed
■ microbes may spread in blood and lymph, leading to widespread infection and the development of numerous small foci throughout the body (miliary tuberculosis)
■ miliary tuberculosis (see above).

Bovine tuberculosis follows the same course but primary complexes develop in the intestines.

Pneumoconioses

This group of lung diseases is caused by inhaling organic or inorganic atmospheric pollutants. To cause pneumoconiosis, particles must be so small that they are carried in inspired air to the level of the respiratory bronchioles and alveoli where they can only be cleared by phagocytosis. Larger particles are trapped by mucus higher up the tract and expelled by ciliary action and coughing. Other contributory factors include:

■ high concentration of pollutants in the air
■ long exposure to pollutants
■ reduced numbers of macrophages and ineffectual phagocytosis
■ cigarette smoking.

Coal workers' pneumoconiosis

This is caused by inhaling dust from soft bituminous coal. It occurs in two forms.

Simple pneumoconiosis
The particles of coal dust lodge mainly in the upper two-thirds of

the lungs and are ingested by macrophages inside the alveoli. Some macrophages remain in the alveoli and some move out into the surrounding tissues and adhere to the outside of the alveolar walls, respiratory bronchioles, blood vessels and to the visceral pleura. Macrophages are unable to digest inorganic particles and when they die they are surrounded by fibrous tissue. Fibrosis is progressive during exposure to coal dust but tends to stop when exposure stops. Early in the disease there may be few clinical signs unless emphysema develops or there is concurrent chronic bronchitis.

Pneumoconiosis with progressive massive fibrosis

This develops in a small number of cases, sometimes after the worker is no longer exposed to coal dust. Masses of fibrous tissue develop and progressively encroach on the blood vessels and bronchioles. Large parts of the lung are destroyed and emphysema is extensive, leading to pulmonary oedema, pulmonary hypertension and right-sided cardiac failure. The reasons for the severity of the disease are not clear. One factor may be hypersensitivity to antigens released by the large number of dead macrophages. About 40% of the patients have tuberculosis.

Silicosis

This may be caused by long-term exposure to dust containing silicon compounds. High-risk industries are:

- quarrying granite, slate, sandstone
- mining hard coal, gold, tin, copper
- stone masonry and sand blasting
- glass and pottery work.

When silica particles are inhaled they accumulate in the alveoli. The particles are ingested by macrophages, some of which remain in the alveoli and some move out into the connective tissues around respiratory bronchioles and blood vessels and close to the pleura. Progressive fibrosis is stimulated which eventually obliterates the blood vessels and respiratory bronchioles. Fibrous adhesions form between the two layers of pleura, and eventually fix the lung to the chest wall. The relationship between the presence of silicon and the production of excess fibrous tissue is not clear. It may be that:

- inflammation is caused by silicic acid which gradually forms when silicon compounds dissolve
- there is an immune reaction in which silicon is the antigen
- fibrosis is stimulated by enzymes released when macrophages containing silicon die.

Silicosis appears to predispose to the development of tuberculosis which rapidly progresses to tubercular bronchopneumonia and possibly to miliary tuberculosis. Gradual destruction of lung tissue leads to pulmonary hypertension and right-sided heart failure.

Asbestos-related diseases

Diseases caused by inhaling asbestos fibres containing silicon usually develop after 10 to 20 years' exposure but sometimes after only 2 years. Asbestos miners and workers involved in making and using some products containing asbestos are at risk. The types associated with disease are crocidolite (blue asbestos), chrysotile (white asbestos) and amosite (brown asbestos).

Asbestosis

This occurs when asbestos fibres are inhaled in dust. In spite of their large size the particles penetrate to the level of respiratory bronchioles and alveoli. Macrophages accumulate in the alveoli and the shorter fibres are ingested. The larger fibres form *asbestos bodies*, consisting of fibres surrounded by macrophages, protein material and iron deposits. Their presence in sputum indicates exposure to asbestos but not necessarily that there is asbestosis. The macrophages that have engulfed fibres move out of the alveoli and accumulate round respiratory bronchioles and blood vessels, stimulating the formation of fibrous tissue. There is progressive destruction of lung tissue, with the development of dyspnoea, chronic hypoxia, pulmonary hypertension and right-sided cardiac failure. The link between inhaled asbestos and fibrosis is not clear. It may be that asbestos stimulates the macrophages to secrete enzymes that promote fibrosis or that it stimulates an immune reaction causing fibrosis.

Pleural mesothelioma (malignant tumour)

The majority of cases of carcinoma of the pleura are linked with previous exposure to asbestos dust, e.g. asbestos workers and people living near asbestos mines and factories. Mesothelioma may develop after widely varying duration of exposure to asbestos, e.g. 3 months to 60 years, and is usually associated with crocidolite fibres (blue asbestos). The latent period between exposure and the appearance of symptoms may range from 10 to 40 years. The tumour involves both layers of pleura and as it grows it obliterates the pleural cavity, compressing the lung. Lymph and blood-spread metastases are commonly found in the hilar and mesenteric lymph nodes, the other lung, liver, thyroid and adrenal glands, bone, skeletal muscle and brain.

Byssinosis

This is caused by the inhalation of fibres of cotton, flax and hemp over a period of years. The fibres cause bronchial irritation and possibly the release of histamine-like substances. At first, breathless attacks similar to asthma occur only when the individual is at work. Later, they become more persistent and chronic bronchitis and emphysema may develop, leading to chronic hypoxia, pulmonary hypertension and right-sided heart failure.

Extrinsic allergic alveolitis

This group of conditions is caused by inhaling materials contaminated by moulds and fungi, e.g.:

Disease	Contaminant
Farmer's lung	Mouldy hay
Bagassosis	Mouldy sugar waste
Bird handler's lung	Moulds in bird droppings
Malt worker's lung	Mouldy barley

The contaminants act as antigens causing antigen/antibody reactions in the walls of the alveoli. There is excess fluid exudate and the accumulation of platelets, lymphocytes and plasma cells. The alveolar walls become thick and there is progressive fibrosis, leading to pulmonary hypertension and right-sided heart failure.

Chemically induced lung diseases

Paraquat (1,1-dimethyl-4,4 bipyridylium chloride)

Within hours of ingestion of this weedkiller it is blood-borne to the lungs and begins to cause irreversible damage. The alveolar membrane becomes swollen, pulmonary oedema develops and alveolar epithelium is destroyed. The kidneys are also damaged and death may be due to combined respiratory and renal failure or cardiac failure.

Cytotoxic drugs (busulphan, bleomycin, methotrexate)

These and other drugs used in cancer treatment may cause inflammation that heals by fibrosis of interstitial tissue in the lungs and is followed by alveolar fibrosis.

Oxygen toxicity

The lungs may be damaged by a high concentration of oxygen administered for several days, e.g. in intensive care units, to premature babies in incubators. The mechanisms involved are unknown but effects include:

- progressive decrease in lung compliance
- pulmonary oedema
- fibrosis of lung tissue
- breakdown of capillary walls.

In severe cases pneumonia may develop followed by pulmonary hypertension and right-sided heart failure.

Retrolental fibroplasia. This affects premature babies requiring high-concentration oxygen therapy. The oxygen may stimulate immature retinal blood vessels to constrict causing fibrosis, retinal detachment and blindness (p. 212).

Bronchial carcinoma

Primary bronchial carcinoma is a common form of malignancy. The tumour usually develops in a main bronchus, forming a large friable mass that projects into the lumen sometimes causing obstruction. Mucus then collects and predisposes to development of infection. As the tumour grows it may erode a blood vessel, causing haemoptysis.

The cause is not known but there is a strong positive association with cigarette smoking and the inhalation of other people's smoke (passive smoking).

Spread of bronchial cancer

This does not follow any particular pattern or sequence. The modes of spread are infiltration of local tissues and the transport of tumour fragments in blood and lymph. If blood or lymph vessels are eroded, fragments may spread while the tumour is quite small. A metastatic tumour may, therefore, cause symptoms before the primary in the lung has been detected.

Local spread may be within the lung, to the other lung or to mediastinal structure, e.g. blood vessels, nerves, oesophagus.

Lymphatic spread. Tumour fragments spread along lymph vessels to successive lymph nodes in which they may cause metastatic tumours. Fragments may enter lymph draining from a tumour or gain access to a larger vessel when its walls have been eroded by a growing tumour. Early symptoms may be due to pressure caused by enlarged lymph nodes in the thorax.

Blood spread. Tumour cells usually enter the blood when a blood vessel is eroded by local spread of the tumour. The most common sites of blood-borne metastases are the liver, brain, adrenal glands, bones and kidneys.

Atelectasis

In atelectasis, expansion of the lungs at birth is defective. There are two types, distinguished by the time of onset.

Immediately after birth

There may be partial or complete lack of expansion of the lungs due to:

- obstruction of the airways by secretions
- incomplete development of the respiratory passages
- lack of stimulation by the respiratory centre in the medulla oblongata due to congenital abnormality or prematurity.

Within minutes or hours of birth

Breathing appears to be normal at first but acute respiratory distress and cyanosis develop later. The condition is associated with prematurity. Normally fluid containing phospholipid surfactant is secreted between the surfaces of the unexpanded alveoli after about the 35th week of gestation (p. 248). Its function is to reduce the tension between the alveolar surfaces, and so reduce the effort needed to expand the lungs at birth. Surfactant deficiency, possibly accompanied by immaturity of the respiratory centre, causes atelectasis. Reasons for its occurrence following caesarian section and in maternal diabetes are not known.

Collapse of lung

(Fig. 10.31)

This may be caused by airway obstruction or by positive pressure in the pleural cavity. The degree of dyspnoea and respiratory distress is determined by the amount of air or fluid in the pleural cavity.

Absorption collapse (airway obstruction)

The amount of lung affected depends on the size of the obstructed air passage. Distal to the obstruction air is trapped and absorbed, the lung collapses and secretions collect. These may become infected, causing abscess formation. Short-term obstruction is usually followed by reinflation of the lung without lasting ill-effects. Prolonged obstruction leads to progressive fibrosis and permanent collapse. Sudden obstruction may be due to inhalation of a foreign body or a mucus plug formed during an asthmatic attack or in chronic bronchitis. Gradual obstruction may be due to a bronchial tumour or pressure on a bronchus by, e.g. enlarged mediastinal lymph nodes, aortic aneurysm.

Pressure collapse

When air or fluid enters the pleural cavity the negative pressure becomes positive, preventing lung expansion. The collapse usually affects only one lung and may be partial or complete. There is no obstruction of the airway.

Pneumothorax

In this condition there is air in the pleural cavity. It may occur spontaneously or be the result of trauma.

Spontaneous pneumothorax is either primary or secondary. *Primary spontaneous pneumothorax* is of unknown cause and occurs in fit and healthy people, usually males between 20 and 40 years. *Secondary spontaneous pneumothorax* occurs when air enters the pleural cavity after the visceral pleura ruptures due to lung disease, e.g. emphysema, asthma, pulmonary tuberculosis, bronchial cancer.

Traumatic pneumothorax is due to a penetrating injury, e.g. compound fracture of rib, stab or gunshot wound, surgery.

Tension pneumothorax occurs as a complication when a flap or one-way valve develops between the lungs and the pleural cavity. Air enters the pleural cavity during inspiration but cannot escape on expiration and steadily accumulates. This causes shift of the mediastinum and compression of the other lung resulting in severe respiratory distress and is often fatal.

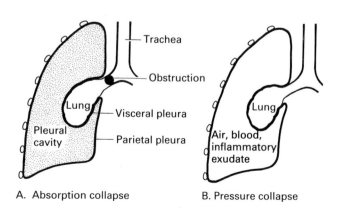

A. Absorption collapse   B. Pressure collapse

Figure 10.31 Collapsed lung.

Haemothorax

This is blood in the pleural cavity. It may be caused by:

- penetrating chest injury involving blood vessels
- ruptured aortic aneurysm
- erosion of a blood vessel by a malignant tumour.

Pleural effusion

This is excess fluid in the pleural cavity and may be caused by:

- increased hydrostatic pressure, e.g. heart failure, increased blood volume
- increased capillary permeability due to local inflammation, e.g. pneumonia, pulmonary tuberculosis, bronchial cancer, mesothelioma
- decreased plasma osmotic pressure, e.g. nephrotic syndrome (p. 350), cirrhosis of the liver (p. 332)
- impaired lymphatic drainage, e.g. malignant tumour involving the pleura.

Fibrous adhesions which limit reinflation may form between the layers of pleura, following haemothorax and pleural effusion.

11
Introduction to nutrition

Before discussing the digestive system it is necessary to have an understanding of the needs of the body regarding nutrition, i.e. the dietary constituents and their functions within the body.

A *nutrient* is any substance that is digested, absorbed and utilised to promote body function. These substances are:

- carbohydrates
- proteins
- fats
- vitamins
- mineral salts
- water.

Many foods contain a number of nutrients, e.g. potatoes and bread are mainly carbohydrate but both contain protein and some vitamins. Foods are described as carbohydrate or protein because they contain a higher proportion of one or the other. *Fibre* consists of indigestible material. It is not a nutrient, as it is not digested, absorbed or utilised, but it has many beneficial effects on the digestive tract.

The *diet* is the selection of foods eaten by an individual. A *balanced diet* is essential for health. It provides the appropriate amounts of all nutrients in the correct proportions to meet the requirements of the body cells. An *essential nutrient* is a substance that cannot be made by the body and must therefore be included in the diet.

Details of digestion, absorption and utilisation of nutrients are presented in Chapter 12.

CARBOHYDRATES

These are found in a wide variety of foods, e.g. sugar, jam, cereals, bread, biscuits, pasta, convenience foods, fruit and vegetables. They consist of carbon, hydrogen and oxygen, the hydrogen and oxygen being in the same proportion as in water. Carbohydrates are classified according to the complexity of the chemical substances of which they are formed.

Monosaccharides

Carbohydrates are digested in the alimentary canal and when absorbed they are in the form of monosaccharides. Examples include: glucose, fructose and galactose. These are, chemically, the simplest form in which a carbohydrate can exist. They are made up of single units or molecules which, if they were broken down further, would cease to be monosaccharides.

Disaccharides

These consist of two monosaccharide molecules chemically combined to form sugars, e.g. sucrose, maltose and lactose.

Polysaccharides

These consist of complex molecules made up of large numbers of monosaccharide molecules in chemical combination, e.g. starches, glycogen, cellulose and dextrins.

Not all polysaccharides can be digested by human beings; e.g. cellulose and other substances present in vegetables, fruit and some cereals pass through the alimentary canal almost unchanged.

The functions of digestible carbohydrates

These include:

- provision of rapidly available energy and heat
- 'protein sparing'; i.e., when there is an adequate supply of carbohydrate in the diet, protein does not need to be used to provide energy and heat
- provision of a store of energy when carbohydrate is eaten in excess of the body's needs as it is converted to fat and deposited in the fat depots, e.g. under the skin.

PROTEINS OR NITROGENOUS FOODS

Proteins are made up of a large number of units called amino acids linked together chemically. Each protein consists of a specific number of different amino acids arranged in a way which is characteristic of that protein.

Proteins are broken down into their constituent amino acids by digestion and it is in this form that they are absorbed through the intestinal wall. Dietary protein is the only source of nitrogen that is usable in the body. If it is absent from the diet the body goes into *negative nitrogen balance*. This is because amino acids are constantly being used to form enzymes, hormones and cell proteins and the turnover of cells is accompanied by the formation of nitrogenous waste materials that are excreted by the kidneys.

Amino acids

These are composed of the elements carbon, hydrogen, oxygen, nitrogen. Some contain minerals such as iron, copper, zinc, iodine, sulphur and phosphorus. They are divided into two categories, *essential* and *non-essential*.

Essential amino acids cannot be synthesised in the body, therefore they must be included in the diet. They are:

isoleucine	methionine	tryptophan
leucine	phenylalanine	valine
lysine	threonine	

Non-essential amino acids are those which can be synthesised in the body. They are:

alanine	cystine	hydroxyproline
arginine	glutamic acid	proline
asparagine	glutamine	serine
aspartic acid	glycine	tyrosine
cysteine	histidine	

The nutritional value of a protein depends on the amino acids of which it is composed.

Complete (first-class) proteins

This term is given to protein foods which contain all the essential amino acids in the proportions required to maintain health. They are derived almost entirely from animal sources and include:

meat	fish	soya beans
milk	eggs	
milk products (excluding butter)		

Incomplete (second-class) proteins

These do not contain all the essential amino acids in the correct proportions; they are mainly of vegetable origin and can be found in the *cereals* and *pulses*, i.e. peas, beans and lentils. A variable proportion of protein is to be found in other vegetables and in some of the mainly carbohydrate foods, such as bread and potatoes. By eating different types of incomplete proteins potential deficiency in the missing amino acids can be avoided.

Functions of proteins

Amino acids are used for:

- growth and repair of body cells and tissues
- synthesis of enzymes, plasma proteins, antibodies (immunoglobulins) and some hormones
- provision of energy, normally a secondary function, this becomes important only when there is not enough carbohydrate in the diet and fat stores are depleted.

When protein is eaten in excess of the body's needs, the nitrogenous part is detached, i.e. it is deaminated, and excreted by the kidneys. The remainder is converted to fat for storage in the fat depots, e.g. in the fat cells of adipose tissue (p. 26).

FATS

Fats consist of carbon, hydrogen and oxygen, but they differ from carbohydrates in that the hydrogen and oxygen are not in the same proportions as in water. Fats are divided into two groups, *saturated* and *unsaturated*.

Saturated or *animal fat*, containing mainly saturated fatty acids and glycerol, is found in milk, cheese, butter, eggs, meat and oily fish such as herring, cod and halibut. All the animal sources of protein contain some saturated fat.

Cholesterol is synthesised in the body and is also taken in the diet from full fat dairy products, fatty meat and egg yolk.

Unsaturated or *vegetable fat*, containing mainly unsaturated fatty acids and glycerol, is found in some margarine and in most vegetable oils.

Linoleic, linolenic and arachidonic acids are polyunsaturated fatty acids that are essential in the diet because they cannot be synthesised in the body. They are the precursors of prostaglandins and some substances which promote blood clotting and others that are anticoagulants.

Functions of fats

These include:

- production of chemical energy and heat
- support of certain body organs, e.g. the kidneys, the eyes
- transport and storage of the fat-soluble vitamins: A, D, E, K
- constituent of nerve sheaths and of sebum, the secretion of sebaceous glands in the skin
- formation of cholesterol and steroid hormones
- storage of energy as fat in adipose tissue under the skin and in the mesentery, when eaten in excess of requirements
- insulation—as a subcutaneous layer it reduces heat loss through the skin
- satiety value—when gastric contents (chyme) containing fat enter the duodenum, the emptying time of the stomach is prolonged, postponing the return of hunger.

VITAMINS

Vitamins are chemical compounds required in very small quantities which are essential for normal metabolism and health. They are found widely distributed in food and are divided into two main groups:

■ fat-soluble vitamins: A, D, E and K
■ water-soluble vitamins: B complex, C.

Fat-soluble vitamins

Vitamin A (retinol)

This vitamin is found in such foods as cream, egg yolk, liver, fish oil, milk, cheese and butter. It is absent from vegetable fats and oils but is added to margarine during manufacture. It can be formed in the body from certain carotenes the main dietary sources of which are green vegetables, fruit and carrots. Vitamin A and carotene are only absorbed from the small intestine satisfactorily if fat absorption is normal. Although some is synthesised in the body the daily dietary requirement is 600 to 700 μg. It is essential for the regeneration of *rhodopsin* (visual purple) which is bleached by bright light, maintaining healthy epithelial cells and the balance between osteoblasts and osteoclasts in bone growth.

Deficiency results in:

■ night blindness when rhodopsin is not regenerated
■ xerophthalmia or drying and ulceration of the cornea
■ atrophy and keratinisation of epithelium, leading to increased incidence of infections of the ear, air sinuses, respiratory, urinary and alimentary tracts
■ slow and faulty development of bones.

Vitamin D

Vitamin D_3, the *antirachitic vitamin*, is found mainly in animal fats such as eggs, butter, cheese, fish liver oils.

Humans and other animals can synthesise *cholecalciferol* (vitamin D) by the action of the ultraviolet rays of the sun on a form of cholesterol in the skin (7-dehydrocholesterol).

Calciferol (vitamin D_2) is formed in plants and is used in therapeutics.

Vitamin D regulates calcium and phosphorus metabolism and is therefore associated with the calcification of bones and teeth. Deficiency causes *rickets* in children and *osteomalacia* in adults, due to deficient absorption and utilisation of calcium and phosphorus.

The daily requirement is 10 μg and stores in fat and muscle are such that deficiency may not be apparent for several years.

Vitamin E

This is a group of substances called *tocopherols*. They are found in nuts, egg yolk, wheat germ, whole cereal, milk and butter and the daily requirement is about 3 to 4 mg. Vitamin E prevents the catabolism of polyunsaturated fats.

Deficiency is associated with mild haemolytic anaemia because of erythrocyte membrane fragility. Chronic deficiency leads to defective prostaglandin synthesis, ataxia, cystic fibrosis and blind spots in the retina (scotomas).

Vitamin K

The sources of vitamin K are fish, liver, leafy green vegetables and fruit. It is synthesised in the large intestine by microbes and significant amounts are absorbed. Absorption is dependent upon the presence of bile salts in the small intestine. The normal daily requirement is 1 μg/kg body weight and only a small amount is stored in the liver and spleen.

It is necessary for the formation by the liver of prothrombin and factors VII, IX and X, all essential for the clotting of blood (p. 61). Deficiency causes defective blood coagulation. It may occur in adults when there is obstruction to the flow of bile, severe liver damage and in malabsorption conditions, such as *coeliac disease*. It may occur in newborn infants before microbes are established in the bowel.

Water-soluble vitamins

Vitamin B complex

This consists of a group of water-soluble vitamins that promote activity of enzymes at various stages in the chemical breakdown (catabolism) of nutrients to release energy.

Vitamin B_1 (thiamine)

This vitamin is present in nuts, yeast, egg yolk, liver, legumes, meat and the germ of cereals. It is rapidly destroyed by heat. The daily requirement is 0.8 to 1 mg and the body stores only about 30 mg. Thiamine is essential for the complete aerobic release of energy from carbohydrate. When it is absent there is accumulation of lactic acid and pyruvate.

Deficiency causes *beriberi* which occurs mainly in countries where polished rice is the chief constituent of the diet. In beriberi there is:

- severe muscle wasting
- stunted growth in children
- polyneuritis, causing degeneration of motor, sensory and some autonomic nerves
- susceptibility to infections.

If untreated, death occurs due to cardiac failure or severe microbial infection.

Vitamin B₂ (riboflavine)

Riboflavine is found in yeast, green vegetables, milk, liver, eggs, cheese and fish roe. The daily requirement is 1.1 to 1.3 mg and only small amounts are stored in the body. It is concerned with carbohydrate and protein metabolism, especially in the eyes and skin. Deficiency leads to:

- blurred vision, cataract formation, corneal ulceration
- cracking of the skin, commonly around the mouth
- lesions of intestinal mucosa.

Folic acid

This is found in liver, kidney, fresh leafy green vegetables and yeast. It is synthesised by bacteria in the large intestine, and significant amounts derived from this source are believed to be absorbed. The daily requirement is 200 μg. and, as only a small amount is stored in the body, deficiency is evident within a short time. It is essential for the maturation of erythrocytes and deficiency causes a type of megaloblastic anaemia (p. 74).

Niacin (nicotinic acid)

This is found in liver, cheese, yeast, whole cereals, eggs, fish and nuts. It is associated with energy-releasing reactions in cells. In fat metabolism it inhibits the production of cholesterol and assists in fat breakdown. Deficiency occurs mainly in areas where maize is the chief constituent of the diet because niacin in maize is in an unusable form. The daily requirement is 12 to 17 mg.

Pellagra develops within 6 to 8 weeks of severe deficiency. It is characterised by:

- redness of the skin in parts exposed to light, especially in the neck
- anorexia, nausea, dysphagia, inflammation of the lining of the mouth
- delirium, mental disturbance, dementia.

Vitamin B₆ (pyridoxine)

This is found in egg yolk, peas, beans, soya beans, yeast, meat and liver. The daily requirement is about 1.2 to 1.4 mg and deficiency is rare. It is associated with amino acid metabolism, especially the production of antibodies.

Vitamin B₁₂ (cyanocobalamin)

Vitamin B_{12} consists of a number of *cobalamin compounds* (containing cobalt). It is found in liver, meat, eggs, milk and fermented liquors. The normal daily requirement is 1.5 μg.

It is essential for the maturation of erythrocytes in red bone marrow and for the formation and maintenance of myelin, the fatty substance that surrounds and protects some nerve fibres. Deficiency causes megaloblastic anaemia (p. 74) and subacute combined degeneration of the spinal cord (p. 186).

Pantothenic acid

This is found in many foods and is associated with amino acid metabolism. The daily safe intake is 3 to 7 mg and no deficiency diseases have been identified.

Biotin

This is found in yeast, egg yolk, liver, kidney and tomatoes and is synthesised by microbes in the intestine. It is associated with the metabolism of carbohydrates. The daily safe intake is 10 to 200 μg. Deficiency is rare.

Vitamin C (ascorbic acid)

This is found in fresh fruit, especially blackcurrants, oranges, grapefruit and lemons, and also in rosehips and green vegetables.

The daily requirement is 40 mg and after 2 to 3 months, deficient intake becomes apparent. Vitamin C is associated with protein metabolism, especially the laying down of collagen in connective tissue. The vitamin is very soluble in water and is easily destroyed by heat, so cooking may be a factor in the development of *scurvy*. Manifestations of deficiency include:

- swollen and spongy gums
- anaemia
- haemorrhage under the skin and into joints
- delayed wound healing.

MINERAL SALTS

Mineral salts (inorganic compounds) are necessary within the body for all body processes. They are usually required in small quantities. They include many compounds some of which are in very small quantities. The main elements involved are:

calcium   phosphorus   sodium
iron   iodine   potassium

Calcium

This is found in milk, cheese, eggs, green vegetables and some fish. An adequate supply should be obtained in a normal, well-balanced diet. It is associated with vitamin D and phosphorus in the hardening of bones and teeth, so an adequate supply in young people is important. It is also involved in the coagulation of blood and the mechanism of muscle contraction.

Phosphorus

Sources of phosphorus include cheese, oatmeal, liver and kidney. If there is sufficient calcium in the diet it is unlikely that there will be a deficiency of phosphorus.

It is associated with calcium and vitamin D in the hardening of bones and teeth and helps to maintain the constant composition of the body fluids. Phosphates are an essential part of systems of energy storage inside cells as adenosine triphosphate (ATP).

Sodium

Sodium is found in most foods, especially fish, meat, eggs, milk, artificially enriched bread and as cooking and table salt. The normal intake of sodium chloride per day varies from 5 to 20 g and the daily requirement is 1.6 g. Excess is excreted in the urine.

It is the most commonly occurring *extracellular cation* and is associated with:

- contraction of muscles
- transmission of nerve impulses in nerve fibres
- maintenance of the electrolyte balance in the body.

Potassium

This substance is to be found widely distributed in all foods, especially fruit and vegetables. The normal intake of potassium chloride is 3.5 g per day and this is in excess of potassium requirements.

It is the most commonly occurring *intracellular cation* and is involved in many chemical activities inside cells including:

- contraction of muscles
- transmission of nerve impulses
- maintenance of the electrolyte balance in the body.

Iron

Iron, as a soluble compound, is found in liver, kidney, beef, egg yolk, wholemeal bread and green vegetables. In normal adults about 1 mg of iron is lost from the body daily. The normal daily diet contains more, i.e. 9 to 15 mg, but the amount absorbed is only equal to the amount lost. Higher intake is needed by women especially during pregnancy. Iron is essential for the formation of *haemoglobin* in the red blood cells. It is necessary for oxidation of carbohydrate (p. 312).

Iodine

Iodine is found in salt-water fish and in vegetables grown in soil containing iodine. In some parts of the world where iodine is deficient in soil very small quantities are added to table salt. The daily requirement of iodine depends upon the individual's metabolic rate. Some people have a higher normal metabolic rate than others and their iodine requirements are greater. The daily requirement is 140 μg.

It is essential for the formation of *thyroxine* and *triiodothyronine*, two hormones secreted by the thyroid gland.

FIBRE

Fibre is the indigestible part of the diet that comes from plants and meat. It consists of bran, cellulose and other polysaccharides. It is widely distributed in wholemeal flour, the husks of cereals and in vegetables. Dietary fibre is partly digested by microbes in the large intestine with gas (flatus) formation. The daily requirement of fibre is not less than 20 g.

Functions

Fibre:

- provides bulk to the diet and helps to satisfy the appetite

- stimulates peristalsis (muscular activity) of the alimentary tract
- attracts water, increasing bulk and softness of faeces
- increases frequency of defaecation preventing constipation
- prevents some gastrointestinal disorders, e.g. diverticular disease (p. 326).

WATER

Water is a liquid compound of hydrogen and oxygen formed by the chemical combination of two parts hydrogen and one part oxygen (H_2O). Water makes up about 70% of the body weight in men and about 60% in women.

A man weighing 65 kg contains about 40 litres of water, 28 of which are intracellular and 12 extracellular. Extracellular water consists of 2 to 3 litres in plasma and the remainder, interstitial fluid (Fig. 11.1).

A large amount of water is lost each day in faeces, sweat and urine. Under normal circumstances this is balanced by intake in food and to satisfy thirst. Dehydration with serious consequences may occur if intake does not balance loss.

Functions

These include:

- provision of the moist internal environment which is required by all living cells in the body, i.e. all

Total body water 40 litres	Extracellular fluid (ECF) 12 litres (Plasma 2.5 l, Interstitial fluid 9.5 l)
	Intracellular fluid (ICF) 28 litres

Figure 11.1 Distribution of body water in a 70 kg person.

the cells except the superficial layers of the skin, the nails, the hair and outer hard layer of the teeth
- participation in all the chemical reactions which occur inside and outside the body cells
- dilution and moistening of food (saliva, p. 290)
- regulation of body temperature—as a constituent of sweat, which is secreted onto the skin, it evaporates, cooling the body surface (p. 363)
- a major constituent of blood and tissue fluid it transports some substances in solution and some in suspension round the body
- dilution of waste products and poisonous substances in the body
- providing the medium for the excretion of waste products, e.g. urine and faeces.

Tables 11.1 and 11.2 summarise the vitamins—their chemical names, sources, stability, functions, deficiency diseases and daily adult requirements.

Table 11.1 Summary—fat-soluble vitamins (DoH 1991)

Vitamin	Chemical name	Source	Stability	Functions	Deficiency diseases	Daily recommended intake (adults)
A	Retinol (carotene provitamin in plants)	Milk, butter, cheese, egg yolk, fish, liver oils, green and yellow vegetables	Some loss at high temperatures and long exposure to light and air	Maintains healthy epithelial tissues and cornea. Formation of visual purple	Keratinisation Xerophthalmia Stunted growth Night blindness	600–700 μg
D	Calciferol	Fish, liver, oils, milk, cheese, egg yolk, irradiated 7-dehydrocholesterol in human skin	Very stable	Facilitates the absorption and utilisation of calcium and phosphorus = healthy bones and teeth	Rickets (children) Osteomalacia (adults)	10 μg
E	Tocopherols	Egg yolk, milk, butter, green vegetables, nuts	Stable in heat but oxidised by exposure to air	Prevents catabolism of polyunsaturated fats	Anaemia Ataxia Cystic fibrosis Scotomas	3–4 mg*
K	Phylloquinone	Leafy vegetables, fish, liver, fruit	Destroyed by light, strong acids and alkalis	Formation of prothrombin and factors VII, IX and X in the liver	Slow blood clotting Haemorrhages in the newborn	60–70 μg*

Bile is necessary for the absorption of these vitamins.
Mineral oils interfere with absorption.
* Daily safe intake (DoH 1991). Data for recommended intake not available.

Table 11.2 Summary—water-soluble vitamins (DoH 1991)

Vitamin	Chemical name	Source	Stability	Functions	Deficiency diseases	Daily recommended intake (adults)
B₁	Thiamin	Yeast, liver, germ of cereals, nuts, pulses, rice polishings, egg yolk, liver, legumes	Destroyed by heat	Metabolism of carbohydrates and nutrition of nerve cells	General fatigue and loss of muscle tone Ultimately leads to beriberi Stunted growth	0.8–1 mg
B₂	Riboflavine	Liver, yeast, milk, eggs, green vegetables, kidney, fish roe	Destroyed by light and alkalis	Carbohydrate and protein metabolism Healthy skin and eyes	Angular stomatitis Cheilosis Dermatitis Eye lesions	1–1.3 mg
B₆	Pyridoxine	Meat, liver, vegetables, bran of cereals, egg yolk, beans	Stable	Protein metabolism Production of antibodies	Very rare	1.2–1.4 mg
B₁₂	Cobalamins	Liver, milk, moulds, fermenting liquors, egg	Destroyed by heat	Maturation of RBCs DNA synthesis	Pernicious anaemia Degeneration of nerve fibres of the spinal cord	1.5 μg
B	Folic acid	Dark green vegetables, liver, kidney, eggs. Synthesised in colon	Destroyed by heat and moisture	Formation of RBCs DNA synthesis	Anaemia	200 μg
B	Niacin (nicotinic acid)	Yeast, offal, fish, pulses, wholemeal cereals. Synthesised in the body from tryptophan	Fairly stable	Necessary for cell respiration Inhibits production of cholesterol	Prolonged deficiency causes pellagra, i.e. dermatitis, diarrhoea, dementia	12–17 mg
B	Pantothenic acid	Liver, yeast, egg yolk, fresh vegetables	Destroyed by excessive heat and freezing	Associated with amino acid metabolism	Unknown	3–7 mg*
B	Biotin	Yeasts, liver, kidney, pulses, nuts	Stable	Carbohydrates and fat metabolism	Dermatitis, conjunctivitis Hypercholesterolaemia	10–200 μg*
C	Ascorbic acid	Citrus fruits, currants, berries, green vegetables, potatoes, liver and glandular tissue in animals	Destroyed by heat, ageing, acids, alkalis, chopping, salting, drying	Formation of collagen Maturation of RBCs	Multiple haemorrhages Slow wound healing Anaemia Gross deficiency causes scurvy	40 mg

Para-aminobenzoic acid and inositol are two vitamins of the B group about which little is known.
* Daily safe intake (DoH 1991). Data for recommended intake not available.

DISORDERS OF NUTRITION

The importance of nutrition is increasingly recognised as essential for health, and illness often alters nutritional requirements.

Malnutrition

This may be due to:

- protein–energy malnutrition (PEM)
- vitamin deficiencies (Tables 11.1 and 11.2)
- both PEM and vitamin deficiencies.

Protein–energy malnutrition (Fig. 11.2)

This is the result of inadequate intake of protein, carbohydrate and fat. Infants and young children are especially susceptible as they need sufficient nutrients to grow and develop normally. If dietary intake is inadequate, it is not uncommon for vitamin deficiency to develop at the same time. Poor nutrition, or malnutrition, reduces the ability to combat other illness and infection.

Kwashiorkor

This is mainly caused by protein deficiency, and occurs in infants and children in some developing countries and when there has been serious drought and crop failure. Reduced plasma proteins lead to ascites and oedema (p. 117) in the lower limbs that masks emaciation. There is severe liver damage. Growth stops and there is loss of weight and loss of pigmentation of skin and hair accompanied by listlessness, apathy and irritability.

Marasmus

This is caused by deficiency of both protein and energy. It is characterised by severe emaciation due to breakdown (catabolism) of muscle and fat. Growth is retarded, the skin becomes wrinkled and hair is lost.

Malabsorption

When this is present, nutritional intake needs to be modified due to impaired intestinal function, e.g. in coeliac disease, tropical sprue (p. 329).

Obesity

This is a very common nutritional disorder in which there is accumulation of excess body fat. Clinically, obesity is present when body weight is 120% of that recommended for the height, age and sex of the individual. It occurs when energy intake exceeds energy expenditure, e.g. when food intake is increased and energy intake is the same, or when energy output is reduced and food intake remains the same or is increased.

Obesity predisposes to the development of a number of conditions:

- gallstones (p. 334)
- cardiovascular diseases, e.g. ischaemic heart disease (p. 120), hypertension (p. 126)
- hernias (p. 327)
- varicose veins (p. 120)
- osteoarthritis (p. 410)
- type II (non-insulin-dependent) diabetes mellitus
- increased incidence of postoperative complications.

Genetic abnormality

Phenylketonuria

See p. 185.

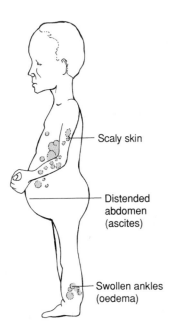
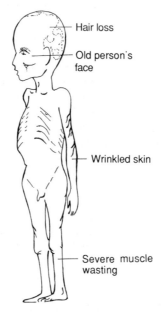

A. Kwashiorkor

B. Marasmus

Figure 11.2 Features of kwashiorkor and marasmus.

12
The digestive system

The digestive system is the collective name used to describe the *alimentary canal,* some *accessory organs* and a variety of *digestive processes* which take place at different levels in the canal to prepare food eaten in the diet for absorption. The alimentary canal begins at the mouth, passes through the thorax, abdomen and pelvis and ends at the anus. It has a general structure which is modified at different levels to provide for the processes occurring at each level. The complex of digestive processes gradually simplifies the foods eaten until they are in a form suitable for absorption. For example, meat, even when cooked, is chemically too complex to be absorbed from the alimentary canal.

It therefore goes through a series of changes which release its constituent nutrients: amino acids, mineral salts, fat and vitamins. Chemical substances or *enzymes** which effect these changes are secreted into the canal by special glands, some of which are in the walls of the canal and some outside the canal, but with ducts leading into it.

* An enzyme is a chemical substance which causes, or speeds up, a chemical change in other substances without itself being changed. Each enzyme is specific to one chemical change and has an optimal pH and temperature for action. The name of an active enzyme may be recognised by the suffix -ase. Sometimes an inactive precursor is secreted; its name has the suffix -ogen.

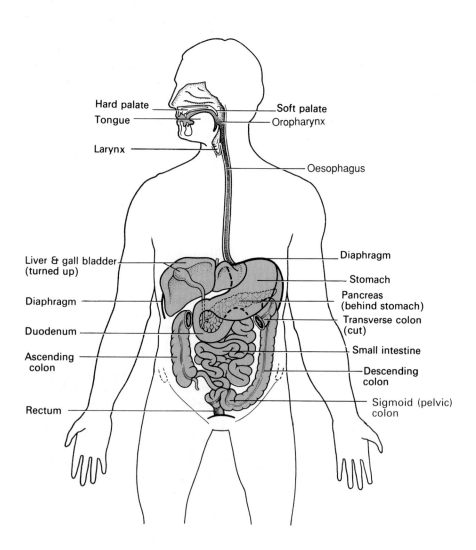

Figure 12.1 The organs of the digestive system.

After they are absorbed, the nutrient materials are used in the synthesis of the constituents of the body. They provide the raw materials for the manufacture of new cells, hormones and enzymes, and the energy needed for these and other processes and for the disposal of waste materials.

The activities in the digestive system can be grouped under five main headings.

Ingestion, taking food into the alimentary tract.

Propulsion moves the contents along the alimentary tract.

Digestion is divided into:

- *mechanical breakdown* of food by, e.g. mastication (chewing)
- *chemical breakdown* of food by *enzymes* present in secretions produced by glands and accessory organs of the digestive system.

Absorption is the process by which digested food substances pass through the walls of some organs of the alimentary canal into the blood and lymph capillaries for circulation round the body.

Elimination Food substances which have been eaten but cannot be digested and absorbed are excreted by the bowel as faeces.

ORGANS OF THE DIGESTIVE SYSTEM (FIG. 12.1)

Alimentary tract

This is a long tube through which food passes. It commences at the mouth and terminates at the anus, and the various parts are given separate names, although structurally they are remarkably similar. The parts are:

- mouth
- pharynx
- oesophagus
- stomach
- small intestine
- large intestine
- rectum and anal canal.

Accessory organs

Various secretions are poured into the alimentary tract, some by glands in the lining membrane of the organs, e.g. gastric juice secreted by glands in the lining of the stomach, and some by glands situated outside the tract. The latter are the accessory organs of digestion and their secretions pass through ducts to enter the tract. They consist of:

- 3 pairs of salivary glands
- pancreas
- liver and the biliary tract.

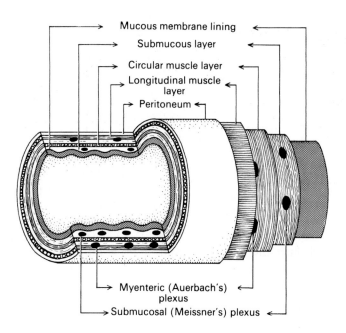

Mucous membrane lining
Submucous layer
Circular muscle layer
Longitudinal muscle layer
Peritoneum
Myenteric (Auerbach's) plexus
Submucosal (Meissner's) plexus

Figure 12.2 General plan of the alimentary canal.

The organs and glands are linked physiologically as well as anatomically in that digestion and absorption occur in stages, each stage being dependent upon the previous stage or stages.

GENERAL PLAN OF THE ALIMENTARY CANAL (FIG. 12.2)

The structure of the alimentary canal follows a consistent pattern from the level of the oesophagus onwards. This *general plan* does not apply so obviously to the mouth and the pharynx so these parts of the tract have been excluded at this stage.

In the different organs from the oesophagus onwards, modifications of structure are found which are associated with special functions. The general plan is described here and the modifications in structure and function are described in the appropriate section.

The walls of the alimentary tract are formed by four layers of tissue:

- adventitia or outer covering
- muscle layer
- submucous layer
- mucosa—lining.

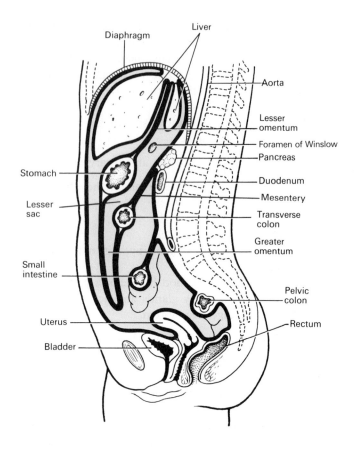

Figure 12.3 The peritoneum (gold) and its association with the abdominal organs of the digestive system and the pelvic organs viewed from the side.

Adventitia (outer covering)

In the thorax this consists of *loose fibrous tissue* and in the abdomen the organs are covered by a serous membrane called *peritoneum*.

Peritoneum (Fig. 12.3)

The peritoneum is the largest serous membrane of the body. It consists of a closed sac, containing a small amount of serous fluid, within the abdominal cavity. It has two layers:

- the *parietal layer*, which lines the abdominal wall
- the *visceral layer*, which covers the organs (viscera) within the abdominal and pelvic cavities.

The arrangement of the peritoneum is such that the organs are invaginated into the closed sac from below, behind and above so that they are at least partly covered by the visceral layer. This means that:

- pelvic organs are covered only on their superior surface
- the stomach and intestines, deeply invaginated from behind, are almost completely surrounded by peritoneum and have a double fold (the *mesentery*) that attaches them to the posterior abdominal wall
- the pancreas, spleen, kidneys and adrenal glands are invaginated from behind but only their anterior surfaces are covered and are therefore *retroperitoneal*
- the liver is invaginated from above and is almost competely covered by peritoneum which attaches it to the inferior surface of the diaphragm
- the main blood vessels and nerves pass close to the posterior abdominal wall and send branches to the organs between folds of peritoneum.

The parietal peritoneum lines the anterior abdominal wall.

The two layers of peritoneum are actually in contact and friction between them is prevented by the presence of serous fluid secreted by the peritoneal cells, thus the *peritoneal cavity* is only a *potential cavity*. In the male it is completely closed but in the female the uterine tubes open into it and the ovaries are the only structures inside (Ch. 18).

Muscle layer

With some exceptions this consists of two layers of *smooth (involuntary) muscle*. The muscle fibres of the outer layer are arranged longitudinally, and those of the inner layer encircle the wall of the tube. Between these two muscle layers there are blood vessels, lymph vessels and a plexus of sympathetic and parasympathetic nerves, called the *myenteric* or *Auerbach's plexus*. These nerves supply the adjacent smooth muscle and blood vessels.

Contraction and relaxation of these muscle layers occurs in waves which push the contents of the tract onwards. This type of contraction of smooth muscle is called *peristalsis* (Fig. 12.4). Muscle contraction also mixes food with the digestive juices. Onward movement of the contents of the tract is controlled at various points by *sphincters* consisting of an increased number of circular muscle fibres. They also act as valves preventing backflow in the tract. The control allows time for digestion and absorption to take place.

Submucous layer

This layer consists of loose connective tissue with some elastic fibres. Within this layer there are plexuses of blood vessels and nerves, lymph vessels and varying

amounts of lymphoid tissues. The blood vessels consist of arterioles, venules and capillaries. The nerve plexus is the *submucosal* or *Meissner's plexus,* consisting of sympathetic and parasympathetic nerves which supply the mucous membrane lining.

Mucosa

This consists of three layers of tissue:

- *mucous membrane* formed by columnar epithelium is the innermost layer and has three main functions: *protection, secretion* and *absorption*
- *lamina propria* consisting of loose connective tissue, which supports the blood vessels that nourish the inner epithelial layer, and varying amounts of lymphoid tissue that has a protective function
- *muscularis mucosa*, a thin outer layer of smooth muscle that provides involutions of the mucosa layer, e.g. gastric glands, villi.

Mucous membrane

In parts of the tract which are subject to great wear and tear or mechanical injury this layer consists of *stratified squamous epithelium* with mucus-secreting glands just below the surface. In areas where the food is already soft and moist and where the secretion of digestive juices and absorption occur, the mucous membrane consists of *columnar epithelial cells* interspersed with mucus-secreting goblet cells (Fig. 12.5). Mucus lubricates the walls of the tract and protects them from digestive enzymes. Below the surface in the part lined by columnar epithelium there are collections of spe-

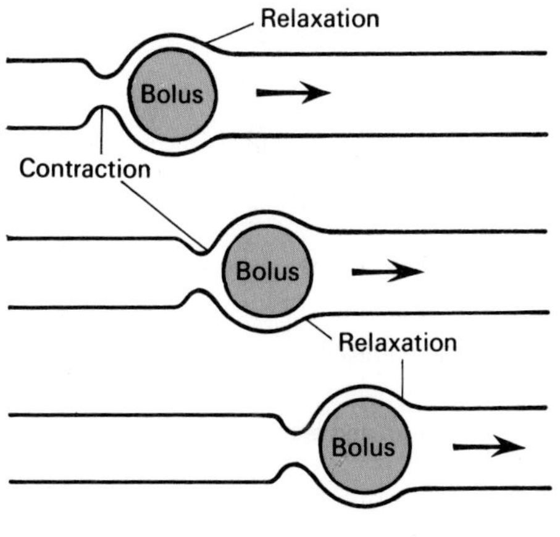

Figure 12.4 Movement of a bolus through the oesophagus by peristalsis.

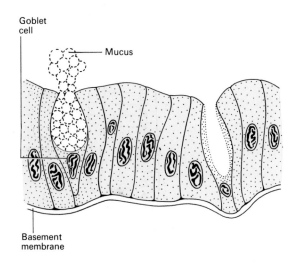

Figure 12.5 Columnar epithelium with goblet cells.

cialised cells, or glands, which pour their secretions into the lumen of the tract. The secretions include:

- *saliva* from the salivary glands
- *gastric juice* from the gastric glands
- *intestinal juice* from the intestinal glands
- *pancreatic juice* from the pancreas
- *bile* from the liver.

These are *digestive juices* and they contain the enzymes which chemically simplify food. Under the epithelial lining there are varying amounts of lymphoid tissue.

Nerve supply

The alimentary tract is supplied by nerves from both parts of the autonomic nervous system, i.e. parasympathetic and sympathetic, and in the main their actions are antagonistic (Fig. 12.6). In the normal healthy state one influence may outweigh the other according to the needs of the body as a whole at a particular time.

The parasympathetic supply to most of the alimentary tract is provided by one pair of cranial nerves, the *vagus nerves*. Stimulation causes smooth muscle contraction and the secretion of digestive juices. The most distal part of the tract is supplied by sacral nerves.

The sympathetic supply is provided by numerous nerves which emerge from the spinal cord in the thoracic and lumbar regions. These form *plexuses* in the thorax, abdomen and pelvis, from which nerves pass to the organs of the alimentary tract. Their action is to reduce smooth muscle contraction and glandular secretion.

Within the walls of the canal there are two nerve plexuses from which both sympathetic and parasympathetic fibres are distributed (Fig. 12.2).

The myenteric or Auerbach's plexus lies between the two layers of smooth muscle that it supplies, e.g. influencing peristalsis.

The submucosal or Meissner's plexus lies in the submucosa and supplies the mucous membrane and secretory glands.

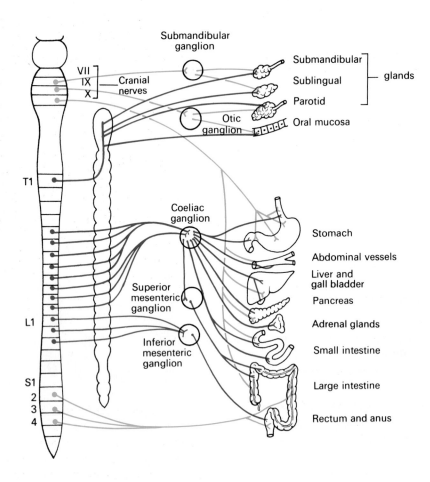

Figure 12.6 Autonomic nerve supply to the digestive system. Parasympathetic—blue; sympathetic—red.

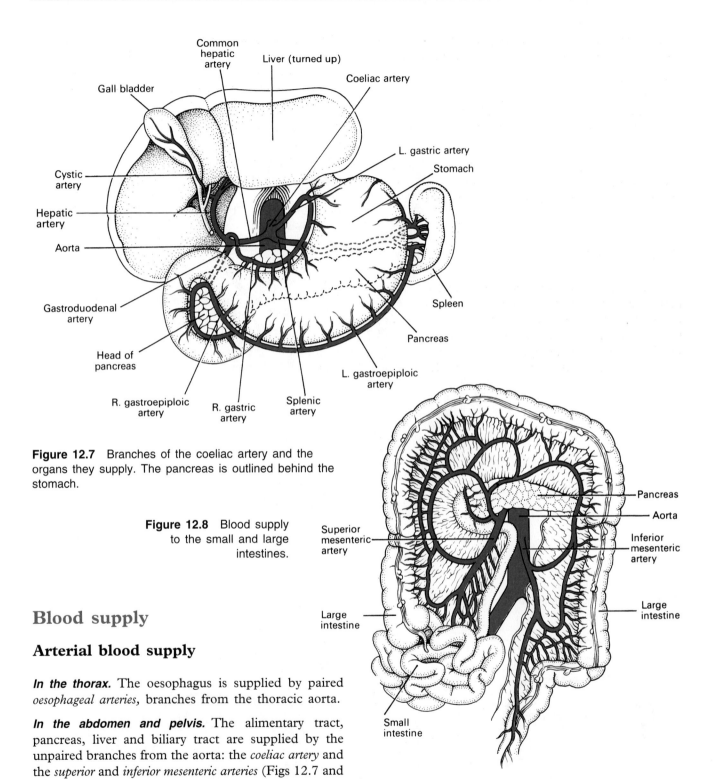

Figure 12.7 Branches of the coeliac artery and the organs they supply. The pancreas is outlined behind the stomach.

Figure 12.8 Blood supply to the small and large intestines.

Blood supply

Arterial blood supply

In the thorax. The oesophagus is supplied by paired *oesophageal arteries*, branches from the thoracic aorta.

In the abdomen and pelvis. The alimentary tract, pancreas, liver and biliary tract are supplied by the unpaired branches from the aorta: the *coeliac artery* and the *superior* and *inferior mesenteric arteries* (Figs 12.7 and 12.8).

The *coeliac artery* divides into three branches which supply the stomach, duodenum, pancreas, spleen, liver, gall bladder and bile ducts. They are:

- left gastric artery
- splenic artery
- hepatic artery.

The *superior mesenteric artery* supplies the whole of the small intestine, the caecum, ascending colon and most of the transverse colon.

The *inferior mesenteric artery* supplies a small part of the transverse colon, the descending colon, pelvic colon and most of the rectum.

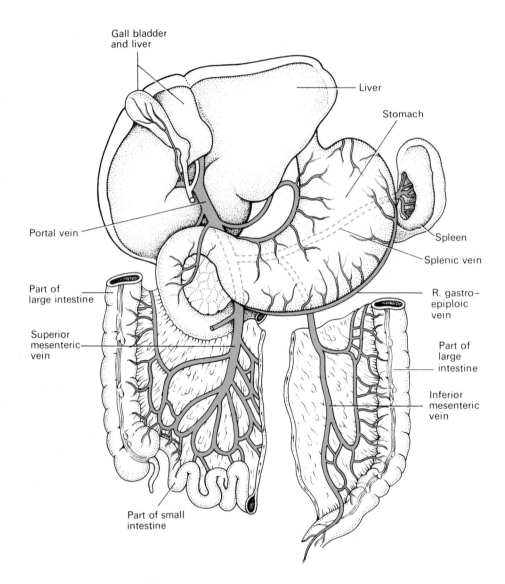

Figure 12.9   Venous drainage from the abdominal part of the digestive system.

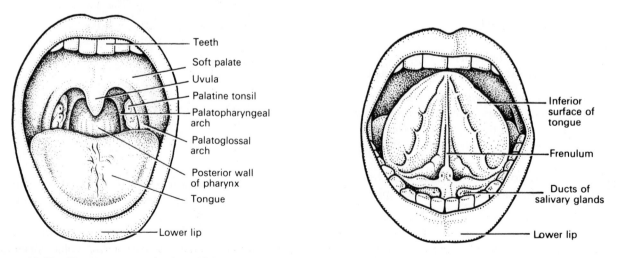

Figure 12.10   Structures seen in the widely open mouth.

Figure 12.11   The inferior surface of the tongue.

The distal part of the rectum and the anus are supplied by the *middle* and *inferior rectal arteries,* branches of the internal iliac arteries.

The arteries supplying the stomach and intestines pass between the layers of peritoneum from the posterior abdominal wall to the organs.

Venous drainage

In the thorax. Venous blood from the oesophagus passes in the oesophageal veins to the *azygos* and *hemiazygos veins.* The azygos vein joins the superior vena cava near the heart, and the hemiazygos joins the left brachiocephalic vein.

Some blood from the lower part of the oesophagus drains into the *left gastric vein.* There are anastomotic vessels between the azygos, hemiazygos and left gastric veins.

In the abdomen and pelvis. The veins that drain blood from the lower part of the oesophagus, the stomach, pancreas, small intestine, large intestine and most of the rectum join to form the *portal vein* (Fig. 12.9). This blood, containing a high concentration of absorbed nutritional materials, is conveyed first to the liver then to the inferior vena cava. The circulation of blood in liver lobules is described later (p. 308).

Blood from the lower part of the rectum and the anal canal drains into the *internal iliac veins.*

MOUTH (FIG. 12.10)

The mouth or oral cavity is bounded by muscles and bones:

Anteriorly — by the lips
Posteriorly — it is continuous with the oropharynx
Laterally — by the muscles of the cheeks
Superiorly — by the bony hard palate and muscular soft palate
Inferiorly — by the muscular tongue and the soft tissues of the floor of the mouth

The oral cavity is lined throughout with *mucous membrane,* consisting of *stratified squamous epithelium* containing small mucus-secreting glands.

The part of the mouth between the gums (alveolar ridges) and the cheeks is the *vestibule* and the remainder of the cavity is the *mouth proper.* The mucous membrane lining of the cheeks and the lips is reflected on to the gums or *alveolar ridges* and is continuous with the skin of the face.

The *palate* forms the roof of the mouth and is divided into the anterior *hard palate* and the posterior *soft palate.* The bones forming the hard palate are the maxilla and the palatine bones. The soft palate is muscular, curves downwards from the posterior end of the hard palate and blends with the walls of the pharynx at the sides.

The *uvula* is a curved fold of muscle covered with mucous membrane, hanging down from the middle of the free border of the soft palate. Originating from the upper end of the uvula there are four folds of mucous membrane, two passing downwards at each side to form membranous arches. The posterior folds, one on each side, are the *palatopharyngeal arches* and the two anterior folds are the *palatoglossal arches.* On each side, between the arches, there is a collection of lymphoid tissue called the *palatine tonsil.*

Tongue

The tongue is a voluntary muscular structure which occupies the floor of the mouth. It is attached by its base to the *hyoid bone* and by a fold of its mucous membrane covering, called the *frenulum,* to the floor of the mouth (Fig. 12.11). The superior surface consists of stratified squamous epithelium, with numerous *papillae* (little projections), containing nerve endings of the sense of taste, sometimes called the *taste buds.* There are three varieties of papillae (Fig. 12.12).

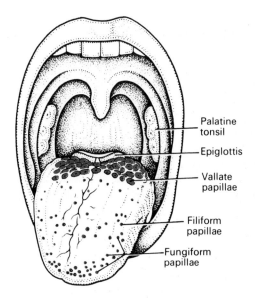

Palatine tonsil

Epiglottis

Vallate papillae

Filiform papillae

Fungiform papillae

Figure 12.12 Diagram of the papillae of the tongue and related structures.

Vallate papillae are usually about 8 to 12 in number and are arranged in an inverted V shape towards the base of the tongue. These are the largest of the papillae and are the most easily seen.

Fungiform papillae are situated mainly at the tip and the edges of the tongue and are more numerous than the vallate papillae.

Filiform papillae are the smallest of the three types. They are most numerous on the surface of the anterior two-thirds of the tongue.

Blood supply

The main arterial blood supply to the tongue is by the *lingual branch* of the *external carotid artery*. Venous drainage is by the *lingual vein* which joins the *internal jugular vein*.

Nerve supply

The nerves involved are:

- the *hypoglossal nerves* (12th cranial nerves) which supply the voluntary muscle tissue
- the *lingual branch of the mandibular nerves* which are the nerves of somatic (ordinary) sensation, i.e. pain, temperature and touch
- the *facial* and *glossopharyngeal nerves* (7th and 9th cranial nerves) which are the nerves of the special sensation of taste.

Functions of the tongue

The tongue plays an important part in:

- mastication (chewing)
- deglutition (swallowing)
- speech (p. 243)
- taste (p. 208).

Nerve endings of the sense of taste are present in the papillae and widely distributed in the epithelium of the tongue, soft palate, pharynx and epiglottis.

Teeth

The teeth are embedded in the alveoli or sockets of the alveolar ridges of the mandible and the maxilla (Fig. 12.13). Each individual has two sets, or *dentitions,* the *temporary* or *deciduous teeth* and the *permanent teeth* (Figs 12.14 and 12.15). At birth the teeth of both dentitions are present in immature form in the mandible and maxilla.

The *temporary teeth* are 20 in number, 10 in each jaw.

They begin to erupt when the child is about 6 *months* old, and should all be present by the end of *24 months* (Table 12.1).

The *permanent teeth* begin to replace the deciduous teeth in the *6th year* of age and this dentition, consisting of 32 teeth, is usually complete by the *24th year*.

Functions

The *incisor* and *canine* teeth are the cutting teeth and are used for biting off pieces of food, whereas the

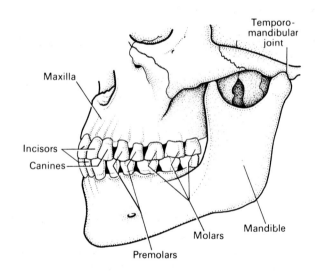

Figure 12.13   The permanent teeth and the jaw bones.

Table 12.1	Deciduous and permanent dentitions							
Jaw	Molars	Premolars	Canine	Incisors	Incisors	Canine	Premolars	Molars
Deciduous teeth								
Upper	2	—	1	2	2	1	—	2
Lower	2	—	1	2	2	1	—	2
Permanent teeth								
Upper	3	2	1	2	2	1	2	3
Lower	3	2	1	2	2	1	2	3

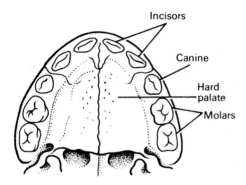

Figure 12.14 The roof of the mouth and the deciduous teeth. Viewed from below.

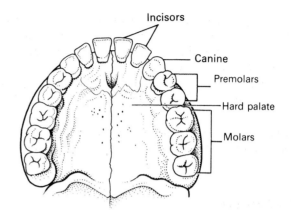

Figure 12.15 The roof of the mouth and the permanent teeth. Viewed from below.

premolar and *molar* teeth, with broad, flat surfaces, are used for grinding or chewing food (Fig. 12.16).

Structure of a tooth (Fig. 12.17)

Although the shapes of the different teeth vary, the structure is the same and consists of:

■ *the crown*—the part which protrudes from the gum
■ *the root*—the part embedded in the bone
■ *the neck*—the slightly constricted part where the crown merges with the root.

In the centre of the tooth there is the *pulp cavity* containing blood vessels, lymph vessels and nerves, and surrounding this there is a hard ivory-like substance called *dentine*. Outside the dentine of the crown there is a thin layer of very hard substance, the *enamel*. The root of the tooth, on the other hand, is covered with a substance resembling bone, called *cement,* which fixes the tooth in its socket. Blood vessels and nerves pass to the tooth through a small foramen at the apex of each root.

Blood supply
Most of the arterial blood supply to the teeth is by branches of the *maxillary arteries*. The venous drainage is by a number of veins which empty into the *internal jugular veins*.

Nerve supply
The nerve supply to the upper teeth is by branches of the *maxillary nerves* and to the lower teeth by branches of the *mandibular nerves.* These are both branches of the *trigeminal nerves* (5th cranial nerves) (see p. 168).

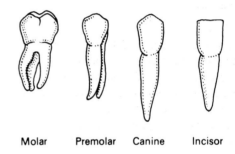

Molar   Premolar   Canine   Incisor

Figure 12.16 The shapes of the permanent teeth.

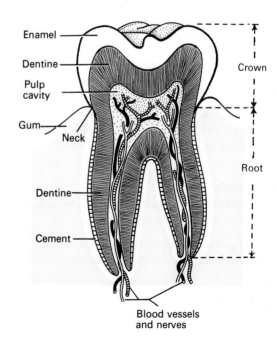

Figure 12.17 A section of a tooth.

SALIVARY GLANDS (FIG. 12.18)

There are three pairs of *compound racemose glands* which pour their secretions into the mouth. They are:

- 2 parotid
- 2 submandibular
- 2 sublingual.

Parotid glands

These are situated one on each side of the face just below the external acoustic meatus. Each gland has a *parotid duct* opening into the mouth at the level of the second upper molar tooth.

Submandibular glands

These lie one on each side of the face under the angle of the jaw. The two *submandibular ducts* open on the floor of the mouth, one on each side of the frenulum of the tongue.

Sublingual glands

These glands lie under the mucous membrane of the floor of the mouth in front of the submandibular glands. They have numerous small ducts that pierce the mucous membrane of the floor of the mouth.

Structure of the salivary glands

The glands are all surrounded by a *fibrous capsule*. They consist of a number of *lobules* made up of small alveoli lined with *secretory cells* (Fig. 12.18B). The secretions are poured into ductules which join up to form larger ducts leading into the mouth.

Nerve supply

All the glands are supplied by parasympathetic and sympathetic nerve fibres:

- parasympathetic supply—stimulates secretion
- sympathetic supply—depresses secretion.

Blood supply

Arterial supply is by various branches from the *external carotid arteries* and venous drainage is into the *external jugular veins*.

Composition of saliva

This is the combined secretions from the salivary glands and the small mucus-secreting glands of the lining of the oral cavity. About 1 to 1.5 l of saliva is produced daily and it consists of:

- water
- mineral salts
- enzyme: salivary amylase (previously called ptyalin)
- mucus
- lysozyme
- immunoglobulins
- blood clotting factors.

Secretion of saliva

Secretion of saliva is under autonomic nerve control. Parasympathetic stimulation causes vasodilatation and profuse secretion of watery saliva with a relatively low content of enzymes and other organic substances. Sympathetic stimulation causes vasoconstriction and secretion of small amounts of saliva rich in organic material, especially from the submandibular glands. Reflex secretion occurs when there is food in the mouth and the reflex can easily become *conditioned* so that the sight, smell and even the thought of food stimulates the flow of saliva.

Functions of saliva

Chemical digestion. The enzyme salivary amylase acts on cooked starches (polysaccharides), changing them to the disaccharide *maltose*. The pH is between 5.4 and 7.5 depending on the rate of flow. The more rapid the flow of saliva the higher the pH. The optimum pH for salivary amylase action is 6.8 (slightly acid). Enzyme action continues after the bolus is swallowed, until it is finally inhibited by the strongly acid reaction of gastric juices—pH 1.5 to 1.8.

Lubrication of food. Dry food entering the mouth is moistened and lubricated by saliva before it can be made into a bolus ready for swallowing.

Cleansing and lubricating. An adequate flow of saliva is necessary to cleanse the mouth and keep its tissues soft, moist and pliable. It helps to prevent damage to the mucous membrane by hard foods that may have sharp edges and it aids chewing.

Non-specific defence. Lysozyme, immunoglobulins and clotting factors combat invading microbes.

Taste. The taste buds are stimulated by particles present in the food which are dissolved in water. Dry foods stimulate the sense of taste only after thorough mixing

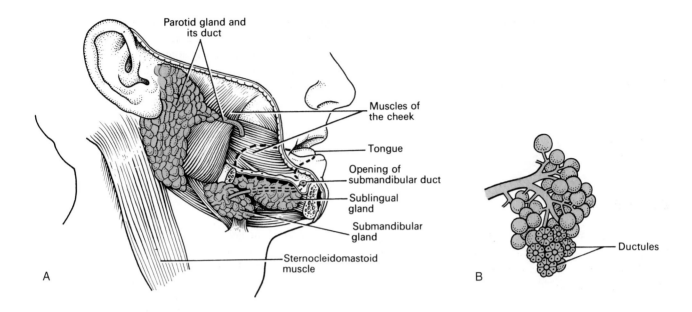

Figure 12.18   A. The position of the salivary glands. B. Enlargement of part of a gland.

with saliva. The senses of taste and smell are closely linked in the enjoyment, or otherwise, of food.

PHARYNX

The pharynx is divided for descriptive purpose into three parts, the nasopharynx, oropharynx and laryngopharynx (see. p. 242). Of these only the oropharynx and laryngopharynx are associated with the alimentary tract. Food passes from the oral cavity to the pharynx then to the oesophagus below, with which it is continuous.

The lining membrane is stratified squamous epithelium, continuous with the lining of the mouth at one end and with the oesophagus at the other.

The middle layer consists of fibrous tissue which becomes thinner towards the lower end, containing blood and lymph vessels and nerves.

The outer layer consists of a number of involuntary *constrictor* muscles which are involved in swallowing. When food reaches the pharynx swallowing is no longer under voluntary control.

Blood supply
The blood supply to the pharynx is by several branches of the *facial arteries*. Venous drainage is into the *facial veins* and the *internal jugular veins*.

Nerve supply
This is from the *pharyngeal plexus* and consists of parasympathetic and sympathetic nerves. Parasympathetic supply is mainly by the *glossopharyngeal* and *vagus nerves* and sympathetic from the *cervical ganglia* (p. 171).

OESOPHAGUS (FIG. 12.19)

The oesophagus or gullet is the first part of the alimentary tract to which the general plan described previously applies (Fig. 12.2). It is about 25 cm long and about 2 cm in diameter and lies in the median plane in the thorax in front of the vertebral column behind the trachea and the heart. It is continuous with the pharynx above and just below the diaphragm it joins the stomach. It passes between muscle fibres of the diaphragm behind the central tendon at the level of the 10th thoracic vertebra. Immediately the oesophagus has passed through the diaphragm it curves upwards before becoming the stomach. This sharp angle is believed to be one of the factors which prevents the regurgitation (backward flow) of gastric contents into the oesophagus. The upper and lower ends of the oesophagus are closed by sphincter muscles. The upper *cricopharyngeal sphincter* prevents air passing into the oesophagus during inspiration and the aspiration of oesophageal contents. The *cardiac* or *lower oesophageal*

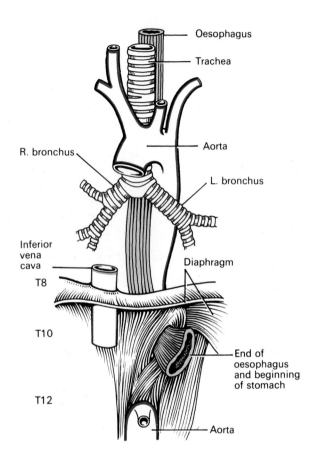

Figure 12.19 Oesophagus and some associated structures.

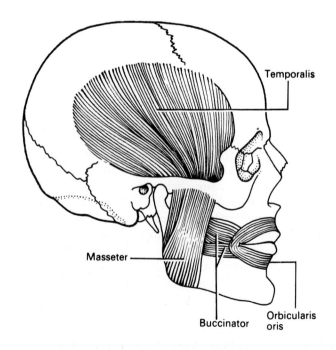

Figure 12.20 The muscles used when chewing.

sphincter prevents the reflux of acid gastric contents into the oesophagus. There is no thickening of the circular muscle in this area and this sphincter is therefore 'physiological', i.e. this region can act as a sphincter without the presence of the anatomical features. When intra-abdominal pressure is raised, e.g. during inspiration and defaecation, the tone of the lower sphincter muscle increases. There is an added pinching effect by the contracting muscle fibres of the diaphragm.

Structure

There are four layers of tissue as described in the general plan. As the oesophagus is almost entirely in the thorax the outer covering, the adventitia, consists of *elastic fibrous tissue*. The proximal third is lined by stratified squamous epithelium and the distal third by columnar epithelium. The middle third is lined by a mixture of the two.

Blood supply

Arterial. The thoracic part of the oesophagus is supplied mainly by the oesophageal arteries, branches from the aorta. The abdominal part is supplied by branches from the inferior phrenic arteries and the left gastric branch of the coeliac artery.

Venous drainage. From the thoracic part venous drainage is into the azygos and hemiazygos veins. The abdominal part drains into the left gastric vein. There is a venous plexus at the distal end that links the upward and downward venous drainage, i.e. the general and portal circulations.

Nerve supply
Sympathetic and parasympathetic nerves terminate in the myenteric and submucosal plexuses. Parasympathetic fibres are branches of the vagus nerves (Fig. 12.6).

Functions of the mouth, pharynx and oesophagus

Formation of a bolus

When food is taken into the mouth it is masticated or chewed by the teeth and moved round the mouth by the tongue and muscles of the cheeks (Fig. 12.20). It is mixed with saliva and formed into a soft mass or *bolus* ready for *deglutition* or swallowing. The length of time that food remains in the mouth depends, to a large extent, on the consistency of the food. Some foods need to the chewed longer than others before the individual feels that the mass is ready for swallowing.

Deglutition or swallowing (Fig. 12.21)

This occurs in three stages after mastication is complete and the bolus has been formed. It is initiated voluntarily but later it is under autonomic nerve control (involuntary).

1. The mouth is closed and the voluntary muscles of the tongue and cheeks push the bolus backwards into the pharynx.
2. The muscles of the pharynx are stimulated by a reflex action initiated in the walls of the oropharynx and coordinated in the medulla and lower pons in the brain stem. Contraction of these muscles propels the bolus down into the oesophagus. All other routes that the bolus could possibly take are closed. The soft palate rises up and occludes the nasal part of the pharynx; the tongue and the pharyngeal folds close the way back into the mouth; and the larynx is lifted up and forward so that its opening is occluded by the overhanging epiglottis coming into contact with the base of the tongue.

3. The presence of the bolus in the pharynx stimulates a wave of peristalsis which propels the bolus through the oesophagus to the stomach (Fig. 12.22).

Peristaltic waves of contraction only pass along the oesophagus after swallowing. Otherwise the walls are relaxed. It is closed at its proximal end by a band of pharyngeal muscle, the *cricopharyngeal sphincter*, and at its distal end by the *lower oesophageal sphincter* (LOS), a 'physiological sphincter'. The LOS relaxes ahead of a peristaltic wave. It prevents regurgitation of acid gastric contents into the oesophagus which would damage the columnar epithelial lining. Other factors that help to prevent reflux of gastric juice include:

- the attachment of the stomach to the diaphragm by the peritoneum
- the maintenance of an acute angle between the oesophagus and the fundus of the stomach, i.e. an acute cardio-oesophageal angle
- increased tone of the LOS when intra-abdominal pressure is increased and the pinching effect of diaphragm muscle fibres.

The walls of the oesophagus are lubricated by mucus which assists the passage of the bolus during the peristaltic contraction of the muscular wall.

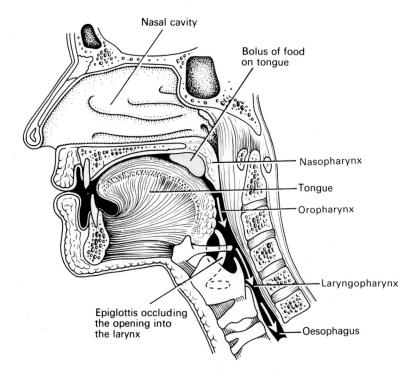

Figure 12.21 Section of the face and neck showing the positions of structures during swallowing.

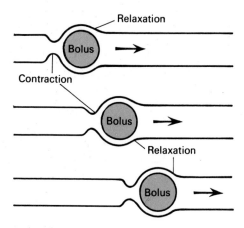

Figure 12.22 Movement of a bolus through the oesophagus by peristalsis.

STOMACH AND GASTRIC JUICE

The stomach is a J-shaped dilated portion of the alimentary tract situated in the epigastric, umbilical and left hypochondriac regions of the abdominal cavity.

Organs associated with the stomach (Fig. 12.23)

Anteriorly — left lobe of liver and anterior abdominal wall

Posteriorly — abdominal aorta, pancreas, spleen, left kidney and adrenal gland

Superiorly — diaphragm, oesophagus and left lobe of liver

Inferiorly — transverse colon and small intestine

To the left — diaphragm and spleen

To the right — liver and duodenum

Structure (Fig. 12.24)

The stomach is continuous with the oesophagus at the *cardiac orifice,* and with the duodenum at the *pyloric sphincter* or, *orifice.* It is described as having two curvatures. The *lesser curvature* is short, lies on the posterior surface of the stomach and is the downwards continuation of the posterior wall of the oesophagus. Just before the pyloric sphincter it curves upwards to complete the J shape. Where the oesophagus joins the stomach the anterior part angles acutely upwards, curves downwards

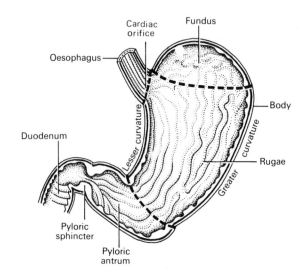

Figure 12.24 Longitudinal section of the stomach.

forming the *greater curvature* then slightly upwards towards the pyloric orifice.

The part of the stomach above the cardiac orifice is the *fundus,* the main part is the *body* and the lower part, the *pyloric antrum* or *pylorus.* At the distal end of the pyloric antrum there is the *pyloric sphincter,* guarding the opening between the stomach and the duodenum. When the stomach is inactive the pyloric sphincter is relaxed and open and when it contains food the sphincter is closed.

Figure 12.23 Stomach and its associated structures.

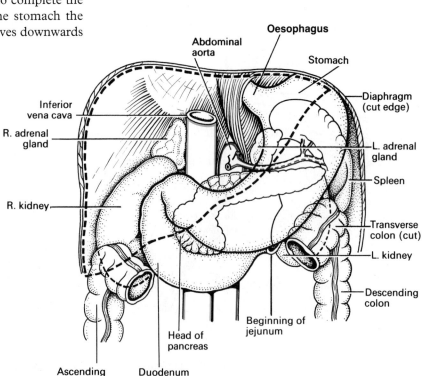

Walls of the stomach

The four layers of tissue described in the *general plan* of the alimentary canal are to be found in the stomach but with some modifications.

Peritoneum

From Figure 12.25 it will be seen that the fold of peritoneum which attaches the stomach to the posterior abdominal wall extends beyond the greater curvature of the stomach. This is the *greater omentum*. It is free at its distal end and hangs down in front of the abdominal organs like an apron.

Functions. The peritoneal fluid allows the digestive organs to glide across each other without friction.

The peritoneum attaches all abdominal organs, except the pancreas, spleen, kidneys and adrenal glands, to the posterior abdominal wall. It is richly supplied with blood and lymph vessels and contains a a considerable number of lymph nodes. It has the ability to isolate an area of slowly developing inflammation, such

as chronic appendicitis, preventing the spread of infection to the peritoneal cavity as a whole.

The greater omentum stores fat which insulates and provides a long-term energy store.

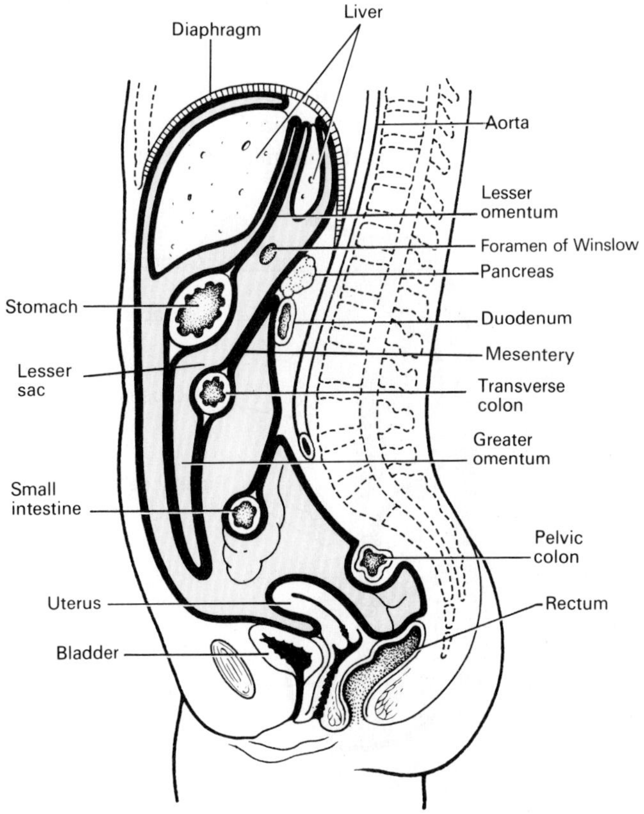

Muscle layer (Fig. 12.26)

This consists of *three layers* of smooth muscle fibres:

- an outer layer of longitudinal fibres
- a middle layer of circular fibres
- an inner layer of oblique fibres.

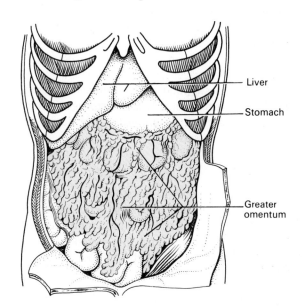

Figure 12.25B   The greater omentum viewed from the front.

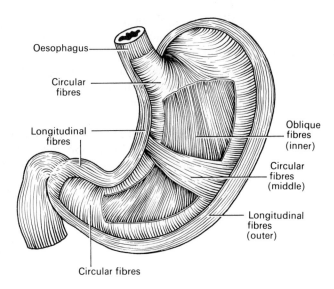

Figure 12.26   The muscle fibres of the stomach wall. Sections have been removed to show the three layers.

Figure 12.25A   The peritoneum viewed from the side.

This arrangement allows for the churning motion characteristic of gastric activity, as well as the peristaltic movement. Circular muscle is strongest in the pyloric antrum and sphincter.

Mucosa

When the stomach is empty the mucous membrane lining is thrown into longitudinal folds or *rugae,* and when full the rugae are 'ironed out' and the surface has a smooth, velvety appearance. There are numerous *gastric glands* situated below the surface in the mucous membrane. They consist of specialised cells that secrete *gastric juice* into the stomach.

Blood supply

Arterial blood is supplied to the stomach by branches of the coeliac artery and venous drainage is into the portal vein. Figures 12.8 and 12.9 give details of the names of these vessels.

Nerve supply

The sympathetic supply to the stomach is mainly from the *coeliac plexus* and the parasympathetic supply is from the *vagus nerves.* Sympathetic stimulation reduces the motility of the stomach and the secretion of gastric juice; vagal stimulation has the opposite effect (Fig. 12.6).

Gastric juice and functions of the stomach

The size of the stomach varies with the amount of food it contains, 1.5 l or more in an adult. When a meal has been eaten the food accumulates in the stomach in layers, the last part of the meal remaining in the fundus for some time. Mixing with the gastric juice takes place gradually and it may be some time before the food is sufficiently acidified to stop the action of salivary amylase.

Gastric muscle contraction consists of a churning movement that breaks down the bolus and mixes it with gastric juice, and peristaltic waves that propel the stomach contents towards the pylorus. When the stomach is active the pyloric sphincter closes. Strong peristaltic contraction of the pyloric antrum forces gastric contents, after they are sufficiently liquefied, through the pylorus into the duodenum in small spurts.

Gastric juice

About 2 to 3 litres of gastric juice are secreted daily by special secretory glands in the mucosa (Fig. 12.27). It consists of:

- water
- mineral salts   } secreted by gastric glands
- mucus secreted by goblet cells in the glands and on the stomach surface
- hydrochloric acid   } secreted by *parietal (oxyntic)*
- intrinsic factor   } *cells* in the gastric glands
- inactive enzyme precursors: pepsinogens secreted by *chief (peptic or zymogen) cells* in the glands.

Functions of gastric juice

- *Water* further liquefies the food swallowed.
- *Hydrochloric acid*:
  —acidifies the food and stops the action of salivary amylase
  —kills many microbes which may be harmful to the body
  —provides the acid environment needed for effective digestion by pepsins.
- *Pepsinogens* are activated to *pepsins* by hydrochloric acid and by pepsins already present in the stomach. They begin the digestion of proteins, breaking them into smaller molecules. Pepsins act most effectively at pH 1.5 to 3.5.
- *Intrinsic factor* (a protein compound) is necessary for the absorption of vitamin B_{12}, the *anti-anaemic factor* (p. 58), from the alimentary tract in the ileum.

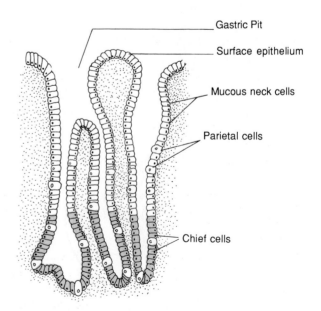

Figure 12.27 Structure of gastric glands.

Figure 12.28
The three phases
of secretion of gastric
juices.

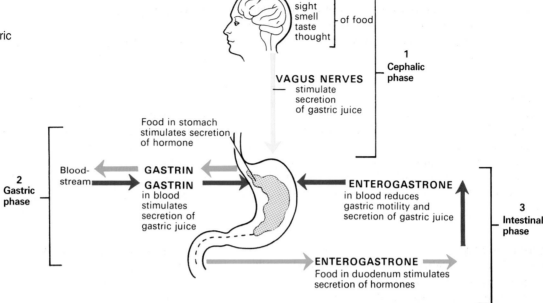

■ *Mucus* prevents mechanical injury to the stomach wall by lubricating the contents. It prevents chemical injury by acting as a barrier between the stomach wall and the other constituents of gastric juice. Hydrochloric acid is present in potentially damaging concentrations and pepsins digest protein.

Secretion of gastric juice

There is always a small quantity of gastric juice present in the stomach, even when it contains no food. This is known as *fasting juice*. Secretion reaches its maximum level about 1 hour after a meal then declines to the fasting level after about 4 hours.

There are three phases of secretion of gastric juice (Fig. 12.28).

1. *Cephalic phase.* This flow of juice occurs *before* food reaches the stomach and is due to reflex stimulation of the vagus nerves initiated by the sight, smell or taste of food. When the vagus nerves have been cut (vagotomy) this phase of gastric secretion stops.
2. *Gastric phase.* When stimulated by the presence of food the *enteroendocrine cells* in the pyloric antrum and duodenum secrete *gastrin*, a hormone which passes directly into the circulating blood. Gastrin, circulating in the blood which supplies the stomach, stimulates the gastric glands to produce more gastric juice. In this way the secretion of digestive juice is continued after the completion of the meal and the end of the cephalic phase. Gastric phase secretion is suppressed when the pH in the pyloric antrum falls to about 1.5.

3. *Intestinal phase.* When the partially digested contents of the stomach reach the small intestine, a hormone complex *enterogastrone** is produced which slows down the secretion of gastric juice and reduces gastric motility. Two hormones forming this complex are *secretin* and *cholecystokinin* (CCK).

By slowing the emptying rate of the stomach, the contents of the duodenum become more thoroughly mixed with bile and pancreatic juice. This phase of gastric secretion is most marked when the meal has had a high fat content.

Functions of the stomach

These include:

■ temporary storage allowing time for the digestive enzymes, pepsins to act
■ chemical digestion—pepsins convert proteins to polypeptides
■ mechanical digestion—the three smooth muscle layers enable the stomach to act as a churn, gastric juice is added and the contents are liquefied to *chyme*
■ limited absorption of water, alcohol and some lipid-soluble drugs

---

* Enterogastrone has been described as any hormone or combination of hormones released by the intestine that inhibits gastric secretion.

- non-specific defence against microbes is provided by hydrochloric acid in gastric juice and *vomiting* may be a response to local irritation, e.g. ingestion of noxious chemicals or microbes, mechanical irritation
- dissolving out of iron from food—this takes place most effectively in the presence of hydrochloric acid although absorption occurs in the small intestine
- production of intrinsic factor needed for absorption of vitamin B_{12} in the terminal ileum
- outward movements of the contents of the pyloric end of the stomach. When they have reached a suitable degree of acidity and liquefaction the pyloric antrum forces small jets of gastric contents through the pyloric sphincter into the duodenum. The rate at which the stomach empties depends to a large extent on the type of food eaten. A carbohydrate meal leaves the stomach in 2 to 3 hours, a protein meal remains longer and a fatty meal remains in the stomach longest.

SMALL INTESTINE
(FIGS 12.29 AND 12.30)

The small intestine is continuous with the stomach at the *pyloric sphincter* and leads into the large intestine at the *ileocaecal valve*. It is a little over 5 metres long and lies in the abdominal cavity surrounded by the large intestine. In the small intestine the chemical digestion of food is completed and most of the absorption of nutrient materials takes place.

The small intestine is described in three parts which are continuous with each other.

The *duodenum* is about 25 cm long and curves around the head of the pancreas. At its midpoint there is an opening, common to the pancreatic duct and the common bile duct, guarded by the *hepatopancreatic sphincter* (of Oddi).

The *jejunum* is the middle part of the small intestine and is about 2 metres long.

The *ileum*, or terminal part, is about 3 metres long and ends at the *ileocaecal valve* which controls the flow of material from the *ileum* to the *caecum*, the first part of the large intestine, and prevents regurgitation.

Structure

The walls of the small intestine are composed of the four layers of tissue described in the *general plan* (Fig.

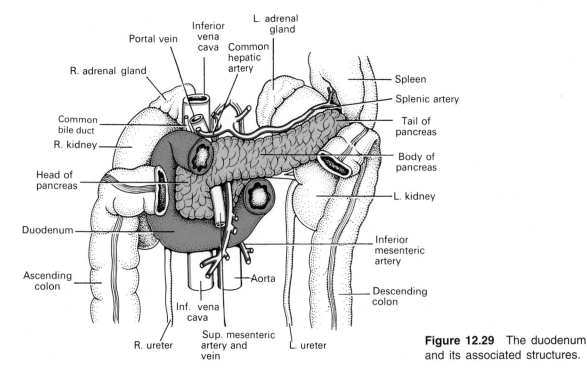

Figure 12.29 The duodenum and its associated structures.

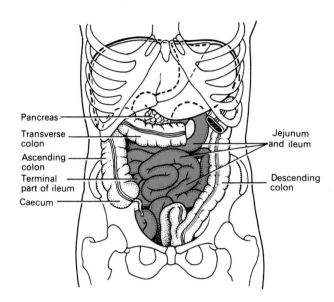

Figure 12.30 The jejunum and ileum and their associated structures.

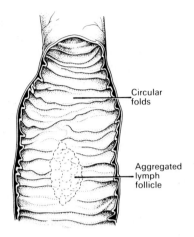

Figure 12.31 Section of a piece of small intestine showing the permanent circular folds.

12.2). There are some modifications of the peritoneum and mucosa (mucous membrane lining).

Peritoneum

A double layer of peritoneum called the *mesentery* attaches the jejunum and ileum to the posterior abdominal wall (Fig. 12.25A). The attachment is quite short in comparison with the length of the small intestine, therefore it is fan-shaped. The large blood vessels and nerves lie on the posterior abdominal wall and the branches to the small intestine pass between the two layers of the mesentery.

Mucosa

The surface area of the small intestine mucosa is greatly increased by permanent circular folds, villi and microvilli.

The *permanent circular folds,* unlike the rugae of the stomach, are not smoothed out when the small intestine is distended (Fig. 12.31). They promote mixing of chyme as it passes along.

The *villi* are tiny finger-like projections of the mucosa layer into the intestinal lumen, about 0.5 to 1 mm long (Fig. 12.32). Their walls consist of columnar epithelial cells, or *enterocytes,* with tiny *microvilli* (1 μm long) on their free border. *Goblet cells* that secrete mucus are interspersed between the enterocytes. These epithelial cells enclose a network of blood and lymph capillaries. The lymph capillaries are called *lacteals* because absorbed fat gives the lymph a milky appearance. Ab-

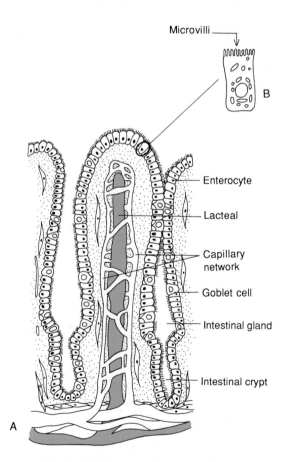

Figure 12.32 A. Highly magnified view of villi in the small intestine. B. Enterocyte showing microvilli.

sorption and some final stages of digestion of nutrient materials take place in the enterocytes before entering the blood and lymph capillaries.

The *intestinal glands* are simple tubular glands situated below the surface between the villi. The cells of the glands migrate upwards to form the walls of the villi replacing those at the tips as they are rubbed off by the intestinal contents. The entire epithelium is replaced every 3 to 5 days. During migration the cells form digestive enzymes that lodge in the microvilli and, together with intestinal juice, complete the chemical digestion of carbohydrates, protein and fats.

The *lymph nodes* are numerous in the mucosa at irregular intervals throughout the length of the small intestine. The smaller ones are known as *solitary lymphatic follicles*, and about 20 or 30 larger nodes situated towards the distal end of the ileum are called *aggregated lymphatic follicles* (Peyer's patches).

Blood supply (Figs 12.8 and 12.9)
The *superior mesenteric artery* supplies the whole of the small intestine, and venous drainage is by the *superior mesenteric vein* which joins other veins to form the portal vein.

Nerve supply
Sympathetic and parasympathetic (Fig. 12.6).

Intestinal juice (succus entericus)

About 3 litres of intestinal juice with pH 7.8 to 8.0 are secreted daily by the glands of the small intestine. It consists of:

- water
- mucus
- mineral salts
- enzyme: enterokinase (enteropeptidases).

Functions of the small intestine

The functions are:

- onward movement of its contents which is produced by peristaltic, segmental and pendular movements
- secretion of intestinal juice
- completion of chemical digestion of carbohydrates, protein and fats in the enterocytes of the villi
- protection against infection by microbes that have survived the antimicrobial action of the hydrochloric acid in the stomach, by the solitary lymph follicles and aggregated lymph follicles

- secretion of the hormones cholecystokinin (CCK) and secretin
- absorption of nutrient materials.

Chemical digestion in the small intestine

When acid chyme passes into the small intestine it is mixed with *pancreatic juice*, *bile* and *intestinal juice*, and is in contact with the enterocytes of the villi. In the small intestine the digestion of all the nutrients is completed:

- carbohydrates to monosaccharides
- proteins to amino acids
- fats to fatty acids and glycerol.

Pancreatic juice

Pancreatic juice enters the duodenum at the hepato-pancreatic ampulla (ampulla of the bile duct) and consists of:

- water
- mineral salts
- enzymes:
  —amylase
  —lipase
- inactive enzyme precursors:
  —trypsinogen
  —chymotrypsinogen
  —procarboxypeptidase.

Pancreatic juice is alkaline (pH 8). When acid stomach contents enter the duodenum they are mixed with pancreatic juice and bile and the pH is raised to between 6 and 8. This is the pH at which the pancreatic enzymes, amylase and lipase, act most effectively.

Functions

Digestion of proteins. *Trypsinogen* and *chymotrypsinogen* are inactive enzyme precursors until they come in contact with *enterokinase* (enteropeptidase), an enzyme in the microvilli, which converts them into the active proteolytic enzymes *trypsin* and *chymotrypsin*. These enzymes convert some polypeptides to amino acids and some to smaller molecule polypeptides (dipeptides and tripeptides). It is important that they are produced as inactive precursors of protein-splitting enzymes that are only activated in the duodenum otherwise they would digest the pancreas.

Digestion of carbohydrates. *Pancreatic amylase* converts *all digestible* polysaccharides (starches) not affected by salivary amylase to disaccharides (sugars).

Digestion of fats. *Lipase* converts fats to fatty acids and glycerol. To aid the action of lipase, *bile salts* emulsify fats, i.e. reduce the size of the globules, increasing their surface area.

Control of secretion

The secretion of pancreatic juice is stimulated by the two hormones *secretin* and CCK produced by cells in the walls of the duodenum. The presence in the duodenum of acid material from the stomach stimulates the production of these hormones.

Bile

Bile, secreted by the liver, is unable to enter the duodenum when the hepatopancreatic sphincter is closed; therefore it passes from the *hepatic duct* along the *cystic duct* to the gall bladder where it is stored.

Bile has a pH of 8 and between 500 and 1000 ml are secreted daily. It consists of:

- water
- mineral salts
- mucus
- bile salts
- bile pigment—bilirubin
- cholesterol.

Functions

- The bile salts, *sodium taurocholate* and *sodium glycocholate,* emulsify fats in the small intestine.
- The bile pigment, *bilirubin*, is a waste product of the breakdown of erythrocytes. Bilirubin is altered by microbes in the large intestine. Some of the resultant *urobilinogen* is reabsorbed and then excreted in the urine, but most is converted to *stercobilin* and excreted in the faeces.
- The presence of bile salts in the small intestine is necessary for the absorption of vitamin K and digested fats.

- Stercobilin colours and deodorises the faeces.
- It has an aperient effect.

Release from the gall bladder

When a meal has been taken the hormone CCK is secreted by the duodenum during the intestinal phase of secretion of gastric juice (p. 297). This stimulates contraction of the gall bladder and relaxation of the *hepatopancreatic sphincter,* enabling the bile and pancreatic juice to pass into the duodenum together. A more marked activity is noted if chyme entering the duodenum contains a high proportion of fat.

Intestinal secretions

About 3 litres of *intestinal juice* with pH 7.8 to 8.0 are secreted daily by the glands of the small intestine. It consists of:

- water
- mucus
- mineral salts
- enzyme: enterokinase (enteropeptidase).

Traces of enzymes found in intestinal juice are believed to be released following the breakdown of cells brushed off the villi.

Most of the digestive enzymes in the small intestine are contained in the enterocytes of the walls of the villi. The digestion of carbohydrate, protein and fat is completed by direct contact between these nutrients and the microvilli and within the enterocytes.

The enzymes involved in completing the chemical digestion of food in the enterocytes of the villi are:

- peptidases
- lipase
- sucrase, maltase and lactase.

Chemical digestion associated with enterocytes

Alkaline intestinal juice assists in raising the pH of the intestinal contents to between 6.5 and 7.5.

Enterokinase activates pancreatic peptidases which convert some polypeptides to amino acids and some to smaller molecule peptides. The final stage of breakdown to amino acids of all peptides occurs inside the cells of the villi.

Lipase completes the digestion of emulsified fats to *fatty acids* and *glycerol* partly in the intestine and partly in the cells of the villi.

Sucrase, maltase and *lactase* complete the digestion of carbohydrates by converting disaccharides, sucrose, maltose and lactose, to *monosaccharides,* inside the cells of the villi.

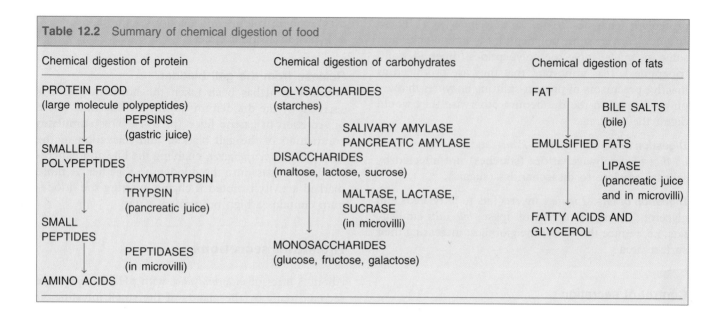

Table 12.2 Summary of chemical digestion of food

Chemical digestion of protein	Chemical digestion of carbohydrates	Chemical digestion of fats
PROTEIN FOOD (large molecule polypeptides)	POLYSACCHARIDES (starches)	FAT
↓ PEPSINS (gastric juice)	↓ SALIVARY AMYLASE PANCREATIC AMYLASE	↓ BILE SALTS (bile)
SMALLER POLYPEPTIDES	DISACCHARIDES (maltose, lactose, sucrose)	EMULSIFIED FATS
↓ CHYMOTRYPSIN TRYPSIN (pancreatic juice)	↓ MALTASE, LACTASE, SUCRASE (in microvilli)	↓ LIPASE (pancreatic juice and in microvilli)
SMALL PEPTIDES	MONOSACCHARIDES (glucose, fructose, galactose)	FATTY ACIDS AND GLYCEROL
↓ PEPTIDASES (in microvilli)		
AMINO ACIDS		

Secretion

Mechanical stimulation of the intestinal glands by chyme is believed to be the main stimulus to the secretion of intestinal juice, although the hormone secretin may be involved.

Absorption of nutritional materials (Fig. 12.33)

The processes involved in the absorption of nutrients include:

■ carbohydrates as monosaccharides, proteins as amino acids and fats as fatty acids and glycerol may be slowly absorbed by diffusion but more rapidly by active transport
■ carbohydrates as disaccharides and proteins as dipeptides and tripeptides are actively transported into the microvilli where chemical digestion is completed to monosaccharides and amino acids before transfer to the capillaries in the villi.

Monosaccharides and amino acids pass into the capillaries in the villi and fatty acids and glycerol into the lacteals.

Some proteins are absorbed unchanged, e.g. antibodies present in mother's milk and oral vaccines, such as poliomyelitis vaccine. The extent of protein absorption is believed to be limited.

Other nutritional materials such as vitamins, mineral salts and water are absorbed from the small intes-

tine into the blood capillaries. Fat-soluble vitamins are absorbed into the lacteals along with fatty acids and glycerol. Vitamin B_{12} combines with intrinsic factor in the stomach and is absorbed in the terminal ileum.

The surface area through which absorption takes place in the small intestine is greatly increased by the

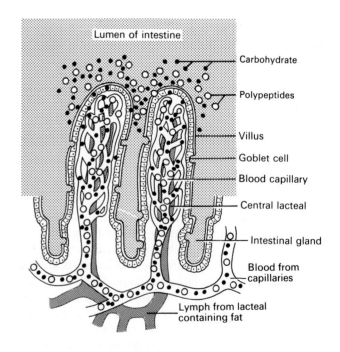

Figure 12.33 Diagram of the absorption of nutrient materials.

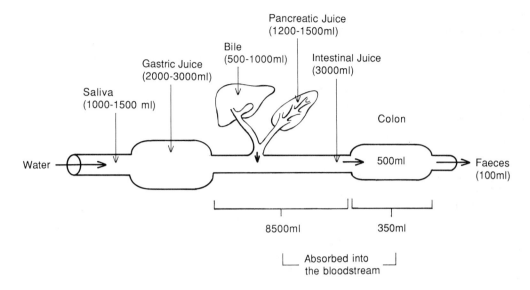

Figure 12.34 Volumes of fluid ingested, secreted, absorbed and eliminated from the gastrointestinal tract daily.

circular folds of mucous membrane and by the very large number of *villi* and *microvilli* present. It has been calculated that the surface area of the small intestine is about five times that of the whole body.

Large amounts of fluid enter the alimentary tract each day (Fig. 12.34). Of this, only about 500 ml is not absorbed by the small intestine, and passes into the large intestine.

LARGE INTESTINE (COLON), RECTUM AND ANAL CANAL

The large intestine is about 1.5 metres long, beginning at the *caecum* in the right iliac fossa and terminating at the *rectum* and *anal canal* deep in the pelvis. Its lumen is larger than that of the small intestine. It forms an arch round the coiled-up small intestine (Fig. 12.35).

For descriptive purposes the colon is divided into the caecum, ascending colon, transverse colon, descending colon, sigmoid or pelvic colon, rectum and anal canal.

The *caecum* is the first part of the colon. It is a dilated portion which has a blind end inferiorly and is continuous with the *ascending colon* superiorly. Just below the junction of the two the *ileocaecal valve* opens from the ileum. The *vermiform appendix* is a fine tube, closed at one end, which leads from the caecum. It is usually about 13 cm long and has the same structure as the walls of the colon but contains more lymphoid tissue (Fig. 12.36).

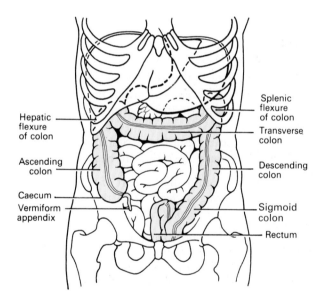

Figure 12.35 The parts of the large intestine (colon) and their positions.

The *ascending colon* passes upwards from the caecum to the level of the liver where it bends acutely to the left at the *hepatic flexure* (right colic flexure) to become the *transverse colon*.

The *transverse colon* is a loop of colon which extends across the abdominal cavity in front of the duodenum and the stomach to the area of the spleen where it forms the *splenic flexure* (left colic flexure) by bending acutely downwards to become the *descending colon*.

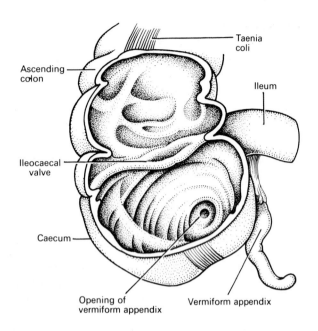

Figure 12.36 Interior of the caecum.

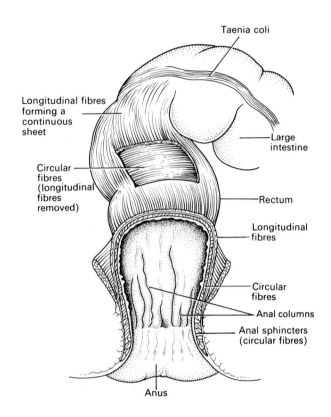

Figure 12.37 The arrangement of muscle fibres in the colon, rectum and anus. Sections have been removed to show the layers.

The *descending colon* passes down the left side of the abdominal cavity then curves towards the midline. After it enters the true pelvis it is known as the *sigmoid* or *pelvic colon.*

The *sigmoid colon* describes an S-shaped curve in the pelvis then continues downwards to become the *rectum.*

The rectum is a slightly dilated part of the colon which is about 13 cm long. It leads from the sigmoid colon and terminates in the *anal canal.*

The anal canal is a short canal about 3.8 cm long in the adult and leads from the rectum to the exterior. There are two sphincter muscles which control the anus; the *internal sphincter,* consisting of smooth muscle fibres, is under the control of the *autonomic nervous system* and the *external sphincter,* formed by striated muscle, is under *voluntary nerve* control (Fig. 12.37).

Structure

The four layers of tissue described in the *general plan* are present in the colon, the rectum and the anal canal. The arrangement of the *longitudinal muscle fibres* is modified in the colon. They do not form a smooth continuous layer of tissue but are collected into three bands, called *taeniae coli,* situated at regular intervals round the colon. They stop at the junction of the sigmoid colon and the rectum. As these bands of muscle

tissue are slightly shorter than the total length of the colon they give a sacculated or puckered appearance to the organ (Fig. 12.37).

The longitudinal muscle fibres spread out as in the general plan and completely surround the rectum and the anal canal. The anal sphincters are formed by thickening of the circular muscle layer.

In the submucous layer there is more lymphoid tissue than in any other part of the alimentary tract, providing non-specific defence against invasion by resident and other microbes.

In the mucosa lining the colon and the upper part of the rectum there are large numbers of goblet cells forming simple tubular glands which secrete mucus. They are not present beyond the junction between the rectum and the anus.

The lining membrane of the *anus* consists of stratified squamous epithelium which is continuous with the mucous membrane lining of the rectum above and merges with the skin beyond the external anal sphincter. In the upper part of the anal canal the mucous membrane is arranged in 6 to 10 vertical folds, the *anal columns*. Each column contains a terminal branch of the superior rectal artery and vein.

Blood supply

Arterial supply is mainly by the superior and inferior mesenteric arteries (Fig. 12.7).

The *superior mesenteric artery* supplies the caecum, ascending and most of the transverse colon.

The *inferior mesenteric artery* supplies the remainder of the colon and the proximal part of the rectum.

The distal part of the rectum and the anus are supplied by branches from the *internal iliac arteries*.

Venous drainage is mainly by the *superior* and *inferior mesenteric veins* which drain blood from the parts supplied by arteries of the same names. These veins join the splenic and gastric veins to form the portal vein (Fig. 12.9). Veins draining the distal part of the rectum and the anus join the *internal iliac veins*.

Functions of the large intestine, rectum and anal canal

Absorption

The contents of the ileum which pass through the ileocaecal valve into the caecum are fluid, even though some water has been absorbed in the small intestine. In the large intestine absorption of water continues until the familiar semisolid consistency of faeces is achieved. Mineral salts, vitamins and some drugs are also absorbed into the blood capillaries from the large intestine.

Microbial activity

There are large numbers of microbes in the colon which synthesise vitamin K and folic acid. They include *Escherichia coli, Enterobacter aerogenes, Streptococcus faecalis, Clostridium perfringens (welchii)*. These microbes are *commensals* in man. They may become pathogenic if transferred to another part of the body, e.g. *Escherichia coli* may cause cystitis if it gains access to the urinary bladder.

Gases in the bowel consist of some of the constituents of air, mainly nitrogen, swallowed with food and drink and as a feature of some anxiety states. Hydrogen, carbon dioxide and methane are produced by bacterial fermentation of unabsorbed nutrients, especially carbohydrate. Gases pass out of the bowel as *flatus*.

Large numbers of microbes are present in the faeces.

Mass movement

The large intestine does not exhibit peristaltic movement as it is seen in other parts of the digestive tract. Only at fairly long intervals does a wave of strong peristalsis sweep along the transverse colon forcing its contents into the descending and sigmoid colons. This is known as *mass movement* and it is often precipitated by the entry of food into the stomach. This combination of stimulus and response is called the *gastrocolic reflex*.

Defaecation

Usually the rectum is empty, but when a mass movement forces the contents of the sigmoid colon into the rectum the nerve endings in its walls are stimulated by stretch. In the infant defaecation occurs by reflex action which is not under voluntary control. However, after the nervous system has fully developed, nerve impulses are conveyed to consciousness when the stretch receptors in the rectum are stimulated, and the brain can inhibit the reflex until such times as it is convenient to defaecate. The external anal sphincter is under conscious control through the *pudendal nerve*. Thus defaecation involves involuntary contraction of the muscle of the rectum and relaxation of the internal anal sphincter. Contraction of the abdominal muscles and lowering of the diaphragm increase the intra-abdominal pressure (Valsalva's manoeuvre) and so assist the process of defaecation. When defaecation is voluntarily postponed the feeling of fullness and need to defaecate tends to fade until the mass movement occurs and the reflex is initiated again. Repeated suppression of the reflex may lead to constipation.

Constituents of faeces The faeces consist of a semisolid brown mass. The brown colour is due to the presence of stercobilin (p. 310 and Fig. 12.43).

Even though absorption of water takes place in the large intestine water still makes up about 60 to 70% of the weight of the faeces. The remainder consists of:

- fibre (indigestible cellular plant and animal material)
- dead and live microbes
- epithelial cells from the walls of the tract
- fatty acids
- mucus secreted by the epithelial lining of the large intestine.

Mucus helps to lubricate the faeces and an adequate amount of roughage in the diet ensures that the contents of the colon are sufficiently bulky to stimulate defaecation.

PANCREAS (FIG. 12.38)

The pancreas is a pale grey gland weighing about 60 grams. It is about 12 to 15 cm long and is situated in the *epigastric* and *left hypochondriac* regions of the abdominal cavity. It consists of a broad head, a body and a narrow tail. The head lies in the curve of the duodenum, the body behind the stomach and the tail lies in front of the left kidney and just reaches the spleen. The abdominal aorta and the inferior vena cava lie behind the gland.

Structure

The pancreas is both an *exocrine* and *endocrine* gland.

The exocrine pancreas
This consists of a large number of *lobules* made up of small *alveoli*, the walls of which consist of *secretory cells*. Each lobule is drained by a tiny duct and these unite eventually to form the *pancreatic duct*, which extends the whole length of the gland and opens into the duodenum at its midpoint. Just before entering the duodenum the pancreatic duct joins the *common bile duct* to form the *hepatopancreatic ampulla*. The duodenal opening of the ampulla is controlled by the *hepatopancreatic sphincter*.

The *function* of the alveoli of the pancreas is to produce *pancreatic juice* containing enzymes that digest carbohydrates, proteins and fats (p. 300).

The endocrine pancreas
This is called the *pancreatic islets* (islets of Langerhans) which consist of groups of specialised cells distributed throughout the gland (p. 274). The islets have no ducts so the hormones pass directly into the blood.

The *function* of the pancreatic islets is to secrete the hormones *insulin* and *glucagon* that are involved in metabolic homeostasis, especially the blood glucose level.

Blood supply
The splenic and mesenteric arteries supply arterial blood to the pancreas and the venous drainage is by the veins of the same names that join other veins to form the portal vein (Figs 12.7 and 12.9).

Nerve supply
As in the alimentary tract, parasympathetic stimulation increases the secretion of pancreatic juice and sympathetic stimulation depresses it.

LIVER

The liver is the largest gland in the body, weighing between 1 and 2.3 kg. It is situated in the upper part of the abdominal cavity occupying the greater part of the *right hypochondriac region*, part of the *epigastric region* and extending into the *left hypochondriac region*. Its upper and anterior surfaces are smooth and curved to fit the under surface of the diaphragm (Fig. 12.39); its posterior surface is irregular in outline (Fig. 12.40).

Organs associated with the liver

Superiorly and anteriorly	— diaphragm and anterior abdominal wall
Inferiorly	— stomach, bile ducts, duodenum, hepatic flexure of the colon, right kidney and adrenal gland
Posteriorly	— oesophagus, inferior vena cava, aorta, gall bladder, vertebral column and diaphragm
Laterally	— lower ribs and diaphragm

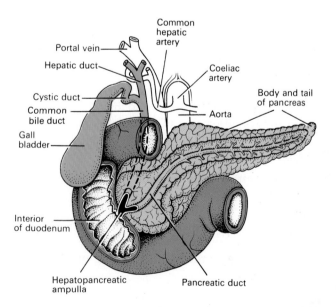

Figure 12.38 The pancreas in relation to the duodenum and biliary tract. Part of the anterior wall of the duodenum removed.

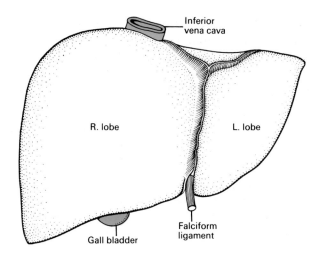

Figure 12.39 The liver: anterior view.

The liver is enclosed in a thin capsule and incompletely covered by a layer of peritoneum. Folds of peritoneum form supporting ligaments attaching the liver to the inferior surface of the diaphragm. It is held in position partly by these ligaments and partly by the pressure of the organs in the abdominal cavity.

The liver is described as having four lobes. The two most obvious are the large *right lobe* and the smaller, wedge-shaped, *left lobe*. The other two, the *caudate* and *quadrate* lobes, are areas on the posterior surface (Fig. 12.40).

The porta hepatis (portal fissure)

This is the name given to the part on the posterior surface of the liver where various structures enter and leave the gland.

The *portal vein* enters, carrying blood from the stomach, spleen, pancreas and the small and large intestines.

The *hepatic artery* enters, carrying arterial blood. It is a branch from the coeliac artery which is a branch from the abdominal aorta.

Nerve fibres, sympathetic and parasympathetic.

The *right* and *left hepatic ducts* leave, carrying bile from the liver to the gall bladder.

Lymph vessels leave the liver, draining some lymph to abdominal and some to thoracic nodes.

Blood supply (Figs 12.7 and 12.9)

The hepatic artery and the portal vein take blood to the liver. Hepatic veins, varying in number, leave the posterior surface and immediately enter the inferior vena cava just below the diaphragm.

Structure

The lobes of the liver are made up of tiny lobules just visible to the naked eye (Fig. 12.41A). These lobules are *hexagonal* in outline and are formed by cubical-shaped cells, the *hepatocytes*, arranged in *pairs* of col-

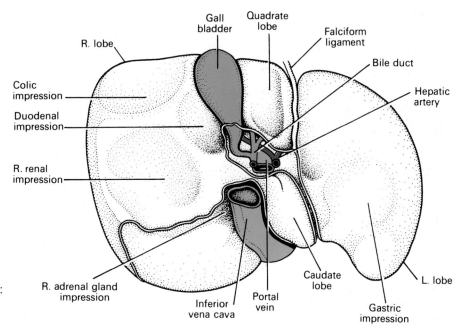

Figure 12.40 The liver: turned up to show the posterior surface.

umns radiating from a *central vein*. Between two pairs of columns of cells there are *sinusoids* (blood vessels with incomplete walls) containing *a mixture of blood from the tiny branches of the portal vein and hepatic artery* (Fig. 12.41B). This arrangement allows the arterial blood and venous blood (with a high concentration of nutritional materials) to mix and come into close contact with the liver cells. Some cells, lining the

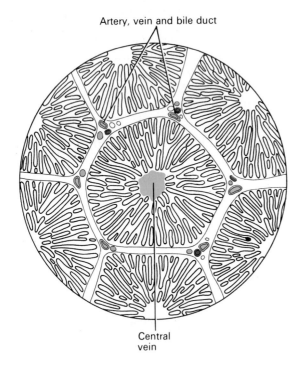

Artery, vein and bile duct

Central vein

Figure 12.41A A magnified transverse section of liver lobules.

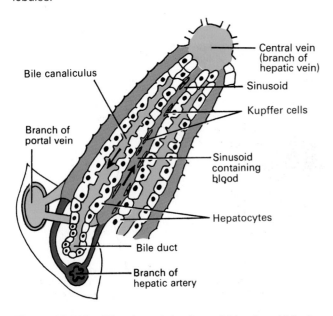

Bile canaliculus

Branch of portal vein

Central vein (branch of hepatic vein)

Sinusoid

Kupffer cells

Sinusoid containing blood

Hepatocytes

Bile duct

Branch of hepatic artery

Figure 12.41B Direction of the flow of blood and bile in a liver lobule.

sinusoids, are *hepatic macrophages* (Kupffer cells).

Blood drains from the sinusoids into *central* or *centrilobular veins*. These then join with veins from other lobules, forming larger veins, until eventually they become the *hepatic veins* which leave the liver and empty blood into the inferior vena cava just below the diaphragm. Figure 12.42 shows the system of blood flow through the liver. One of the functions of the liver is to secrete *bile*. In Figure 12.41B it will be seen that *bile canaliculi* run between the columns of liver cells. This means that each column of hepatocytes has a blood sinusoid on one side and a bile canaliculus on the other. The canaliculi join up to form larger bile canals until eventually they form the *right and left hepatic ducts* which drain bile from the liver.

Lymphoid tissue and a system of lymph vessels are present in each lobule.

Functions of the liver

The liver is an extremely active organ. Some of its functions have already been described, and they will only be mentioned here.

Carbohydrate metabolism

■ *Conversion of glucose to glucogen* in the presence of *insulin*, and changing liver glycogen back to glucose in the presence of *glucagon*. These changes are important regulators of the blood glucose level. After a meal the blood in the portal vein has a high glucose content and insulin converts some to glycogen. Glucagon converts this glycogen back to glucose as it is needed to maintain the blood glucose level within relatively narrow limits.

Fat metabolism

■ *Desaturation of fat*, i.e. converts stored fat to a form in which it can be used by the tissues to provide energy.

Protein metabolism

■ *Deamination of amino acids*
—Removes the nitrogenous portion from the amino acids not required for the formation of new protein. Forms *urea* from this nitrogenous portion which is excreted in urine.
—Breaks down nucleoprotein of worn-out cells of the body to form *uric acid* which is excreted in the urine.
■ *Transamination*—removes the nitrogenous portion of amino acids and adds it to other carbohydrate molecules forming new non-essential amino acids.

■ *Synthesis of plasma proteins*, and most of the *blood clotting factors* from the available amino acids.

Breakdown of erythrocytes and *defence against microbes* is carried out by phagocytic Kupffer cells in the sinusoids.

Detoxification of drugs and noxious substances, such as toxins produced by microbes.

Metabolism of ethanol in alcoholic drinks.

Inactivation of hormones, including insulin, glucagon, cortisol, aldosterone, thyroid and sex hormones.

Synthesis of vitamin A from carotene, the provitamin found in some plants, e.g. carrots and green leaves of vegetables.

Production of heat. The liver uses a considerable amount of energy, has a high metabolic rate and produces a great deal of heat. It is the main heat-producing organ of the body.

Secretion of bile. The hepatocytes synthesise the constituents of bile from the mixed arterial and venous blood in the sinusoids. These include bile salts, bile pigments and cholesterol.

Storage of:

■ fat-soluble vitamins: A, D, E, K
■ iron, copper
■ some water-soluble vitamins, e.g. riboflavine, niacin, pyridoxine, folic acid and vitamin B_{12} (antianaemic factor).

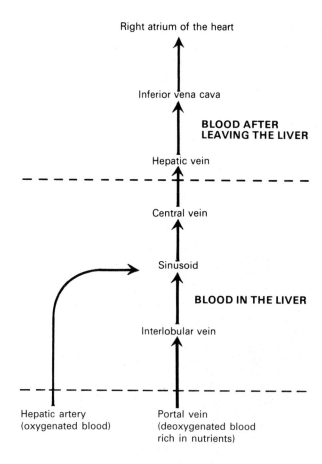

Figure 12.42 Scheme of blood flow through the liver.

Composition of bile

Between 500 and 1000 ml of bile are secreted by the liver daily. It consists of:

■ water
■ mineral salts
■ mucus
■ bile pigment: bilirubin
■ bile salts: derived from cholic and chenodeoxycholic acid
■ cholesterol.

The bile acids, *cholic* and *chenodeoxycholic acid*, are synthesised by hepatocytes, conjugated (combined) with either glycine or taurine, then secreted into bile as sodium or potassium salts. In the small intestine they emulsify fats, aiding their digestion. In the terminal ileum most of the bile salts are reabsorbed and return to the liver in the portal vein. This *enterohepatic circulation*, or recycling of bile salts, ensures that large amounts of bile salts enter the small intestine daily from a relatively small bile acid pool (Fig. 12.43).

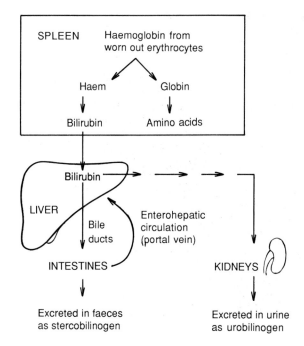

Figure 12.43 Fate of bilirubin from breakdown of worn out erythrocytes.

Bilirubin is one of the products of haemolysis of erythrocytes by Kupffer cells in the liver and by other macrophages in the spleen and bone marrow. In its original form bilirubin is insoluble in water and is bound to albumin. In hepatocytes it is conjugated to glucuronic acid and becomes water soluble before being excreted in bile. Bacteria in the intestine change the form of bilirubin and most is excreted as *stercobilin* in the faeces. A small amount is reabsorbed and excreted in urine as *urobilinogen* (Fig. 12.43). Jaundice is yellow pigmentation of the tissues, seen in the skin and conjunctiva, caused by excess blood bilirubin (p. 334).

BILIARY TRACT

Bile ducts (Fig. 12.44)

The *right and left hepatic ducts* join to form the *common hepatic duct* just outside the portal fissure. The hepatic duct passes downwards for about 3 cm where it is joined at an acute angle by the *cystic duct* from the gall bladder. The cystic and hepatic ducts together form the *common bile duct* which passes downwards behind the head of the pancreas to be joined by the main pancreatic duct at the *hepatopancreatic ampulla*. The opening of the combined ducts into the duodenum is controlled by the *hepatopancreatic sphincter*. The common bile duct is about 7.5 cm long and has a diameter of about 6 mm.

Structure
The walls of the bile ducts have the same layers of tissue as those described in the *general plan* of the alimentary canal (Fig. 12.2). In the cystic duct the mucous membrane lining is arranged in irregularly situated circular folds which have the effect of a *spiral valve*. Bile passes through the cystic duct twice—on its way into the gall bladder and again when it is expelled from the gall bladder to the common bile duct and thence to the duodenum.

Gall bladder

The gall bladder is a pear-shaped sac attached to the posterior surface of the liver by connective tissue. It has a *fundus* or expanded end, a *body* or main part and a *neck* which is continuous with the cystic duct.

Structure
The gall bladder has the same layers of tissue as those

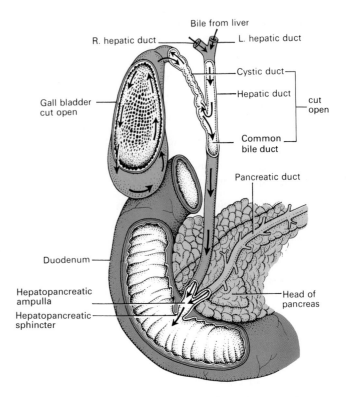

Figure 12.44   Direction of the flow of bile from the liver to the duodenum.

described in the *general plan* of the alimentary canal, with some modifications.

Peritoneum covers only the inferior surface. The gall bladder is in contact with the posterior surface of the right lobe of the liver and is held in place by the visceral peritoneum of the liver (Fig. 12.40).

Muscle layer. There is an additional layer of oblique muscle fibres.

Mucous membrane displays small rugae when the gall bladder is empty that disappear when it is distended with bile.

Blood supply
The *cystic artery*, a branch of the hepatic artery, supplies blood to the gall bladder. Blood is drained away by the *cystic vein* which joins the portal vein.

Nerve supply
Nerve impulses are conveyed by sympathetic and parasympathetic nerve fibres. There are the same autonomic plexuses as those described in the *general plan* (p. 283).

Functions of the gall bladder

- Reservoir for bile.
- Secretion of mucus into the bile.

- Absorption of water so that it is 10 to 15 times more concentrated than liver bile.
- Release of stored bile.

When the muscle wall of the gall bladder contracts bile passes through the bile ducts to the duodenum. Contraction is stimulated by:

- the hormone *cholecystokinin* (CCK), secreted by the duodenum
- the presence of fat and acid chyme in the duodenum.

Relaxation of the hepatopancreatic sphincter is caused by CCK and as a reflex response to contraction of the gall bladder.

METABOLISM

This refers to all the chemical reactions that occur in the body, using absorbed nutrients to:

- provide energy by chemical oxidation of nutrients
- make new or replacement body substances.

Two types of processes are involved:

Catabolism breaks down large molecules into smaller ones releasing *chemical energy* that is stored as adenosine triphosphate (ATP), and *heat*. Heat is used to maintain the body at the optimum level for chemical activity (36.8°C or 98.4°F). Excess heat is disposed of through the skin and excreta (p. 363).

Anabolism is building up, or synthesis, of large molecules from smaller ones and utilises the energy stored as ATP.

Anabolism and catabolism usually involve a series of chemical reactions, known as *metabolic pathways*. These enable efficient and gradual transfer of energy from ATP rather than large intracellular 'explosions'. Metabolic pathways are switched on and off by hormones, providing control of metabolism and meeting individual requirements.

Both processes occur continually in all cells maintaining a 'balance of energy'. In cells that are very active, there must be an adequate energy supply produced from chemical breakdown of nutrients to meet the demand posed by activity.

Energy
The energy produced in the body may be measured and expressed in units of work (*joules*) or units of heat (*Calories*).

A *Calorie* (capital C) is the amount of heat required to raise the temperature of 1 litre of water through 1 degree Celsius (1°C).

1 Calorie = 4184 joules (J) = 4.184 kilojoules (kJ)

The nutritional value of carbohydrates, protein and fats eaten in the diet may be expressed in *kilojoules per gram* or *Calories per gram*.

1 gram of carbohydrate provides 17 kilojoules (4 Calories)
1 gram of protein provides 17 kilojoules (4 Calories)
1 gram of fat provides 38 kilojoules (9 Calories).

Energy balance
Body weight remains constant when energy intake in the form of nutrients is equal to energy utilisation. When intake exceeds requirement body weight increases. Conversely, body weight decreases when nutrient intake does not meet energy requirements.

Metabolic rate
The metabolic rate is the rate at which energy is released from the nutrients inside cells. As most of the processes involved require oxygen and produce carbon dioxide as waste, the metabolic rate can be estimated by measuring oxygen uptake or carbon dioxide excretion.

The *basal metabolic rate* (BMR) is the rate of metabolism when the individual is at rest in a warm environment and is in the *post-absorptive state*, i.e. has not had a meal for at least 12 hours. In this state the release of energy is sufficient to meet only the essential needs of vital organs, such as the heart, lungs, nervous system, kidneys. The post-absorptive state is important because the intake of food, especially protein, stimulates an increase in metabolic rate, possibly due to increased energy utilisation by the liver. This is called the *specific dynamic action* (SDA) of food. In measuring the BMR, the surface area of the body is taken into account because energy in the form of heat is lost through the skin. Surface area in square metres is calculated from the height and weight of the individual. Some of the wide variety of factors that affect the metabolic rate are shown in Table 12.3.

Most foods contain a mixture of different amounts of carbohydrate, protein, fat, minerals, vitamins, roughage and water. Carbohydrates, proteins and fats are the sources of energy and they are obtained from the variety of food, usually in the following proportions:

Protein   10–15%
Fat   15–30%
Carbohydrate 55–75%

Table 12.3 Factors affecting metabolic rate

Factor	Effect on metabolic rate
Age	Gradually reduced with age
Gender	Higher in men than women
Height, weight	Relatively higher in small people
Pregnancy, menstruation, lactation	Increased
Ingestion of food	Increased
Muscular activity	Increased
Elevated body temperature	Increased
Excess thyroid hormones	Increased
Starvation	Decreased

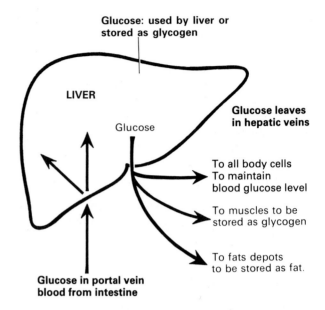

Figure 12.45 Summary of the sources, distribution and utilisation of glucose.

Metabolism of carbohydrate

Erythrocytes and neurones can only use glucose for fuel and therefore homeostasis of blood glucose levels is needed to provide a constant energy source to these cells. Most other cells can also use other sources of fuel.

Digested carbohydrate, mainly glucose, is absorbed into the blood capillaries of the villi of the small intestine. It is transported by the portal circulation to the liver, where it is dealt with in several ways (Fig. 12.45):

■ glucose may be oxidised to provide the chemical energy, in the form of ATP, necessary for the considerable metabolic activity which takes place in the liver (p. 308).
■ some of the glucose may remain in the circulating blood to maintain the normal blood glucose of about 2.5 to 5.3 millimoles per litre (mmol/l) (45 to 95 mg/100 ml).
■ some of the glucose in excess of the above requirements may be converted to the insoluble polysaccharide, *glycogen*, in the liver and in skeletal muscles. *Insulin* is the hormone necessary for this change to take place. The formation of glycogen inside cells is a means of storing carbohydrate without upsetting the osmotic equilibrium. Before it can be used to maintain blood levels or to provide ATP it must be broken down again into its constituent glucose units. Liver glycogen constitutes a store of glucose used for liver activity and to maintain the blood glucose level. Muscle glycogen provides the

glucose requirement of muscle activity. *Adrenaline, thyroxine* and *glucagon* are the main hormones associated with the conversion of glycogen to glucose.
■ carbohydrate in excess of that required to maintain the blood glucose level and glycogen level in the tissues is converted to fat and stored in the fat depots.

All the cells of the body require energy to carry out their metabolic processes including: multiplication of cells for replacement of worn out cells, contraction of muscle fibres, synthesis of secretions produced by the cells of glands. The oxidation of carbohydrate and fat provides most of the energy required by the body. When glycogen stores are low and more glucose is needed, the body can make glucose from non-carbohydrate sources, e.g. amino acids, glycerol. This is called *gluconeogenesis* (formation of new glucose).

Oxidation of carbohydrate

Complete oxidation of glucose requires an adequate supply of oxygen. This is the process by which energy is released during prolonged physical activity, e.g. the man who runs 1500 metres in 4 minutes depends upon *aerobic oxidation*. The energy release takes place slowly and is balanced by oxygen intake. Complete oxidation of carbohydrate in the body results in the production of energy, carbon dioxide and water (called *metabolic water*).

Some energy can be provided by glucose in the absence of oxygen. This *anaerobic process* does not release all the energy from the glucose molecule and, using this process, effort can be maintained for only a limited period of time. This is the energy used in a sudden spurt of activity over a very short period of time, e.g. the man who runs 100 metres in 10 seconds could not take in enough oxygen in that time to provide energy by complete oxidation of glucose, so he has to depend on the anaerobic process. One of the end products of this process is lactic acid, and if it accumulates in excess in the muscle it causes the pain associated with unaccustomed exercise.

Catabolism of glucose occurs in a series of steps with a little energy being released at each stage. One series of reactions converts monosaccharides into pyruvic acid, a process that is anaerobic and occurs in the cytoplasm. The fate of pyruvic acid depends on the availability of oxygen (Fig. 12.46). In the presence of oxygen, complete oxidative phosphorylation takes place in the mitochondria. This occurs through a pathway called the *citric acid cycle* or *Krebs cycle* and is the most efficient method of energy storage in ATP. When there is inadequate oxygen, pyruvic acid is converted to lactic acid and much less ATP is formed.

Fate of the end products of carbohydrate metabolism

Lactic acid. Some of the lactic acid produced by anaerobic catabolism of glucose may be oxidised in the cells to carbon dioxide and water but first it must be changed back to pyruvic acid. If complete oxidation does not take place lactic acid passes to the liver in the circulating blood where it is converted to glucose and may then take any of the pathways open to glucose (Fig. 12.45).

Carbon dioxide is excreted from the body as a gas by the lungs.

Water. The water of metabolism is added to the considerable amount of water already present in the body; excess is excreted as urine by the kidneys.

Metabolism of protein

Protein foods taken as part of the diet consist of a number of amino acids (p. 270). About *20 amino acids* have been named and about 8 of these are described as *essential* because they cannot be synthesised in the body. The remainder are described as *non-essential* amino acids because they can be synthesised by many tissues. The enzymes involved in this process are called *transaminases*. Digestion breaks down the protein of the diet to its constituent amino acids in preparation for transfer into the blood capillaries of the villi in the wall of the small intestine. In the portal circulation amino acids are transported to the liver then into the general circulation, thus making them available to all the cells and tissues of the body. Different cells choose from those available the particular amino acids required for building or repairing their specific type of tissue and for synthesising their secretions, e.g. antibodies, enzymes, hormones.

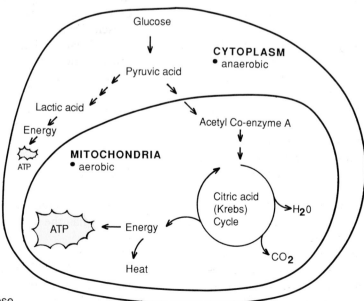

Figure 12.46 Oxidation of glucose.

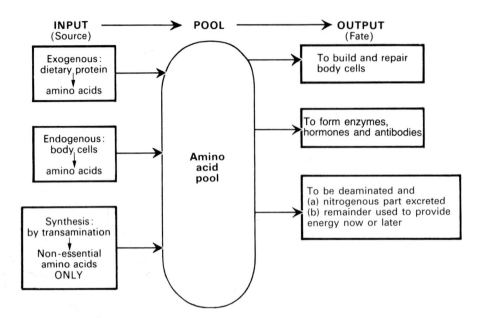

Figure 12.47 Sources and utilisation of amino acids in the body.

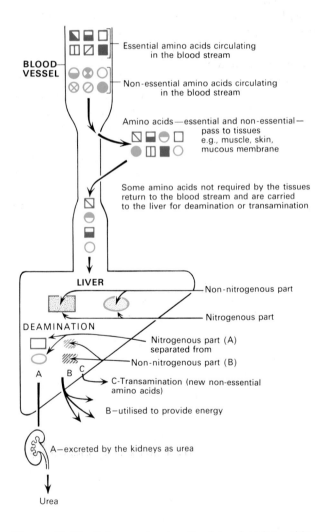

Figure 12.48 Scheme showing the fate of amino acids in the body.

Amino acids not required for building and repairing body tissues cannot be stored and are broken down in the liver:

- the *nitrogenous part*, the amino group (NH_2) is converted to ammonia (NH_3) and then combined with carbon dioxide forming *urea* by the process of *deamination* and excreted in the urine.
- the remaining part is used to provide energy, as glucose by gluconeogenesis, or stored as fat, if in excess of immediate requirements.

Amino acid pool (Fig. 12.47)

A pool of amino acids is maintained within the body. This is the source from which the different cells of the body draw the amino acids they need to synthesise their own materials, e.g. new cells, secretions such as enzymes and hormones, plasma proteins.

Sources of amino acids

Exogenous. These are derived from the protein eaten in the diet.

Endogenous. These are obtained from the breakdown of body protein. In an adult about 80 to 100 g of protein are broken down and replaced each day. Intestinal mucosa has the most rapid turnover of cells.

Loss of amino acids

Deamination. Amino acids not needed by the body are deaminated, mainly in the liver. The nitrogenous part,

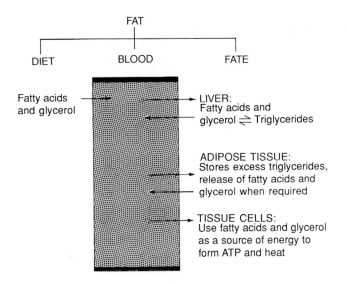

Figure 12.49 Sources, distribution and utilisation of fats in the body.

or amino group (NH_2) is converted to ammonia (NH_3) and then to urea before being excreted by the kidneys. The remainder is used to provide energy and heat.

Excretion. The faeces contain a considerable amount of protein consisting of desquamated cells from the lining of the alimentary tract.

Endogenous and exogenous amino acids are mixed in the 'pool' and the body is said to be in *nitrogen balance* when the rate of removal from the pool is equal to the additions to it. Unlike carbohydrates, the body has no

capacity for the storage of amino acids except for this relatively small pool. Figure 12.48 depicts what happens to amino acids in the body.

Metabolism of fat (Fig. 12.49)

Fats which have been digested and absorbed as fatty acids and glycerol into the *lacteals* are transported via the cisterna chyli and the thoracic duct to the bloodstream and so, by a circuitous route, to the liver. Fatty acids and glycerol circulating in the blood are used by the cells of organs and glands to provide energy and in the synthesis of some of their secretions. In the liver some fatty acids and glycerol are used to provide energy and heat, and some are recombined forming *triglycerides*, the form in which fat is stored. A triglyceride consists of three fatty acids chemically combined with a glycerol molecule. When required, triglycerides are converted back to fatty acids and glycerol and used to provide energy. The end products of fat metabolism are energy, heat, carbon dioxide and water.

Ketone bodies are the *keto acids* produced during the process of oxidation of fats and are always present in the blood in very small amounts. They are excreted in the urine and in the expired air as *acetone*. Fat is used in increased amounts when there is not enough carbohydrate available for metabolism. For complete oxidation of fatty acids and glycerol, oxygen and glucose are required. If there is inadequate glucose, excess keto acids are formed and a state of *ketosis* develops (Fig. 12.50). This may occur in starvation or diabetes mellitus when there is deficiency of insulin which facilitates the

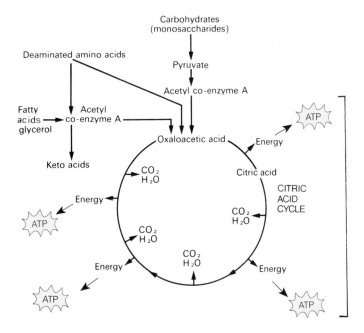

Figure 12.50 The relationship between carbohydrate, deaminated amino acids and fats as energy-releasing substances.

movement of glucose into cells. Excess keto acids have a toxic effect on brain cells.

Fat is synthesised from carbohydrates and proteins which are taken into the body in excess of its needs and stored in the fat depots, i.e. under the skin, in the omentum, around the kidneys.

Relationships between carbohydrates, fatty acids, glycerol and deaminated amino acids as energy-releasing substances

The degradation of carbohydrates, fatty acids, glycerol and the residue after amino acids are deaminated occurs inside the cells, releasing heat and chemical energy (ATP) and forming the waste products *carbon dioxide* and *water*. The catabolism of these molecules occurs in a series of steps, a little energy being released at each stage. Up to a certain point each nutrient passes through a series of separate and distinct stages but thereafter, they all follow a *common pathway of degradation*. This final common pathway is called the *citric acid cycle* or *Krebs cycle*.

Figure 12.50 provides a diagrammatic representation of the processes involved and only a few of the many steps are shown.

Glucose goes through a series of stages to *pyruvate* and *acetyl co-enzyme A*. It is in this form that it joins *oxaloacetic acid* in the citric acid cycle.

Fatty acids pass through a series of oxidative stages to *acetyl co-enzyme A* and, under normal circumstances, progress to oxaloacetic acid and the citric acid cycle. If, however, an excessive amount of acetyl co-enzyme A is produced some of it develops into *keto acids*.

Deaminated amino acids are of two types: those which go through a series of stages to *oxaloacetic acid* and so to the citric acid cycle and those which follow a different series of changes to become *acetyl co-enzyme A* and thereafter take the pathway either to oxaloacetic acid or to keto acids.

The formation of abnormal amounts of keto acids occurs in starvation and in *diabetes mellitus* when excessive amounts of fat and amino acids are used to provide energy. In both these examples there is an insufficiency of carbohydrate inside the cells. In diabetes this is due to a shortage in the supply of the hormone *insulin* which facilitates the transport of glucose from the extracellular fluid across the cell membrane and its subsequent metabolism. Excess keto acids are excreted in the urine and in expired air as acetone.

SUMMARY OF DIGESTION, ABSORPTION AND UTILISATION OF CARBOHYDRATES, PROTEINS AND FATS

Carbohydrates

Digestion

Organ	Digestive juice	Enzyme and action
Mouth	Saliva	Amylase converts cooked starches to *disaccharides*
Stomach	Gastric juice	Hydrochloric acid stops the action of salivary amylase
Small intestine	Pancreatic juice	Amylase converts all starches to *disaccharides* (sugars)
Small intestine	In microvilli	Sucrase Maltase Lactase } Convert all sugars to *monosaccharides*, mainly *glucose* also fructose, galactose

Absorption

Glucose is absorbed into the capillaries of the villi and transported in the portal circulation to the liver.

Utilisation of monosaccharides

Monosaccharides provide energy needed by all cells. To achieve this a fairly constant blood glucose level is maintained. Oxygen is needed to obtain all the energy they contain and the waste products are carbon dioxide and water. In addition:

- some of the excess is converted to glycogen in the presence of insulin and stored in the liver and in muscle
- any remaining glucose is converted into fat and stored in the fat depots (adipose tissue).

Proteins

Digestion

Organ	Digestive juice	Enzyme and action
Mouth	Saliva	No action
Stomach	Gastric juice	Hydrochloric acid converts pepsinogen to *pepsins* Pepsins convert all proteins to smaller molecule *polypeptides*
Small intestine	Pancreatic juice	Enterokinase of intestinal mucosa converts trypsinogen and chymotrypsinogen to *trypsin* and *chymotrypsin* which convert all polypeptides to *di- and tripeptides*
Small intestine	In microvilli	Peptidases complete the conversion of peptides to *amino acids*

Absorption

Amino acids are absorbed into the capillaries of the villi and transported in the portal circulation to the liver.

Utilisation of amino acids

- In the liver to synthesise albumin, globulin, prothrombin and fibrinogen.
- In various combinations by cells of the body for protein synthesis for cell replacement, cell repair, the production of secretions, e.g. hormones, enzymes, antibodies
- To maintain the amino acid pool.
- Amino acids not required are deaminated in the liver. The nitrogenous part is converted into urea and excreted in the urine. The remainder is used to provide energy and heat or deposited as fat in the fat depots.

Fats

Digestion

Organ	Digestive juice	Enzyme and action
Mouth	Saliva	No action
Stomach	Gastric juice	No action
Small intestine	Bile	Bile salts emulsify fats
Small intestine	Pancreatic juice	Lipase converts fats to *fatty acids* and *glycerol*
Small intestine	In microvilli	Lipase completes the digestion of fats to *fatty acids* and *glycerol*

Absorption

Fatty acids and glycerol are absorbed into the lacteals of the villi and are transported via the cisterna chyli and the thoracic duct to the left subclavian vein. In this way they are transported by the circulating blood to the liver where fatty acids and glycerol are combined forming triglycerides.

Utilisation of fats

- Fatty acids and glycerol are utilised in the presence of oxygen to provide energy and heat, the waste products carbon dioxide and water being produced.
- Excess fat is stored as triglycerides in the fat depots.

DISEASES OF THE MOUTH

Inflammation

This may be caused by solids or liquids taken into the mouth, or by infection.

The injury may be due to:

- excessive heat or cold
- the rough texture of the materials
- corrosion by chemical substances.

Corrosive chemicals are the most likely to cause serious tissue damage and acute inflammation. The outcome depends on the extent and depth of the injury.

Thrush (oral candidiasis)

This acute fungal infection of the lining epithelium of the mouth is caused by *Candida albicans*. In adults it causes infection mainly in debilitated people and in those whose immunity is suppressed by steroids, antibiotics or cytotoxic drugs. In babies it may be a severe infection, sometimes causing epidemics in nurseries by cross-infection. It occurs most commonly in bottle-fed babies. *Chronic thrush* may develop, affecting the roof of the mouth in people who wear dentures. The fungus survives in the fine grooves on the upper surface of the denture and repeatedly reinfects the epithelium.

Angular cheilitis

Painful cracks develop in folds of tissue at the corners of the mouth, usually occurring in elderly debilitated people, especially if they do not wear their dentures and the folds remain moist. The usual causal organisms are *Candida albicans* and *Staphylococcus aureus*.

Dietary deficiency of iron and vitamins in the B group predispose to this condition.

Acute gingivitis (Vincent's infection)

This is an acute infection with severe ulceration of the lips, gums, mouth, throat and the palatine tonsil. It is caused by two commensal organisms acting together, *Borrelia vincenti* and a fusiform bacillus. Both organisms may be present in the mouth and only cause the disease in the presence of:

- malnutrition
- debilitating disease
- poor mouth hygiene
- injury caused by previous infection.

Aphthous stomatitis (recurrent oral ulceration)

Extremely painful ulcers occur singly or in crops inside the mouth. They are often found in association with iron and vitamin B group deficiency but a link has not been established.

Virus infections

Acute herpetic gingivostomatitis
This is caused by *Herpes simplex* virus and is the commonest oral virus infection. It is characterised by extensive and very painful ulceration.

Secondary or recurrent herpes lesions (cold sores)
Lesions, caused by *Herpes simplex* virus, occur round the nose and on the lips. After an outbreak the viruses remain alive in the cells, but inactive. Later outbreaks, usually at the same site, are believed to be precipitated by a variety of stimuli not yet clearly identified but failing immune response is a major factor in old age.

Tumours of the mouth

Squamous cell carcinoma
This is the most common type of malignant tumour in the mouth. The usual sites are the lower lip and the edge of the tongue. Ulceration occurs frequently and there is early spread to surrounding tissues and cervical lymph nodes.

Developmental defects

Cleft palate and cleft lip (harelip)
Before birth the right and left halves of the palate develop separately then fuse with the midline nasal septum. One or both lines of fusion may be incomplete, leaving an opening between the mouth and the nose. The membranous soft palate also develops in two parts and fuses in the midline. Thus the lines of fusion extend from the uvula posteriorly to the upper lip anteriorly. The extent of defective fusion varies from bilateral cleft palate and cleft lip to cleft uvula. The causes may be:

- genetic abnormality
- defective development between the 8th and 12th week of gestation caused by, e.g. maternal nutritional disturbances or hypoxia.

DISEASES OF THE PHARYNX

Tonsillitis and diphtheria are described on page 259.

DISEASES OF THE SALIVARY GLANDS

Mumps

This is an acute inflammatory condition of the salivary glands, especially the parotids. It is caused by the mumps virus, one of the para-influenza group. The virus is inhaled in infected droplets and during the 18- to 21-day incubation period viruses multiply elsewhere in the body before spreading to the salivary glands. The virus is present in saliva for about 7 days before and after symptoms appear so infection may spread to others during this 2-week period. They may also spread to:

- the pancreas, causing pancreatitis

- the testes, causing orchitis after puberty and sometimes atrophy of the glands and sterility
- the brain, causing meningitis or meningoencephalitis.

Calculus formation

Calculi (stones) are formed in the salivary glands by the crystallisation of mineral salts in saliva. They may partially or completely block the ducts, leading to swelling of the gland, a predisposition to infection and, in time, atrophy. The causes are not known.

Tumours

Mixed tumours (pleomorphic salivary adenoma)

This benign tumour consists of epithelial and connective tissue cells and occurs mainly in the parotid gland. A second tumour may develop in the same gland several years after the first has been removed. It rarely undergoes malignant change.

Carcinoma

Malignant tumours occur in any salivary gland or duct. Some forms have a tendency to infiltrate nerves in the surrounding tissues, causing severe pain. Lymph spread is to the cervical nodes.

DISEASES OF THE OESOPHAGUS

Oesophageal varices
(Fig. 12.51)

Varicosities of the venous plexus at the distal end of the oesophagus occur when there is impairment of the flow of portal vein blood through the liver. This causes venous congestion in its tributaries, including the gastric veins draining blood from the oesophageal plexus. The anastomotic veins between the venous plexus and the azygos vein become distended, causing valvular incompetence. The distended thin-walled veins may be ruptured by increased venous pressure or by bulky food passing through the oesophagus. This may result in steady slow blood loss causing iron-deficiency anaemia, or in severe cases acute haemorrhage.

Inflammatory conditions

Peptic reflux oesophagitis

This condition is caused by persistent regurgitation of acid gastric juice into the oesophagus, causing irritation and painful ulceration. Haemorrhage occurs when blood vessels are eroded. Persistent reflux leads to chronic inflammation and if damage is extensive, secondary healing with fibrosis occurs. Shrinkage of ageing fibrous tissue may cause stric-

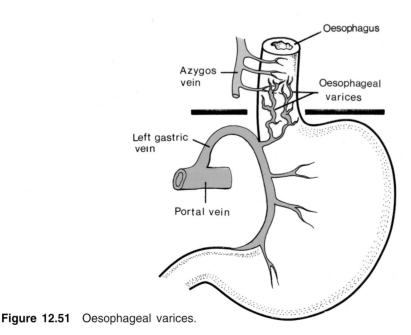

Figure 12.51 Oesophageal varices.

ture of the oesophagus. Reflux of gastric contents is associated with:

- increase in the intra-abdominal pressure, e.g. in pregnancy, constipation and obesity
- high acid content of gastric juice
- low levels of secretion of the hormone gastrin, leading to reduced sphincter action at the lower end of the oesophagus
- the presence of hiatus hernia (p. 328).

Swallowing caustic materials

When swallowed, caustic materials burn the walls of the oesophagus causing an inflammatory reaction. The extent of the damage depends on the concentration and amount swallowed. Following severe injury, healing causes fibrosis, and there is a risk of oesophageal stricture developing later, as the fibrous tissue shrinks.

Microbial infections

Infections are relatively rare and are usually spread from the mouth or pharynx. The microbes most commonly involved are *Candida albicans*, which causes thrush, and herpes viruses. Bottle-fed babies and adults with diminished immunity are most susceptible.

Achalasia

This disease tends to occur in young adults. The cardiac end of the oesophagus is constricted and there is dilatation and muscle hypertrophy proximal to the stricture. This is caused by peristaltic waves of contraction that are not preceded by the normal waves of relaxation. There is an abnormal autonomic

nerve supply to the oesophageal muscle but the cause is not known.

The condition may lead to dysphagia, regurgitation of gastric contents and possibly aspiration pneumonia.

Spontaneous rupture of oesophagus

This may occur, usually at the distal end, if the oesophagus is suddenly distended:

- during a vomiting attack
- by ingestion of foreign bodies
- by passage of an instrument.

Gastric contents pass into the mediastinum, causing acute inflammation. The cause of weakness in the wall of the oesophagus is not known.

Tumours

Benign tumours rarely occur.

Malignant tumours

These occur more often in males than females. The most common sites are the distal end of the oesophagus and at the levels of the larynx and bifurcation of the trachea. The tumours are mainly of two types, both of which may eventually lead to oesophageal obstruction.

Scirrhous (fibrous) tumours. These spread round the circumference and along the oesophagus. They cause thickening of the wall and loss of elasticity.

Soft tissue tumours. These grow into the lumen and spread along the wall.

The causes of malignant change are not known but may be associated with diet and the temperature of swallowed food.

Spread of a malignant tumour at the level of the bifurcation of the

trachea may ulcerate the wall of the oesophagus, the trachea or a bronchus, leading to aspiration pneumonia. Other local spread may involve adjacent mediastinal structures, such as lymph nodes. Death is usually due to oesophageal obstruction before metastases have had time to grow.

Congenital abnormalities

The most common congenital abnormalities of the oesophagus are:

- oesophageal atresia in which the lumen is narrow or blocked
- tracheo-oesophageal fistula in which there is an opening between the oesophagus and the trachea through which milk or regurgitated gastric contents are aspirated.

One or both abnormalities may be present. The causes of these developmental deficiencies are not known.

DISEASES OF THE STOMACH

Gastritis

This is a common condition which occurs when an imbalance between the corrosive action of gastric juice and the protective effect of mucus on the gastric mucosa develops. The amount of mucus in the stomach is insufficient to protect the surface epithelium from the destructive effects of hydrochloric acid. It may be acute or chronic.

Acute gastritis

Gastritis occurs with varying degrees of severity. The most severe form is *acute haemorrhagic gastritis*. When the surface epithelium of the stomach is exposed to acid gastric juice the cells absorb hydrogen ions which increase their internal acidity, disrupt their metabolic processes and trigger the inflammatory reaction. The causes of acute gastritis include:

- regular prolonged use of aspirin and other anti-inflammatory drugs, especially the non-steroids
- regular excessive alcohol consumption
- food poisoning caused by, e.g., *Staphylococcus aureus, Salmonella paratyphi*, viruses
- heavy cigarette smoking
- treatment with cytotoxic drugs and ionising radiation
- ingestion of corrosive poisons, acids and alkalis
- regurgitation of bile into the stomach.

The outcome depends on the extent of the damage. In many cases recovery is uneventful after the cause is removed. In the most severe forms there is ulceration of the mucosa that may be followed by haemorrhage, perforation of the stomach wall and peritonitis. Where there has been extensive tissue damage, healing is by fibrosis causing reduced elasticity and peristalsis.

Chronic gastritis

Chronic gastritis is a milder longer-lasting form. It may follow repeated acute attacks or be an autoimmune disease and is more common in later life.

Helicobacter-associated gastritis

The microbe *Helicobacter pylori* is known to be associated with gastric conditions especially chronic gastritis. Antibodies to this microbe develop in early adulthood although lesions of gastritis occur later in life.

Autoimmune chronic gastritis

This is a progressive form of the disease. There are destructive inflammatory changes that begin on the surface of the mucous membrane and may extend to affect its whole thickness, including the gastric glands. When this stage is reached the secretion of digestive enzymes, hydrochloric acid and intrinsic factor are markedly reduced. The antigens are the *acid-secreting cells* and the *intrinsic factor* they secrete. When these cells are destroyed the inflammation subsides. The initial causes of the autoimmunity are not known but there is a familial predisposition and an association with chronic thyroiditis, thyrotoxicosis and atrophy of the adrenal glands. Secondary effects include:

- Addisonian pernicious anaemia due to lack of intrinsic factor (p. 74)
- impairment of digestion due to lack of enzymes
- microbial infection due to lack of hydrochloric acid.

Peptic ulceration

Ulceration of the gastrointestinal mucosa is caused by disruption of the normal balance of the corrosive effect of gastric juice and the protective effect of mucus on the gastric epithelial cells. It may be viewed as an extension of the cell damage found in acute gastritis. The most common sites for ulcers are the stomach and the first few centimetres of the duodenum. More rarely they occur in the oesophagus, following reflux of gastric juice, and round the anastomosis of the stomach and small intestine, following gastrectomy. The underlying causes are not known but, if factors associated with the maintenance of healthy mucosa are defective, acid gastric juice gains access to the epithelium, causing the initial cell

damage that leads to ulceration. The main factors are: normal blood supply, mucus secretion and cell replacement.

Blood supply

Reduced blood flow and ischaemia may be caused by excessive cigarette smoking and stress, physical or mental. In a stressful situation there is an increase in the secretion of the hormones noradrenaline and adrenaline and these cause constriction of the blood vessels supplying the alimentary tract.

Secretion of mucus

The composition and the amount of mucus may be altered, e.g.:

- by regular and prolonged use of aspirin and other anti-inflammatory drugs
- by the reflux of bile acids and salts
- in chronic gastritis.

Epithelial cell replacement

There is normally a rapid turnover of gastric and intestinal epithelial cells. This may be reduced:

- by raised levels of steroid hormones, e.g. in response to stress or when they are used as drugs
- in chronic gastritis
- by irradiation and the use of cytotoxic drugs.

The microbe *Helicobacter pylori* has been isolated from many peptic ulcer cases, but the mechanism involved is unknown.

Acute peptic ulcers

The tissues involved are the mucous and submucous layers and the ulcers may be single or multiple. They are found in many sites in the stomach and in the first few centimetres of the duodenum. The underlying causes are unknown but their development is often associated with severe stress, e.g. severe illness, shock, burns, severe emotional disturbance and following surgery. Healing without the formation of fibrous tissue usually occurs when the cause of the stress is removed.

Chronic peptic ulcers

These ulcers penetrate through the epithelial and muscle layers of the stomach wall and may include the adjacent pancreas or liver. In the majority of cases they occur singly in the pyloric antrum of the stomach and in the duodenum. Occasionally there are two ulcers facing each other in the duodenum, called kissing ulcers. Healing occurs with the formation of fibrous tissue and subsequent shrinkage may cause:

■ stricture of the lumen of the stomach
■ stenosis of the pyloric sphincter
■ adhesions to adjacent structures, e.g. pancreas, liver, transverse colon.

Complications of peptic ulcers

Haemorrhage. Acid gastric juice may cause the development of many tiny ulcers, or *gastric erosions*, leading to multiple capillary bleeding points and possibly iron-deficiency anaemia (p. 73).

When a major artery is eroded a serious and possibly life-threatening haemorrage may occur causing:

■ shock (p. 114)
■ haematemesis—vomiting of blood
■ melaena—blood in the faeces.

Perforation. When an ulcer erodes through the full thickness of the wall of the stomach or duodenum their contents enter the peritoneal cavity, causing acute peritonitis (p. 323).

Infected inflammatory material may collect under the diaphragm, forming a *subphrenic abscess* and the infection may spread through the diaphragm to the pleural cavity.

Pyloric stenosis. Fibrous tissue formed as an ulcer in the pyloric region heals may cause narrowing of the pylorus, obstructing outflow from the stomach and resulting in persistent vomiting.

Development of a malignant tumour. This may complicate gastric ulceration.

Tumours of the stomach

Benign tumours of the stomach rarely occur.

Malignant tumours

This is a relatively common form of malignancy and it occurs more frequently in men than women. The local growth of the tumour gradually destroys the normal tissue so that achlorhydria and pernicious anaemia are frequently secondary features. The causes have not been established but there appears to be:

■ a familial predisposition
■ an association with environmental factors, e.g. foods, methods of cooking
■ the presence of other diseases, e.g. chronic gastritis, chronic ulceration, pernicious anaemia.

Spread of gastric carcinoma

Local spread. These tumours spread locally to the remainder of the stomach, to the oesophagus, duodenum, omentum, liver and pancreas. The spleen is seldom affected.

As the tumour grows, the surface may ulcerate and become infected,

especially when achlorhydria develops.

Lymphatic spread. This occurs early in the disease. At first the spread is within the lymph channels in the stomach wall then to lymph nodes round the stomach, in the mesentery, omentum and walls of the small intestine and colon.

Blood spread. The common sites for blood-spread metastases are the liver, lungs, brain and bones.

Peritoneal spread. When a tumour includes the full thickness of the stomach wall, small groups of cells may break off and spread throughout the peritoneal cavity. Metastases may develop in any tissue in the abdominal or pelvic cavity where the fragments settle.

Congenital pyloric stenosis

In this condition there is spasmodic constriction of the pyloric sphincter, characteristic projective vomiting and lack of weight increment. In an attempt to overcome the spasms, hypertrophy of the muscle of the pyloric antrum develops, causing obstruction of the pylorus 2 to 3 weeks after birth. The reason for the excess stimulation or neuromuscular abnormality of the pylorus is not known but there is a familial tendency and it is more common in males.

DISEASES OF THE INTESTINES

Diseases of the small and large intestines will be described together because they have certain characteristics in common and some conditions affect both.

Appendicitis

The lumen of the appendix is very small and there is little scope for swelling when it becomes inflamed. The initial cause of inflammation is not always clear. Microbial infection is commonly superimposed on obstruction by, e.g. hard faecal matter (faecoliths), kinking, a foreign body. Inflammatory exudate, with fibrin and phagocytes, causes swelling and ulceration of the mucous membrane lining. In mild cases the inflammation subsides and healing takes place. In more severe cases microbial growth progresses, leading to suppuration, abscess formation and further congestion. The rising pressure inside the appendix occludes first the veins, then the arteries and ischaemia develops, followed by gangrene and rupture.

Complications of appendicitis

Peritonitis. The peritoneum becomes acutely inflamed, the blood vessels dilate and excess serous fluid is secreted. It occurs as a complication of appendicitis when:

- microbes spread through the wall of the appendix and infect the peritoneum
- an appendix abscess ruptures and pus enters the peritoneal cavity
- the appendix becomes gangrenous and ruptures, discharging its contents into the peritoneal cavity.

Abscess formation. The most common abscesses are (Fig. 12.52):

- subphrenic abscess, between the liver and diaphragm, from which infection may spread upwards to the pleura, pericardium and mediastinal structures

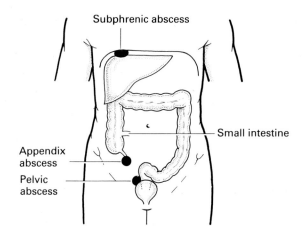

Figure 12.52
Abscess formation: complication of appendicitis.

- pelvic abscess from which infection may spread to adjacent structures.

Fibrous adhesions. When healing takes place fibrous tissue forms and later shrinkage may cause:

- stricture or obstruction of the bowel
- limitation of the movement of a loop of bowel which may twist around the adhesion, causing a type of bowel obstruction called a *volvulus* (p. 328).

Microbial diseases
(Fig. 12.53)

Typhoid fever

This type of enteritis is caused by the microbe *Salmonella typhi*, ingested in food and water. Man is its only host so the source of contamination is an individual who is either suffering from the disease or is a carrier.

After ingestion of microbes there is an incubation period of about 14 days before signs of the disease appear. During this period the microbes invade lymphoid tissue in the walls of the small and large intestine, especially the aggregated lymph follicles (Peyer's patches) and solitary lymph nodes. The microbes then enter the blood vessels and spread to the liver, spleen and gall bladder. In the bacteraemic period acute inflammation develops with necrosis of intestinal lymphoid tissue and ulceration of overlying mucosa. Other effects of *Salmonella typhi* or their endotoxins include:

- typhoid cholecystitis in which the microbes multiply in the gall bladder and are excreted in bile, reinfecting the intestine
- red spots on the skin, especially of the chest and abdomen
- enlargement of the spleen
- myocardial damage and endocarditis
- liver and kidney damage
- reduced resistance to other infections, especially of the respiratory tract, e.g. laryngitis, bronchitis, pneumonia.

Uncomplicated recovery takes place in about 5 weeks with healing of intestinal ulcers and very little fibrosis.

Complications

- The ulcers may penetrate a blood vessel, causing haemorrhage, or erode the intestinal wall, leading to acute peritonitis.
- The individual may become a carrier. When this happens the typhoid fever becomes a chronic, asymptomatic infection

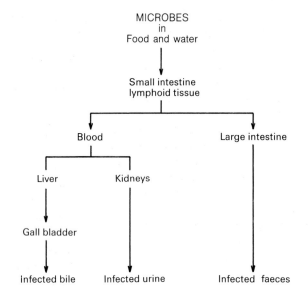

MICROBES
in
Food and water

Small intestine
lymphoid tissue

Blood   Large intestine

Liver   Kidneys

Gall bladder

Infected bile   Infected urine   Infected faeces

Figure 12.53
The routes of
excretion of
microbes in
enteric fever.

of the biliary and urinary tracts. Microbes continue to be excreted indefinitely in urine and faeces. Contamination of food and water by carriers is the usual source of infection.

Paratyphoid fever

This disease is caused by *Salmonella paratyphi A* or *B* spread in the same way as typhoid fever, i.e. in food and drink contaminated by infected urine or faeces. The infection, causing inflammation of the intestinal mucosa, is usually confined to the ileum. Other parts of the body are not usually affected but occasionally chronic infection of the urinary and biliary tracts occurs and the individual becomes an asymptomatic carrier, excreting the microbes in urine and faeces.

Other salmonella infections

Salmonella typhimurium and *S. enteritidis* are the most common infecting microbes in this group. In addition to man their hosts are domestic animals and birds. The microbes may be present in meat,

poultry, eggs and milk, causing infection if cooking does not achieve sterilisation. Mice and rats also carry the organisms and may contaminate food before or after cooking.

The infection is usually of short duration but may be accompanied by acute abdominal pain and diarrhoea, causing dehydration and electrolyte imbalance. In children and debilitated elderly people the infection may be severe or even fatal. Chronic infection of the biliary and urinary tracts may develop and the individual becomes a carrier, excreting the organisms in urine and faeces (Fig. 12.53).

Staphylococcal food poisoning

This is not an infection in the true sense. Acute gastroenteritis is caused by exotoxins produced by the *Staphylococcus aureus* before the ingestion of the contaminated food. The organisms are usually killed by cooking but the toxins can withstand higher temperatures and remain unchanged.

There is usually short-term acute inflammation with violent vomiting

and diarrhoea, causing dehydration and electrolyte imbalance. In most cases recovery is uneventful after the toxin has been removed.

Clostridium perfringens (Cl. welchii) food poisoning

These microbes, although normally present in the intestines of man and animals, cause food poisoning when ingested in large numbers. Meat may be contaminated at any stage between slaughter and the consumer. Outbreaks of food poisoning are associated with large-scale cooking, e.g. in institutions. The spores survive the initial cooking and if the food is cooled slowly they change to the vegetative phase and multipy between the temperatures of 50°C and 20°C. Following refrigeration the microbes multiply if the food is reheated slowly. After being eaten, microbes that remain vegetative die and release endotoxins that cause gastroenteritis.

Campylobacter food poisoning

These Gram-negative bacilli are a common cause of gastroenteritis accompanied by fever, acute pain and sometimes bleeding. They affect mainly young adults and children under 5 years. The microbes are present in the intestines of birds and animals and are spread in undercooked poultry and meat. They may also be spread in water and milk. Pets, such as cats and dogs, may be a source of infection.

Cholera

The disease is caused by *Vibrio cholerae* and is spread by contaminated water, food, hands and fomites. The only known host is man. A very powerful exotoxin is produced which stimulates the intestinal glands to secrete large quantities of water, bicarbonates and chlorides, leading to persistent diarrhoea, severe dehydration and electrolyte imbalance, and may cause death due to hypovolaemic shock. The microbes occasionally spread to the gall bladder where they multiply. They are then excreted in bile and faeces. This carrier state usually lasts for a maximum of about 4 years providing a reservoir for spread of infection.

Dysentery

Bacillary dysentery

This infection of the colon is caused by microbes of the *Shigella* group. The severity of the condition depends on the organisms involved. In Britain it is usually a relatively mild condition caused by *Shigella sonnei*. Outbreaks may reach epidemic proportions, especially in institutions. Children and elderly debilitated adults are particularly susceptible. The only host is man and the organisms are spread by faecal contamination of food, drink, hands and fomites.

There is inflammation, ulceration and oedema of the intestinal mucosa with excess mucus secretion. In severe infections, the acute diarrhoea, containing blood and excess mucus, causes dehydration, electrolyte imbalance and anaemia. When healing occurs the mucous membrane is fully restored. Occasionally a chronic infection develops and the individual becomes a carrier, excreting the microbes in faeces. *Shigella dysenteriae* causes the most severe type of infection. It occurs mainly in tropical countries.

Amoebic dysentery

This disease is caused by *Entamoeba histolytica*. The only known host is man and it is spread by faecal contamination of food, water, hands and fomites. Before ingestion the amoebae are inside resistant cysts. When these reach the colon they grow and divide and invade the cells of the mucosa, causing inflammation and ulceration. Further development of the disease may result in destruction of the mucosa over a large area and sometimes perforation occurs. Diarrhoea containing mucus and blood is persistent and debilitating.

The disease may progress in a number of ways:

- healing may produce fibrous adhesions, causing partial or complete obstruction
- the amoebae may spread to the liver, causing amoebic hepatitis and abscesses
- chronic dysentery may develop with intermittent diarrhoea and amoebae in the faeces.

Although most infected people do not develop symptoms they may become carriers.

Inflammatory bowel disease

Crohn's disease (regional ileitis)

This chronic inflammatory condition of the alimentary tract usually occurs in young adults. The terminal ileum and the rectum are most commonly affected but the disease may be more widespread. There is chronic patchy inflammation with oedema of the full thickness of the intestinal wall, causing partial obstruction of the lumen, sometimes described as *skip lesions*. There are periods of remission of varying duration. The cause of Crohn's disease is not entirely clear but it may be that immunological abnormality renders the individual susceptible to infection, especially by viruses. Complications include:

- secondary infections, occurring when inflamed areas ulcerate
- fibrous adhesions and subsequent intestinal obstruction caused by the healing process
- fistulae between intestinal lesions and adjacent structures, e.g. loops of bowel, surface of the skin (p. 71)
- peri-anal fistula formation
- megaloblastic anaemia due to malabsorption of vitamin B_{12} and folic acid
- cancer of the small or large intestine.

Ulcerative colitis

This is a chronic inflammatory disease of the mucosa of the colon and rectum which may ulcerate and become infected. It usually occurs in young adults and begins in the rectum and sigmoid colon. From there it may spread to involve a variable proportion of the colon and, sometimes, the entire colon. There are periods of remission lasting weeks, months or years. The cause is not known but there is an association with arthritis, iritis, some skin lesions, haemolytic anaemia and some drug sensitivities. In long-standing cases cancer sometimes develops.

Fulminating ulcerative colitis

This is also called *toxic megacolon*. The colon loses its muscle tone and dilates, the wall becomes thinner and perforation, which may be fatal, may follow. There is a sudden onset of acute diarrhoea, with severe blood loss, leading to dehydration, electrolyte imbalance, perforation, hypovolaemic shock and possibly death.

Diverticular disease

Diverticula are small pouches of mucosa that protrude into the peritoneal cavity through the circular muscle fibres of the colon between the taeniae coli (Fig. 12.54). The walls consist of mucous membrane with a covering of visceral peritoneum. They occur at the weakest points of the intestinal wall, i.e. where the blood vessels enter, most commonly in the sigmoid colon. *Diverticulitis* arises when faeces impact in the diverticula and the walls become inflamed and oedematous as secondary infection develops. This reduces the blood supply causing ischaemic pain. Occasionally, rupture occurs resulting in peritonitis.

The causes of *diverticulosis* (presence of diverticuli) are not known but it is associated with low-residue diet and abnormally active peristalsis. In Western countries diverticulosis is fairly common after the age of 60 but diverticulitis affects only a small proportion.

Tumours of the small and large intestines

Benign and malignant tumours of the small intestine are rare, compared with their occurrence in the stomach and colon.

Benign tumours

Benign neoplasms may form a broad-based mass or develop a pedicle. Occasionally those with pedicles twist upon themselves, causing ischaemia, necrosis and possibly gangrene. Malignant changes may occur.

Malignant tumours

Small intestine. Malignant tumours tend not to obstruct the lumen and may remain unnoticed until symptoms caused by metastases appear. The most common sites of metastases are local lymph nodes, the liver, lungs and brain.

The colon is the most common site of malignancy in the alimentary tract in Western countries. The tumour may be:

- a soft friable mass, projecting into the lumen of the colon with a tendency to ulceration, infection and haemorrhage
- a hard fibrous mass encircling the colon, causing reduced elasticity and peristalsis and narrowing of the lumen
- a gelatinous mucoid mass that thickens the wall and tends to ulcerate and become infected.

The causes of cancer of the colon are not known but environmental factors including dietary constituents may be implicated. Slow movement of bowel contents may result in the conversion of as yet unknown substances that are present into carcinogenic agents. Predisposing diseases include ulcerative colitis and some benign tumours.

Local spread of intestinal tumours occurs early but may not be evident until there is severe ulceration and haemorrhage or obstruction. Spread can be outwards through the wall into the peritoneal cavity and adjacent structures.

Lymph-spread metastases occur in

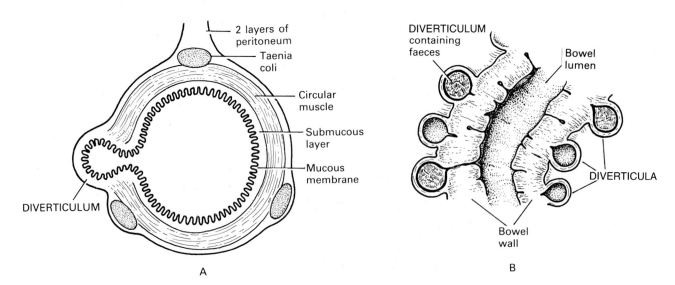

Figure 12.54 Intestinal diverticula. A. Cross-section of bowel showing one diverticulum. B. Longitudinal section of bowel showing numerous diverticula.

mesenteric lymph nodes, the peritoneum and other abdominal and pelvic organs. Pressure caused by enlarged lymph nodes may cause obstruction or damage other structures.

Blood-spread metastases are most common in the liver, brain and bones.

Carcinoid tumours (argentaffinomas)

These tumours are considered, on clinical evidence, to be benign but they spread into the tissues around their original site. They grow very slowly and rarely metastasise. The parent cells are hormone-secreting cells widely dispersed throughout the body, not situated in endocrine glands. Some of these tumours secrete hormones while others do not. They are called APUD cells, an acronym for some of their chemical characteristics. The cells react with silver compounds, hence the name argentaffinomas. Common sites in the intestines for these *apudomas* are the appendix, ileum, stomach, colon and rectum. The tumours are frequently multiple and may spread locally, causing obstruction.

Carcinoid syndrome

This is the name given to the effects of the variety of substances secreted by apudomas in the intestine and elsewhere. The secretions include serotonin (5-hydroxytryptamine), histamine and bradykinin, and the effects include flushing attacks, tachycardia, sweating, anxiety and diarrhoea.

Hernias

A hernia is a protrusion of bowel through a weak point in the musculature of the anterior abdominal wall or an existing opening (Fig. 12.55). It occurs when there are intermittent increases in intra-abdominal pressure, most commonly in men who lift heavy loads at work. The underlying causes of the abdominal

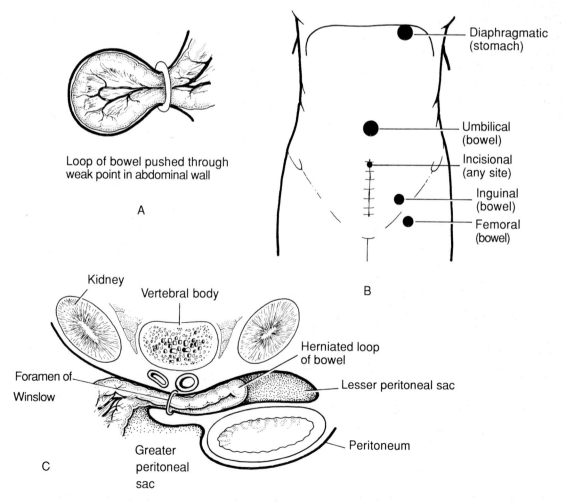

Figure 12.55 A. Hernia formation. B. and C. Common sites.

wall weakness are not known. Possible outcomes include:

- spontaneous reduction, i.e. the loop of bowel slips back to its correct place when the intra-abdominal pressure returns to normal
- manual reduction, i.e. by applying slight pressure over the abdominal swelling
- strangulation, when the venous drainage from the herniated loop of bowel is impaired, causing congestion, ischaemia and gangrene. In addition there is intestinal obstruction.

Sites of hernias

Inguinal hernia. The weak point is the inguinal canal which contains the spermatic cord in the male and the round ligament in the female. It occurs more commonly in males than in females.

Femoral hernia. The weak point is the femoral canal through which the femoral artery, vein and lymph vessels pass from the pelvis to the thigh.

Umbilical hernia. The weak point is the umbilicus where the umbilical blood vessels from the placenta enter the fetus.

Incisional hernia. This is caused by repeated stretching of the fibrous tissue formed during the repair of a surgical wound.

Diaphragmatic or hiatus hernia. This is the protrusion of a part of the fundus of the stomach through the oesophageal opening in the diaphragm. The main complication is irritation caused by reflux of acid gastric juice, especially when the individual lies flat or bends down. The long-term effects may be oesophagitis, fibrosis and narrowing of the oesophagus, causing dysphagia. Strangulation does not occur.

Sliding hiatus hernia. An unusually short oesophagus that ends above the diaphragm pulls a part of the stomach upwards into the thorax. The abnormality may be congenital or be caused by shrinkage of fibrous tissue formed during healing of a previous oesophageal injury. The sliding movement of the stomach in the oesophageal opening is due to normal shortening of the oesophagus by muscular contraction during swallowing.

Rolling hiatus hernia. An abnormally large opening in the diaphragm allows a pouch of stomach to 'roll' upwards into the thorax beside the oesophagus. This is associated with obesity and increased intra-abdominal pressure.

Peritoneal hernia. A loop of bowel may herniate through the foramen of Winslow, the opening in the lesser omentum that separates the greater and lesser peritoneal sacs.

Volvulus

This occurs when a loop of bowel twists through 180 degrees, cutting off its blood supply, causing gangrene and obstruction. It occurs in parts of the intestine that are attached to the posterior abdominal wall by a long double fold of visceral peritoneum, the mesentery. The most common site in adults is the sigmoid colon and in children the small intestine. The causes are unknown but predisposing factors include:

- an unusually long mesocolon or mesentery
- heavy loading of the pelvic colon with faeces
- a slight twist of a loop of bowel, causing gas and fluid to accumulate and promote further twisting
- adhesions formed following surgery or peritonitis.

Intussusception

In this condition a length of intestine is invaginated into itself (Fig. 12.56). It occurs most commonly in children when a piece of terminal ileum is pushed through the ileocaecal valve. In a child, infection, usually by viruses, causes swelling of the lymphoid tissue in the intestinal wall. The overlying mucosa bulges into the lumen, creating a partial obstruction and a rise in pressure inside the intestine proximal to the swelling. Strong peristaltic waves develop in an attempt to overcome the partial obstruction. These push the swollen piece of bowel into the lumen of the section immediately distal to it, creating the intussusception. The pressure on the veins in the invaginated portion is increased, causing congestion, fur-

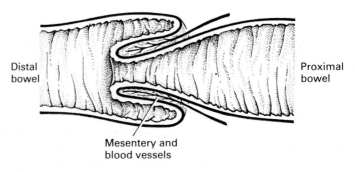

Distal bowel

Proximal bowel

Mesentery and blood vessels

Figure 12.56 Intussusception.

ther swelling, ischaemia and possibly gangrene. Complete intestinal obstruction may occur. In adults tumours that bulge into the lumen, e.g. polypi, together with the strong peristalsis, may be the cause.

Intestinal obstruction

This is not a disease in itself. The following is a summary of the main causes of obstruction with some examples.

Mechanical causes of obstruction

- Constriction of the intestine by, e.g. strangulated hernia, intussusception, volvulus, peritoneal adhesions. Partial obstruction may suddenly become complete.
- Stenosis and thickening of the intestinal wall, e.g. in diverticulosis, Crohn's disease and malignant tumours. There is usually a gradual progression from partial to complete obstruction.
- Obstruction by, e.g. a large gallstone or a tumour growing into the lumen.
- Pressure on the intestine from outside, e.g. a large tumour in any pelvic or abdominal organ, such as a uterine fibroid. This type is most likely to occur inside the confined space of the bony pelvis.

Neurological causes of obstruction

Partial or complete loss of peristaltic activity produces the effects of obstruction. *Paralytic ileus* is the most common form but the paralysis may be more widespread. The cause is either excessive sympathetic stimulation or lack of parasympathetic stimulation. The mechanisms are not clear but there are well-recognised predisposing conditions including:

- general peritonitis, especially when large amounts of exotoxin are released from dead microbes
- following surgery when there has been a considerable amount of handling of the intestines
- severe intestinal infection, especially if there is acute toxaemia, e.g. following ruptured appendix.

Secretion of water and electrolytes continues although intestinal mobility is lost and absorption impaired. This causes distension and electrolyte imbalance, leading to hypovolaemic shock. There is also growth and multiplication of microbes.

Vascular causes of obstruction

When the blood supply to a segment of bowel is cut off, ischaemia is followed by infarction, gangrene and obstruction. The causes may be:

- atheromatous changes in the blood vessel walls, with thrombosis
- embolism
- mechanical obstruction of the bowel, e.g. strangulated hernia.

Malabsorption

Impaired absorption of nutrient materials and water from the intestines is not a disease in itself. It is the result of diseases causing one or more of the following changes:

- atrophy of the villi of the mucosa of the small intestine
- incomplete digestion of food
- interference with the transport of absorbed nutrients from the small intestine to the blood.

Primary malabsorption

Disease of the intestinal mucous membrane

Atrophy of the villi is the main cause, varying in severity from minor abnormality to almost complete loss of function. The most common underlying diseases are coeliac disease and tropical sprue.

Coeliac disease (idiopathic steatorrhoea). This disease is believed to be due to a genetically determined abnormal immunological reaction to the protein *gluten*, present in wheat. When it is removed from the diet, recovery is complete. There is marked villous atrophy and malabsorption characterised by the passage of loose, pale coloured, fatty stools.

There may be abnormal immune reaction to other antigens. Atrophy of the spleen is common and malignant lymphoma of the small intestine may develop. It often presents in infants after weaning but can affect any age.

Tropical sprue. In this disease there is partial villous atrophy with malabsorption, chronic diarrhoea, severe wasting and pernicious anaemia due to deficient absorption of vitamin B_{12} and folic acid. The cause is unknown but it may be that bacterial growth in the small intestine is a factor. The disease is endemic in subtropical and tropical countries except Africa south of the Sahara. After leaving the endemic area most people suffering from sprue recover, but others may not develop symptoms until months or even years later.

Secondary malabsorption

This is associated with incomplete digestion of food, impaired transport of absorbed nutrients and following extensive small bowel resection.

Defective digestion. This occurs in a variety of conditions:

- disease of the liver and pancreas
- following a resection of small intestine
- following surgery if microbes grow in a blind end of intestine.

Impaired transport of nutrients

This occurs when there is:

- lymphatic obstruction by, e.g., lymph node tumours, removal of nodes at surgery, tubercular disease of lymph nodes
- impairment of mesenteric blood flow by, e.g., arterial or venous thrombosis, pressure caused by a tumour
- obstruction of blood flow through the liver, e.g. in cirrhosis of liver.

DISEASES OF THE PANCREAS

Acute pancreatitis

Protein-splitting enzyme precursors are activated while still in the pancreas and digest the parenchymal cells, i.e. by autodigestion. The severity of the disease is directly related to the amount of pancreatic tissue destroyed.

Mild forms may damage only those cells near the ducts.

Severe forms cause widespread damage with necrosis and haemorrhage. Common complications include infection, suppuration, and local venous thrombosis. Pancreatic enzymes, especially amylase, enter and circulate in the blood, causing similar damage to other structures. In severe cases there is a high mortality rate.

The causes of acute pancreatitis are not clear but known predisposing factors are gallstones and alcoholism. When a gallstone obstructs the hepatopancreatic ampulla there is reflux of bile into the pancreas and the spread of infection from cholangitis. Alcoholism is known to be present in a large number of cases but the mechanisms by which it causes pancreatitis are not clear. Other associated conditions include:

- cancer of the ampulla or head of pancreas
- virus infections, notably mumps
- chronic renal failure
- renal transplantation
- hyperparathyroidism
- hypothermia
- drugs, e.g. corticosteroids, cytotoxic agents
- diabetes mellitus
- cholecystitis.

Chronic pancreatitis

This is due to repeated attacks of acute pancreatitis or may arise gradually without evidence of pancreatic disease. It is frequently associated with fibrosis and distortion of the main pancreatic duct.

There is obstruction of the tiny acinar ducts by protein material secreted by the acinar cells. This eventually leads to the formation of cysts which may rupture into the peritoneal cavity. Intact cysts may cause obstruction of the:

- common bile duct, causing jaundice
- portal vein, causing venous congestion in the organs drained by its tributaries.

The causes of these changes are not known but they are associated mainly with heavy wine drinking.

Cystic fibrosis (mucoviscidosis)

This is one of the most common genetic diseases. It is estimated that almost 20% of people carry the abnormal recessive gene which must be present in *both parents* to cause the disease.

The secretions of all exocrine glands have abnormally high viscosity but the most severely affected are those of the pancreas, intestines, biliary tract, lungs and the reproductive system in the male. Sweat glands secrete abnormally large amounts of salt during excessive sweating. In the pancreas highly viscous mucus is secreted by the walls of the ducts and causes obstruction, parenchymal cell damage, the formation of cysts and defective enzyme secretion. In the newborn, intestinal obstruction may be caused by a plug of meconium and viscid mucus, leading to perforation and meconium peritonitis which is often fatal. In less acute cases there may be impairment of protein and fat digestion resulting in malabsorption, steatorrhoea and failure to thrive in infants. In older children:

- digestion of food and absorption of nutrients is impaired
- there may be obstruction of bile ducts in the liver, causing cirrhosis
- bronchitis, bronchiectasis and pneumonia may develop.

Chronic lung disease and *cor pulmonale* are the commonest causes of death.

Tumours of the pancreas

Benign tumours of the pancreas are very rare.

Malignant tumours are relatively common and affect men more than women. They occur most frequently in the head of the pancreas, obstructing the flow of bile and pancreatic juice into the duodenum. Jaundice and acute pancreatitis usually develop. Weight loss is the result of impaired digestion and absorption of fat. Tumours in the body and tail of the gland rarely cause symptoms until the disease is advanced. Metastases are often recognised before the primary tumour. The causes of the malignant changes are not known but it is believed that there may be an association with:

- cigarette smoking
- diet high in fats and carbohydrates
- diabetes mellitus.

DISEASES OF THE LIVER

New liver cells develop only when needed to replace damaged cells. Capacity for regeneration is considerable and damage is usually extensive before it is evident. The effects of disease or toxic agents are seen when:

- regeneration of hepatocytes (liver cells) does not keep pace with damage, leading to hepatocellular failure
- there is a gradual replacement of damaged cells by fibrous tissue, leading to portal hypertension.

In most liver disease both conditions are present.

Acute hepatitis

Areas of necrosis develop as groups of hepatocytes die and the eventual outcome depends on the size and number of these areas. Causes of the damage may be a variety of conditions, including:

- infections
- toxic substances
- circulatory disturbances.

Viral hepatitis

Virus infections are the commonest cause of acute liver injury and include Type A, Type B, Type C and Type non-A and non-B (NANB). The types are distinguished serologically, i.e. by the antibodies produced to combat the infection. The severity of the ensuing disease caused by the different virus types varies considerably but the pattern is similar. The viruses enter the liver cells, causing degenerative changes by mechanisms not yet understood. An inflammatory reaction ensues, accompanied by production of an exudate containing lymphocytes, plasma cells and granulocytes. There is reactive hyperplasia of the reticuloendothelial Kupffer cells in the walls of the sinusoids.

As groups of cells die, necrotic areas of varying sizes develop, phagocytes remove the necrotic material and the lobules collapse. The basic lobule framework (Fig. 12.41) becomes distorted and blood vessels develop kinks. These changes interfere with the circulation of blood to the remaining hepatocytes and the resultant hypoxia causes further damage. Fibrous tissue develops in the damaged area, and adjacent hepatocytes proliferate. The effect of these changes on the overall functioning of the liver depends on the size of the necrotic areas, the amount of fibrous tissue formed and the extent to which the blood and bile channels are distorted.

Type A virus (infectious hepatitis)

This virus has only one known serological type. It occurs endemically, affecting mainly children, causing a mild illness. Infection is spread by hands, food, water and fomites contaminated by infected faeces. The incubation period is 15 to 40 days and the viruses are excreted in the faeces for 7 to 14 days before clinical symptoms appear and for about 7 days after. Antibodies develop and immunity persists after recovery. Subclinical disease may occur but carriers do not develop.

Type B virus (serum hepatitis)

This virus has a number of serological types. Infection occurs at any age, but mostly in adults. The incubation period is 50 to 180 days. The virus enters the blood and is spread by blood and blood products. People at greatest risk of infection are those who come in contact with blood and blood products in their daily work, e.g. people in the health, ambulance and fire services. The virus is also spread by body fluids, i.e. saliva, semen, vaginal secretions and from mother to fetus. Others at risk include intravenous drug addicts and male homosexuals. Antibodies are formed and immunity persists after recovery. Infection usually leads to severe illness lasting 2 to 6 weeks, often followed by a protracted convalescence. Carriers may, or may not, have had clinical disease. Type B virus may cause massive liver necrosis and death. In less severe cases recovery may be complete. In chronic hepatitis which may develop, live viruses continue to circulate in the blood and other body fluids. The condition may predispose to liver cancer. Hepatitis D (delta agent) aggravates hepatitis B.

Hepatitis C

This virus is spread by blood and blood products. It is prevalent in drug addicts and sometimes occurs as a complication of blood transfusion. The infection can be asymptomatic as a carrier state occurs. When hepatitis develops, it is often recurrent and may result in chronic liver disease, especially cirrhosis.

Type non-A and non-B hepatitis (NANB)

These viruses are known to exist because of the occurrence of virus hepatitis that cannot be attributed to Type A, Type B or Type C viruses. Serological identity has not yet been established. One known method of spread is transfusion of infected blood. The incubation period is 10 to 90 days. Clinical illness of varying severity occurs and it may be followed by complete recovery but a high proportion develop chronic hepatitis. Carriers may, or may not, have had clinical disease.

Toxic substances

Many drugs undergo chemical change in the liver before excretion in bile or by other organs. They may damage the liver cells in their original form or while in various intermediate stages. Some substances always cause liver damage (predictably toxic) while others only do so when hypersensitivity develops (unpredictably toxic). In both types the extent of the damage depends on the size of the dose and/or the duration of intake. Examples include:

Predictable group (dose related)	Unpredictable group (individual idiosyncrasy)
Chloroform	Phenothiazine
Tetracyclines	compounds
Cytotoxic	Halothane
drugs	Methyldopa
Anabolic	Phenylbutazone
steroids	Indomethacin
Alcohol	Chlorpropamide
Paracetamol	Thiouracil
Some	Sulphonamides
hydrocarbons	
Some fungi	

Circulatory disturbances

The intensely active hepatocytes are particularly vulnerable to damage by hypoxia which is usually due to deficient blood supply caused by:

- fibrosis in the liver following inflammation
- compression of the portal vein, hepatic artery or vein by a tumour
- acute general circulatory failure and shock
- venous congestion caused by acute or chronic right-sided heart failure.

Chronic hepatitis

This is defined as any form of hepatitis which persists for more than 6 months. It may be caused by viruses or drugs, but in some cases the cause is unknown.

Chronic persistent hepatitis

This is a mild, persistent inflammation following acute viral hepatitis. There is usually little or no fibrosis.

Chronic active hepatitis

This is a continuing progressive inflammation with cell necrosis and the formation of fibrous tissue that may lead to cirrhosis of the liver. There is distortion of the liver blood vessels and hypoxia, leading to further hepatocyte damage. This condition is commonly associated with Type B virus hepatitis, with some forms of autoimmunity and unpredictable drug reactions.

Non-viral inflammation of the liver

Pyogenic

Ascending cholangitis

Infection, usually by *Escherichia coli*, may spread from the biliary tract. The most common predisposing factor is obstruction of the common bile duct by gallstones.

Liver abscess

Septic emboli from septic foci in the abdomen and pelvis may lodge in branches of the portal vein and cause multiple abscesses or infect the vein, causing *portal pylephlebitis*. Common sources of this type of infection are acute appendicitis, diverticulitis and inflamed haemorrhoids.

Cirrhosis of the liver

This is the result of long-term inflammation caused by a wide variety of agents. The most common causes are:

- alcohol abuse
- hepatitis B and C virus infections
- the effects of bile retained in hepatocytes due to obstruction of bile flow or chronic inflammation
- congenital metabolic abnormalities.

As the inflammation subsides:

- destroyed liver tissue is replaced by fibrous tissue
- there is hyperplasia of hepatocytes adjacent to the damaged area, in an attempt to compensate for the destroyed cells. This leads to the formation of nodules consisting of hepatocytes confined within sheets of fibrous tissue.

As the condition progresses there is the development of:

- portal hypertension, leading to congestion in the organs drained by the tributaries of the portal vein, to ascites and possibly to the development of oesophageal varices (p. 120)
- liver failure when hyperplasia is unable to keep pace with cell destruction
- possibly cancer of the liver.

Liver failure

This occurs when liver function is reduced to such an extent that other body activities are impaired. It may be acute or chronic and may be the outcome of a wide variety of disorders, e.g.:

- acute viral hepatitis
- extensive necrosis due to poisoning, e.g. some drug overdoses, hepatotoxic chemicals, adverse drug reactions
- cirrhosis of the liver
- following some medical procedures, e.g. abdominal paracentesis, portacaval shunt operations.

Liver failure has serious effects on other parts of the body.

Hepatic encephalopathy

The cells affected are the astrocytes in the brain. The condition is characterised by apathy, disorientation, muscular rigidity, delirium and coma. Several factors may be involved, e.g.:

- nitrogenous bacterial metabolites absorbed from the colon, normally detoxicated in the liver, reach the brain via the blood
- metabolites, normally present in trace amounts, e.g. ammonia, may reach toxic concentrations

and change the permeability of the cerebral blood vessels and the effectiveness of the blood–brain barrier
- hypoxia and electrolyte imbalance.

Blood coagulation defects

The liver fails to synthesise substances needed for blood clotting, i.e. prothrombin, fibrinogen and factors II, V, VII, IX and X. Platelet production is impaired but the cause is unknown. Purpura and bleeding may occur.

Oliguria and renal failure

Portal hypertension may cause the development of oesophageal varices. If these rupture, bleeding may lead to a fall in blood pressure sufficient to reduce the renal blood flow, causing progressive oliguria and renal failure.

Oedema and ascites

These may be caused by the combination of two factors:

- portal hypertension raises the capillary hydrostatic pressure in the organs drained by the tributaries of the portal vein (Fig. 12.9)
- diminished production of serum albumin and clotting factors reduces the plasma osmotic pressure.

Together these changes cause the movement of excess fluid into the interstitial spaces where it causes *oedema*. Eventually free fluid accumulates in the peritoneal cavity and the resultant *ascites* may be severe (p. 117).

Anaemia

This is usually due to the combined effect of a number of factors:

- upset in the metabolism of folic acid and vitamin B_{12}

- chronic blood loss from oesophageal varices, causing iron-deficiency anaemia
- increased breakdown of red blood cells in the congested spleen, causing haemolytic anaemia.

Jaundice

The following factors may cause jaundice as liver failure develops:

- inability of the hepatocytes to conjugate and excrete bilirubin
- obstruction to the movement of bile through the bile channels by fibrous tissue that has distorted the structural framework of liver lobules.

Tumours of the liver

Benign tumours of the liver are very rare.

Malignant tumours

In many cases cancer of the liver is associated with cirrhosis but the relationship between them is not clear. It may be that both cirrhosis and cancer are caused by the same agents or that the carcinogenic action of other agents is promoted by cirrhotic changes. Malignancy develops in a number of cases of acute hepatitis caused by Type B virus. The most common sites of metastases are the abdominal lymph nodes, the peritoneum and the lungs.

Secondary malignant tumours in the liver are common, especially from primary tumours in the gastrointestinal tract, the lungs and the breast. The metastases tend to grow rapidly and are often the cause of death.

DISEASES OF THE GALL BLADDER AND BILE DUCTS

Gallstones (Cholelithiasis)

Gallstones consist of deposits of the constituents of bile, most commonly cholesterol. Many small or one large stone may form. The causes are not clear but predisposing factors include:

- changes in the composition of bile that affect the solubility of its constituents
- high levels of blood and dietary cholesterol
- cholecystitis
- diabetes mellitus when associated with high blood cholesterol levels
- haemolytic disease
- female gender
- obesity
- long-term use of oral contraceptives
- high parity in young women especially when accompanied by obesity.

Complications

Biliary colic
If a gallstone gets stuck in the cystic or common bile duct there is strong spasmodic contraction of the wall of the duct in an effort to move the stone onwards. The severe pain associated with biliary colic is due to ischaemia of the duct wall over the stone during the spasmodic muscle contraction.

Inflammation
Gallstones cause irritation and inflammation of the walls of the gall bladder and the cystic and common bile ducts. There may be superimposed microbial infection.

Impaction
Blockage of the cystic duct by a gallstone leads to distension of the gall bladder and *cholecystitis*. This does not cause jaundice because liver bile can pass directly into the duodenum. Obstruction of the common bile duct leads to retention of bile, jaundice and *cholangitis* (infection of the bile ducts).

Acute cholecystitis

This is usually a complication of gallstones or an exacerbation of chronic cholecystitis, especially if there has been partial or intermittent obstruction of the cystic duct. Inflammation develops followed by secondary microbial infections spread from a focus of infection elsewhere in the body, e.g. they may be blood-borne or pass directly from the adjacent colon. Those most commonly involved are *Escherichia coli* and *Streptococcus faecalis*. In severe cases there may be fibrinous exudate into the gall bladder, suppuration, gangrene, perforation, peritonitis, local abscess formation, disruption of gall bladder activity, gallstone formation and the infection may spread to the bile ducts and the liver.

Chronic cholecystitis

The onset is usually insidious, sometimes following repeated acute attacks. Gallstones are usually present and there may be accompanying biliary colic. Pain is due to the spasmodic contraction of muscle, causing ischaemia when the gall bladder is packed with gallstones. There is usually secondary infection with suppuration. Ulceration of the tissues between the gall bladder and the duodenum or colon may occur with fistula formation and, later, fibrous adhesions.

Tumours of the biliary tract

Benign tumours are rare.

Malignant tumours are relatively rare but when they do occur the most common sites are:

- the neck of the gall bladder
- the junction of the cystic and bile ducts
- the ampulla of the bile duct.

Local spread to the liver, the pancreas and other adjacent organs is common. Lymph and blood spread lead to widespread metastases. Early sites include the liver, lungs, abdominal lymph nodes and the peritoneum.

Jaundice

This is not a disease in itself. It is a sign of abnormal bilirubin metabolism and excretion. Serum bilirubin may rise to 34 μmol/l before the yellow colouration of jaudice is evident in the skin and conjunctiva (normal 3 to 13 μmol/l).

Jaundice develops when there is an abnormality at some stage in the metabolic sequence caused by one or more factors, e.g.:

- excess haemolysis of red blood cells with the production of more bilirubin than the liver can deal with
- abnormal liver function that may cause:
  —incomplete uptake of unconjugated bilirubin by hepatocytes
  —ineffective conjugation of bilirubin
  —interference with bilirubin secretion
- obstruction to the flow of bile from the liver to the duodenum.

Types of jaundice

Haemolytic jaundice (acholuric)

This is due to increased haemolysis of red blood cells in the spleen. The amount of bilirubin is increased and if hypoxia develops the efficiency of hepatocyte activity is reduced.

Neonatal haemolytic jaundice occurs in many babies, especially in prematurity where the normal high haemolysis is coupled with shortage of conjugating enzymes in the hepatocytes.

Unconjugated bilirubin which is fat soluble has a toxic effect on brain cells. However, it is unable to cross the blood–brain barrier until the plasma level rises above 340 μmol/l, but when it does, it may cause neurological damage, fits and mental handicap.

Obstructive jaundice

Obstruction to the flow of bile in the biliary tract is caused by, e.g.:

- gallstones
- tumour of the head of the pancreas
- fibrosis of the bile ducts, following inflammation or injury by cholangitis or the passage of gallstones.

Effects include:

- pruritus caused by the irritating effects of bile salts on the skin
- pale faeces due to absence of stercobilin (p. 310)
- dark urine due to the presence of increased amounts of bilirubin.

Hepatocellular jaundice

This is the result of damage to the liver by, e.g.:

- viral infection
- toxic substances, such as drugs
- amoebiasis (amoebic dysentery)
- cirrhosis of the liver.

The damaged cells may be unable to:

- remove unconjugated bilirubin from the blood
- conjugate the bilirubin
- secrete bilirubin into the bile canaliculi.

13
The urinary system

The urinary system is one of the excretory systems of the body. It consists of the following structures:

- 2 *kidneys* which secrete urine
- 2 *ureters* which convey the urine from the kidneys to the urinary bladder
- 1 *urinary bladder* where urine collects and is temporarily stored
- 1 *urethra* through which the urine is discharged from the urinary bladder to the exterior.

Figure 13.1 shows an overview of the urinary system.

The urinary system plays a vital part in maintaining homeostasis of water and electrolyte concentrations within the body. The kidneys produce urine that contains metabolic waste products, especially the nitrogenous compounds urea and uric acid, excess ions and some drugs. The kidneys also have functions mediated by hormones:

- stimulation of erythropoiesis (erythrocyte production, p. 59)
- control of blood volume.

Urine is stored in the bladder and excreted by the process of *micturition*.

KIDNEYS

The kidneys lie on the posterior abdominal wall, one on each side of the vertebral column, behind the peritoneum and below the diaphragm. They extend from the level of the 12th thoracic vertebra to the 3rd lumbar vertebra. The right kidney is usually slightly lower than the left, probably because of the considerable space occupied by the liver.

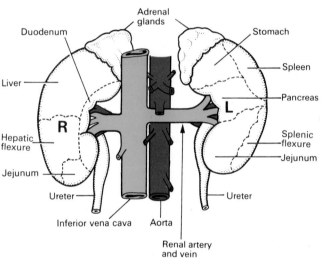

Figure 13.2 Anterior view of the kidneys showing the areas of contact with associated structures.

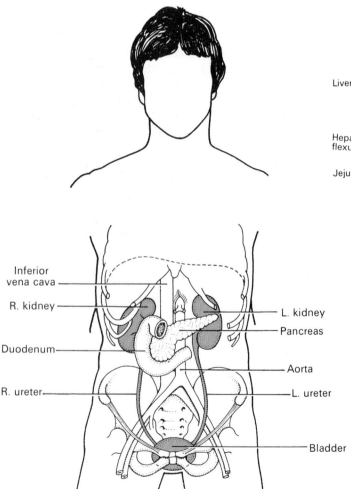

Figure 13.1 The parts of the urinary system (excluding the urethra) and some associated structures.

Kidneys are bean-shaped organs, about 11 cm long, 6 cm wide, 3 cm thick and weigh 150 g. They are embedded in, and held in position by, a mass of fat. A sheath of fibroelastic *renal fascia* encloses the kidney and the renal fat.

Organs associated with the kidneys (Figs 13.1, 13.2 and 13.3)

As the kidneys lie on either side of the vertebral column each is associated with a different group of structures.

Right kidney

Superiorly — the right adrenal gland
Anteriorly — the right lobe of the liver, the duodenum and the hepatic flexure of the colon
Posteriorly — the diaphragm, and muscles of the posterior abdominal wall

Left kidney

Superiorly — the left adrenal gland
Anteriorly — the spleen, stomach, pancreas, jejunum and splenic flexure of the colon
Posteriorly — the diaphragm and muscles of the posterior abdominal wall

Gross structure of the kidney

There are three areas of tissue which can be distinguished when a longitudinal section of the kidney is viewed with the naked eye (Fig. 13.4):

- *a fibrous capsule*, surrounding the kidney
- *the cortex* is the reddish-brown layer of tissue immediately under the capsule and between the pyramids
- *the medulla* is the innermost layer, consisting of pale conical-shaped striations, the *renal pyramids*.

The hilum is the concave medial border of the kidney where the renal blood and lymph vessels and nerves enter.

The renal pelvis is the funnel-shaped structure which acts as a receptacle for the urine formed by the kidney (Fig. 13.4). It has a number of branches called *calyces* at its upper end, each of which surrounds the apex of a renal pyramid. Urine formed in the kidney passes through a *papilla* at the apex of a pyramid into a minor calyx, then into a major calyx before passing through

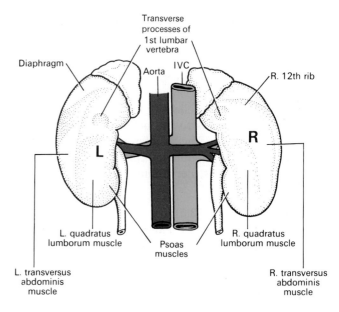

Figure 13.3 Posterior view of the kidneys showing the areas of contact with associated structures.

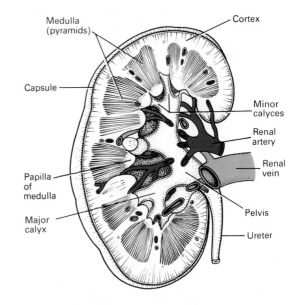

Figure 13.4 A longitudinal section of the right kidney.

the pelvis into the ureter. The walls of the pelvis contain smooth muscle and are lined with transitional epithelium. A peristaltic wave of contraction of the smooth muscle originating in pacemaker cells in the walls of the calyces, propels urine through the pelvis and ureters to the bladder. This is an intrinsic function not under nerve control.

Microscopic structure of the kidney

The kidney substance is composed of about 1 million functional units, the *nephrons*, and a smaller number of *collecting tubules*. The collecting tubules transport urine through the pyramids to the pelvis giving them their striped appearance. The uriniferous tubules are supported by a small amount of connective tissue, containing blood vessels, nerves and lymph vessels.

The nephron (Fig. 13.5)

The nephron consists of a tubule closed at one end, the other end opening into a collecting tubule. The closed or blind end is indented to form the cup-shaped *glomerular capsule* (Bowman's capsule) which almost completely encloses a network of arterial capillaries, the *glomerulus*. Continuing from the glomerular capsule

the remainder of the nephron is about 3 cm long and is described in three parts:

- the *proximal convoluted tubule*
- the *medullary loop* (loop of Henle)
- the *distal convoluted tubule*, leading into a *collecting tubule*.

The collecting tubules unite forming larger tubules that empty into the minor calyces.

After entering the kidney at the hilum the renal artery divides into smaller arteries and arterioles. In the cortex an arteriole, the *afferent arteriole*, enters each glomerular capsule then subdivides into a cluster of capillaries, forming the glomerulus. Between the capillary loops there are connective tissue phagocytic *mesangial cells*. The blood vessel leading away from the glomerulus is the *efferent arteriole*; it breaks up into a second capillary network to supply oxygen and nutritional materials to the remainder of the nephron. Venous blood drained from this capillary bed eventually leaves the kidney in the renal vein which empties into the inferior vena cava (Fig. 13.6). The blood pressure in the glomerulus is higher than in other capillaries because the diameter of the afferent arteriole is greater than that of the efferent arteriole.

The walls of the glomerulus and the glomerular capsule consist of a single layer of *flattened epithelial cells* (Fig. 13.7). The glomerular walls are more permeable than those of other capillaries. The remainder of the nephron and the collecting tubule are formed by a single layer of highly specialised cells.

The nerve supply consists of sympathetic and parasympathetic nerves.

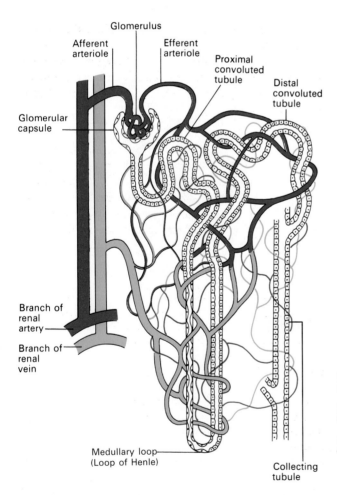

Figure 13.5 Diagram of a nephron including the arrangement of the blood vessels.

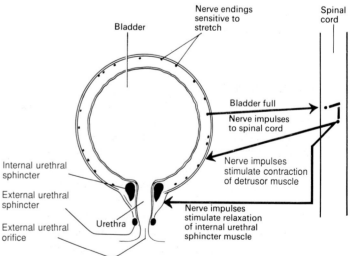

Figure 13.6 Diagram of the series of blood vessels in the kidney.

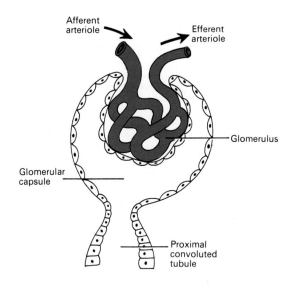

Figure 13.7 Diagram of the glomerulus and glomerular capsule.

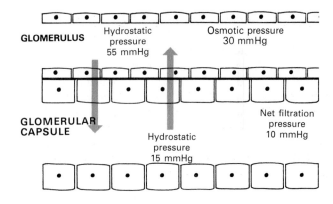

Figure 13.8 Diagram of filtration in the nephron.

Functions of the kidney

Formation of urine

The kidneys form urine which passes through the ureters to the bladder for excretion. The composition of urine reflects the activities of the nephrons in the maintenance of homeostasis. Waste products of protein metabolism are excreted, electrolyte balance is maintained and the acid–base balance is influenced by the excretion of hydrogen ions. There are three phases in the formation of urine:

■ simple filtration
■ selective reabsorption
■ secretion.

Simple filtration (Fig. 13.8)

Filtration takes place through the *semipermeable* walls of the glomerulus and glomerular capsule. Water and a large number of small molecules pass through, some of which are reabsorbed later. Blood cells, plasma proteins and other large molecules are unable to filter through and remain in the capillaries (see right).

Filtration is assisted by the difference between the blood pressure in the glomerulus and the pressure of the filtrate in the glomerular capsule. Because the diameter of the efferent arteriole is less than that of the afferent arteriole, a *capillary hydrostatic pressure* of about 55 mmHg builds up in the glomerulus. This pressure is opposed by the *osmotic pressure* of the blood, about 30 mmHg, and by *filtrate hydrostatic pressure* of about

15 mmHg in the glomerular capsule. The net *filtration pressure* is, therefore:

$$55 - (30 + 15) = 10 \text{ mmHg}$$

About 125 ml/min, i.e. 180 litres of dilute filtrate are formed each day by the two kidneys. Of these 1 to 1.5 litres are excreted as urine. The difference in volume and concentration is due to selective reabsorption of some constituents of the filtrate and secretion by tubular cells of others.

Autoregulation of filtration. Hydrostatic pressure in the glomeruli remains fairly constant because constriction or dilatation of the afferent arterioles maintains pressure which compensates for changes in systemic blood pressure. When the blood pressure falls to below 80 mmHg, e.g. in severe shock, autoregulation fails and the hydrostatic pressure decreases impairing the function of the nephrons.

Blood constituents in glomerular filtrate	Blood constituents remaining in the glomerulus
Water	Leukocytes
Mineral salts	Erythrocytes
Amino acids	Platelets
Ketoacids	Blood proteins
Glucose	
Hormones	
Creatinine	
Urea	
Uric acid	
Toxins	
Drugs	

Selective reabsorption (Fig. 13.9)

Selective reabsorption is the process by which the composition and volume of the glomerular filtrate are altered during its passage through the convoluted tubules, the medullary loop and the collecting tubule. The general purpose of this process is to reabsorb those filtrate constituents needed by the body to maintain fluid and electrolyte balance and blood alkalinity. Active transport is carried out at carrier sites in the epithelial membrane which use chemical energy to transport substances against their concentration gradients (p. 22).

Some constituents of glomerular filtrate do not normally appear in urine because they are completely reabsorbed unless they are present in blood in excessive quantities. The kidneys' maximum capacity for reabsorption of a substance is the *transport maximum*, or renal threshold, e.g. normal blood glucose level is 2.5 to 5.3 mmol/l (45 to 95 mg/100 ml). If the level rises above the transport maximum of about 9 mmol/l (160 mg/100 ml) glucose appears in the urine because all the carrier sites are occupied and the mechanism for active transfer out of the tubules is overloaded. Other substances reabsorbed by active transport include amino acids and sodium, calcium, potassium, phosphate and chloride ions.

Some ions, e.g. sodium and chloride, can be absorbed by both active and passive mechanisms depending on the site in the nephron.

The transport maximum, or renal threshold, of some substances varies according to the body's need for them

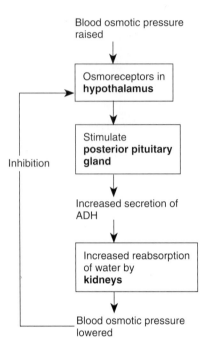

Figure 13.10 The feedback mechanism that controls the secretion of antidiuretic hormone (ADH).

at the time, i.e. in order to maintain homeostasis. In some cases reabsorption is regulated by hormones.

Parathormone from the parathyroid glands and *calcitonin* from the thyroid gland together regulate reabsorption of calcium and phosphate.

Antidiuretic hormone (ADH) from the posterior lobe of the pituitary gland increases the permeability of the distal convoluted tubules and collecting tubules, increasing water reabsorption. (Fig. 13.10).

Aldosterone, secreted by the cortex of the adrenal gland, increases the reabsorption of sodium and excretion of potassium (Fig. 13.11).

Nitrogenous waste products, such as urea and uric acid, are reabsorbed only to a slight extent.

Substances that are not normal blood constituents are not reabsorbed. If the blood passes through the glomerulus too quickly for filtration to clear such substances from the blood, the tubules secrete them into the filtrate. Substances of no physiological significance are sometimes injected into the body to evaluate the kidneys' excretory efficiency.

Secretion (Fig. 13.9)

Filtration occurs as the blood flows through the glomerulus. Substances not required and foreign materials, e.g. drugs, may not be cleared from the blood by filtration because of the short time it remains in the glomerulus. Such substances are cleared by *secretion*

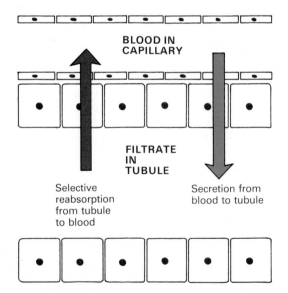

Figure 13.9 Diagram of selective reabsorption and secretion in the nephron.

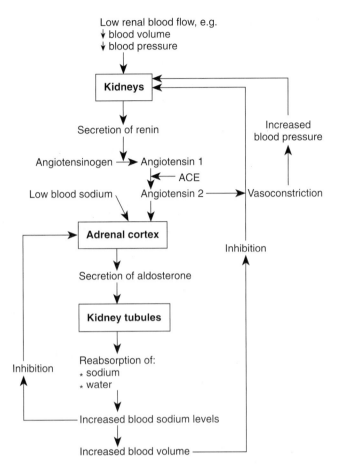

Figure 13.11   The mechanism that maintains renal blood flow and blood volume.
ACE = Angiotensin converting enzyme.

into the convoluted tubules and excreted from the body in the urine.

Composition of urine

Water	96%
Urea	2%
Uric acid	
Creatinine	
Ammonia	
Sodium	
Potassium	2%
Chlorides	
Phosphates	
Sulphates	
Oxalates	

Urine is amber in colour due to the presence of urobilin, a bile pigment altered in the intestine, reabsorbed then excreted by the kidneys. The specific gravity is between 1020 and 1030, and the reaction is acid. A healthy adult passes 1000 to 1500 ml per day.

The amount of urine secreted and the specific gravity vary according to the fluid intake and the amount of solute excreted. During sleep and muscular exercise urine production is decreased.

Water balance and urine output

Water is taken into the body through the alimentary tract and a small amount is formed by the metabolic processes. Water is excreted in saturated expired air, as a constituent of the faeces, through the skin as sweat and as the main constituent of urine. The amount lost in expired air and in the faeces is fairly constant and the amount of sweat produced is associated with the maintenance of normal body temperature (p. 363).

The balance between fluid intake and output is controlled by the kidneys. The minimum urinary output, consistent with the essential removal of waste material, is about 500 ml per day. The amount produced in excess of this is controlled mainly by the *antidiuretic hormone* (ADH) released into the blood by the *posterior lobe of the pituitary gland*. There is a close link between the posterior pituitary and the *hypothalamus* in the brain (Fig. 9.3).

There are cells in the hypothalamus (*osmoreceptors*) sensitive to changes in the osmotic pressure of the blood. Nerve impulses from the osmoreceptors stimulate the posterior lobe of the pituitary gland to release ADH. When the osmotic pressure is raised, ADH output is increased and as a result, water reabsorption by the cells in distal convoluted tubules and collecting ducts is increased, reducing the blood osmotic pressure and ADH output. This feedback mechanism maintains the blood concentration within normal limits (Fig. 13.10).

The feedback mechanism may be overridden when there is an excessive amount of a dissolved substance in the blood so that it can be removed from the body, e.g. in diabetes mellitus when the blood glucose level is above the transport maximum of the renal tubules, excess water is excreted with the excess glucose. This *polyuria* may lead to dehydration in spite of increased production of ADH but it is usually accompanied by acute thirst and increased water intake.

Electrolyte balance

Changes in the *concentration of electrolytes* in the body fluids may be due to changes in the amounts of water or of electrolytes. There are several methods of maintaining the balance between water and electrolyte concentration.

Sodium and potassium concentration

Sodium is the most common cation (positively charged ion) in extracellular fluid and potassium is the most common intracellular cation.

Sodium is a constituent of almost all foods and it is often added to food during cooking. This means that the intake is usually in excess of the body's needs. It is excreted mainly in urine and sweat.

Sodium is a normal constituent of urine and the amount excreted is regulated by the hormone *aldosterone*, secreted by the cortex of the *adrenal gland* (suprarenal gland). Cells in the afferent arteriole of the nephron are stimulated to produce the enzyme *renin* by sympathetic nerves or by low arterial blood pressure. Renin converts the plasma protein *angiotensinogen*, produced by the liver, to *angiotensin 1*. Aldosterone converting enzyme (ACE), formed in small quantities in the lungs, proximal convoluted tubules and other tissues, converts angiotensin 1 into angiotensin 2 which causes vasoconstriction and increases blood pressure. It also stimulates the adrenal gland to secrete aldosterone. Water is reabsorbed with sodium and together they increase the blood volume, leading to reduced renin secretion (Fig. 13.11). When *sodium reabsorption* is increased *potassium excretion* is increased, indirectly reducing intra-cellular potassium. The amount of sodium excreted in sweat is insignificant except when sweating is excessive. This may occur when there is a high environmental temperature or during sustained physical exercise. Normally the renal mechanism described above maintains the cation concentration within physiological limits. When excessive sweating is sustained, e.g. living in a hot climate or working in a hot environment, acclimatisation occurs in about 7 to 10 days and the amount of electrolyte lost in sweat is reduced.

Sodium and potassium occur in high concentrations in digestive juices—sodium in gastric juice and potassium in pancreatic and intestinal juice. Normally these ions are reabsorbed by the colon but following acute and prolonged diarrhoea they may be excreted in large quantities with resultant electrolyte imbalance.

In order to maintain the normal blood pH, hydrogen ions are secreted by the cells of the convoluted tubules and are excreted in urine. They are secreted in combination with bicarbonate as carbonic acid, with ammonia as ammonium chloride and with hydrogen phosphate as dihydrogen phosphate. The normal pH of urine varies from 4.5 to 7.8 depending on diet, time of day and a number of other factors. Individuals whose diet contains a large amount of animal proteins tend to produce urine of a lower pH (toward the lower end of normal) than vegetarians.

URETERS (FIGS 13.12 AND 13.13)

The ureters are the tubes that convey urine from the kidneys to the urinary bladder. They are about 25 to 30 cm long with a diameter of about 3 mm.

The ureter is continuous with the funnel-shaped *renal pelvis*. It passes downwards through the abdominal cavity, behind the peritoneum in front of the psoas muscle into the pelvic cavity, and passes obliquely through the posterior wall of the bladder (Fig. 13.13). Because of this arrangement the ureters are compressed and the opening occluded when urine accumulates and the pressure rises in the bladder. This prevents reflux of urine as the bladder fills and during micturition, when pressure increases as the bladder wall contracts.

Structure

The ureters consist of three layers of tissue:

■ an outer covering of *fibrous tissue*, continuous with the fibrous capsule of the kidney

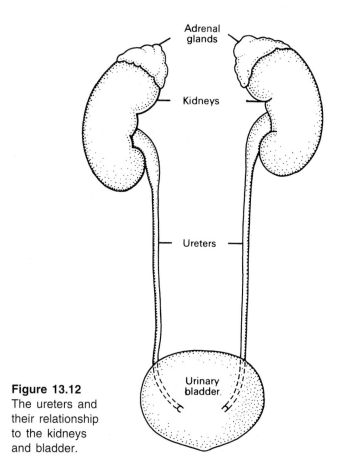

Figure 13.12
The ureters and their relationship to the kidneys and bladder.

- a middle *muscular layer* consisting of interlacing smooth muscle fibres that form a syncytium spiralling round the ureter, some in clockwise and some in anticlockwise directions and an additional outer longitudinal layer in the lower third
- an inner layer of transitional epithelium.

Function

The ureters propel the urine from the kidneys into the bladder by peristaltic contraction of the muscular wall. This is an intrinsic function not under nerve control. The waves of contraction originate in a pacemaker in the minor calyces. Peristaltic waves occur at about 10-second intervals, sending little spurts of urine into the bladder.

URINARY BLADDER

The urinary bladder is a reservoir for urine. It lies in the pelvic cavity and its size and position vary, depending on the amount of urine it contains. When distended the bladder rises into the abdominal cavity.

Organs associated with the bladder

In the female (Fig. 13.14A)
Anteriorly — the symphysis pubis
Posteriorly — the uterus and upper part of the vagina
Superiorly — the small intestine
Inferiorly — the urethra and the muscles forming the pelvic floor

In the male (Fig. 13.14B)
Anteriorly — the symphysis pubis
Posteriorly — the rectum and seminal vesicles
Superiorly — the small intestine
Inferiorly — the urethra and prostate gland

Structure (Fig. 13.15)

The bladder is roughly pear-shaped, but becomes more oval as it fills with urine. It has anterior, superior and posterior surfaces. The posterior surface is the *base*. The bladder opens into the urethra at its lowest point, *the neck*.

Peritoneum covers only the superior surface before it is reflected upwards to become the parietal peritoneum,

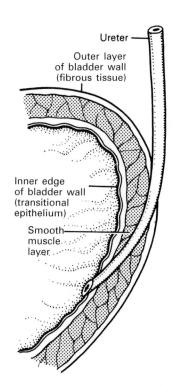

Figure 13.13 Diagram of the position of the ureter in relation to the bladder wall.

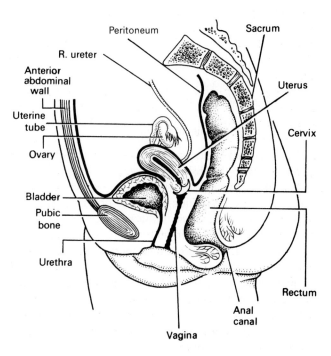

Figure 13.14A The pelvic organs associated with the bladder and the urethra in the female.

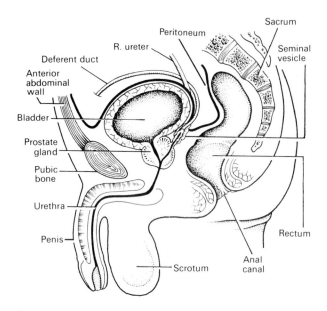

Figure 13.14B The pelvic organs associated with the bladder and the urethra in the male.

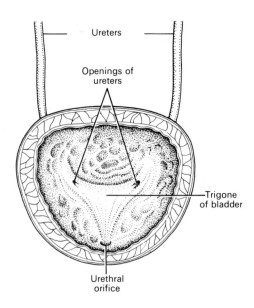

Figure 13.15 Section of the bladder showing the trigone.

lining the anterior abdominal wall. Posteriorly it is reflected on to the uterus in the female and the rectum in the male (Fig. 10.3).

The bladder wall is composed of three layers:

- the outer layer of loose connective tissue, containing blood and lymphatic vessels and nerves, covered on the upper surface by the peritoneum.
- the middle layer, consisting of a mass of interlacing smooth muscle fibres and elastic tissue loosely arranged in three layers. This is called the *detrusor muscle* and it empties the bladder when it contracts.
- the lining of transitional epithelium.

When the bladder is empty or contracted the inner lining is arranged in folds, or rugae, and these gradually disappear as the bladder fills. The bladder is distensible but when it contains 300 to 400 ml the awareness of the desire to urinate is initiated. The total capacity is rarely more than about 600 ml.

The three orifices in the bladder wall form a triangle or *trigone* (Fig. 13.15). The upper two orifices on the posterior wall are the openings of the ureters. The lower orifice is the point of origin of the urethra. Where the urethra commences there is a thickening of the smooth muscle layer which acts as a sphincter and controls the passage of urine from the bladder into the urethra. This *internal sphincter*, like the muscle layer, is under autonomic nerve control.

URETHRA

The urethra is a canal extending from the neck of the bladder to the exterior, at the external urethral orifice. Its length differs in the male and in the female. The male urethra is associated with the urinary and the reproductive systems, and is described in Chapter 18.

The female urethra is approximately 4 cm long. It runs downwards and forwards behind the symphysis pubis and opens at the external urethral orifice just in front of the vagina. The external urethral orifice is guarded by the *external urethral sphincter* which is under voluntary control. Except during the passage of urine, the walls of the urethra are in close apposition.

The male urethra is described in detail in Chapter 18, but in both sexes the basic structure is the same. Its walls consist of three layers of tissue:

- a *muscle layer*, continuous with that of the bladder. At its origin there is an *internal urethral sphincter*, consisting mainly of elastic tissue and smooth muscle fibres, under autonomic nerve control. Slow and continuous contraction of this sphincter keeps the urethra closed. In the middle third there is striated muscle surrounding the urethra, under voluntary nerve control, that forms the *external urethral sphincter*.

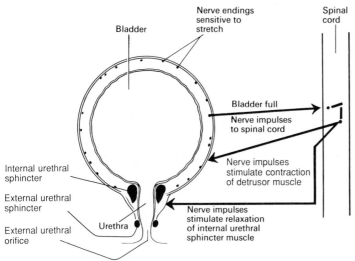

Figure 13.16 Diagram of simple reflex control of micturition when conscious effort cannot override the reflex action.

■ a *submucous spongy layer*, containing blood vessels and nerves.

■ a *mucous membrane lining* which is continuous with that of the bladder in the upper part. In the lower part the lining consists of stratified squamous epithelium, continuous externally with the skin of the vulva.

FUNCTIONS OF THE BLADDER AND MICTURITION

The urinary bladder acts as a reservoir for urine. When 300 to 400 ml of urine have accumulated, afferent autonomic nerve fibres in the bladder wall sensitive to stretch are stimulated. In the infant this initiates a *spinal reflex action* (see p. 160) and micturition occurs (Fig. 13.16). Micturition occurs when autonomic efferent fibres convey impulses to the bladder causing relaxation of the detrusor muscle and relaxation of the internal urethral sphincter.

When the nervous system is fully developed the micturition reflex is stimulated but sensory impulses pass upwards to the brain and there is an awareness of the desire to micturate. By conscious effort, reflex contraction of the bladder wall and relaxation of the internal sphincter can be inhibited for a limited period of time (Fig. 13.17).

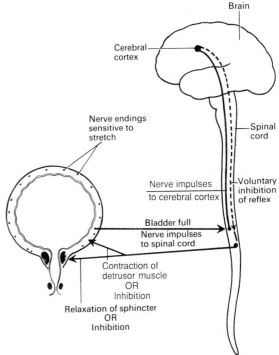

Figure 13.17 Diagram of the nerve control of micturition when conscious effort overrides the reflex action.

In adults, micturition occurs when the detrusor muscle contracts, there is reflex relaxation of the internal sphincter and voluntary relaxation of the external sphincter. It can be assisted by increasing the pressure within the pelvic cavity, achieved by lowering the diaphragm and contracting the abdominal muscles (Valsalva's manoeuvre). Over-distension of the bladder is extremely painful, and when this stage is reached there is a tendency for involuntary relaxation of the external sphincter to occur and a small amount of urine to escape, provided there is no mechanical obstruction.

DISEASES OF THE KIDNEYS

Acute glomerulonephritis

This term suggests inflammatory conditions of the glomerulus, but inflammatory changes are not found in all types. Glomerulonephritis is classified according to microscopic abnormalities:

- the extent of damage
  —diffuse: affecting all glomeruli
  —focal: affecting some glomeruli
- appearance
  —proliferative: increased numbers of cells in glomeruli
  —membranous: thickening of the glomerular basement membrane.

The damage to the glomerulus is believed to be caused by antigen/antibody (immune) complexes being deposited in the walls of the glomerular capillaries, glomerular capsule and/or mesangial cells,* causing local inflammatory reactions. About 7 days after the initial encounter with an antigen, antibodies appear in the blood and combine with the antigen. As more antibodies are produced, the number of immune complexes increases, until all the antigen is used up. Immune complexes are deposited in the walls of the glomeruli and usually cause an inflammatory reaction (Fig. 13.18). Although these complexes circulate widely in the blood they cause more damage to the glomeruli than to other tissues because the blood flows relatively slowly over their large surface area, allowing more contact between immune complexes and the glomeruli.

---

* Mesangial cells are connective tissue cells that lie between capillary loops in the glomeruli.

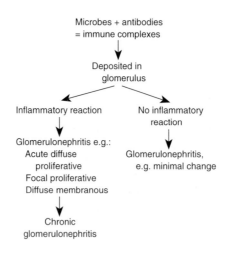

Figure 13.18 Stages of development of glomerulonephritis.

The effects of glomerulonephritis depend on the type and include asymptomatic proteinuria, haematuria, hypertension, nephrotic syndrome (p. 350) and renal failure.

Acute diffuse proliferative glomerulonephritis

This type usually follows 1 to 4 weeks after infection of the pharynx, middle ear or skin by group A beta-haemolytic streptococci, and all the glomeruli are affected. Immune complexes deposited in the glomerular wall stimulate an inflammatory reaction and the walls become swollen and infiltrated with granulocytes. There is increased permeability with leakage of plasma proteins and red blood cells into the filtrate, leading to haematuria and proteinuria. If the glomeruli are obstructed by inflammatory swelling, renal blood flow and the production of filtrate are reduced, causing oliguria, fluid retention, hypertension, oedema and raised blood urea. More rarely this condition follows an initial infection by *Staphylococcus aureus* or *Streptococcus pnuemoniae* or it may be a complication of falciparum malaria, toxo-

plasmosis, schistosomiasis and some acute viral infections.

There are various outcomes, e.g.:

- complete recovery, especially in children, after the immune complexes have either been phagocytosed or have passed through the glomerular membrane into the filtrate and been excreted in urine
- a persistent mild form of the disease of varying duration, followed either by complete recovery or chronic glomerulonephritis
- death due to:
  —hypertension, leading to heart failure or acute renal failure early in the disease
  —infection and hypertension after 1 to 2 years
  —chronic glomerulonephritis several years later.

Focal proliferative glomerulonephritis

This is a relatively rare condition that accompanies systemic diseases, e.g. systemic lupus erythematosus, Henoch–Schönlein purpura, subacute bacterial endocarditis, in which proliferation of mesangial cells occurs. Only parts of some glomeruli are affected. In time, adhesions form between the glomerular loops and the Bowman's capsule, and the associated tubules atrophy. There is short-term haematuria and proteinuria but repeated recurrences may lead to renal failure. No specific antigen/antibody complexes have been identified.

Diffuse membranous glomerulonephritis

Immune complexes of unknown origin pass through the glomerular epithelium and are deposited in the base-ment membrane. No inflammatory reaction occurs but there is diffuse thickening of the walls of the glomeruli. This reduces the amount of filtrate and increases the membrane permeability, causing proteinuria, oliguria, marked progressive oedema and pleural and pericardial effusion. Slow recovery may occur but in the majority of cases there is increased development of glomerular sclerosis, leading to the nephrotic syndrome, chronic renal failure and death.

Minimal-change glomerulonephritis

This occurs mainly in children between 1 and 4 years of age, often following a chest infection, but it is not associated with specific antigen/antibody complexes. There is usually spontaneous recovery but recurrences are fairly common. In children this is the most common cause of *nephrotic syndrome* (p. 350). In adults it may lead to chronic glomerulonephritis.

Chronic glomerulonephritis

This condition may develop:

- with no previous history of kidney disease
- following acute post-streptococcal membranous and recurrent focal glomerulonephritis
- in association with viral diseases elsewhere in the body.

The nephrons gradually become sclerosed and there is progressive loss of kidney function. The rate at which the disease progresses may vary considerably. Hypertension develops which may be either malignant and lead to early renal failure or benign, leading to cardiac

failure, cerebral haemorrhage or chronic renal failure.

Diabetic kidney

Renal failure is the cause of death in many diabetics, especially early-onset insulin-dependent (type I) diabetes mellitus (p. 233). The underlying cause is not known but there may be an immune reaction to insulin that results in damage to large and small blood vessels in many parts of the body. The effects include:

- progressive glomerulosclerosis followed by atrophy of the tubules
- pyelonephritis with papillary necrosis
- atheroma of the renal arteries and their branches, leading to renal ischaemia and hypertension
- development of nephrotic syndrome.

Hypertension and the kidneys

The types of hypertension that affect the kidneys are:

- benign (chronic) essential hypertension
- malignant (accelerated) essential hypertension
- persistent secondary hypertension.

In all cases there is renal arteriosclerosis and arteriolosclerosis, causing ischaemia. The reduced blood flow stimulates the *renin–angiotensin–aldosterone* mechanism (Fig. 13.11), raising the blood pressure still further.

Benign hypertension
This causes gradual and progressive sclerosis and fibrosis of the

glomeruli, leading to renal failure or, more commonly, to malignant hypertension.

Malignant hypertension
This causes rapidly developing arteriolosclerosis which spreads to the glomeruli with subsequent destruction of nephrons, leading to:

- further rise in blood pressure
- reduction in renal blood flow and the amount of filtrate
- increased permeability of the glomeruli, with the passage of plasma proteins and red blood cells into the filtrate resulting in proteinuria and haematuria
- progressive oliguria and renal failure.

Persistent secondary hypertension
This is caused by kidney diseases such as chronic glomerulonephritis and pyelonephritis and leads to renal ischaemia, further hypertension and renal failure.

Acute pyelonephritis

This is an acute microbial infection of the kidney pelvis and calyces, spreading to the kidney substance causing kidney damage and in some cases abscess formation. The infection may travel up the urinary tract from the perineum or be blood-borne. It is accompanied by fever, malaise and loin pain.

Ascending infection
This is the most common route of infection, usually by microbes that are commensals of the bowel, e.g. *Escherichia coli*, *Streptococcus faecalis*, *Pseudomonas pyocyanea*. Pyelonephritis is preceded by cystitis (inflammation of the bladder). Reflux of infected urine into the ureters when the bladder contracts during micturition allows infection

to spread upwards to the renal pelves and kidney substance. The bladder may be infected by:

- microbes from the perineum, especially in females because of the wide short urethra, its proximity to the anus and the moist perineal conditions
- blood-borne microbes, especially if there is stasis of urine in the bladder due to urethral obstruction
- a urinary catheter or other instrument.

Blood-borne infection

The source of microbes may be:

- elsewhere in the body, e.g. boils, carbuncles, wound infections, abscesses
- the lower urinary tract, especially following surgical procedures to relieve urethral strictures due to, e.g. fibrosis following previous infection or enlarged prostate gland in the male.

When the infection spreads into the kidney substance there is suppuration and destruction of nephrons. The outcome depends on the amount of healthy kidney remaining after the infection subsides. Necrotic tissue is eventually replaced by fibrous tissue but there may be some hypertrophy of healthy nephrons. This is a common cause of fluid and electrolyte imbalance when tubular absorption and secretion are disturbed, eventually leading to renal failure.

Chronic pyelonephritis

This usually follows repeated attacks of acute pyelonephritis with scar tissue formation. The progressive loss of functioning nephrons leads to renal failure and uraemia. Concurrent hypertension is common.

Nephrotic syndrome

This is not a disease in itself but is an important feature of several kidney diseases. The main characteristics are:

- proteinuria
- hypoalbuminaemia
- generalised oedema
- hyperlipidaemia.

When glomeruli are damaged, the permeability of the glomerular membrane is increased and plasma proteins pass through in the filtrate. Albumin is the main protein lost because it is the most common and also has the smallest plasma protein molecule. When the amount lost per day exceeds the rate of production by the liver there is a significant fall in the total plasma protein level. The consequent low plasma osmotic pressure leads to widespread oedema and reduced plasma volume. This reduces the renal blood flow and stimulates the renin–angiotensin–aldosterone mechanism, causing increased reabsorption of water and sodium from the renal tubules. The reabsorbed water further reduces the osmotic pressure, increasing the oedema. The key factor is the loss of albumin across the glomerular membrane and as long as this continues the vicious circle is perpetuated (Fig. 13.19). Levels of nitrogenous waste products, i.e.

Figure 13.19 Stages of development of nephrotic syndrome.

uric acid, urea and creatinine, usually remain normal. Hyperlipidaemia also occurs but the cause is unknown.

The nephrotic syndrome occurs in a number of diseases. In children the most common cause is minimal-change glomerulonephritis, although it may follow acute diffuse proliferative and focal proliferative glomerulonephritis. In adults it may complicate:

- most forms of glomerulonephritis
- diabetes mellitus
- systemic lupus erythematosus
- rheumatoid arthritis
- infections, e.g. malaria, infective endocarditis
- drugs and toxins.

Acute renal failure

There is severe reduction in glomerular filtrate, occurring as a complication of a variety of conditions not primarily associated with the kidneys. The causes of acute renal failure are:

- *pre-renal*: the result of reduced renal blood flow, especially severe and prolonged shock
- *renal*, or parenchymal: damage to the kidney itself due to, e.g. acute tubular necrosis, glomerulonephritis

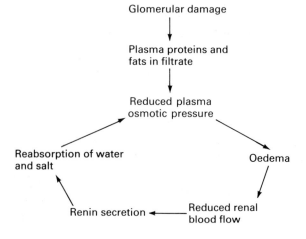

- *post-renal*: obstruction to the outflow of urine, e.g. tumour of the bladder, uterus or cervix, large calculus in the renal pelvis.

Acute tubular necrosis (ATN)

In this condition there is severe damage to the tubular epithelial cells caused by ischaemia or nephrotoxicity.

Ischaemic ATN

This is caused by severe and prolonged shock due to, e.g. haemorrhage, severe trauma, marked dehydration, acute intestinal obstruction, prolonged and complicated surgical procedures, extensive burns.

Nephrotoxic ATN
This is caused by:

- toxic chemicals, e.g. carbon tetrachloride (used in dry cleaning), chromic acid, ethylene glycol (anti-freeze), mercurial compounds, ionising radiation
- drugs, e.g. trilene, aminoglycosides, paracetamol overdose
- endogenous substances, e.g. myoglobin (from damaged muscle), haemoglobin (from incompatible blood transfusion).

Oliguria (less than 400 ml of urine per day in adults), *severe oliguria* (less than 100 ml of urine per day in adults) or *anuria* may last for a few weeks, followed by diuresis. There is reduced glomerular filtrate and tubular selective reabsorption and secretion, leading to:

- generalised and pulmonary oedema

- accumulation of urea (uraemia) and other metabolic waste products
- electrolyte imbalance which may be exacerbated by the retention of potassium (hyperkalaemia) released from cells following severe injury and extensive tissue damage elsewhere in the body
- acidosis due to disrupted excretion of hydrogen ions.

Profound diuresis (the diuretic phase) occurs during the healing process when the epithelial cells of the tubules have regenerated but are still incapable of selective reabsorption and secretion. Diuresis may lead to acute dehydration, complicating the existing high plasma urea, acidosis and electrolyte imbalance. If the patient survives the initial acute phase, a considerable degree of renal function is usually restored over a period of months.

End-stage kidney (chronic renal failure)

This is reached when irreversible damage to nephrons is so severe that 75% of renal function has been lost and the kidneys cannot function effectively. The main causes are chronic glomerulonephritis, diabetes mellitus, chronic pyelonephritis and hypertension. The effects are a reduced filtration rate, selective reabsorption and secretion, and glomerular fibrosis which interferes

with blood flow. These changes have a number of effects on the body.

Uraemia develops after about 7 days of anuria because of the reduced glomerular filtration rate and impaired tubular secretion of urea. Increased blood urea usually leads to confusion and mental disorientation.

Polyuria is caused by defective reabsorption of water in spite of the reduced glomerular filtration rate (GFR) (Table 13.1). This may cause thirst and polydipsia.

Fixed specific gravity. The specific gravity of the urine is similar to that of glomerular filtrate, i.e. about 1.010 (normal = 1.020 to 1.030). It remains low and fixed because of defective tubular reabsorption of water.

Acidosis. Control of the pH of body fluids is defective mainly because the tubules fail to remove hydrogen ions by forming ammonia and hydrogen phosphates.

Electrolyte imbalance occurs as tubular reabsorption and secretion are impaired.

Anaemia caused by deficiency in the hormone erythropoietin occurs when the chronic state extends over a period of months and is often associated with dialysis. It results in fatigue, dyspnoea and cardiac failure.

Hypertension is often a consequence if not the cause of renal failure.

Table 13.1 End-stage kidney polyuria

	Normal kidney	End-stage kidney
GFR	125 ml/min or 180 l/day	10 ml/min or 14 l/day
Reabsorption of water	>99%	Approx. 0.7%
Urine output	<1 ml/min or 1.5 l/day	Approx 7 ml/min or 10 l/day

In the late stages, anorexia, nausea, vomiting and pruritus develop as uraemia progresses. Confusion and impaired mental function also occur.

Renal calculi

Stones form in the kidneys and bladder when urinary constituents normally in solution are precipitated. The solutes involved are oxalates, phosphates, urates and uric acid, and stones usually consist of more than one substance, deposited in layers. Most originate in collecting tubules or in renal papillae. They then pass into the pelvis of the kidney where they may increase in size. Some become too large to pass through the ureter and may obstruct the flow of urine causing renal failure. Others pass to the bladder and are either excreted or increase in size and obstruct the urethra. Occasionally stones originate in the bladder. Predisposing factors include:

Dehydration. This leads to increased reabsorption of water from the tubules but does not change solute reabsorption, resulting in a reduced volume of highly concentrated filtrate in the collecting tubules.

pH of urine. When the normally acid filtrate becomes alkaline some substances may be precipitated, e.g. phosphates. This occurs when the kidney buffering system is defective, and in some infections.

Infection. Necrotic material and pus provide foci upon which solutes in the filtrate may be deposited and the products of infection may alter the pH of the urine.

Tumours. Pressure caused by tumours in the kidney or adjacent to the urinary tract may restrict the flow of urine. This may cause ischaemia and necrosis or predispose to infection. Necrotic debris and tumour fragments provide foci for the deposition of solutes in the urine.

Small calculi

These may pass through or become impacted in a ureter and damage the epithelium, leading to haematuria then fibrosis and stricture. In ureteric obstruction, usually unilateral, there is excessive spasmodic peristaltic contraction of the ureter, causing acute intermittent ischaemic pain (*renal colic*) as the ureter contracts over the stone. Stones reaching the bladder may be passed in urine or increase in size and eventually block the urethra, leading to retention of urine and bilateral hydronephrosis, infection proximal to the blockage, pyelonephritis and severe kidney damage.

Large calculi (staghorn calculus)

One large stone may form, filling the renal pelvis and the calyces. It causes stagnation of urine, predisposing to infection, and kidney tumours. It may cause irreversible kidney damage.

Congenital abnormalities of the kidneys

Misplaced (ectopic) kidney

One or both kidneys may develop in abnormally low positions. Misplaced kidneys function normally if the blood vessels are long enough to provide an adequate blood supply but a kidney in the pelvis may cause problems during pregnancy by compression of the renal blood vessels or the ureters. If the ureters become kinked there is increased risk of infection as there is a tendency for reflux and backflow to the kidney. There may also be difficulties during parturition.

Polycystic disease

This disease, caused by genetic abnormality, occurs in infantile and adult forms. The infantile form is very rare and the child usually dies soon after birth.

Adult polycystic kidney disease. This inherited condition usually becomes apparent at between 30 and 50 years of age. Both kidneys are affected. Dilatations (cysts) form at the junction of the distal convoluted and collecting tubules. The cysts slowly enlarge and pressure causes ischaemia and necrosis of nephrons, resulting in their destruction. The disease is progressive and secondary hypertension usually develops. Death may be due to chronic renal failure, uraemia, cardiac failure, cerebral haemorrhage or subarachnoid haemorrhage due to increased incidence of berry aneurysms of the circulus arteriosus (p. 102). Other associated abnormalities include polycystic liver disease, cysts in the spleen, pancreas and lungs and berry aneurysms in cerebral arteries.

Tumours of the kidney

Benign tumours of the kidney are relatively uncommon.

Malignant tumours

Renal clear cell carcinoma (Grawitz's tumour or hypernephroma)

This is a tumour of tubular epithelium. Local spread involves the renal vein and leads to early blood-spread of tumour fragments, most commonly to the lungs and bones. The causes of the malignant changes are not known but cigarette smoking is believed to be a predisposing factor.

Nephroblastoma (Wilms' tumour)

This is one of the most common malignant tumours in children, occurring in the first 3 years. It is usually unilateral but rapidly becomes very large and invades the renal blood vessels, causing early blood-spread of the malignancy to the lungs and bones. It is believed that the cell abnormalities occur before birth but the cause is not known.

DISEASES OF THE RENAL PELVIS, URETERS, BLADDER AND URETHRA

These structures are considered together because their combined functions are to collect and store urine and discharge it from the body. Obstruction and infection are the main causes of dysfunction.

Obstruction to the flow of urine

Hydronephrosis

This is dilatation of the kidney pelvis and calyces caused by accumulation of urine, leading to destruction of the nephrons, fibrosis and atrophy of the kidney. One or both kidneys may be involved, depending on the cause, e.g. obstruction of a ureter or the urethra or disturbance of bladder nerve supply (Fig. 13.20).

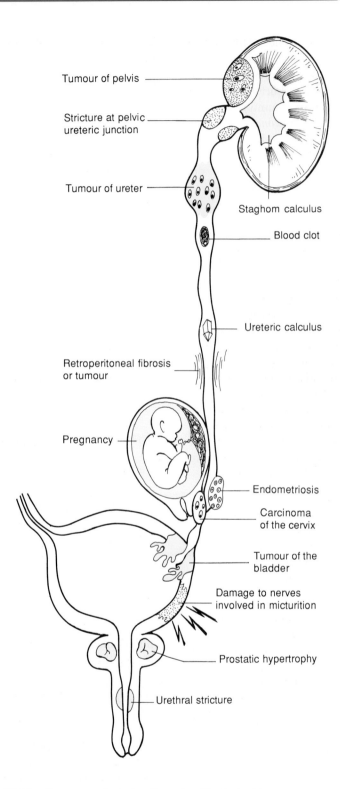

Tumour of pelvis

Stricture at pelvic ureteric junction

Tumour of ureter

Staghom calculus

Blood clot

Ureteric calculus

Retroperitoneal fibrosis or tumour

Pregnancy

Endometriosis

Carcinoma of the cervix

Tumour of the bladder

Damage to nerves involved in micturition

Prostatic hypertrophy

Urethral stricture

Figure 13.20   Summary of obstruction of outflow of urine.

Complete sustained obstruction

In this condition hydronephrosis develops quickly, pressure in the nephrons rises and urine production stops. The most common causes are a *large calculus* or *tumour*. The outcome depends on whether one or both kidneys are involved (homeostasis can be maintained by one kidney).

Partial or intermittent obstruction

This may lead to progressive hydronephrosis caused by, e.g.:

- a succession of renal calculi in a ureter, eventually moved onwards by peristalsis
- a calculus that only partially blocks the ureter
- constriction of a ureter or the urethra by fibrous tissue, following epithelial inflammation caused by the passage of a stone or by infection
- pressure caused by:
  —a tumour in the tract or in the abdominal or pelvic cavity
  —an enlarged prostate gland in the male.

Spinal lesions

The immediate effect of transverse spinal cord lesions that damage the nerve supply to the bladder is that micturition does not occur. When the bladder fills the rise in pressure causes overflow incontinence, back pressure into the ureters and hydronephrosis. Reflex micturition is usually re-established after a time, but loss of voluntary control may be irreversible. Pressure on the spinal cord and other abnormalities, e.g. spina bifida, can also impair micturition.

Complications of urinary tract obstruction

Infection. Urine stasis predisposes to infection and pyelonephritis. The microbes usually spread upwards in the walls of the urinary tract or are blood-borne.

Calculus formation. Infection and urine stasis predispose to calculus formation when:

- the pH of urine changes from acid to alkaline, promoting the precipitation of some solutes, e.g. phosphates
- cell debris and pus provide foci upon which solutes in the urine may be deposited.

Infections of the urinary tract

Infection of any part of the tract may lead to pyelonephritis (p. 349) and severe kidney damage.

Ureteritis

This is usually due to the upward spread of infection in cystitis.

Acute cystitis

This is inflammation of the bladder and may be due to:

- spread of coliform microbes (*Escherichia coli*, *Streptococcus faecalis* and *Pseudomonas pyocyanea*) from the perineum, especially in women because of the short wide urethra, its proximity to the anus and the moist perineal conditions
- blood-borne infection
- a mixed infection of coliform and other organisms which may follow the passage of a catheter or other instrument.

The effects are:

- inflammation, small haemorrhages and oedema of the mucosa
- hypersensitivity of sensory nerve endings in the bladder wall, stimulated by inflammation before the bladder has filled to its usual capacity, leading to *frequency of micturition* accompanied by pain, *dysuria*, and sometimes *haematuria*.

Predisposing factors

The most important predisposing factors are coliform microbes in the perineal region and stasis of urine in the bladder. In the female, hormones associated with pregnancy cause relaxation of perineal muscle. Towards the end of pregnancy pressure caused by the fetus may obstruct the flow of urine. In the male, prostatitis provides a focus of local infection or an enlarged prostate gland may cause progressive urethral obstruction.

Chronic cystitis

This may follow repeated attacks of acute cystitis. It occurs most commonly in males when compression of the urethra by an enlarged prostate gland prevents the bladder from emptying completely. Calculus formation is common, especially if the normally acid urine becomes alkaline due to microbial action or kidney damage.

Urethritis

A common cause is *Neisseria gonorrhoeae* (gonococcus) spread by sexual intercourse directly to the urethra in the male and indirectly from the perineum in the female. Many cases of urethritis have no known cause, i.e. *non-specific urethritis* (Ch. 18).

Tumours of the bladder

It is not always clear whether bladder tumours are benign or malignant. The causes of both types are not known but predisposing factors include cigarette smoking, taking high doses of analgesics over a long period and exposure to chemicals used in some industries, e.g. manufacture of aniline dyes, rubber industry, benzidine-based industries.

Papillomas

These tumours arise from transitional epithelium and are usually benign. They consist of a stalk with fine-branching fronds which tend to break off, causing bleeding and haematuria. Papillomas commonly recur, even when they are benign. Although the cells are well differentiated some papillomas behave as carcinomas and invade surrounding blood and lymph vessels.

Solid tumours

These are all malignant to some degree. At an early stage the more malignant and solid tumours rapidly invade the bladder wall and spread in lymph and blood to other parts of the body. If the surface ulcerates there may be haemorrhage and necrosis.

Urinary incontinence

In this condition there is involuntary passage of urine due to defective voluntary control of the external urethral sphincter.

Stress incontinence
This is leakage of urine when intra-abdominal pressure is raised, e.g. on coughing, sneezing or lifting. It usually affects women, often after childbirth or as part of the ageing process.

Overflow incontinence
This occurs when there is retention of urine due to obstruction of urinary outflow, e.g. enlarged prostate gland. The bladder becomes distended and when the pressure inside overcomes the resistance of the urethral sphincter, urine dribbles from the urethra. The individual may be unable to initiate and/or maintain micturition.

Neurological incontinence
This occurs when there is damage to the nerves involved in bladder control in the brain, spinal cord or at the peripheral nerves. It may be associated with, e.g. stroke, spinal cord injury or multiple sclerosis.

Urge incontinence
This follows a sudden and intense urge to void and may be due to a urinary tract infection, calculus, tumour or sudden stress.

Section 4
Protection and survival

14
The skin

The skin completely covers the body and is continuous with the membranes lining the body orifices. It:

- protects the underlying structures from injury and from invasion by microbes
- contains sensory (*somatic*) nerve endings of pain, temperature and touch
- is involved in the regulation of the body temperature.

STRUCTURE OF THE SKIN

The skin has a surface area of about 1.5 to 2 m^2 in adults and it contains glands, hair and nails. There are two main layers:

- epidermis
- dermis or corium.

Between the skin and underlying structures there is a layer of subcutaneous fat.

Epidermis (Fig. 14.1)

The epidermis is the most superficial layer of the skin and is composed of *stratified epithelium* which varies in thickness in different parts of the body. It is thickest on the palms of the hands and soles of the feet. There are no blood vessels or nerve endings in the epidermis, but its deeper layers are bathed in interstitial fluid from the dermis, which provides oxygen and nutrients, and is drained away as lymph.

There are several layers of cells in the epidermis which extend from the deepest *germinative layer* to the surface *stratum corneum* (horny layer). The cells on the surface are flat, thin, non-nucleated, dead cells in which the cytoplasm has been replaced by *keratin*. These cells are constantly being rubbed off and replaced by cells which originated in the germinative layer and have undergone gradual change as they progressed towards the surface. Complete replacement of the epidermis takes about 40 days.

The maintenance of healthy epidermis depends upon three processes being synchronised:

- desquamation of the keratinised cells from the surface
- effective keratinisation of the cells approaching the surface
- continual cell division in the deeper layers with cells being pushed to the surface.

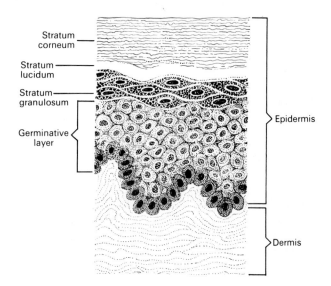

Figure 14.1   The skin showing the main layers of the epidermis.

Hairs, secretion from sebaceous glands and ducts of sweat glands pass through the epidermis to reach the surface.

The surface of the epidermis is ridged by projections of cells in the dermis called the *papillae*. The pattern of ridges is different in every individual and the impression made by them is the 'fingerprint'. The downward projections of the germinative layer between the papillae are believed to aid nutrition of epidermal cells and stabilise the two layers, preventing damage due to shearing forces. *Blisters* develop when acute trauma causes separation of the dermis and epidermis and serous fluid collects between the two layers.

The colour of the skin is affected by three main factors:

- *melanin*, a dark pigment secreted by *melanocytes* in the deep germinative layer, is absorbed by surrounding epithelial cells. The amount varies between different parts of the body, between members of the same race and between races. The number of melanocytes is fairly constant so the differences in colour depend on the amount of melanin secreted. It protects the skin from the harmful effects of sunlight. Exposure to sunlight promotes synthesis of increased amounts of melanin.
- *the level of oxygenation of haemoglobin* and the amount of blood circulating in the dermis give the skin its pink colour.
- *bile pigments* in blood and *carotenes* in subcutaneous fat give the skin a yellowish colour.

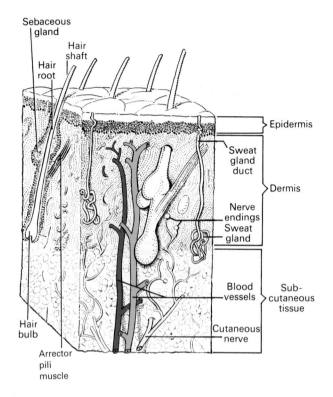

Sebaceous
gland
Hair
shaft
Hair
root

Epidermis

Sweat
gland
duct

Dermis

Nerve
endings
Sweat
gland

Blood
vessels

Sub-
cutaneous
tissue

Cutaneous
nerve

Hair
bulb

Arrector
pili
muscle

Figure 14.2 The skin showing the main structures in the dermis.

Dermis (Fig. 14.2)

The dermis is tough and elastic. It is composed of *collagen fibres* interlaced with *elastic fibres*. Rupture of elastic fibres occurs when the skin is over-stretched, resulting in permanent *striae*, or stretch marks, that may be found in pregnancy and obesity. Collagen fibres bind water and give skin its tensile strength, but as this ability declines with age, wrinkles develop. There are fibroblasts and mast cells in the dermis. Underlying its deepest layer there is areolar tissue and varying amounts of fat. The structures in the dermis are:

- blood vessels
- lymph vessels
- sensory (somatic) nerve endings
- sweat glands and their ducts
- hair roots, hair follicles and hairs
- the arrectores pilorum—involuntary muscles attached to the hair follicles
- sebaceous glands.

Blood vessels. Arterioles form a fine network with capillary branches supplying sweat glands, sebaceous glands, hair follicles and the dermis. The epidermis has no blood supply. It obtains nutrition and oxygen from interstitial fluid derived from blood vessels in the papillae of the dermis.

Lymph vessels form a network throughout the dermis and the deeper layers of the epidermis.

Sensory nerve endings. Nerve endings which are sensitive to *touch, change in temperature, pressure and pain* are widely distributed in the dermis. The skin is an important sensory organ through which individuals are aware of their environment. Nerve impulses, generated in the nerve endings in the dermis, are conveyed to the spinal cord by sensory (*somatic cutaneous*) nerves, then to the sensory area of the cerebrum where the sensations are perceived (Ch. 7).

Sweat glands

Sweat glands are found widely distributed throughout the skin and are most numerous in the palms of the hands, soles of the feet, axillae and groins. They are composed of epithelial cells. The bodies of the glands lie coiled in the subcutaneous tissue. Some ducts open on to the skin surface at tiny depressions, or pores, and others open into hair follicles. Glands opening into hair follicles do not become active until puberty. In the axilla they secrete an odourless milky fluid which, if decomposed by surface microbes, causes an unpleasant odour. The functions of this secretion are not known. Sweat glands are stimulated by sympathetic nerves in response to raised body temperature and fear.

The most important function of sweat secreted by glands opening on to the skin surface is in the regulation of body temperature. Evaporation of sweat on the surface takes heat from the body and the amount produced is governed by the temperature-regulating centre in the hypothalamus. Excessive sweating may lead to dehydration and serious depletion of body sodium chloride unless intake of water and salt is appropriately increased. After 7 to 10 days' exposure to high environmental temperatures the amount of salt lost is substantially reduced but water loss remains high.

Hairs

These are formed by a down-growth of epidermal cells into the dermis or subcutaneous tissue called *hair follicles*. At the base of the follicle there is a cluster of cells called the *bulb*. The hair is formed by the multiplication of cells of the bulb and as they are pushed upwards, away from their source of nutrition, the cells die and become keratinised. The part of the hair above the skin is the *shaft* and the remainder, the *root* (Fig. 14.3).

The colour of the hair is genetically determined and depends on the amount of melanin present. White hair

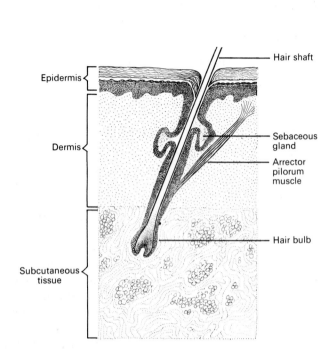

Figure 14.3 A hair in the skin.

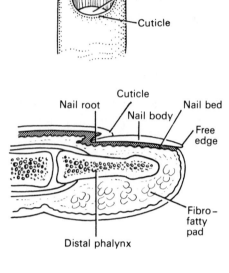

Figure 14.4 The nail and related skin.

is the result of the replacement of melanin by tiny air bubbles.

The arrectores pilorum (sing. arrector pili, Fig. 14.3) are little bundles of involuntary muscle fibres attached to the hair follicles. Contraction makes the hair stand erect and raises the skin around the hair, causing 'goose flesh'. The muscles are stimulated by sympathetic nerve fibres in response to fear and cold. Although each muscle is very small the contraction of a large number generates an appreciable amount of heat, especially when accompanied by shivering, i.e. involuntary contraction of the skeletal muscles.

The sebaceous glands (Fig. 14.3) consist of secretory epithelial cells derived from the same tissue as the hair follicles. They pour their oily secretion, *sebum*, into the hair follicles so they are present in the skin of all parts of the body except the palms of the hands and the soles of the feet. They are most numerous in the skin of the scalp, face, axillae and groins. In regions of transition from one type of superficial epithelium to another, such as lips, eyelids, nipple, labia minora and glans penis, there are sebaceous glands that are independent of hair follicles, secreting sebum directly on to the surface.

Sebum is an oily substance that keeps the hair soft

and pliable and gives it a shiny appearance. On the skin it provides some waterproofing and acts as a bactericidal and fungicidal agent, preventing the successful invasion of microbes. It also prevents drying and cracking of skin, especially on exposure to heat and sunshine. The activity of these glands increases at puberty and is less at the extremes of age, rendering infants and the elderly prone to the effects of excessive moisture, e.g. nappy rash in infants.

Nails (Fig. 14.4)

The nails in human beings are equivalent to the claws, horns and hoofs of animals. They are derived from the same cells as epidermis and hair and consist of a hard, horny type of keratinised dead cell. They protect the tips of the fingers and toes.

The root of the nail is embedded in the skin, is covered by the *cuticle* and forms the hemispherical pale area called the *lunula*.

The body of the nail is the exposed part which has grown out from the germinative zone of the epidermis called the *nail bed*.

Finger nails grow more quickly than toe nails and growth is quicker when the environmental temperature is high.

FUNCTIONS OF THE SKIN

Protection

The skin is one of the main protective organs of the body. It forms a relatively waterproof layer that protects the deeper and more delicate structures and acts as the main barrier against:

- invasion by microbes
- chemicals
- physical agents, e.g. mild trauma, ultraviolet light
- dehydration.

Due to the presence of the sensory nerve endings in the skin the body reacts by reflex action to unpleasant or painful stimuli, protecting it from further injury (p. 159).

Regulation of body temperature

The temperature of the body remains fairly constant at about 36.8°C (98.4°F). In health, variations are usually limited to between 0.5 and 0.75°C, although it is raised slightly in the evening, during exercise and in women just before ovulation. If the temperature is raised the metabolic rate is increased and if it is lowered the rate of metabolism is reduced. To ensure this constant temperature a fine balance is maintained between heat produced in the body and heat lost to the environment.

Heat production

Some of the energy released in the cells when carbohydrates, fats and deaminated amino acids are metabolised is in the form of heat. Because of this the most active organs, chemically and physically, produce the most heat. The principal organs involved are:

- *the muscles*. Contraction of voluntary muscles produces a large amount of heat and the more strenuous the muscular exercise the greater the heat produced. Shivering involves muscle contraction and produces heat when there is the risk of the body temperature falling below normal.
- *the liver* is very chemically active, and heat is produced as a by-product.
- *the digestive organs* produce heat by the contraction of the smooth muscle of the alimentary tract and by the chemical reactions involved in digestion.

- *the specific dynamic action*, i.e. the increase in the metabolic rate that occurs when food is eaten, produces heat.

Heat loss

Most of the heat loss from the body occurs through the skin. Small amounts are lost in expired air, urine and faeces.

Only the heat lost through the skin can be regulated to maintain a constant body temperature. There is no control over heat lost by the other routes.

Heat loss through the skin is affected by the difference between body and environmental temperatures, the amount of the body surface exposed to the air and the type of clothes worn. Air is a poor conductor of heat and when layers of air are trapped in clothing and between the skin and clothing they act as effective insulators against excessive heat loss. For this reason several layers of lightweight clothes provide more effective insulation against a low environmental temperature than one heavy garment. A fine balance is maintained between heat production and heat loss. Control is achieved mainly by thermoreceptors in the hypothalamus.

Control of body temperature

Nervous control
The *temperature regulating centre* in the hypothalamus is responsive to the temperature of circulating blood. This centre affects body temperature through autonomic nerve stimulation of the sweat glands.

The *vasomotor centre* in the medulla oblongata controls the diameter of the small arteries and arterioles, and they control the amount of blood which circulates in the capillaries in the dermis. The vasomotor centre is influenced by the temperature of its blood supply and by nerve impulses from the hypothalamus. When the skin capillaries are dilated the extra blood near the surface increases heat loss by radiation, conduction and convection. The skin is warm and pink in colour. Arteriolar constriction conserves heat and the skin is whiter and feels cool.

Activity of the sweat glands
If the temperature of the body is increased by 0.25 to 0.5°C the sweat glands are stimulated to secrete sweat, which is conveyed to the surface of the body by ducts. The body is cooled by loss of the heat used to *evaporate* the water in sweat. When sweat droplets can be seen

on the skin the rate of production is exceeding the rate of evaporation. This is most likely to happen when the environmental air is humid and the temperature high.

Loss of heat from the body by *evaporation* also occurs by *insensible water loss*. In this case heat is being continuously lost by evaporation, even though the sweat glands are not active. Water diffuses upwards from the deeper layers of the skin to the surface of the body and evaporates into the air. The individual is unaware of this process.

Effects of vasodilatation

The amount of heat lost from the skin depends to a great extent on the amount of blood in the vessels in the dermis. As heat production increases, the arterioles become dilated and more blood pours into the capillary network in the skin. In addition to increasing the amount of sweat produced the *temperature of the skin is raised* and there is an increase in the amount of heat lost by radiation, conduction and convection.

In *radiation* the exposed parts of the body radiate heat away from the body.

In *conduction* the clothes and other objects in contact with the skin take up heat.

In *convection* the air passing over the exposed parts of the body is heated and rises, cool air replaces it and convection currents are set up. Heat is also lost from the clothes by convection.

If the external environmental temperature is low or if heat production is decreased, vasoconstriction occurs, stimulated by sympathetic nerves. This decreases the blood flow near the body surface, conserving heat.

Hypothermia

This is present when core temperature, e.g. the rectal temperature, is below 35°C (95°F). At a rectal temperature below 32°C (89.6°F), compensatory mechanisms to restore body temperature usually fail, e.g. shivering is replaced by muscle rigidity and cramps, vasoconstriction fails to occur and there is lowered blood pressure, pulse and respiration rates. Mental confusion and disorientation occur. Death usually occurs when the temperature falls below 25°C (77°F).

Individuals at the extremes of age are prone to hypothermia.

Formation of vitamin D

There is a fatty substance, *7-dehydrocholesterol*, in the skin and ultraviolet light from the sun converts it to vitamin D. This circulates in the blood and is used, with calcium and phosphorus, in the formation and maintenance of bone. Any vitamin D in excess of immediate requirements is stored in the liver.

Sensation

Sensory receptors consist of nerve endings in the dermis that are sensitive to touch, pressure, temperature or pain. They are stimulated by changes in the external environment and generate nerve impulses that travel to the cerebral cortex. Some areas have more sensory receptors than others causing them to be especially sensitive, e.g. the lips and fingertips (Fig. 7.20B).

Absorption

This property is limited but substances that can be absorbed include:

- some drugs, in transdermal patches, e.g. hormones used as replacement therapy in postmenopausal women, nicotine as an aid to stopping smoking
- some toxic chemicals, e.g. mercury.

Excretion

The skin is a minor excretory organ for some substances including:

- sodium chloride in sweat and excess sweating may lead to abnormally low blood sodium levels
- urea, especially when kidney function is impaired
- aromatic substances, e.g. garlic and other spices.

WOUND HEALING

Conditions required for wound healing

Systemic factors include good nutritional status and general health. Infection, impaired immunity, poor blood supply and some conditions, e.g. diabetes mellitus, cancer, reduce the rate of wound healing.

Local factors that facilitate wound healing include:

- good blood supply providing oxygen and nutrient materials and removing waste products
- freedom from contamination by, e.g. microbes, foreign bodies, toxic chemicals.

Primary healing (healing by first intention)

This method of healing follows minimal destruction of tissue when the damaged edges of a wound are in close apposition. There are several overlapping stages in the repair process (Fig. 14.5):

1. The cut surfaces become inflamed and blood clot and cell debris fill the gap between them (first few hours).
2. Phagocytes and fibroblasts migrate into the blood clot:
   a. phagocytes begin to remove the clot and cell debris stimulating fibroblast activity
   b. fibroblasts secrete collagen fibres which begin to bind the surfaces together
   c. epithelial cells of the dermis begin to spread across the gap through the clot, and the clot above the new skin cells becomes the scab (stage 2 takes 3 to 5 days).
3. The clot between the cut surfaces is completely removed and the scab separates.
4. Layers of epithelial cells grow upwards until the full thickness of skin is restored.
5. Fibrous tissue continues to grow, binding the edges of the wound more strongly.
6. The inflammation resolves but scar tissue remains vascular (stages 3, 4, 5 and 6 progress concurrently and take 2 to 4 weeks).

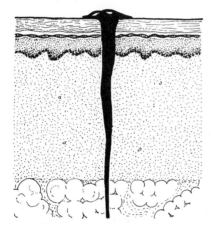

A. Cut surfaces separated by blood clot and cell debris

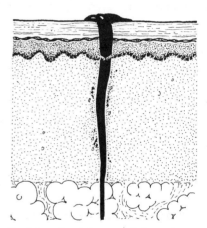

B. Cut surfaces become inflamed
Phagocytosis of clot begins
Epidermal cells spread through clot
Fibrous tissue begins to form

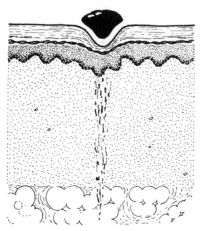

C. Epidermal cells bridge gap
Scab separates
Fibrous tissue binds surfaces together

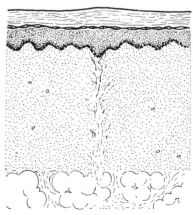

D. Full thickness of epidermis is restored
Wound becomes stronger
Fibrous tissue gradually absorbed

Figure 14.5 Some stages in primary wound healing.

7. After 2 to 4 weeks the wound gradually becomes stronger, the fibrous tissue is reduced by the action of fibrolytic enzymes, the scar becomes less vascular, appearing after a few months as a pale line.

The channels left when stitches are removed heal by the same process.

Secondary healing (healing by second intention)

This method of healing follows destruction of a large amount of tissue or when the edges of a wound cannot be brought into apposition, e.g. following chronic inflammation or in deep bed sores (decubitus ulcers). The time taken for healing depends on the effective removal of the cause and on the size of the wound. There are several recognised stages in the repair process, e.g. of decubitus ulcers (Fig. 14.6):

1. Acute inflammation develops on the surface of the healthy tissue and separation of necrotic tissue (*slough*) begins, due mainly to the action of phagocytes in the inflammatory exudate.
2. Granulation tissue, consisting of new budding capillaries and fibroblasts, begins to develop at the base of the cavity and grows towards the surface, probably stimulated by macrophages in the inflamed area.
3. Phagocytes in the plentiful blood supply tend to prevent infection of the wound after separation of the slough.
4. For unknown reasons some fibroblasts at the edges of the wound develop a limited ability to contract, reducing the size of the wound and the healing time.
5. When granulation tissue reaches the level of the

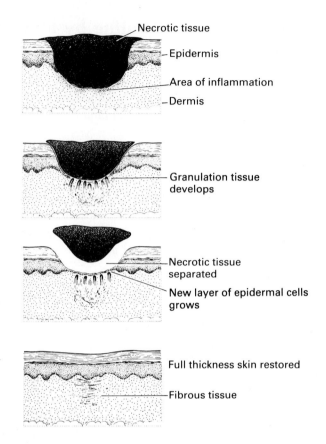

Figure 14.6 Some stages in secondary wound healing.

dermis, epithelial cells at the edges proliferate and grow towards the centre, forming a single layer of cells which gradually increase in number until, several months later, the full thickness of skin is restored.
6. In time the scar tissue shrinks and becomes less vascular.

DISORDERS OF THE SKIN

Infections

Impetigo

This is a highly infectious condition commonly caused by *Staphylococcus aureus*. Superficial pustules develop, usually round the nose and mouth. It is spread by direct contact and affects mainly children and immuno-suppressed individuals. When caused by *Streptococcus haemolyticus* the infection may be complicated, a few weeks later, by an immune reaction causing glomerulonephritis (p. 348).

Cellulitis

This is a spreading infection caused by some anaerobic microbes or by *Streptococcus perfringens*. The spread of infection is facilitated by the formation of substances that break down the connective tissue that normally isolates an area of inflammation. The microbes enter the body through a break in the skin. If untreated, the products of inflammation may enter the blood causing septicaemia.

Ringworm and tinea pedis

These are superficial infections of the skin caused by fungi. In ringworm there is an outward spreading ring of inflammation. It most commonly affects the scalp and is found in cattle from which infection is spread.

Tinea pedis (athlete's foot) affects the area between the toes. Both infections are spread by direct contact.

Non-infective inflammatory conditions

Eczema and dermatitis

In acute dermatitis there is redness, swelling and exudation of serous fluid usually accompanied by itching. This is often followed by crusting and scaling. If the condition becomes chronic, the skin thickens and may become leathery due to long-term scratching. Infection may complicate scratching.

Atopic dermatitis is caused by allergens and commonly affects atopic individuals. Children who may also suffer from asthma (p. 260) or hay fever are often affected.

Contact dermatitis may be caused by:

- direct contact with irritants, e.g. cosmetics, soap, detergent, strong acids or alkalis, industrial chemicals
- a hypersensitivity reaction to, e.g. synthetic rubber, nickel, dyes and other chemicals.

Psoriasis

This condition is genetically determined and characterised by exacerbations and periods of remission of varying duration. There is proliferation of the cells of the basal layers of the epidermis and the more rapid upward progress of these cells through the epidermis results in incomplete maturation of the upper layer. The skin is shiny, silver coloured and scaly. Bleeding may occur when scales are scratched or rubbed off. The elbows, knees and scalp are common sites but other parts can be affected. Triggering factors that lead to exacerbation of the condition include trauma, infection and sunburn.

Acne vulgaris

This is a common condition in adolescents that is thought to be caused by increased levels of male sex hormones after puberty. It occurs when sebaceous glands in hair follicles become blocked. *Blackheads* are formed and these may become infected leading to the development of inflammation and pustule formation. In severe cases permanent scarring may result. The most common sites are the face, chest and upper back.

Pressure sores (decubitus ulcers)

These occur over 'pressure points', areas where the skin is compressed between a bony prominence and a hard surface. When this occurs, blood flow to the affected area is impaired and ischaemia develops. Initially the skin reddens, and later as ischaemia and necrosis occur the skin sloughs and an ulcer forms that may enlarge into a cavity. If infection occurs, this can result in septicaemia. Healing takes place by secondary intention (p. 266).

Predisposing factors

These may be:

- extrinsic, e.g. pressure, shearing forces, trauma, immobility, moisture, infection
- intrinsic, e.g. poor nutritional status, emaciation, incontinence, infection, concurrent illness, sensory impairment, poor circulation, old age.

Burns

These may be caused by many types of trauma including: heat, cold, electricity, ionising radiation and chemicals, including strong acids or alkalis.

Local damage occurs disrupting the structure and functions of the skin. Infection is a common complication of any burn as the outer barrier formed by the epidermis is lost.

Burns are classified according to their depth:

- *partial thickness* (superficial)— only the epidermis is involved
- *full thickness* (deep)—the epidermis, and dermis are destroyed. After a few days the destroyed tissue coagulates and forms an *eschar*, or thick scab, which sloughs off after 2 to 3 weeks. In burns which encircle any area of the body complications may arise from constriction of the part by eschar, e.g. respiratory impairment may follow circumferential burns of the chest, the circulation to the distal part of an affected limb may be seriously impaired. Skin grafting is required except for small injuries. Otherwise, healing, which is prolonged, occurs by secondary intention (p. 366) and there is no regeneration of sweat glands, hair follicles or sebaceous glands. These burns are usually relatively painless as the sensory nerve endings in the dermis are destroyed.

The extent of burns in adults is roughly estimated using the 'rule of nines' (Fig. 14.7). In adults, hypovolaemic shock usually develops when 15% of the surface area is affected. Fatality is likely in adults with full thickness burns if the surface area affected is added to the patient's age and the total is greater than 80.

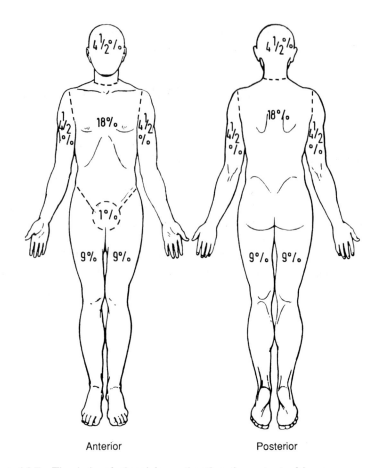

Figure 14.7 The 'rule of nines' for estimating the extent of burns.

Burns complications

Dehydration and hypovolaemia may occur in extensive burns due to excessive leakage of water and plasma proteins from the surface of the damaged skin.

Shock may accompany severe hypovolaemia.

Hypothermia develops when thermoregulation is impaired and excessive heat is lost.

Infection of the surface of a burn may result in septicaemia.

Renal failure occurs when the kidney tubules cannot deal with the amount of waste from haemolysed erythrocytes and damaged tissue.

Contractures may develop later as fibrous scar tissue contracts distorting the limbs, e.g. the hands, and impairing function.

Benign tumours

Viral warts

These are caused by the human papilloma virus spread by direct contact, e.g. from another lesion, or another infected individual. There is proliferation of the epidermis and the development of a small firm growth. The common sites are the hands, the face and the soles of the feet (*plantar warts* or *verrucas*). *Anogenital warts* are larger and affect the genitalia and/or anus; they are spread during sexual intercourse.

Malignant tumours

Basal cell carcinoma

This is sometimes associated with long-term exposure to sunlight and often affects the skin of the face. It appears as a nodule and later this breaks down becoming an ulcer, commonly called a *rodent ulcer*. This is locally invasive but it seldom metastasises.

Malignant melanoma

This is dysplasia of melanocytes, usually originating in a mole that may have an irregular outline. It may ulcerate with bleeding and most commonly affects young and middle-aged adults. Predisposing factors are believed to be a fair skin and recurrent episodes of excessive exposure to sunlight. Metastases develop early and are frequently found in lymph nodes. The most common sites of blood-spread metastases are the liver, brain, lungs, bowel and bone marrow.

Kaposi's sarcoma

In this condition a small red-blue patch or nodule develops usually on the lower limbs.

It is also an AIDS-related disease and has thus become more common. In such cases, multiple lesions affect many sites of the body.

15
The skeleton

BONES

Bone is the hardest tissue in the body and when fully developed it is composed of:

Water	20%
Organic material	30 to 40%
Inorganic material	40 to 50%

Inorganic (non-carbon-containing) constituents are mineral salts, mainly calcium, and phosphorus. The organic component includes the bone cells and part of the matrix.

There are two types of bone tissue, *compact* and *cancellous*.

Compact bone (Fig. 15.1)

To the naked eye, compact bone appears to be solid but on microscopic examination large numbers of *Haversian systems* can be seen. These consist of a central Haversian canal, containing blood and lymph vessels and nerves, surrounded by concentric plates of bone (*lamellae*). Between these there are *lacunae* or spaces, containing lymph and *osteocytes*. *Canaliculi* link the lacunae with the lymph vessels in the Haversian canal and the osteocytes obtain nourishment from the lymph. This 'tubular' arrangement of lamellae gives bone greater strength than a solid structure of the same size would have.

Cancellous bone

To the naked eye, cancellous bone looks spongy. Microscopically, the Haversian canals are much larger than in compact bone and there are fewer lamellae, giving a honeycomb appearance. *Red bone marrow* is always present in cancellous bone.

Periosteum

Bones are almost completely covered by this vascular fibrous membrane. In the deeper layers of the periosteum there are *osteogenic cells* that increase the thickness of compact tissue and maintain the shape of the bones. It gives attachment to muscles and tendons and protects the bone from injury. Periosteum is replaced by hyaline cartilage on the articular surfaces of synovial joints and by dura mater on the inner surface of the cranial bones.

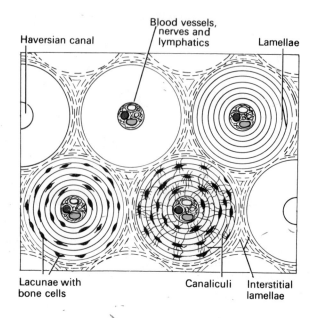

A. Cross section.

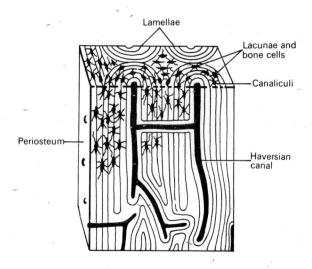

B. Longitudinal section.

Figure 15.1 Microscopic structure of bone.

Types of bones

Bones are classified as long, short, irregular, flat and sesamoid.

Long bones have a *diaphysis* or shaft and two *epiphyses* or extremities. The diaphysis is composed of compact bone with a central *medullary canal*, containing fatty *yellow bone marrow*. The epiphyses consist of an outer covering of compact bone with cancellous bone inside. The diaphysis and epiphyses are separated by *epiphyseal*

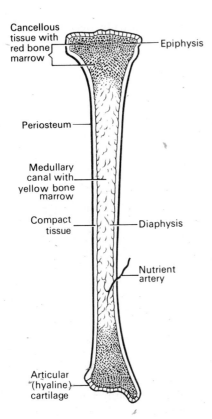

Figure 15.2 A mature long bone—longitudinal section.

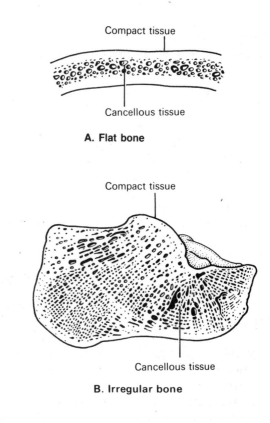

Figure 15.3 Flat and irregular bones.

cartilages. A bone grows in length by ossification of the diaphyseal surface of these cartilages and growth is complete when the cartilages stop growing and are completely ossified (Fig. 15.2). The focal points from which ossification begins are small concentrations of osteogenic cells, or *centres of ossification.* There is a primary centre in the diaphysis and one or more secondary centres in each epiphysis. Growth in thickness occurs by the deposition of bone under the periosteum.

Irregular, flat and sesamoid bones are composed of a relatively thin outer layer of compact bone with cancellous bone inside, containing red bone marrow (Fig. 15.3). Examples include:

- irregular bones—vertebrae and some skull bones
- flat bones—sternum, ribs and most skull bones
- sesamoid bones—patella (kneecap).

Development of bone tissue (osteogenesis or ossification)

This begins before birth and is not complete until about the 25th year of life (Fig. 15.4). Long, short and irregular bones develop from cartilage models, flat bones

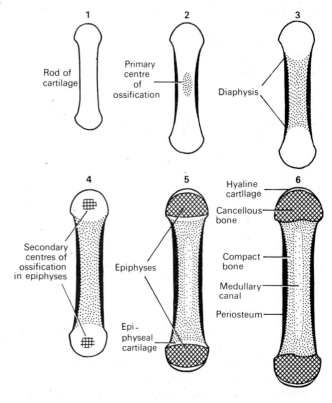

Figure 15.4 Diagram of the stages of development of long bones.

from membrane and sesamoid bones from tendon. Bone development consists of two processes:

- the secretion by osteoblasts of *osteoid*, i.e. collagen fibres in a mucopolysaccharide matrix which gradually replaces the original cartilage and membrane models
- calcification of the osteoid immediately after its deposition.

There are two types of arrangement of collagen in osteoid.

Non-lamellar bone (woven bone)
The collagen fibres are deposited in bundles, then ossified. This occurs in:

- ossification of bones that originate as membrane models, e.g. skull bones
- healing of fractures, when collagen fibres are deposited in the granulation tissue that grows between the broken ends.

Lamellar bone
The collagen fibres are deposited as in non-lamellar bone, organised into the characteristic Haversian systems then ossified. This occurs when cartilage models are replaced by bone and in fracture healing.

Growth of bones

Hormones that regulate the growth and consistency of size and shape of bones are:

- *growth hormone* and the thyroid hormones, *thyroxine* and *triiodothyronine* are important during infancy and childhood; deficient or excessive secretion of these results in abnormal development of the skeleton (Ch. 9).
- *testosterone* and *oestrogens* influence the physical changes that occur at puberty, i.e. the growth spurt and masculinising or feminising changes of specific parts of the skeleton, e.g. the pelvis
- *calcitonin* from the thyroid gland and *parathormone* from the parathyroid glands are involved in maintaining the homeostasis of blood and bone calcium levels required for bone development.

Although the length and shape of bones does not normally change after ossification is complete, bone tissue is continually being replaced. Osteoblasts continue to lay down osteoid and osteoclasts reabsorb it. The rate in different bones varies, e.g. the distal part of the femur is replaced gradually over a period of 5 to 6 months.

Bone cells

The cells responsible for bone formation are *osteoblasts* (these later develop into *osteocytes*). Osteoblasts and *chondrocytes* (cartilage-forming cells) develop from the same parent fibrous tissue cells. Differentiation into *osteogenic cells*, rather than *chondroblasts*, is believed to depend upon an adequate oxygen supply. This may be a factor affecting healing of fractures, i.e. if the oxygen supply is deficient there may be a preponderance of chondroblasts, resulting in a cartilaginous union of the fracture.

Osteoclasts are involved in resorption of bone.

Osteoblasts
These are the bone-forming cells and are present:

- in the deeper layers of periosteum
- in the centres of ossification of immature bone
- at the ends of the diaphysis adjacent to the epiphyseal cartilages of long bones
- at the site of a fracture.

As bone develops, osteoblasts become trapped and remain isolated in lacunae. They stop forming new bone at this stage and are called *osteocytes*. Osteocytes receive nourishment from lymph in the canaliculi that radiate from the Haversian canals. Their functions are not clear but they may be associated with the movement of calcium between the bones and the blood.

Osteoclasts
Their function is resorption of bone to maintain the optimum shape. This takes place at bone surfaces:

- under the periosteum, to maintain the shape of bones during growth and to remove excess callus formed during healing of fractures
- round the walls of the medullary canal, to maintain the correct ratio of canal to lamellar bone during growth, and to canalise callus during healing.

A fine balance of osteoblast and osteoclast activity maintains normal bone.

Functions of bones

Bones have a variety of functions. They:

- provide the framework of the body
- give attachment to muscles and tendons
- permit movement of the body as a whole and of parts of the body, by forming joints that are moved by muscles
- form the boundaries of the cranial, thoracic and pelvic cavities, protecting the organs they contain
- contain red bone marrow in which blood cells develop: haematopoiesis (see Fig. 4.4)
- provide a reservoir of calcium, phosphorus and fat.

Bones of the skeleton

Most bones have rough surfaces, raised protuberances and ridges which give attachment to muscle tendons and ligaments. These are not included in the following descriptions of individual bones unless they are of particular note, but many are marked on illustrations. Related terminology is explained on page 33.

The bones of the skeleton are divided into two groups (Figs 15.5 and 15.6): the *axial skeleton* and the *appendicular skeleton*.

AXIAL SKELETON

This part consists of the *skull, vertebral column, ribs* and *sternum*. Together the bones forming these structures constitute the central bony core of the body, the axis.

Skull (Figs 15.7 and 15.8)

The skull rests on the upper end of the vertebral column and its bony structure is divided into two parts: the cranium and the face.

Cranium

The cranium is formed by a number of flat irregular bones that provide a bony protection for the brain. It has a *base* upon which the brain rests and a *vault* that surrounds and covers it. The periosteum inside the skull bones consists of the outer layer of dura mater. In the mature skull the joints (*sutures*) between the bones are immovable (fibrous). The bones have numerous perforations through which nerves, blood and lymph vessels pass. The bones of the cranium are:

- 1 frontal bone
- 2 parietal bones
- 2 temporal bones
- 1 occipital bone
- 1 sphenoid bone
- 1 ethmoid bone.

Frontal bone

This is the bone of the forehead. It forms part of the orbital cavities and the prominent ridges above the eyes, the *supraorbital margins*. Just above the supraorbital margins, within the bone, there are two air-filled cavities or *sinuses* lined with ciliated mucous membrane which have openings into the nasal cavities.

The *coronal suture* joins the frontal and parietal bones and other fibrous joints are formed with the sphenoid, zygomatic, lacrimal, nasal, and ethmoid bones. The bone originates in two parts joined in the midline by the *frontal suture* (Fig. 15.15).

Parietal bones

These bones form the sides and roof of the skull. They articulate with each other at the *sagittal suture*, with the frontal bone at the coronal suture, with the occipital bone at the *lambdoidal suture* and with the temporal bones at the *squamous sutures*. The inner surface is concave and is grooved by the brain and blood vessels.

Temporal bones (Fig. 15.9)

These bones lie one on each side of the head and form immovable joints with the parietal, occipital, sphenoid and zygomatic bones. Each temporal bone is divided into four parts.

The squamous part is the thin fan-shaped part that articulates with the parietal bone.

The mastoid process is a thickened part behind the ear. It contains a large number of very small air sinuses which communicate with the middle ear and are lined with squamous epithelium.

The petrous portion forms part of the base of the skull and contains the organ of hearing, the spiral organ (of Corti).

The zygomatic process articulates with the zygomatic bone to form the zygomatic arch.

The temporal bone articulates with the mandible at the *temporomandibular joint*, the only movable joint of the skull. Immediately behind this articulating surface is the *auditory meatus* which passes inwards towards the petrous portion of the bone.

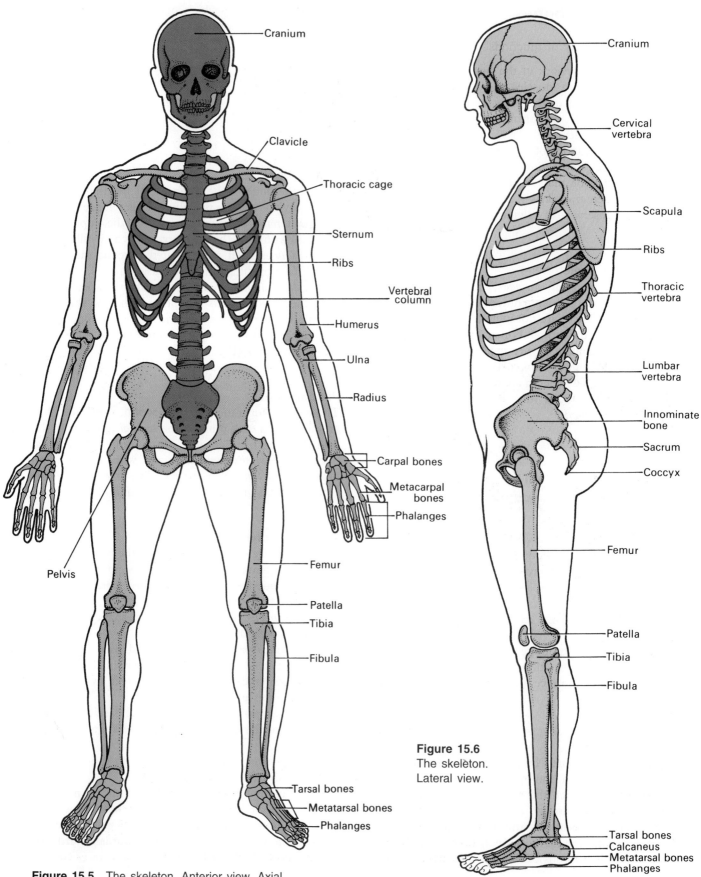

Figure 15.5 The skeleton. Anterior view. Axial skeleton—brown; appendicular skeleton—gold.

Figure 15.6
The skeleton.
Lateral view.

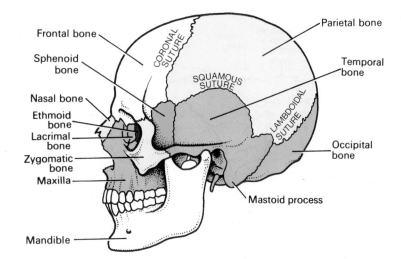

Figure 15.7 labels: Frontal bone, CORONAL SUTURE, SQUAMOUS SUTURE, Parietal bone, Temporal bone, LAMBDOIDAL SUTURE, Sphenoid bone, Nasal bone, Ethmoid bone, Lacrimal bone, Zygomatic bone, Maxilla, Mandible, Occipital bone, Mastoid process

Figure 15.7 The bones of the skull and their joints or sutures.

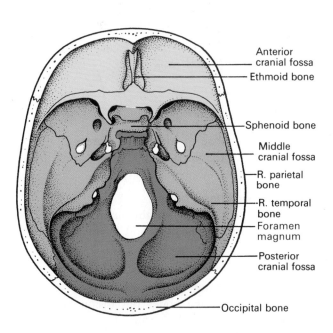

Figure 15.8 labels: Anterior cranial fossa, Ethmoid bone, Sphenoid bone, Middle cranial fossa, R. parietal bone, R. temporal bone, Foramen magnum, Posterior cranial fossa, Occipital bone

Figure 15.8 The bones forming the base of the skull and the cranial fossae. Viewed from above. Anterior cranial fossa—green. Middle cranial fossa—gold. Posterior cranial fossa—purple.

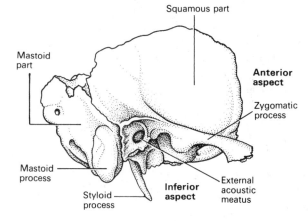

Figure 15.9 labels: Squamous part, Mastoid part, Anterior aspect, Zygomatic process, Mastoid process, Styloid process, Inferior aspect, External acoustic meatus

Figure 15.9 The right temporal bone. Lateral view.

Occipital bone (Fig. 15.10)

This bone forms the back of the head and part of the base of the skull. It has immovable joints with the parietal, temporal and sphenoid bones. Its inner surface is deeply concave and the concavity is occupied by the occipital lobes of the cerebrum and by the cerebellum. The occiput has two articular condyles that form hinge joints with the first bone of the vertebral column, the *atlas*. Between the condyles there is the *foramen magnum* through which the spinal cord passes.

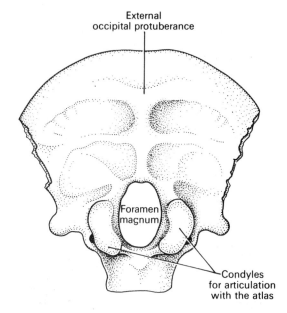

Figure 15.10 labels: External occipital protuberance, Foramen magnum, Condyles for articulation with the atlas

Figure 15.10 The occipital bone viewed from below.

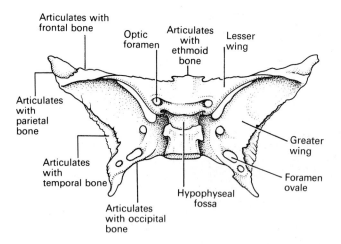

Figure 15.11   The sphenoid bone viewed from above.

Sphenoid bone (Fig. 15.11)

This bone occupies the middle portion of the base of the skull and it articulates with the temporal, parietal and frontal bones. On the superior surface in the middle of the bone there is a little saddle-shaped depression, the *hypophyseal fossa* (*sella turcica*) in which the *pituitary gland* rests. The body of the bone contains some fairly large air sinuses lined by ciliated mucous membrane with openings into the nasal cavities.

Ethmoid bone (Fig. 15.12)

The ethmoid bone occupies the anterior part of the base of the skull and helps to form the orbital cavity, the nasal septum and the lateral walls of the nasal cavity.

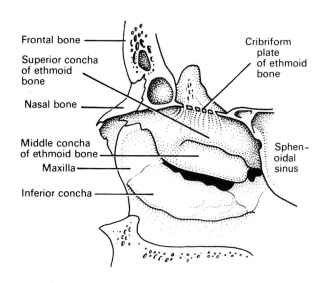

Figure 15.12   The right ethmoid bone and its related structures.

On each side there are two projections into the nasal cavities, the *upper* and *middle conchae* or *turbinated processes*. It is a very delicate bone containing many air sinuses lined with ciliated epithelium and with openings into the nasal cavities. The horizontal flattened part, the *cribriform plate*, forms the roof of the nasal cavities and has numerous small foramina through which nerve fibres of the *olfactory nerve* (the nerve of the sense of smell) pass upwards from the nasal cavities to the brain. There is also a very fine *perpendicular plate* of bone that forms the upper part of the *nasal septum*.

Face

The skeleton of the face is formed by 13 bones in addition to the frontal bone, already described. Figure 15.13 shows the relationships between the bones:

- 2 zygomatic or cheek bones
- 1 maxilla (originated as 2)
- 2 nasal bones
- 2 lacrimal bones
- 1 vomer
- 2 palatine bones
- 2 inferior conchae or turbinated bones
- 1 mandible (originated as 2).

Zygomatic or cheek bone

The zygomatic bones form the prominences of the cheeks and part of the floor and lateral walls of the orbital cavities.

Maxilla or upper jaw bone

This originates as two bones but fusion takes place before birth. The maxilla forms the upper jaw, the anterior part of the roof of the mouth, the lateral walls of the nasal cavities and part of the floor of the orbital cavities. The *alveolar ridge*, or *process*, projects downwards and carries the upper teeth. On each side there is a large air sinus, the *maxillary sinus*, lined with ciliated mucous membrane and with openings into the nasal cavities.

Nasal bones

These are two small flat bones which form the greater part of the lateral and superior surfaces of the bridge of the nose.

Lacrimal bones

These two small bones are posterior and lateral to the nasal bones and form part of the medial walls of

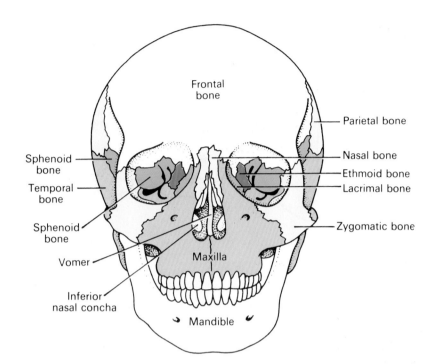

Figure 15.13 The bones of the face. Anterior view.

the orbital cavities. Each is pierced by a foramen for the passage of the *nasolacrimal duct* which carries the tears from the medial canthus of the eye to the nasal cavity.

Vomer

The vomer is a thin flat bone which extends upwards from the middle of the hard palate to form the main part of the nasal septum. Superiorly it articulates with the perpendicular plate of the ethmoid bone.

Palatine bones

These are two L-shaped bones. The horizontal parts unite to form the posterior part of the hard palate and the perpendicular parts project upwards to form part of the lateral walls of the nasal cavities. At their upper extremities they form part of the orbital cavities.

Inferior conchae or turbinated bones

Each concha is a scroll-shaped bone which forms part of the lateral wall of the nasal cavity and projects into it below the middle concha. The superior and middle conchae are parts of the ethmoid bone.

Mandible (Fig. 15.14)

This is the only movable bone of the skull. It originates as two parts which unite at the midline. Each half consists of two main parts: a *curved body* with the *alveolar ridge* containing the lower teeth and a *ramus* which projects upwards almost at right angles to the posterior end of the body.

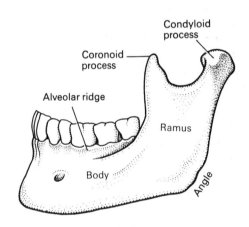

Figure 15.14 The mandible. Lateral view.

At the upper end the ramus divides into the *condyloid process* which articulates with the temporal bone to form the *temporomandibular* joint and the *coronoid process* that gives attachment to muscles and ligaments. The point where the ramus joins the body is the *angle* of the jaw.

Hyoid bone

This is an isolated horse-shoe-shaped bone lying in the soft tissues of the neck just above the *larynx* and below the *mandible*. It does not articulate with any other bone but is attached to the styloid process of the temporal bone by ligaments. It gives attachment to the base of the tongue.

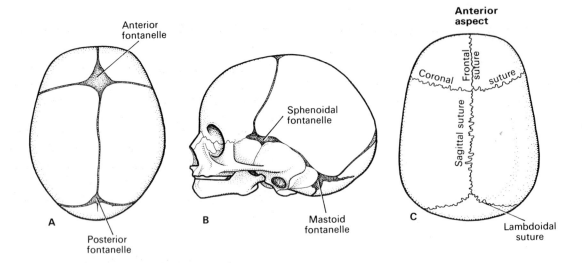

Figure 15.15   The skull showing the fontanelles and sutures. A. Fontanelles viewed from above. B. Fontanelles viewed from the side. C. Main sutures viewed from above when ossification is complete.

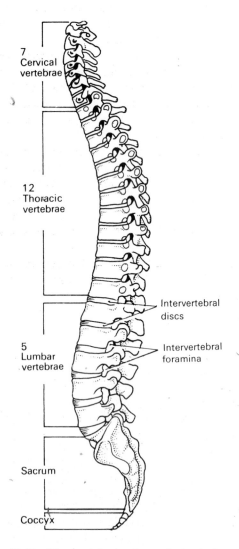

Figure 15.16   The vertebral column. Lateral view.

Sinuses

Sinuses containing air are present in the sphenoid, ethmoid, maxillary and frontal bones. They all communicate with the nose and are lined with ciliated mucous membrane. Their functions are:

- to give resonance to the voice
- to lighten the bones of the face and cranium, making it easier for the head to balance on top of the vertebral column.

Fontanelles of the skull (Fig. 15.15)

At birth, ossification of the cranial sutures is incomplete. Where three or more bones meet there are distinct membranous areas, or *fontanelles*. The two largest are: the *anterior fontanelle*, not fully ossified until the child is 12 to 18 months old and the *posterior fontanelle*, usually ossified 2 to 3 months after birth. Some moulding of the skull occurs as the baby's head passes through the birth canal.

Vertebral column (Fig. 15.16)

The vertebral column consists of 24 separate movable, irregular bones, the *sacrum* (five fused bones) and the *coccyx* (four fused bones). The 24 separate bones are in three groups: 7 cervical, 12 thoracic and 5 lumbar.

The movable vertebrae have many characteristics in common but some groups have distinguishing features.

Characteristics of a typical vertebra
(Fig. 15.17)

The body of each vertebra is situated anteriorly. The size varies with the site. They are smallest in the cervical region and become larger towards the lumbar region.

The neural arch encloses a large *vertebral foramen*. The ring of bone consists of *two pedicles* that project backwards from the body and *two laminae*. Where the pedicles and laminae unite, *transverse processes* project laterally and where the two laminae meet in the midline posteriorly they form a *spinous process*. The neural arch has four articular surfaces: two articulate with the vertebra above and two with the one below. The vertebral foramina form the neural canal that contains the spinal cord.

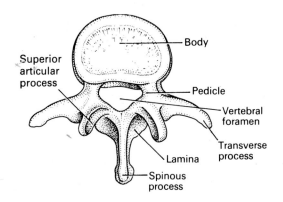

Figure 15.17 A lumbar vertebra showing the features of a typical vertebra—viewed from above.

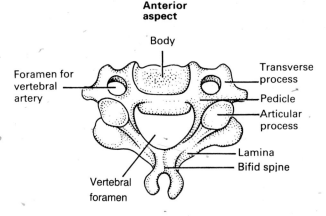

Figure 15.18 A cervical vertebra viewed from above.

Special features of vertebrae in different parts of the vertebral column

Cervical vertebrae (Fig. 15.18)
The transverse processes have a foramen through which a vertebral artery passes upwards to the brain. The first two cervical vertebrae are atypical.

The atlas (Fig. 15.19A) is the 1st cervical vertebra and it consists simply of a ring of bone with two short transverse processes. The anterior part of the large vertebral foramen is occupied by the *odontoid process* of the axis, which is held in position by a *transverse ligament* (Fig. 15.20).

Thus the odontoid process represents the body of the atlas. The posterior part is the true vertebral foramen and is occupied by the spinal cord. On its superior surface the bone has two articular facets which form joints with the condyles of the occipital bone of the skull. The nodding movement of the head takes place at these joints.

The axis (Fig. 15.19B) is the 2nd cervical vertebra. The body is small and has the upward projecting

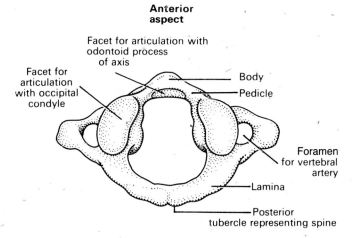

Figure 15.19A The atlas viewed from above.

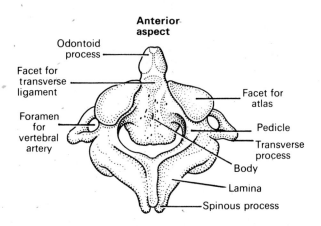

Figure 15.19B The axis viewed from above.

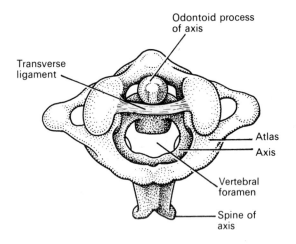

Figure 15.20 The atlas and axis in position showing the transverse ligament. Viewed from above.

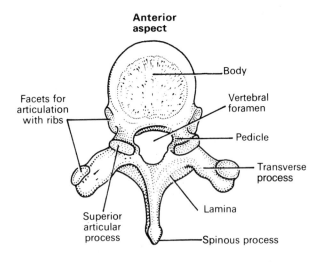

Figure 15.21A A thoracic vertebra. Viewed from above.

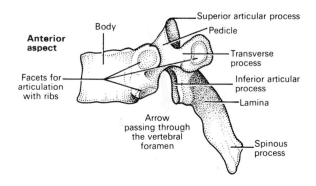

Figure 15.21B A thoracic vertebra. Viewed from the side.

odontoid process or *dens* that articulates with the first cervical vertebra, the atlas. The movement at this joint is turning the head from side to side.

Thoracic vertebrae (Fig. 15.21A and B)
The bodies and transverse processes have facets for articulation with the ribs.

Lumbar vertebrae
These have no special features.

Sacrum (Fig. 15.22)
This consists of five rudimentary vertebrae fused to form a wedge-shaped bone with a concave anterior surface. The upper part, or base, articulates with the 5th lumbar vertebra. On each side it articulates with the ilium to form a *sacroiliac joint*, and at its inferior tip it articulates with the *coccyx*. The anterior edge of the base, the *promontory*, protrudes into the pelvic cavity. The vertebral foramina are present, and on each side of the bone there is a series of foramina for the passage of nerves.

Coccyx (Fig. 15.22)
This consists of the four terminal vertebrae fused to form a very small triangular bone, the broad base of which articulates with the tip of the sacrum.

The vertebral column as a whole

Intervertebral discs
The bodies of adjacent vertebrae are separated by *intervertebral discs*, consisting of an outer rim of fibrocartilage (*annulus fibrosus*) and a central core of soft gelatinous material (*nucleus pulposus*). They are thinnest in the cervical region and become progressively thicker towards the lumbar region. The posterior longitudinal ligament in the vertebral canal helps to keep them in place. They have a shock-absorbing function and the cartilaginous joints they form contribute to the flexibility of the vertebral column as a whole.

Intervertebral foramina
When two adjacent vertebrae are viewed from the side, a foramen can be seen. Half of the wall is formed by the vertebra above and half by the one below (Fig. 15.23).

Throughout the length of the column there is an intervertebral foramen on each side between every pair

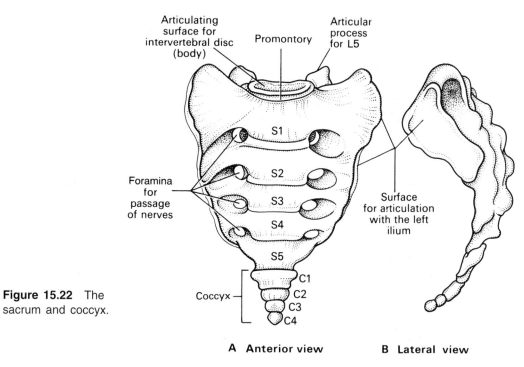

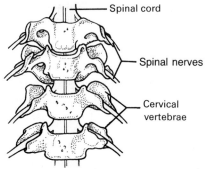

Figure 15.22 The sacrum and coccyx.

A Anterior view   B Lateral view

Figure 15.23 Lower cervical vertebra separated to show the spinal cord and spinal nerves emerging through the intervertebral foramina.

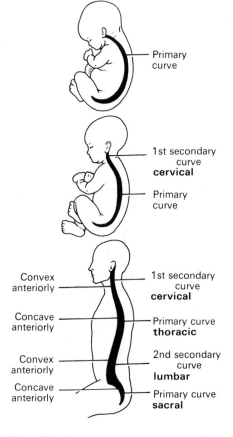

of vertebrae, through which the spinal nerves, blood vessels and lymph vessels pass.

Curves of the vertebral column (Fig. 15.24)
When viewed from the side the vertebral column presents four curves, two *primary* and two *secondary*.

The fetus in the uterus lies curled up so that the head and the knees are more or less touching. This position shows the *primary curvature*. The secondary *cervical curve* develops when the child can hold up his head (after about 3 months) and the secondary *lumbar curve* develops when he stands upright (after 12 to 18 months). The thoracic and sacral primary curves are retained.

Figure 15.24 Diagram showing the order of development of the curves of the spine.

Ligaments of the vertebral column (Fig. 15.25)

These ligaments hold the vertebrae together and help to maintain the intervertebral discs in position.

The *transverse ligament* maintains the odontoid process of the axis in the correct position in relation to the atlas (Fig. 15.20).

The anterior longitudinal ligament extends the whole length of the column and lies in front of the vertebral bodies.

The posterior longitudinal ligament lies inside the vertebral canal and extends the whole length of the vertebral column in close contact with the posterior surface of the bodies of the bones.

The ligamenta flava connect the laminae of adjacent vertebrae.

The ligamentum nuchae and the *supraspinous ligament* connect the spinous processes, extending from the occiput to the sacrum.

Movements of the vertebral column

The movements between the individual bones of the vertebral column are very limited. However, the movements of the column as a whole are quite extensive and include *flexion* (bending forward), *extension* (bending backward), *lateral flexion* (bending to the side) and *rotation*. There is more movement in the cervical and lumbar regions than elsewhere.

Functions of the vertebral column

- Collectively the vertebral foramina form the vertebral canal which provides a strong bony protection for the delicate spinal cord lying within it.
- The pedicles of adjacent vertebrae form intervertebral foramina, one on each side, through which spinal nerves, blood vessels and lymph vessels pass.
- Because of the numerous individual bones, a certain amount of movement is possible.
- It supports the skull.
- The intervertebral discs act as shock absorbers, protecting the brain.
- It forms the axis of the trunk, giving attachment to the ribs, shoulder girdle and upper limbs, and the pelvic girdle and lower limbs.

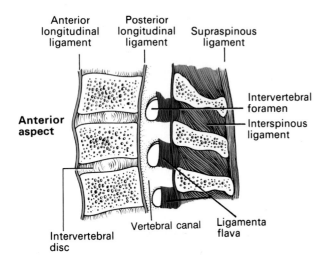

Figure 15.25   Section of the vertebral column showing the ligaments, intervertebral discs and intervertebral foramina.

Thoracic cage (Fig. 15.26)

The bones of the thorax or thoracic cage are:

- 1 sternum
- 12 pairs of ribs
- 12 thoracic vertebrae.

Sternum or breast bone (Fig. 15.27)

This *flat bone* can be felt just under the skin in the middle of the front of the chest.

The manubrium is uppermost and articulates with

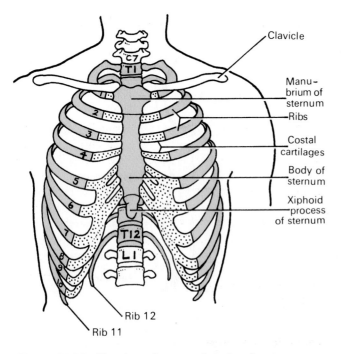

Figure 15.26   The thoracic cage. Anterior view.

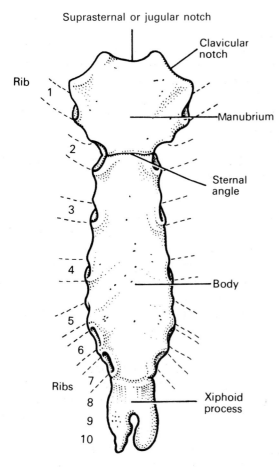

Figure 15.27 The sternum and its attachments.

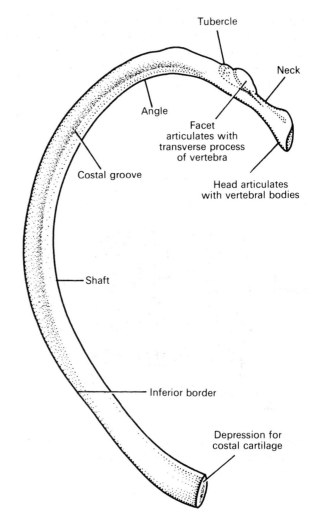

Figure 15.28 A typical rib viewed from below.

the clavicles at the *sternoclavicular joints* and with the first two pairs of ribs.

The body or middle portion gives attachment to the ribs.

The xiphoid process is the tip of the bone. It gives attachment to the diaphragm, muscles of the anterior abdominal wall and the *linea alba*.

Ribs

There are 12 pairs of ribs which form the bony lateral walls of the thoracic cage and articulate posteriorly with the thoracic vertebrae. The first 10 pairs are attached anteriorly to the sternum by *costal cartilages*, some directly and some indirectly (Fig. 15.26).

The last two pairs (*floating ribs*) have no anterior attachment.

Characteristics of a rib (Fig. 15.28). The head articulates posteriorly with the bodies of two adjacent tho-

racic vertebrae and the tubercle articulates with the transverse process of one. The sternal end is attached to the sternum by a costal cartilage, i.e. a band of hyaline cartilage. The superior border is rounded and smooth while the inferior border has a marked groove occupied by the intercostal blood vessels and nerves.

The first rib does not move during respiration.

The spaces between the ribs are occupied by the intercostal muscles. During inspiration, when these muscles contract, the ribs and sternum are lifted upwards and outwards increasing the capacity of the thoracic cavity (see Fig. 10.24).

Thoracic vertebrae

The 12 thoracic vertebrae have already been described.

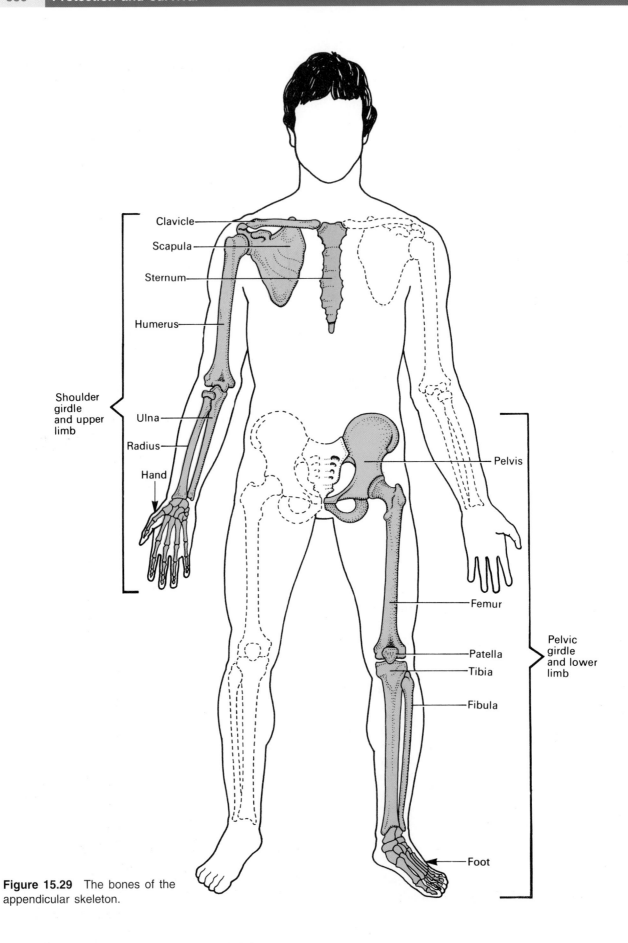

Figure 15.29 The bones of the
appendicular skeleton.

APPENDICULAR SKELETON

The appendicular skeleton consists of the shoulder girdle with the upper limbs and the pelvic girdle with the lower limbs (Fig. 15.29).

Shoulder girdle and upper limb

Each shoulder girdle consists of 1 clavicle and 1 scapula.
Each upper extremity consists of the following bones:

- 1 humerus
- 1 radius
- 1 ulna
- 8 carpal bones
- 5 metacarpal bones
- 14 phalanges.

Clavicle or collar bone (Fig. 15.30)
The clavicle is a long bone which has a double curve. It articulates with the manubrium of the sternum at the *sternoclavicular joint* and forms the *acromioclavicular joint* with the *acromion process* of the scapula. The clavicle provides the only bony link between the upper extremity and the axial skeleton.

Scapula or shoulder blade (Fig. 15.31)
The scapula is a flat triangular-shaped bone, lying on the posterior chest wall superficial to the ribs and separated from them by muscles.

At the lateral angle there is a shallow articular surface, the *glenoid cavity* which, with the *head of the humerus*, forms the *shoulder joint*.

On the posterior surface there is a *spinous process* that projects beyond the lateral angle of the bone that overhangs the shoulder joint, called the *acromion process*. It articulates with the clavicle at the *acromioclavicular joint*. The *coracoid process*, a projection from the upper border of the bone, gives attachment to muscles that move the shoulder joint.

Humerus (Fig. 15.32)
This is the bone of the upper arm. The head articulates with the glenoid cavity of the scapula, forming the

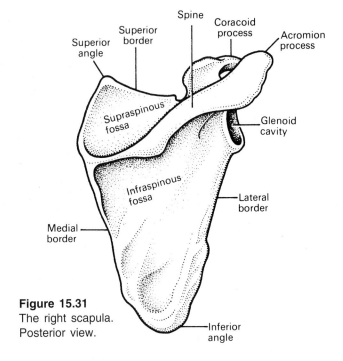

Figure 15.31
The right scapula.
Posterior view.

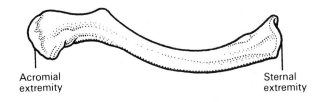

Acromial extremity

Sternal extremity

Figure 15.30 The right clavicle.

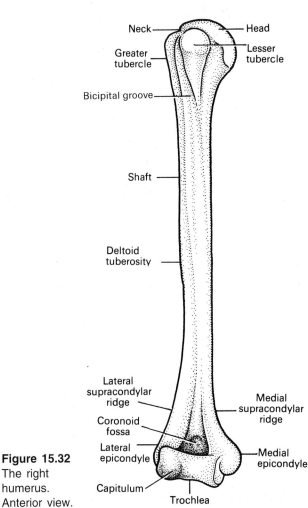

Figure 15.32
The right humerus.
Anterior view.

Figure 16.32 The right humerus. Anterior view.

shoulder joint. Distal to the head there are two roughened projections of bone, the *greater* and *lesser tubercles* and between them there is a deep groove, the *bicipital groove* or *intertubercular sulcus*, occupied by one of the tendons of the biceps muscle.

The distal end of the bone presents two surfaces that articulate with the radius and ulna to form the elbow joint.

Ulna and radius (Fig. 15.33)

These are the two bones of the forearm. The ulna is medial to the radius and when the arm is in the anatomical position, i.e. with the palm of the hand facing forward, the two bones are parallel. They articulate with the humerus at the *elbow joint*, the carpal bones at the *wrist joint* and with each other at the *superior* and *inferior radioulnar* joints.

Carpal or wrist bones (Fig. 15.34)

There are eight carpal bones arranged in two rows of four. From without inwards they are:

- *proximal row*: scaphoid, lunate, triquetral, pisiform
- *distal row*: trapezium, trapezoid, capitate, hamate.

These bones are closely fitted together and held in position by ligaments which allow a certain amount of movement between them. The bones of the proximal row are associated with the wrist joint and those of the distal row form joints with the metacarpal bones. Tendons of muscles lying in the forearm cross the wrist and are held close to the bones by strong fibrous bands, called retinacula (Fig. 16.8).

Metacarpal bones or the bones of the hand

These five bones form the palm of the hand. They are numbered from the thumb side inwards. The proximal ends articulate with the carpal bones and the distal ends with the phalanges.

Phalanges or finger bones

There are 14 phalanges, three in each finger and two in the thumb. They articulate with the metacarpal bones and with each other.

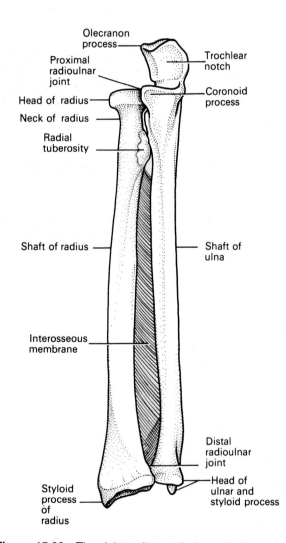

Figure 15.33 The right radius and ulna with the interosseous membrane. Anterior view.

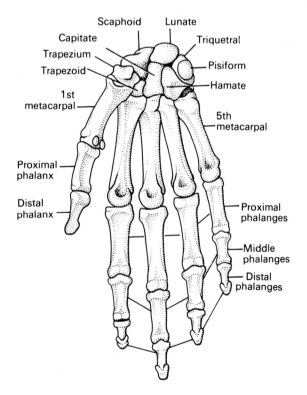

Figure 15.34 The bones of the wrist, hand and fingers. Anterior aspect.

Pelvic girdle and lower limb

The bones of the pelvic girdle are 2 innominate bones and 1 sacrum.

The bones of the lower extremity are:

- 1 femur
- 1 tibia
- 1 fibula
- 1 patella
- 7 tarsal bones
- 5 metatarsal bones
- 14 phalanges.

Innominate or hip bones (Fig. 15.35)

Each hip bone consists of three fused bones, the *ilium, ischium* and *pubis.* On its outer surface there is a deep depression, the *acetabulum,* which forms the hip joint with the almost-spherical head of femur.

The *ilium* is the upper flattened part of the bone and it presents the *iliac crest,* the anterior point of which is called the *anterior superior iliac spine.*

The *pubis* is the anterior part of the bone and it articulates with the pubis of the other hip bone at a cartilaginous joint, the *symphysis pubis.*

The *ischium* is the inferior and posterior part.

The union of the three parts takes place in the *acetabulum.*

The pelvis (Fig. 15.36)

The pelvis is formed by the two innominate bones which articulate anteriorly at the symphysis pubis and posteriorly with the sacrum at the *sacroiliac joints* which are

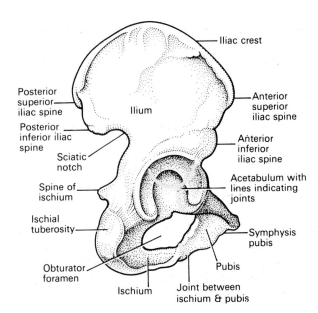

Figure 15.35 The right innominate bone. Lateral view.

synovial joints. It is divided into two parts by the *brim of the pelvis,* consisting of the promontory of the sacrum and the *iliopectineal lines* of the innominate bones. The *greater* or *false pelvis* is above the brim and the *lesser* or *true pelvis* is below.

Differences between male and female pelves (Fig. 15.37)

The shape of the female pelvis allows for the passage of the baby during childbirth. In comparison with the

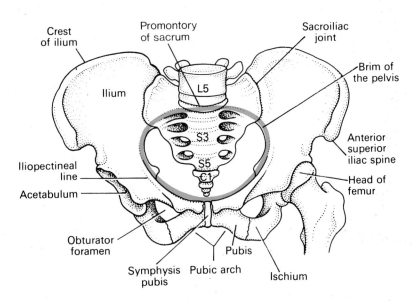

Figure 15.36 The bones of the pelvis and the upper part of the left femur.

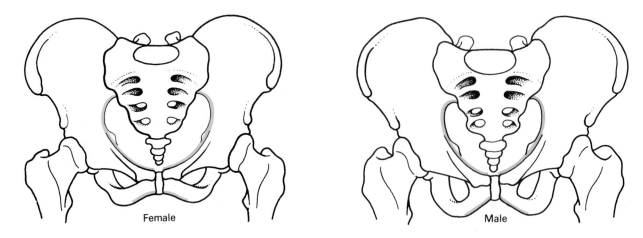

Figure 15.37 Diagram showing the difference in shape of the male and female pelves.

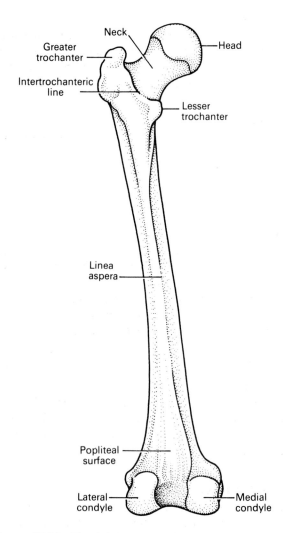

Figure 15.38 The left femur. Posterior aspect.

male pelvis, the female pelvis has lighter bones, is more shallow and rounded and is generally more roomy.

Femur or thigh bone (Fig. 15.38)

The femur is the longest and strongest bone of the body. The head is almost spherical and fits into the *acetabulum* of the hip bone to form the *hip joint*. In the centre of the head there is a small depression for the attachment of the *ligament of the head of the femur*. This extends from the acetabulum to the femur and contains a blood vessel that supplies blood to an area of the head of the bone. The neck extends outwards and slightly downwards from the head to the shaft and most of it is within the capsule of the hip joint.

The posterior surface of the lower third forms a flat triangular area called the *popliteal surface*. The distal extremity has two articular *condyles* which, with the tibia and patella, form the knee joint.

Tibia or shin bone (Fig. 15.39)

The tibia is the medial of the two bones of the lower leg. The proximal extremity is broad and flat and presents two *condyles* for articulation with the femur at the *knee joint*. The head of the fibula articulates with the inferior aspect of the lateral condyle, forming the *superior tibiofibular* joint.

The distal extremity of the tibia forms the *ankle joint* with the *talus* and the fibula. The *medial malleolus* is a downward projection of bone medial to the ankle joint.

Fibula

The fibula is the long slender lateral bone in the leg. The head or upper extremity articulates with the lat-eral condyle of the tibia and the lower extremity articu-

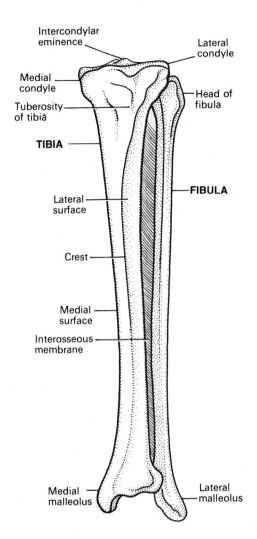

Figure 15.39 The left tibia and fibula with the interosseous membrane.

lates with the tibia then projects beyond it to form the *lateral malleolus*.

Patella or knee cap
This is a roughly triangular-shaped *sesamoid* bone associated with the knee joint. Its posterior surface articulates with the patellar surface of the femur in the knee joint and its anterior surface is in the *patellar tendon*, i.e. the tendon of the quadriceps femoris muscle.

Tarsal or ankle bones (Fig. 15.40)
There are seven tarsal bones which form the posterior part of the foot. They are:

- 1 talus
- 1 calcaneus
- 1 navicular
- 3 cuneiform
- 1 cuboid.

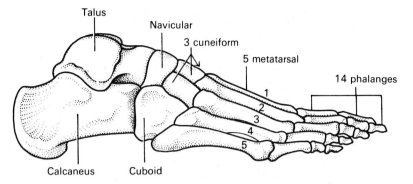

Figure 15.40 The bones of the foot. Lateral view.

The talus articulates with the tibia and fibula at the ankle joint. The other bones articulate with each other and with the metatarsal bones.

Metatarsal bones
These are five bones, numbered from within outwards, which form the greater part of the dorsum of the foot. At their proximal ends they articulate with the tarsal bones and at their distal ends, with the phalanges.

Phalanges
There are 14 phalanges arranged in a similar manner to those in the fingers, i.e. two in the great toe and three in each of the other toes.

Arches of the foot

The arrangement of the bones of the foot is such that it is not a rigid structure. This point is well illustrated by comparing a normal foot with a 'flat' foot. The bones have a bridge-like arrangement and are supported by muscles and ligaments so that four arches are formed, a *medial* and *lateral longitudinal arch* and two *transverse arches*.

Medial longitudinal arch
This is the highest of the arches and is formed by the calcaneus, navicular, three cuneiform and first three metatarsal bones. Only the calcaneus and the distal end of the metatarsal bones should touch the ground.

Lateral longitudinal arch
The lateral arch is much less marked than its medial counterpart. The bony components are the calcaneus, cuboid and the two lateral metatarsal bones. Again

only the calcaneus and metatarsal bones should touch the ground.

Transverse arches

These run across the foot and can be more easily seen by examining the skeleton than the live model. They are most marked at the level of the three cuneiform and cuboid bones.

Muscles and ligaments which support the arches of the foot (Fig. 15.41)

As there are movable joints between all the bones of the foot, very strong muscles and ligaments are necessary to maintain the strength, resilience and stability of the foot during walking, running and jumping.

Posterior tibialis muscle

This is the most important muscular support of the medial longitudinal arch. It lies on the posterior aspect of the lower leg, originates from the middle third of the tibia and fibula and its tendon passes behind the medial malleolus to be inserted into the navicular, cuneiform, cuboid and metatarsal bones. It acts as a sling or 'suspension apparatus' for the arch.

Short muscles of the foot

This group of muscles is mainly concerned with the maintenance of the lateral longitudinal and transverse arches. They make up the fleshy part of the sole of the foot.

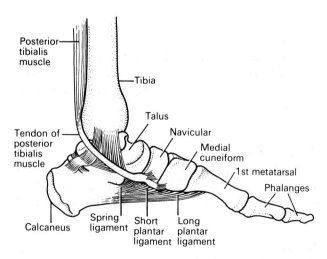

Figure 15.41 The tendons and ligaments supporting the arches of the foot. Medial view.

Plantar calcaneonavicular ligament or 'spring' ligament

This is a very strong thick ligament stretching from the calcaneus to the navicular bone. It plays an important part in supporting the medial longitudinal arch.

Plantar ligaments and interosseous membranes

These structures support the lateral and transverse arches.

HEALING OF BONES

Bone fractures are classified as:

- *simple:* the bone ends do not protrude through the skin
- *compound:* the bone ends protrude through the skin
- *pathological:* fracture of a bone weakened by disease.

Following a fracture, the broken ends of bone are joined by the deposition of new bone. This occurs in several stages (Fig. 15.42):

- formation of a haematoma between the ends of bone and in surrounding soft tissues
- development of acute inflammation and accumulation of macrophages which phagocytose the haematoma, inflammatory exudate and small fragments of bone without blood supply (this takes about 5 days)
- growth of granulation tissue and new blood vessels
- development of large numbers of osteoblasts that secrete non-lamellar osteoid which is quickly organised into lamellar osteoid and calcified, forming *callus* (in about 3 weeks)
- shaping of new bone by osteoclasts which remove excess callus and open up a medullary canal in the callus (in weeks or months).

Factors that delay healing of fractures

Infection

Microbes usually gain access through broken skin, although they may be blood-borne if healing is delayed. Inflammatory swelling increases pressure in the bone, leading to ischaemia and necrosis.

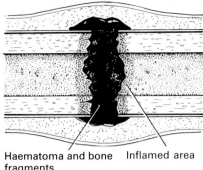

Haematoma and bone fragments   Inflamed area

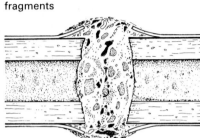

Phagocytosis of clot and debris. Growth of granulation tissue begins

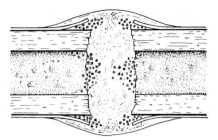

Osteoblasts begin to form new bone or callus

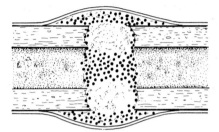

Gradual spread of new bone to bridge gap

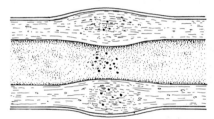

Bone healed. Osteoclasts reshape and canalise new bone

Figure 15.42   Stages in bone healing.

Fat embolism

Emboli, consisting of fat from the medullary canal, may enter torn veins. They are most likely to lodge in the lungs.

Tissue fragments between the ends of bone

Splinters of dead bone (*sequestra*) and soft tissue fragments not removed by phagocytosis delay osteogenesis.

Deficient blood supply

This delays growth of granulation tissue and new blood vessels. Hypoxia also reduces the number of osteoblasts and increases the number of chondroblasts that develop from their common parent cells. This may lead to cartilaginous union of the fracture. The most vulnerable sites, because of their normally poor blood supply, are the neck of femur, the scaphoid and the shaft of tibia.

Continued mobility

Continuous movement of the broken ends of bone tends to prevent osteogenesis. Fibrosis of the granulation tissue occurs, resulting in fibrous union of the fracture.

Old age

Healing of bones, like healing elsewhere, becomes slower with advancing age.

DISEASES OF BONES

Osteoporosis

In this condition the amount of bone tissue is reduced because its deposition does not keep pace with resorption, which may be due to diminished deposition or increased resorption. The imbalance may be continuously progressive or the balance may be temporarily or permanently restored. Cancellous bone is usually affected before compact bone, and the disease may be localised or general. The cause is not known.

Osteoporosis associated with immobility

Localised osteoporosis

This occurs in limbs and is secondary to lack of movement. The bones return to normal when mobility is restored. Immobility may be due to:

- treatment of a fracture
- paralysis
- protracted severe pain that results in voluntary immobilisation, e.g. in arthritis.

Generalised osteoporosis

This is usually secondary to prolonged unconsciousness. Excess calcium is resorbed from bone and raises the blood and urine calcium levels, predisposing to calculus formation in the kidneys which may lead to renal failure.

Ideopathic generalised osteoporosis

This is believed to be due to acceleration of the normal generalised reduction in bone substance that occurs in post-menopausal women and elderly men. It also occurs in some younger women, following oophorectomy. The cause is not entirely clear but one factor may be disturbance of the hormone balance between *anabolic steroids* (oestrogen and androgens) and *anti-anabolic steroids* (glucocorticoids). Fractures caused by relatively minor trauma or prolonged immobility may increase the rate of decalcification.

Paget's disease

In this disease there is hyperactivity of osteoblasts and osteoclasts and an abnormally rapid turnover of bone tissue. Bones become soft, thick and enlarged, and weight-bearing causes bowing. The bones most commonly affected are the pelvis, femur, tibia, lumbar vertebrae and the skull, usually in people over 40 years. The cause is not known. Complications may include:

- bone pain
- compression of cranial nerves in the diminished cranial foramina due to thickening of the bones, e.g. compression of the vestibulocochlear nerve, causing deafness
- fractures that may be spontaneous or follow minor trauma, occurring in spite of thickening of bones
- osteoarthritis, e.g. in the hip joint the acetabulum and head of the femur become soft and weight-bearing alters their shape; stresses in the misshapen joint damage the articular cartilage and, eventually, the underlying bone
- development of osteosarcoma (p. 395).

Rickets and osteomalacia

Rickets occurs in children and osteo- malacia in adults after ossification is complete. They are caused by deficiency of vitamin D which promotes calcification of bone and absorption of calcium in the small intestine. Vitamin D is present in some foods and is formed in the skin by the action of ultraviolet light on 7-dehydrocholesterol. Deficiency may be due to:

- a diet deficient in foods containing vitamin D, e.g. dairy products, fish, meat
- malabsorption syndromes, e.g. in association with coeliac disease or following gastrointestinal surgery
- lack of exposure to sunlight, e.g. in housebound people or because of cultural modes of dress
- excretion of excess vitamin D or its precursors, e.g. in chronic renal disease or long continued renal dialysis
- long continued use of some anticonvulsant drugs that convert vitamin D to inactive substances.

In *rickets* osteoid is deposited but calcification is incomplete. Although growth of the epiphyseal cartilage continues, growth generally is stunted. The bones remain soft and those of the lower limbs become bowed by the weight of the body.

In *osteomalacia* the normal processes of resorption and replacement of bone tissue are defective. As in rickets, osteoid is not calcified, the bones becoming soft, bowed and prone to fractures.

Infection of bones

Osteomyelitis

Microbes gain access to bones:

- through the skin in compound fractures
- by spread from a local focus of

infection, e.g. from a tooth abscess to the mandible or maxilla

- blood-borne from elsewhere in the body, commonly from a boil or paronychia (infection of the nail bed)
- during a surgical procedure.

The most common infecting organism is *Staphylococcus aureus* although mixed infection of the soft tissues of the feet, common in elderly diabetics, may spread to the bones. Infection of bone may lead to:

- necrosis, which prevents healing if pieces of dead bone (sequestra) are too large to be removed by phagocytosis
- pus formation in bone which causes considerable congestion in the confined space, and severe pain
- formation of a *subperiosteal abscess* that may rupture through the skin and drain through a sinus.

The outcome may be:

- resolution and complete repair
- delayed repair due to the presence of sequestrae
- chronic infection, often with acute exacerbations
- septicaemia and pyaemia if microbes or pus enter the bloodstream, leading to abscess formation elsewhere in the body, most commonly in the lungs, kidneys, myocardium and endocardium
- spread of the infection to joints, especially if the part of the bone infected is inside the joint capsule, e.g. neck of femur.

Developmental abnormalities of bone

Achondroplasia
This is caused by a genetic abnormality. There is defective growth of cartilage, especially the epiphyseal cartilage of long bones, leading to dwarfism and under-development of the bones of the base of the skull.

Osteogenesis imperfecta ('brittle bone syndrome')
This is a group of conditions in which there is a congenital defect of osteoblasts, resulting in failure of ossification. The bones are brittle and fracture easily, either spontaneously or following very slight trauma.

Tumours of bone

Benign tumours

Single or multiple tumours may develop for unknown reasons in:

- bone—*exostosis*
- cartilage—*endochondromas*.

They may cause pathological fractures or pressure damage to soft tissues, e.g. a vertebral exostosis may damage the spinal cord or a spinal nerve. Endochondromas have a tendency to undergo malignant change.

Malignant tumours

Metastatic tumours
The most common malignancies of bone are metastases of primary carcinomas of the breast, lungs, thyroid, kidneys and prostate gland. The usual sites are those with the best blood supply, i.e. cancellous bone, especially the bodies of the lumbar vertebrae and the epiphyses of the humerus and femur. Tumour fragments are spread in blood, and possibly along the walls of the veins from pelvic tumours to vertebrae. The effects of the malignancy may be:

- destruction of bone, leading to pathological fractures
- fibrosis of bone
- anaemia, leukopenia and thrombocytopenia but in most cases the link is not known
- collapse of vertebrae causing damage to the spinal cord and/ or spinal nerves.

Primary tumours

Osteosarcoma. This is a rapidly growing tumour believed to develop from the precursors of osteogenic cells. In young people between 10 and 25 years of age the tumour develops most commonly in the medullary canal of long bones, especially the femur. It is usually well advanced before it becomes evident. In older people, usually over 60 years of age, it is often associated with Paget's disease and the bones most commonly affected are the vertebrae, skull and pelvis.

Chondrosarcoma. These relatively slow-growing tumours are usually the result of malignant change in benign tumours of cartilage cells (endochondromas). They occur mainly between the ages of 40 and 70 years.

16
The joints

A joint is the site at which any two or more bones come together. Some joints have no movement (*fibrous*), some only slight movement (*cartilaginous*) and some are freely movable (*synovial*).

FIBROUS OR FIXED JOINTS (FIG. 16.1)

These immovable joints have fibrous tissue between the bones, e.g. joints between the bones of the skull (sutures) and those between the teeth and the maxilla and mandible.

CARTILAGINOUS OR SLIGHTLY MOVABLE JOINTS (FIG. 16.2)

There is a pad of *fibrocartilage* between the ends of the bones making up the joint which allows for very slight movement caused by compression of the pad of cartilage. Examples include the symphysis pubis and the joints between the bodies of the vertebrae.

SYNOVIAL OR FREELY MOVABLE JOINTS

Movements possible at synovial joints are:

- *flexion* or bending, usually forward but occasionally backward, e.g. knee joint
- *extension* means straightening or bending backward
- *abduction* is movement away from the midline of the body
- *adduction* is movement towards the midline of the body
- *circumduction* is the combination of flexion, extension, abduction and adduction
- *rotation* is movement round the long axis of a bone
- *pronation* means turning the palm of the hand down
- *supination* means turning the palm of the hand up
- *inversion* is turning the sole of the foot inwards
- *eversion* is turning the sole of the foot outwards.

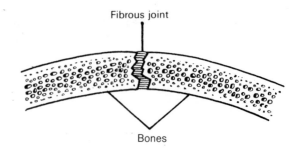

Figure 16.1 A fibrous or fixed joint, e.g. the sutures of the skull.

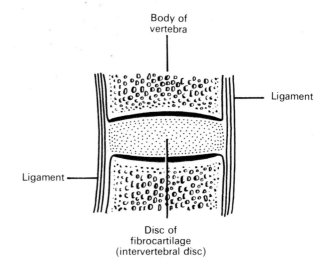

Figure 16.2 A cartilaginous or slightly movable joint, e.g. between the bodies of the vertebrae.

Synovial joints are classified according to the range of movement possible or to the shape of the articulating parts of the bones involved.

Ball and socket. The shape of the bones allows for a wide range of movement. Those possible are flexion, extension, abduction, adduction, rotation and circumduction. The joints are the shoulder and hip.

Hinge joints. These allow the movements of flexion and extension only. They are the elbow, knee, ankle, the joints between the atlas and the occipital bone, and the interphalangeal joints of the fingers and toes.

Gliding joints. The articular surfaces glide over each other, e.g. sternoclavicular joints, acromioclavicular joints and joints between the carpal bones and those between the tarsal bones.

Pivot joints. Movement is round one axis (rotation), e.g. proximal and distal radioulnar joints and the joint between the atlas and the odontoid process of the axis.

Condyloid and saddle joints. Movements take place round two axes, permitting flexion, extension, abduction, adduction and circumduction, e.g. the wrist, temporomandibular, metacarpophalangeal and metatarsophalangeal joints.

Characteristics of a synovial joint
(Fig. 16.3)

All synovial joints have certain characteristics in common.

Articular or hyaline cartilage. The parts of the bones which are in contact are always covered with hyaline cartilage. It provides a smooth articular surface and is strong enough to bear the weight of the body.

Capsule or capsular ligament. The joint is surrounded and enclosed by a sleeve of fibrous tissue which holds the bones together. It is sufficiently loose to allow freedom of movement but strong enough to protect it from injury.

Synovial membrane. This is found:

- lining the capsule
- covering those parts of the bones within the joint not covered by articular cartilage
- covering all intracapsular structures that do not bear weight.

It is composed of epithelial cells which secrete a thick sticky fluid, of egg-white consistency, *synovial fluid.* This is found inside the *synovial cavity,* and it:

- provides nutrient materials for the structures within the joint cavity
- contains phagocytes which remove microbes and cellular debris
- acts as a lubricant
- maintains joint stability
- prevents the ends of the bones from being separated as does a little water between two glass surfaces.

Little sacs of synovial fluid or *bursae* are present in some joints, e.g. the knee. They act as cushions to prevent friction between a bone and a ligament or tendon, or skin where a bone in a joint is near the surface.

Other intracapsular structures. Some joints have structures within the capsule, but outside the synovial membrane, which assist in maintenance of stability. When these structures do not bear weight they are covered by synovial membrane.

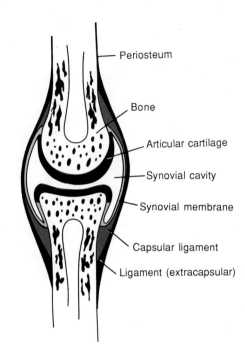

Figure 16.3   Diagram of simple synovial joint.

Extracapsular structures:

- *Ligaments* that blend with the capsule provide additional stability at most joints.
- *Muscles* or their *tendons* stretch across the joints they move. When the muscle contracts it shortens, pulling one bone towards the other.

Nerve and blood supply. Nerves and blood vessels crossing a joint usually supply the capsule and the muscles that move it.

MAIN SYNOVIAL JOINTS OF THE LIMBS

Individual synovial joints have the characteristics described above so only their distinctive features are included in this section.

Shoulder joint (Fig. 16.4)

This *ball and socket joint* is formed by the glenoid cavity of the scapula and the head of the humerus. The capsular ligament is very loose inferiorly to allow for the free movement normally possible at this joint. The

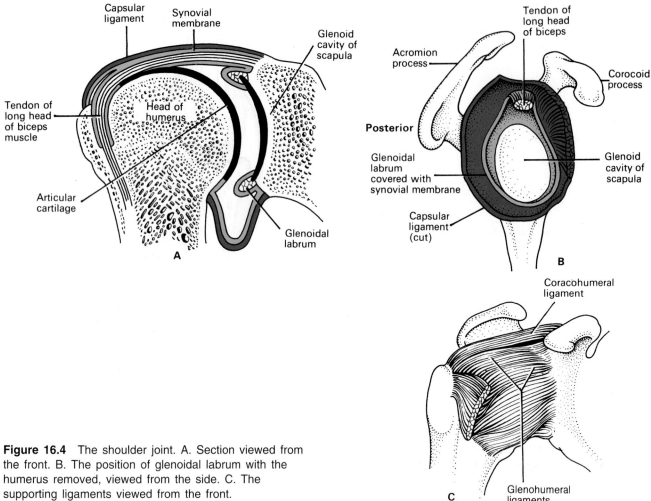

Figure 16.4 The shoulder joint. A. Section viewed from the front. B. The position of glenoidal labrum with the humerus removed, viewed from the side. C. The supporting ligaments viewed from the front.

glenoid cavity is deepened by a rim of fibrocartilage, the *glenoidal labrum*, which provides additional stability without limiting movement. The tendon of the long head of the *biceps muscle*, lying in the bicipital (intertubercular) groove of the humerus, extends through the joint cavity and is attached to the upper rim of the glenoid cavity. It has an important stabilising effect on the joint.

Synovial membrane forms a sleeve round the part of the tendon of the long head of the biceps muscles within the capsular ligament and covers the glenoidal labrum.

Extracapsular structures consist of:

- the *coracohumeral ligament*, extending from the coracoid process of the scapula to the humerus
- the *glenohumeral ligament* blends with and strengthens the capsule
- the *transverse humeral ligament*, retaining the biceps tendon in the intertubercular groove.

The stability of the joint may be reduced if these struc-

tures, together with the tendon of the biceps muscle, are stretched by repeated dislocations of the joint.

Muscles and movements (Fig. 16.5)

- *Flexion*: coracobrachialis, anterior fibres of deltoid and pectoralis major.
- *Extension*: teres major, latissimus dorsi and posterior fibres of deltoid.
- *Abduction*: deltoid.
- *Adduction*: combined action of flexors and extensors.
- *Circumduction*: flexors, extensors, abductors and adductors acting in series.
- *Medial rotation*: pectoralis major, latissimus dorsi, teres major and anterior fibres of deltoid.
- *Lateral rotation*: posterior fibres of deltoid.

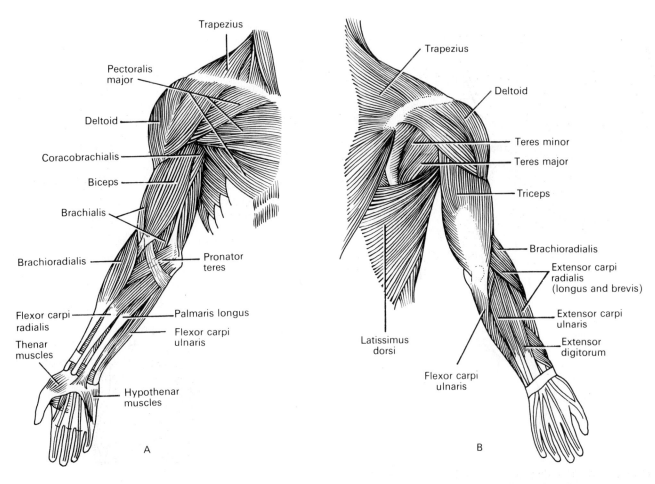

Figure 16.5 The main muscles which move the joints of the upper limb. A. Anterior view. B. Posterior view.

Coracobrachialis muscle lies on the upper medial aspect of the arm. It arises from the coracoid process of the scapula, stretches across in front of the shoulder joint and is inserted into the middle third of the humerus. It flexes the shoulder joint.

Deltoid muscle fibres originate from the clavicle, acromion process and spine of scapula and radiate over the shoulder joint to be inserted into the deltoid tuberosity of the humerus. The anterior fibres cause flexion, the middle or main part, abduction and the posterior fibres extend the shoulder joint.

Pectoralis major lies on the anterior thoracic wall. The fibres originate from the middle third of the clavicle and from the sternum and are inserted into the lip of the bicipital groove of the humerus. It draws the arm forward and towards the body, i.e. flexes and adducts.

Latissimus dorsi arises from the posterior part of the iliac crest and the spinous processes of the lumbar and lower thoracic vertebrae. It passes upwards across the back then under the arm to be inserted into the bicipital groove of the humerus. It adducts, medially rotates and extends the arm.

Teres major originates from the inferior angle of the scapula and is inserted into the humerus just below the shoulder joint. It extends and adducts the arm.

Elbow joint (Fig. 16.6)

This *hinge* joint is formed by the trochlea and the capitulum of the humerus and the trochlear notch of the ulna and the head of the radius.

Extracapsular structures consist of anterior, posterior, medial and lateral strengthening ligaments.

Muscles and movements (Fig. 16.5)

- *Flexion*: biceps and brachialis.
- *Extension*: triceps.

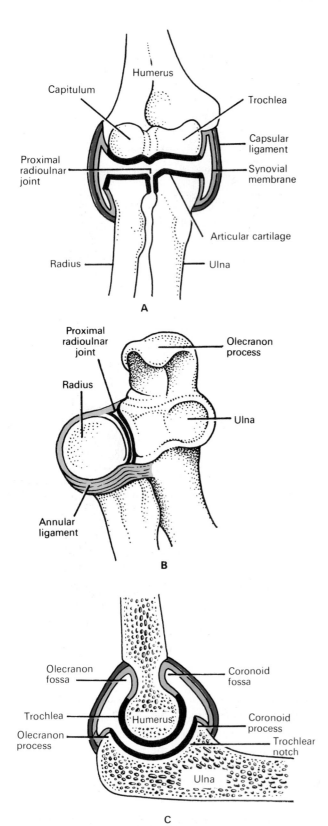

Figure 16.6 The elbow and proximal radioulnar joints. A. Section viewed from the front. B. The proximal radioulnar joint, viewed from above. C. Section of the elbow joint, partly flexed, viewed from the side.

Biceps muscle lies on the anterior aspect of the upper arm. At its proximal end it is divided into two parts (heads) each of which has its own tendon. The short head rises from the coracoid process of the scapula and passes in front of the shoulder joint to the arm. The long head originates from the rim of the glenoid cavity and its tendon passes through the joint cavity and the bicipital groove to the arm. It is retained in the bicipital groove by a transverse ligament which stretches across the groove. The distal tendon crosses the elbow joint and is inserted into the radial tuberosity. It helps to stabilise and flex the shoulder joint and at the elbow joint it assists with flexion and supination.

Brachialis lies on the anterior aspect of the upper arm deep to the biceps. It originates from the shaft of the humerus, extends across the elbow joint and is inserted into the ulna just distal to the joint capsule. It is the main flexor of the elbow joint.

Triceps muscle lies on the posterior aspect of the humerus. It arises from three heads, one from the scapula and two from the posterior surface of the humerus. The insertion is by a single tendon to the olecranon process of the ulna. It extends the elbow joint.

Proximal and distal radioulnar joints

The *proximal radioulnar joint*, formed by the rim of the head of the radius rotating in the radial notch of the ulna, is in the same capsule as the elbow joint. The *annular ligament* is a strong extracapsular ligament which encircles the head of the radius and keeps it in contact with the radial notch of the ulna (Fig. 16.6).

The distal *radioulnar joint* is a pivot joint between the distal end of the radius and the head of the ulna (Fig. 16.7).

Muscles and movements (Fig. 16.5)

- *Pronation*: pronator teres.
- *Supination*: supinator and biceps.

Pronator teres lies obliquely across the upper third of the front of the forearm. It arises from the medial epicondyle of the humerus and the coronoid process of the ulna, passes obliquely across the forearm to be inserted into the lateral surface of the shaft of the radius. It rotates the radioulnar joints, changing the hand from the anatomical to the writing position, i.e. pronation.

Supinator muscle lies obliquely across the posterior and lateral aspects of the forearm. Its fibres arise from the lateral epicondyle of the humerus and the upper part of the ulna and are inserted into the lateral surface of the upper third of the radius. It rotates the radioulnar joints, changing the hand from the writing to the anatomical position, i.e. supination. It lies deep to the muscles shown in Figure 16.5.

Wrist joint (Fig. 16.7)

This is a *condyloid* joint between the distal end of the radius and the proximal ends of the scaphoid, lunate and triquetral. A disc of *fibrocartilage* separates the ulna from the joint cavity and articulates with the carpal bones. It also separates the inferior radioulnar joint from the wrist joint.

Extracapsular structures consist of medial and lateral ligaments and anterior and posterior radiocarpal ligaments.

Muscles and movements (Fig. 16.5)

- *Flexion*: flexor carpi radialis and the flexor carpi ulnaris.
- *Extension*: extensors carpi radialis (longus and brevis) and the extensor carpi ulnaris.
- *Abduction*: flexor and extensors carpi radialis.
- *Adduction*: flexor and extensor carpi ulnaris.

Flexor carpi radialis lies on the anterior surface of the forearm. It originates from the medial epicondyle of the humerus and is inserted into the second and third metacarpal bones. It flexes the wrist joint, and when acting with the extensor carpi radialis, abducts the joint.

Flexor carpi ulnaris lies on the medial aspect of the forearm. It originates from the medial epicondyle of the humerus and the upper parts of the ulna and is inserted into the pisiform, the hamate and the fifth metacarpal bones. It flexes the wrist, and when acting with the extensor carpi ulnaris, adducts the joint.

Extensor carpi radialis longus and brevis lie on the posterior aspect of the forearm. The fibres originate from the lateral epicondyle of the humerus and are inserted by a long tendon into the second and third metacarpal bones. They extend and abduct the wrist.

Extensor carpi ulnaris lies on the posterior surface of the forearm. It originates from the lateral epicondyle of the humerus and is inserted into the fifth metacarpal bone. It extends and adducts the wrist.

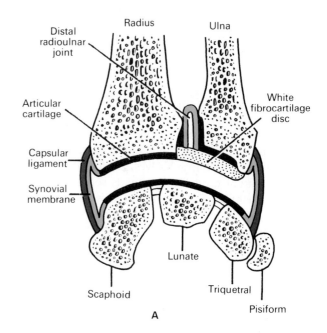

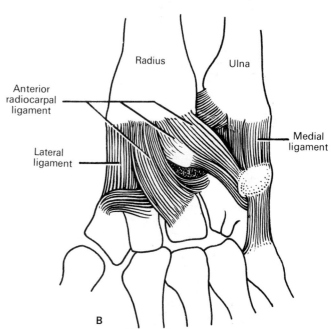

Figure 16.7 The wrist and distal radioulnar joints. Anterior view. A. Section. B. Supporting ligaments.

Joints of the hands and fingers

There are synovial joints between the carpal bones, between the carpal and metacarpal bones, between the metacarpal bones and proximal phalanges and between the phalanges. The powerful movements that occur at these joints are produced by muscles in the forearm which have tendons extending into the hand. Many of the finer movements of the fingers are produced by numerous small muscles in the hand.

The flexor retinaculum is a strong fibrous band that stretches across the front of the carpal bones, enclosing their concavity and forming the *carpal tunnel*. The tendons of flexor muscles of the wrist joint and the fingers and the median nerve pass through the carpal tunnel, the retinaculum holding them close to the bones. Synovial membrane forms sleeves around these tendons in the carpal tunnel and extends some way into the palm of the hand. Synovial sheaths also enclose the tendons on the flexor surfaces of the fingers. Synovial fluid prevents friction that might damage the tendons as they move over the bones (Fig. 16.8).

The extensor retinaculum is a strong fibrous band that extends across the back of the wrist. Tendons of muscles that extend the wrist and finger joints are encased in synovial membrane under the retinaculum. The synovial sheaths are less extensive than on the flexor aspect. The synovial fluid secreted prevents friction.

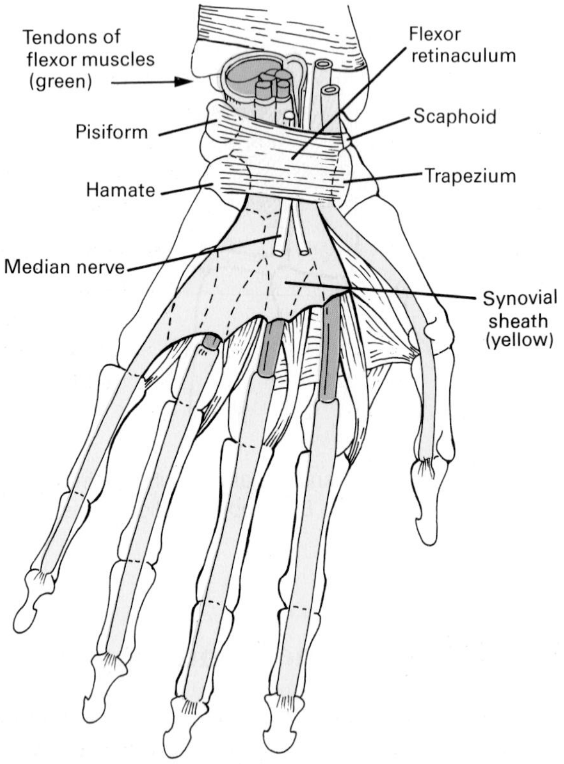
Tendons of flexor muscles (green)
Flexor retinaculum
Pisiform
Scaphoid
Hamate
Trapezium
Median nerve
Synovial sheath (yellow)

Figure 16.8 The carpal tunnel and synovial sheaths in the wrist and hand in yellow; tendons in green.

Hip joint (Fig. 16.9)

This *ball* and *socket* joint is formed by the cup-shaped acetabulum of the innominate bone and the almost spherical head of the femur. The capsular ligament includes most of the neck of the femur. The cavity is deepened by the *acetabular labrum*, a ring of fibrocartilage attached to the rim of the acetabulum. This adds stability to the joint without limiting its range of movement. The ligament of the head of the femur extends from the shallow depression in the middle of the head of the femur to the acetabulum. It conveys a blood vessel to the head of the femur. Synovial membrane covers both sides of the acetabular labrum and forms a sleeve around the ligament of the head of the femur. There are three important ligaments that surround and strengthen the capsule. They are the iliofemoral, ischiofemoral and pubofemoral ligaments.

Muscles and movements (Figs 16.10 and 16.11)

- *Flexion*: psoas, iliacus, rectus femoris and sartorius.
- *Extension*: gluteus maximus and the hamstrings.
- *Abduction*: gluteus medius and minimus, sartorius and others.
- *Adduction*: adductor group.
- *Lateral rotation*: mainly gluteal muscles and adductor group.
- *Medial rotation*: gluteus medius and minimus and others.

Psoas muscle arises from the transverse processes and bodies of the lumbar vertebrae. It passes across the flat part of the ilium and behind the inguinal ligament to be inserted into the femur. Together with the iliacus it flexes the hip joint (Fig. 16.10).

Iliacus muscle lies in the iliac fossa of the innominate bone. It originates from the iliac crest, passes over the iliac fossa and joins the tendon of the psoas muscle to be inserted into the femur. The combined action of iliacus and psoas flexes the hip joint.

Quadriceps femoris is a group of four muscles lying on the front of the thigh. They are *rectus femoris* and *three vasti*. The rectus femoris originates from the ilium and the three vasti from the upper end of the femur. Together they pass over the front of the knee joint to be inserted into the tibia by the patellar tendon. Only the rectus femoris flexes the hip joint. Together the group acts as a very strong extensor of the knee joint.

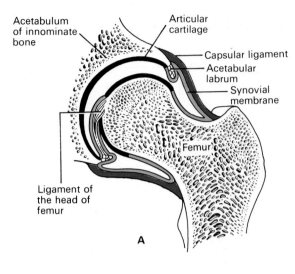

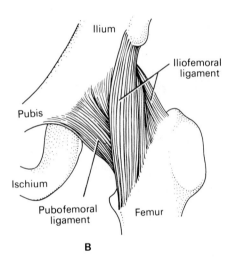

Figure 16.9 The hip joint. Anterior view. A. Section. B. Supporting ligaments. C. Head of femur and acetabulum separated to show acetabular labrum and ligament of head of femur.

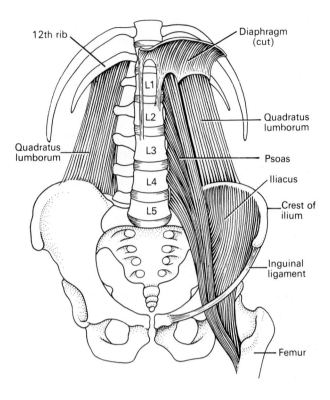

Figure 16.10 The muscles of the posterior abdominal wall and pelvis which flex the hip joint.

Gluteal muscles consist of the gluteus maximus, medius and minimus which together form the fleshy part of the buttock. They originate from the ilium and sacrum and are inserted into the femur. They cause extension, abduction and medial rotation at the hip joint.

Sartorius is the longest muscle in the body. It originates from the anterior superior iliac spine and passes obliquely across the hip joint, thigh and knee joint to be inserted into the medial surface of the upper part of the tibia. It is associated with flexion and abduction at the hip joint and flexion at the knee.

Adductor group lies on the medial aspect of the thigh. They originate from the pubic bone and are inserted into the linea aspera of the femur. They adduct the thigh.

Knee joint (Fig. 16.12)

This *hinge* joint is formed by the condyles of the femur, the condyles of the tibia and the posterior surface of the patella. The anterior part of the capsule consists of the tendon of the quadriceps femoris muscle which also supports the patella. Intracapsular structures in-

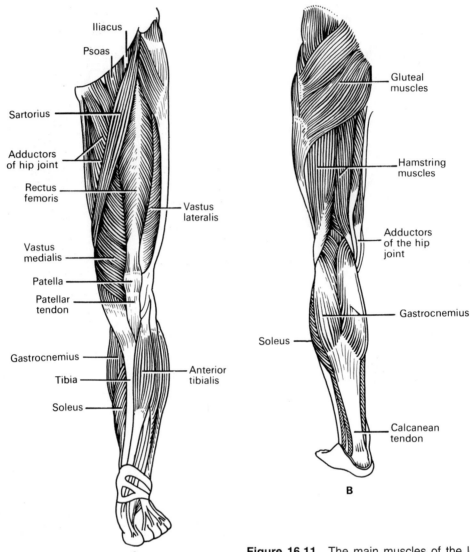

Figure 16.11 The main muscles of the lower limb.
A. Anterior view. B. Posterior view.

clude two cruciate ligaments which cross each other, extending from the intercondylar notch of the femur to the intercondylar eminence of the tibia. They help to stabilise the joint.

Semilunar cartilages or *menisci* are incomplete discs of white fibrocartilage lying on top of the articular condyles of the tibia. They are wedge-shaped, being thicker at their outer edges. They help to stabilise the joint by preventing lateral displacement of the bones.

Bursae and *pads of fat* are numerous. They prevent friction between a bone and a ligament or tendon and between the skin and the patella. Synovial membrane covers the cruciate ligaments and the pads of fat. The menisci are not covered with synovial membrane because they are weight-bearing. The most important strengthening ligaments are the medial and lateral ligaments.

Muscles and movement (Fig. 16.11)

The movements are flexion, extension and a rotatory movement which 'locks' the joint when it is fully extended. When the joint is locked, balance is maintained with less muscular effort than when it is flexed.

- *Flexion* (bending backwards): gastrocnemius and hamstrings.
- *Extension* (straightening): quadriceps femoris muscle.

Hamstring muscles lie on the posterior aspect of the thigh. They originate from the ischium and are inserted into the upper end of the tibia. They are *biceps femoris*, *semimembranosus* and *semitendinosus muscles*. They flex the knee joint.

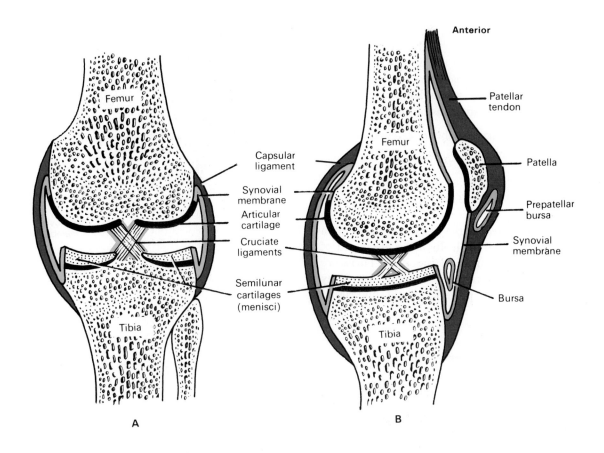

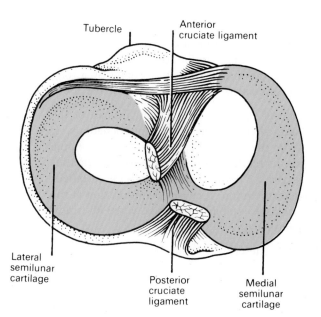

Figure 16.12 The knee joint. A. Section viewed from the front. B. Section viewed from the side. C. The superior surface of the tibia showing the semilunar cartilages and the cruciate ligaments.

Gastrocnemius forms the bulk of the calf of the leg. It arises by two heads, one from each condyle of the femur, and passes down behind the tibia to be inserted into the calcaneus by the *calcanean tendon (Achilles tendon)*. It crosses both knee and ankle joints, causing flexion at the knee and plantarflexion at the ankle.

Quadriceps femoris (described above) extends the knee joint.

Ankle joint (Fig. 16.13)

This *hinge* joint is formed by the distal end of the tibia and its malleolus (medial malleolus), the distal end of the fibula (lateral malleolus) and the talus. There are four important ligaments strengthening this joint. They are the deltoid and anterior, posterior, medial and lateral ligaments.

Muscles and movements (Fig. 16.11)

- *Flexion (dorsiflexion)*: anterior tibialis assisted by the muscles which extend the toes.
- *Extension (plantarflexion)*: gastrocnemius and soleus assisted by the muscles which flex the toes.

The movements of *inversion* and *eversion* occur between the tarsal bones and not at the ankle joint.

Anterior tibialis muscle originates from the upper end of the tibia, lies on the anterior surface of the leg and is inserted into the middle cuneiform bone by a long tendon. It is associated with dorsiflexion of the foot.

Soleus is one of the main muscles of the calf of the leg, lying immediately deep to the gastrocnemius. It originates from the heads and upper parts of the fibula and the tibia. Its tendon joins that of the gastrocnemius so that they have a common insertion into the calcaneus by the calcanean tendon. It causes plantarflexion at the ankle and helps to stabilise the joint when the individual is standing up.

Gastrocnemius (described above) is a powerful plantarflexor.

Joints of the foot and toes

There are a number of synovial joints between the tarsal bones, between the tarsal and metatarsal bones, between the metatarsals and proximal phalanges and be-

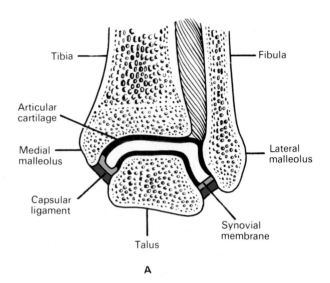

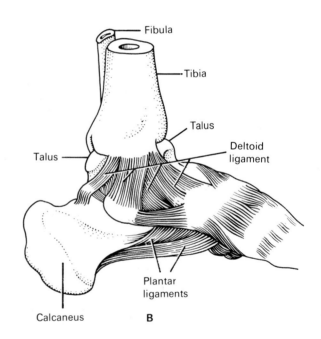

Figure 16.13 The left ankle joint. A. Section viewed from the front. B. Supporting ligaments. Medial view.

tween the phalanges. Movements are produced by muscles in the leg with long tendons which cross the ankle joint, and by muscles of the foot. The tendons crossing the ankle joint are encased in synovial sheaths and are held close to the bones by strong transverse ligaments. They move smoothly within their sheaths as the joints move. In addition to moving the joints of the foot these muscles support the arches of the foot and help to maintain body balance.

DISORDERS OF JOINTS

The tissues involved in diseases of the synovial joints are synovial membrane, hyaline cartilage and bone.

Inflammatory diseases of joints (arthritis)

Rheumatoid arthritis (RA, rheumatoid disease)

This is a chronic progressive inflammatory autoimmune disease. It is a systemic disorder where inflammatory changes not only affect synovial joints but also many other sites including:

- blood vessels
- the heart
- the skin.

It is more common in females than males and can affect all ages, including children, although it usually develops between the ages of 35 and 55 years. The cause is not clearly understood but it may be that development of the autoimmunity is initiated by microbial infection, possibly by viruses, in genetically susceptible people. Antigen/antibody complexes (*rheumatoid factors*) are formed and are often found in the blood and synovial fluid (*seropositive RA*). Seropositive individuals tend to have a more aggressive form of RA than those without rheumatoid factors, i.e. seronegative RA. Rheumatoid factors appear early in severe cases of sudden onset, and later when the disease develops gradually.

RA is an acute febrile condition, usually with periods of remission and exacerbation of varying lengths of time. The joints most commonly affected are those of the hands and feet, but in severe cases most of the synovial joints may be involved.

With each febrile exacerbation of the disease there is additional and cumulative damage to the joints, leading to increasing deformity, pain and loss of function. The primary changes that may be *reversible* include hypertrophy and hyperplasia of synovial cells and fibrinous inflammatory effusion into the joint. If the disease progresses there are further secondary changes which may be *irreversible*, including:

- erosion of articular cartilage and the growth of granulation tissue (*pannus*) that separates the bones and distorts the shape of the joint
- fibrosis of pannus which causes adhesions between the bones, limiting movement
- ossification of the fibrosed pannus, further restricting joint movement
- spread of granulation tissue to tendons
- weakening and atrophy of muscles possibly due to limited exercise
- development of collagen rheumatoid nodules outside the joints, e.g. in pressure areas such as the elbows, over the knuckles and in the lungs, pleura, heart and eyes
- enlargement of lymph nodes and spleen.

In the later stages of the disease the inflammation and fever are less marked and movement is limited by deformity of the joint, muscle weakness and pain.

Other types of polyarthritis

This group of autoimmune inflammatory arthritic diseases has many characteristics similar to rheumatoid arthritis but the rheumatoid factor is absent. The causes are not known but genetic features may be involved.

The joints affected are mainly those of the axial skeleton. The diseases include:

- *ankylosing spondylitis* in which the sacroiliac and vertebral joints become ossified
- *psoriatic arthritis* that occurs in a proportion of people who suffer from psoriasis, especially if the nails are involved
- *Reiter's syndrome* (polyarthritis with urethritis and conjunctivitis) which, it is believed, may be precipitated by infection with *Chlamydia trachomatis*; the affected joints are usually those of the lower limb
- arthritis that complicates acute rheumatic fever.

Acute infective arthritis

Many commonly occurring microbes may be carried in the blood to the joints from foci of infection elsewhere in the body. In most cases the joint has been damaged by previous injury or arthritic disease. The outcome may be:

- resolution of the infection with no residual ill-effects
- suppuration followed by healing with the formation of fibrous tissue that may become ossified
- development of chronic infection, especially in brucellosis, gonorrhoea and tuberculosis.

Traumatic injury to joints

Sprains, strains and dislocations

These damage the soft tissues, tendons and ligaments round the joint without penetrating the joint capsule. In dislocations there may be additional damage to intracapsular structures by stretching, e.g. long head of biceps muscle in the shoulder joint, cruciate ligaments in the knee joint, ligament of head of femur in the hip joint. If repair is incomplete there may be some loss of stability which increases the risk of repeated injury.

Penetrating injuries

These may be caused by a compound fracture of one of the articulating bones, or trauma caused by, e.g. gun shot. Healing may be uneventful or it may be delayed by:

- the presence in the joint of tissue fragments or sequestra too large to be removed by phagocytes
- incomplete healing of torn ligaments inside the capsule
- infection that may be blood-borne or enter through broken skin.

When healing is incomplete there is a tendency for irreversible degenerative changes to occur.

Osteoarthritis (osteoarthrosis, OA)

This is a degenerative non-inflammatory disease that results in pain and restricted movement of affected joints. Osteoarthrosis is the more appropriate name but is less commonly used. Articular cartilage gradually becomes thinner because its replacement does not keep pace with its removal. Eventually the bony articular surfaces come in contact and the bones begin to degenerate. There is abnormal bone repair and the articular surfaces become misshapen. Chronic inflammation develops with effusion into the joint, possibly due to irritation caused by tissue debris not removed by phagocytes. Sometimes there is

abnormal outgrowth of cartilage at the edges of bones which becomes ossified, forming *osteophytes*.

Primary osteoarthritis

In this type the cause is unknown. Changes may be due to acceleration of the normal ageing process in joints that have had excessive use. It usually develops in late middle age and affects large weight-bearing joints, i.e. the hips, knees and joints of the cervical and lower lumbar spine. In many cases only one joint is involved.

Osteoarthritis of spine
This condition is relatively common in the elderly. Degenerative changes cause narrowing of intervertebral discs and osteophytes may develop round the margins of joints of the vertebral column, commonly in the cervical region. They may cause damage to the nervous system, varying from compression of individual spinal nerves to spinal cord injury.

Secondary osteoarthritis

This occurs in joints in which cartilage has already been damaged due to:

- congenital deformity of bones, e.g. in congenital dislocation of the hip there are unusual stresses in the joint
- trauma, e.g. intracapsular fracture of a bone, injury to intracapsular structures
- disease, e.g. inflammatory diseases, incomplete repair following injury, haemophilia with repeated haemorrhages into the joints, peripheral nerve lesions, gout, acromegaly (p. 227), diabetic neuropathy in which the joints of the feet are most commonly involved.

Gout

This is caused by the deposition of sodium urate crystals in joints and tendons. Acute inflammation is due to chemotaxic substances released by phagocytes that have ingested the crystals. It occurs in some people whose blood uric acid is abnormally high due to either overproduction or defective excretion by the kidneys. Uric acid is a waste product of the breakdown of nucleic acids, i.e. DNA and RNA, and is produced in excess when there is large-scale cell destruction, e.g. following trauma or treatment with cytotoxic drugs and in anaemia, starvation and malignancy. Defective excretion occurs in some kidney conditions. Episodes of arthritis lasting days or weeks are interspersed with periods of remission. After repeated acute attacks permanent damage may occur. The joints most commonly affected are the metatarsophalangeal joint of the big toe, the ankle, knee, wrist and elbow. In many cases only one joint is affected. It is more prevalent in males than females.

Connective tissue diseases

This group of disorders has common features. They:

- affect many systems of the body, especially the joints, skin and subcutaneous tissues
- tend to occur in early adult life
- usually affect more females than males
- are chronic conditions
- are autoimmune diseases in which abnormal autoantibodies are formed that attack the individual's tissues.

These disorders include:

- *systemic lupus erythematosus* (SLE) in which the affected joints are usually the hands, knees and ankles. A characteristic red 'butterfly' rash may occur on the face. Kidney involvement is common and can result in glomerulonephritis that may be complicated by chronic renal failure.

■ *systemic sclerosis* (scleroderma) is a progressive thickening of connective tissue. There is increased production of collagen that affects many organs. In the skin there is dermal fibrosis and tightness that impairs the functioning of joints, especially the hands. It also affects the walls of blood vessels, intestinal tract and other organs.

■ *polyarteritis nodosa* (p. 118).
■ *rheumatoid arthritis* (p. 409).
■ *ankylosing spondylitis, Reiter's disease* (p. 409).

The muscular system

The three types of muscle tissue, their features and the nomenclature of skeletal muscles are described on page 28.

This chapter considers the skeletal muscles not involved in the movements of the joints of the limbs:

■ muscles of the face and neck
■ muscles of the back
■ muscles of the abdominal wall
■ muscles of the pelvic floor.

Muscles of respiration are described on page 252. The muscles that move the joints are described in Chapter 16.

MUSCLES OF THE FACE AND NECK (FIG. 17.1)

Muscles of the face

There are many muscles involved in changing facial expression and with movement of the lower jaw during chewing and speaking. Only the main muscles are described here. Except where indicated the muscles are present in pairs, one on each side.

Occipitofrontalis (unpaired) consists of a posterior muscular part over the occipital bone, an anterior part over the frontal bone and an extensive flat tendon or *aponeurosis* that stretches over the dome of the skull and joins the two muscular parts. It raises the eyebrows.

Levator palpebrae superioris extends from the posterior part of the orbital cavity to the upper eyelid. It raises the eyelid.

Orbicularis oculi surrounds the eye, eyelid and orbital cavity. It closes the eye and when strongly contracted 'screws up' the eyes.

Buccinator. This flat muscle of the cheek draws the cheeks in towards the teeth in chewing and in forcible expulsion of air from the mouth ('the trumpeter's muscle').

Orbicularis oris (unpaired) surrounds the mouth and blends with the muscles of the cheeks. It closes the lips and, when strongly contracted, shapes the mouth for whistling.

Masseter is a broad muscle, extending from the zygomatic arch to the angle of the jaw. In chewing it draws the mandible up to the maxilla and exerts considerable pressure on the food.

Temporalis covers the squamous part of the temporal bone. It passes behind the zygomatic arch to be inserted into the coronoid process of the mandible. It closes the mouth and assists with chewing.

Pterygoid muscle extends from the sphenoid bone to the mandible. It closes the mouth and pulls the lower jaw forward.

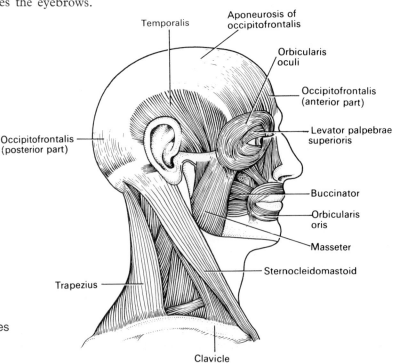

Figure 17.1 The main muscles on the right side of the face, head and neck.

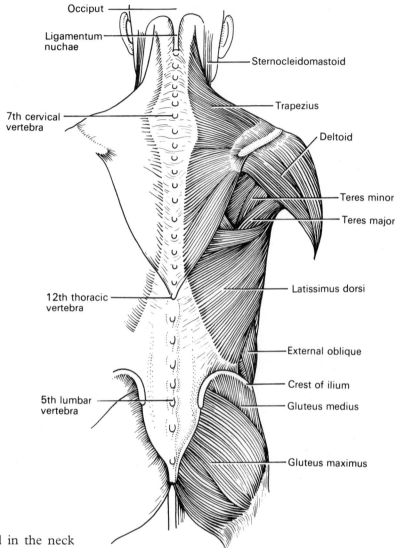

Occiput

Ligamentum nuchae

7th cervical vertebra

12th thoracic vertebra

Figure 17.2 The main muscles of the back.

5th lumbar vertebra

Sternocleidomastoid

Trapezius

Deltoid

Teres minor

Teres major

Latissimus dorsi

External oblique

Crest of ilium

Gluteus medius

Gluteus maximus

Muscles of the neck

There are a great many muscles situated in the neck but only the two largest are considered here.

Sternocleidomastoid muscle arises from the manubrium of the sternum and the clavicle and extends upwards to the mastoid process of the temporal bone. It assists in turning the head from side to side. When the muscle on one side contracts it draws the head towards the shoulder. When both contract at the same time they flex the cervical vertebrae or draw the sternum and clavicle upwards when the head is maintained in a fixed position, e.g. in forced respiration.

Trapezius muscle covers the shoulder and the back of the neck. The upper attachment is to the occipital protuberance, the medial attachment is to the transverse processes of the cervical and thoracic vertebrae and the lateral attachment is to the clavicle and to the spinous and acromion processes of the scapula. It pulls the head backwards, squares the shoulders and controls the movements of the scapula when the shoulder joint is in use.

MUSCLES OF THE BACK
(FIG. 17.2)

There are six pairs of large muscles in the back in addition to those that form the posterior abdominal wall. The arrangement of these muscles is the same on each side of the vertebral column. They are:

- trapezius
- teres major
- psoas

  } described in Chapter 16 in association with joints

- quadratus lumborum
- sacrospinalis
- latissimus dorsi.

Quadratus lumborum originates from the crest of the ilium then it passes upwards, parallel and close to the vertebral column and it is inserted into the 12th rib. Together the two muscles fix the lower rib during respiration and cause extension of the vertebral column (bending backwards). If one muscle contracts it causes lateral flexion of the lumbar region of the vertebral column.

Sacrospinalis is a group of muscles, lying between the spinous and transverse processes of the vertebrae. They originate from the sacrum and are finally inserted into the occipital bone. Their contraction causes extension of the vertebral column.

MUSCLES OF THE ABDOMINAL WALL (FIGS 17.3, 17.4 AND 17.5)

There are six pairs of muscles that form the abdominal wall. From the surface inwards they are:

- rectus abdominis
- external oblique
- internal oblique
- transversus abdominis
- quadratus lumborum } described in
- psoas } Chapter 16.

The anterior abdominal wall is divided longitudinally by a very strong midline tendinous cord, the *linea alba*, which extends from the xiphoid process of the sternum to the symphysis pubis. The structure of the abdominal wall on each side of the linea alba is identical.

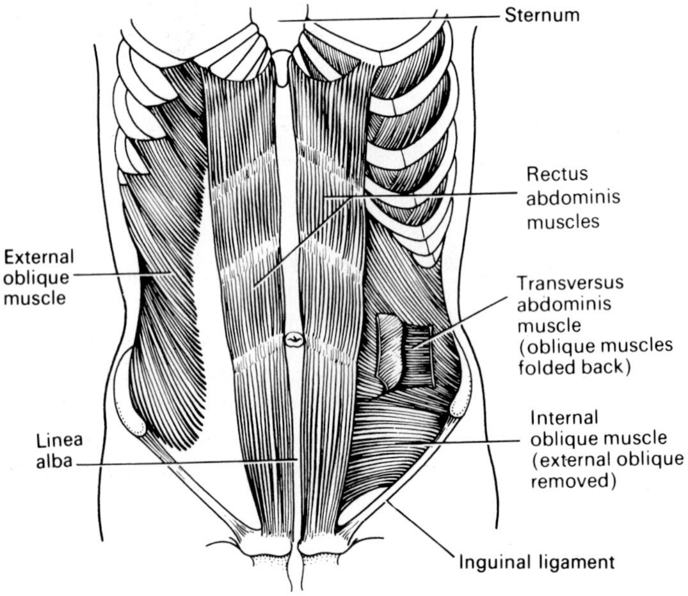

Sternum

Rectus abdominis muscles

External oblique muscle

Transversus abdominis muscle (oblique muscles folded back)

Internal oblique muscle (external oblique removed)

Linea alba

Inguinal ligament

Figure 17.3 The muscles of the abdominal wall.

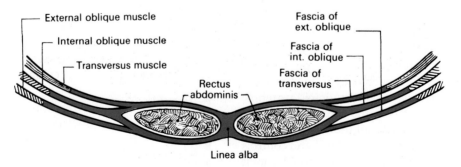

External oblique muscle

Internal oblique muscle

Transversus muscle

Rectus abdominis

Fascia of ext. oblique

Fascia of int. oblique

Fascia of transversus

Linea alba

Figure 17.4 Diagram of the arrangement of the fascia of the muscles of the anterior abdominal wall. Cross-section.

Rectus abdominis is the most superficial muscle. It is broad and flat, originating from the transverse part of the pubic bone then passing upwards to be inserted into the lower ribs and the xiphoid process of the sternum. Medially the two muscles are attached to the linea alba.

External oblique extends from the lower ribs *downwards* and *forward* to be inserted into the iliac crest and, by an aponeurosis, to the linea alba.

Internal oblique lies deep to the external oblique. Its fibres arise from the crest of the ilium and by a broad band of fascia from the spinous processes of the lumbar vertebrae. The fibres pass *upwards towards the midline* to be inserted into the lower ribs and, by an aponeurosis, into the linea alba. The fibres are at right angles to those of the external oblique.

Transversus abdominis is the deepest muscle of the abdominal wall. The fibres arise from the iliac crest and the lumbar vertebrae and pass across the abdominal wall to be inserted into the linea alba by an aponeurosis. The fibres are at right angles to those of the rectus abdominis.

Functions

The main function of the four pairs of muscles is to form the strong muscular anterior wall of the abdominal cavity. When the muscles contract together they:

- compress the abdominal organs
- flex the vertebral column in the lumbar region.

Contraction of the muscles on one side only bends the trunk towards that side. Contraction of the oblique muscles on one side rotates the trunk.

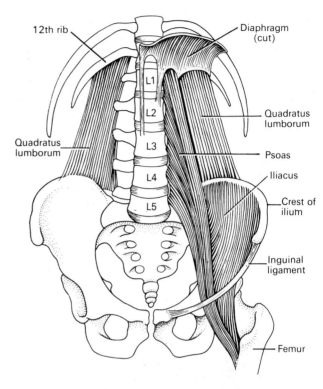

Figure 17.5 The deep muscles of the posterior abdominal wall.

Inguinal canal

This canal is 2.5 to 4 cm long and passes obliquely through the abdominal wall. It runs parallel to and immediately in front of the transversalis fascia and part of the inguinal ligament. In the male it contains the *spermatic cord* and in the female, the *round ligament*. It

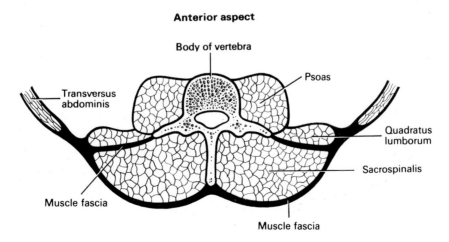

Figure 17.6 Transverse section of a lumbar vertebra and its associated muscles.

consitutes a weak point in the otherwise strong abdominal wall through which herniation may occur (see p. 327).

MUSCLES OF THE PELVIC FLOOR
(FIG. 17.7)

The pelvic floor is divided into two identical parts at the midline. Each half is made up of muscles and fascia which unite in the midline. The muscles are:

- levator ani
- coccygeus.

Levatores ani are broad flat muscles, forming the anterior part of the pelvic floor. They originate from the inner surface of the true pelvis and unite in the midline. Together they form a sling which supports the pelvic organs.

Coccygei are triangular sheets of muscle and tendinous fibres situated behind the levator ani. They originate from the medial surface of the ischium and are inserted into the sacrum and coccyx. They complete the formation of the pelvic floor which is perforated in the male by the urethra and anus, and in the female by the urethra, vagina and anus.

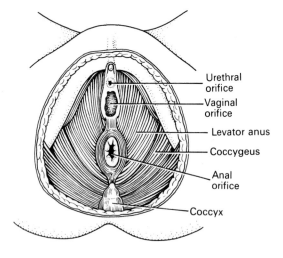

Figure 17.7 The muscles of the pelvic floor.

Urethral orifice
Vaginal orifice
Levator anus
Coccygeus
Anal orifice
Coccyx

Functions
The pelvic floor supports the organs of the pelvis and maintains continence, i.e. it plays a part in micturition and defaecation.

HEALING OF MUSCLE FIBRES

Muscle fibres may be damaged accidentally or be cut during surgery. The extent of the damage determines the mode and effectiveness of healing. In all cases, damaged tissue is removed by phagocytosis and replaced by granulation tissue.

In *slight injury* the small gap in the muscle fibre is bridged by outgrowths from the surviving ends of the fibre, completely restoring its integrity.

In *more extensive injury* the muscle fibre outgrowths may not be able to extend far enough into the granulation tissue to restore it completely. When this happens the remaining granulation tissue becomes fibrosed and scar tissue forms. In time this contracts and may restrict joint movement.

In *very extensive injury* repair is by fibrosis. In some cases, such as following the crushing of a limb, there may be systemic effects (*crush syndrome*).

REPAIR OF NERVES SUPPLYING MUSCLES

A *motor unit* consists of a lower motor neurone (LMN) and the muscle fibres it supplies. When the nerve supply is cut the muscle ceases to contract and gradually atrophies but, if the nerve regenerates, muscle fibre function is restored. The axon of the LMN in a peripheral nerve divides into numerous terminal branches each of which supplies a muscle fibre. In a bundle of muscle fibres the nerve supply is derived from several LMNs (see Fig. 7.10). Nerve supply to muscle fibres may be restored by:

- regeneration of the nerve if cut near the parent cell and if the cut ends are in close apposition (Fig. 17.8)
- the outgrowth of new terminal nerve fibres from the other axons supplying adjacent muscle fibres in the same bundle (Fig. 17.9)

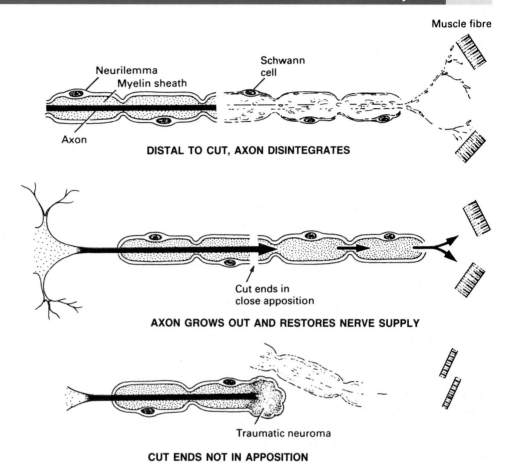

Figure 17.8   Regrowth of a peripheral nerve.

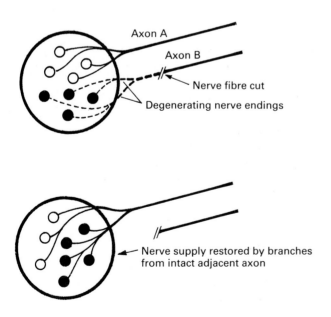

○ = bundles of muscle fibres supplied by Axon A
● = bundles of muscle fibres normally supplied by Axon B

Figure 17.9   Restoration of nerve supply to muscle.

DISEASES OF MUSCLES

Myasthenia gravis

This condition affects more women than men and usually those between 20 and 40 years. It is an auto-immune disease of unknown origin in which there is defective muscle stimulation. Antibodies develop which damage the acetylcholine receptors of neuromuscular junctions, blocking the transmission of the nerve impulses to muscle fibres (Fig. 7.7). This causes progressive and extensive muscle weakness. Extraocular and eyelid muscles are affected first causing *ptosis* (drooping of the eyelid) or *diplopia* (double vision), followed by those of the neck and limbs. There are periods of remission, relapses being precipitated by, e.g. severe muscular exercise, infections, emotional disturbances, pregnancy.

Myopathies

Progressive muscular dystrophies

In this group of inherited diseases there is progressive degeneration of groups of muscles. The main differences in the types are:

- age of onset
- rate of progression
- groups of muscles involved.

Duchenne type

Inheritance of this condition is sex linked from female carriers whose offspring may be affected if they are males (50% chance) or carriers if they are females (50% chance). See Figure 4.19.

The muscle abnormality is present before birth but may not be evident until the child is about 5 years of age. Wasting and weakness begin in muscles of the lower limbs then spread to the upper limbs, progressing rapidly without remission. Death usually occurs in adolescence, often from respiratory failure, cardiac arrhythmias or cardiomyopathy.

Facio-scapulo-humeral dystrophy

This disease usually begins in adolescence and the younger the age of onset the more rapidly it progresses. Muscles of the face and upper limbs are affected first. This is a chronic condition that usually progresses slowly and may not cause complete disability.

Myotonic dystrophy

This disease usually begins in adult life. Muscles contract and relax slowly, often seen as difficulty in releasing an object held in the hand. Muscles of the tongue and the face are first affected then muscles of the limbs. Systemic conditions associated with myotonic dystrophy include:

- premature cataract
- atrophy of the gonads
- cardiomyopathy
- endocrine disturbances, e.g. in insulin utilisation.

The disease progresses without remission and with increasing disability. Death usually occurs in middle age from respiratory or cardiac failure.

Crush syndrome

Sustained pressure, e.g. on a limb, causes ischaemia resulting in massive muscle necrosis. When pressure is relieved and the circulation is restored, myoglobin and other necrotic products enter the blood and pass to the kidneys. If there is too much of this material for the kidneys to cope with, death may result from acute renal failure. A common complication of this type of injury is infection, especially by anaerobic microbes, e.g. *Clostridium perfringens* (*Cl. welchii*) and other clostridia causing *gas gangrene*.

Healing of such extensive injury is by fibrosis.

18
The reproductive systems

The ability to reproduce is one of the properties which distinguishes living from non-living matter. The more primitive the animal, the simpler the process of reproduction. In human beings the process is one of sexual reproduction in which the male and female organs differ anatomically and physiologically.

Both males and females produce specialised reproductive germ cells, called *gametes*. In the male they are *spermatozoa* and in the female, *ova*. The gametes contain the genetic material, or *genes*, on *chromosomes*, which pass it on to the next generation. In other body cells there are 46 chromosomes arranged in 23 pairs but in the gametes there are only 23, one from each pair. Gametes are formed by *meiosis* (p. 21). When the ovum is fertilised by a spermatozoon the resultant *zygote* contains 23 *pairs* of chromosomes, one of each pair obtained from the father and one from the mother.

The zygote embeds itself in the wall of the uterus where it grows and develops during the 40-week *gestation period* before birth.

The functions of the female reproductive system are:

■ formation of female gametes, ova
■ reception of male gametes, spermatozoa
■ provision of suitable environments for fertilisation of the ovum by spermatozoa and development of the resultant fetus
■ parturition (childbirth)
■ lactation, nourishment of the baby with breast milk until it can take a mixed diet.

The functions of the male reproductive system are:

■ production of male gametes, spermatozoa
■ transmission of spermatozoa to the female.

FEMALE REPRODUCTIVE SYSTEM

The female reproductive organs, or genitalia, are divided into external and internal organs (Fig. 18.1).

External genitalia (Fig. 18.2)

The external genitalia are known collectively as the *vulva* which consists of:

■ labia majora   ■ vestibule
■ labia minora   ■ hymen
■ clitoris   ■ greater vestibular glands.

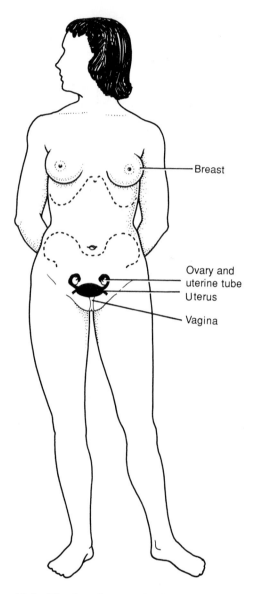

Figure 18.1   The female reproductive organs. Broken lines denote the positions of the lower ribs and the pelvis.

Labia majora

These are the two large folds which form the boundary of the *vulva*. They are composed of skin, fibrous tissue and fat and contain large numbers of sebaceous glands. Anteriorly the folds join in front of the symphysis pubis, and posteriorly they merge with the skin of the perineum. At puberty hair grows on the mons pubis and on the lateral surfaces of the labia majora.

Labia minora

These are two smaller folds of skin between the labia majora, containing numerous sebaceous glands. Poster-

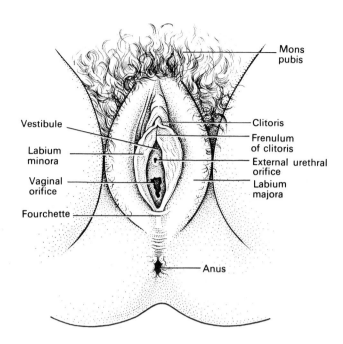

Figure 18.2   The external genitalia in the female.

iorly they fuse to form the *fourchette*.

The cleft between the labia minora is the *vestibule*. The vagina, urethra and ducts of the greater vestibular glands open into the vestibule.

Clitoris
The clitoris corresponds to the penis in the male and contains sensory nerve endings and erectile tissue but it has no reproductive significance.

Hymen
The hymen is a thin layer of mucous membrane which partially occludes the opening of the vagina.

Greater vestibular glands
The greater vestibular glands (Bartholin's glands) are situated one on each side near the vaginal opening. They are about the size of a small pea and have ducts, opening into the vestibule immediately lateral to the attachment of the hymen. They secrete mucus that keeps the vulva moist.

Blood supply, lymph drainage and nerve supply of the external genitalia
Arterial supply is by branches from the *internal pudendal arteries* that branch from the internal iliac arteries and by *external pudendal arteries* that branch from the femoral arteries.

Veins form a large plexus which eventually drains into the internal iliac veins.

Lymph drainage is through the superficial inguinal nodes.

Nerve supply is by branches from pudendal nerves.

Perineum
The perineum is the area extending from the fourchette to the anal canal. It is roughly triangular and consists of connective tissue, muscle and fat. It gives attachment to the muscles of the pelvic floor (p. 418).

Internal organs (Figs 18.3 and 18.4)

The internal organs of the female reproductive system lie in the pelvic cavity and consist of the vagina, uterus, two uterine tubes and two ovaries.

Vagina

The vagina is a fibromuscular tube lined with stratified epithelium, connecting the external and internal organs of reproduction. It runs obliquely upwards and backwards at an angle of about 45° between the bladder in front and rectum and anus behind. In the adult the anterior wall is about 7.5 cm (3 inches) long and the posterior wall about 9 cm long. The difference is due to the protrusion of the cervix through the anterior wall.

Structure

The vagina has an outer covering of *areolar tissue*, a middle layer of *smooth muscle* and an inner lining of *stratified squamous epithelium* that forms ridges or *rugae*. It has no secretory glands but the surface is kept moist by cervical secretions. Between puberty and the menopause *Lactobacillus acidophilus* microbes are normally present and they secrete *lactic acid*, maintaining the pH between 4.9 and 3.5. The acidity inhibits the growth of most microbes that may enter the vagina from the perineum.

Blood supply, lymph drainage and nerve supply
An *arterial plexus* is formed round the vagina, derived from the uterine and vaginal arteries which are branches of the internal iliac arteries.

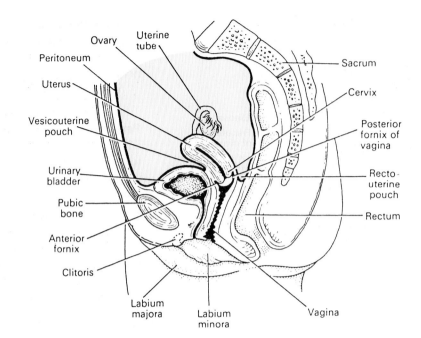

Figure 18.3 The female reproductive organs in the pelvis and their associated structures. Lateral view.

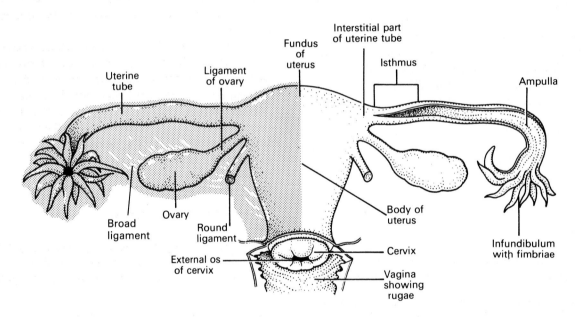

Figure 18.4 The female reproductive organs in the pelvis: posterior walls of the vagina and right uterine tube removed. Hatched area shows the arrangement of the peritoneum.

A *venous plexus*, situated in the muscular wall, drains into the internal iliac veins.

The lymph drainage is through the deep and superficial iliac glands.

The nerve supply consists of parasympathetic fibres from the sacral outflow, sympathetic fibres from the lumbar outflow and somatic sensory fibres from the pudendal nerves.

Uterus

The uterus is a hollow muscular pear-shaped organ, flattened anteroposteriorly. It lies in the pelvic cavity between the urinary bladder and the rectum in an anteverted anteflexed position.

Anteversion means that the uterus *leans forward*.

Anteflexion means that it is bent forward almost at right angles to the vagina with its anterior surface resting

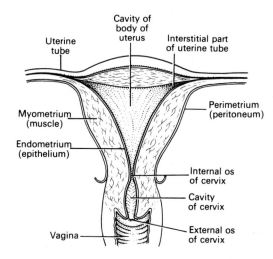

Figure 18.5 Diagram of a section of the uterus.

on the urinary bladder. As the bladder fills the degree of anteflexion is reduced slightly.

When the body is in the upright position the uterus lies in an almost horizontal position. It is about 7.5 cm long, 5 cm wide and its walls are about 2.5 cm thick. It weighs from 30 to 40 grams. The parts of the uterus are the fundus, body and cervix (Fig. 18.5).

The fundus is the dome-shaped part of the uterus above the openings of the uterine tubes.

The body is the main part. It is narrowest inferiorly at the *internal os* where it is continuous with the cervix.

The cervix protrudes through the anterior wall of the vagina, opening into it at the *external os*.

Structure

The walls of the uterus are composed of three layers of tissue: perimetrium, myometrium and endometrium.

Perimetrium consists of peritoneum, which is distributed differently on the various surfaces of the uterus (Fig. 18.3).

Anteriorly it extends over the fundus and the body where it is reflected on to the upper surface of the urinary bladder. This fold of peritoneum forms the *vesicouterine pouch.*

Posteriorly the peritoneum extends over the fundus, the body and the cervix, then it is reflected on to the rectum to form the *rectouterine pouch.*

Laterally only the fundus is covered because the peritoneum forms a double fold with the uterine tubes in the upper free border. This double fold is the *broad ligament* which, at its lateral ends, attaches the uterus to the sides of the pelvis.

Myometrium is the thickest layer of tissue in the uterine wall. It consists of a mass of smooth muscle fibres interlaced with areolar tissue, blood vessels and nerves.

Endometrium consists of columnar epithelium. It contains a large number of mucus-secreting tubular glands. The thickness of this layer varies during the monthly menstrual cycle. The upper two-thirds of the cervical canal is lined with mucous membrane. The lower third is lined with squamous epithelium, continuous with that of the vagina.

Blood supply, lymph drainage and nerve supply

The *arterial supply* is by the *uterine arteries* which are branches of the internal iliac arteries. They pass up the lateral aspects of the uterus between the two layers of the broad ligaments. They supply the uterus and uterine tubes and join with the ovarian arteries to supply the ovaries. Branches pass downwards to anastomose with the vaginal arteries to supply the vagina.

Venous drainage. The veins follow the same route as the arteries and eventually drain into the internal iliac veins.

Lymph drainage. There are deep and superficial lymph vessels which drain lymph from the uterus and the uterine tubes to the aortic lymph nodes and groups of nodes associated with the iliac blood vessels.

Nerve supply. The nerves supplying the uterus and the uterine tubes consist of parasympathetic fibres from the sacral outflow and sympathetic fibres from the lumbar outflow.

Supports of the uterus

The uterus is supported in the pelvic cavity by: surrounding organs, muscles of the pelvic floor and ligaments that suspend it from the walls of the pelvis.

Supporting structures (Fig. 18.6)

Two broad ligaments are formed by a double fold of peritoneum, one on each side of the uterus. They hang down from the uterine tubes as though draped over them and at their lateral ends they are attached to the sides of the pelvis. The uterine tubes are enclosed in the upper free border and near the lateral ends they penetrate the posterior wall of the broad ligament and open into the peritoneal cavity. The ovaries are attached to the posterior wall, one on each side. Blood and lymph vessels and nerves pass to the uterus and uterine tubes between the layers of the broad ligaments.

The round ligaments are bands of fibrous tissue between the two layers of broad ligament, one on each

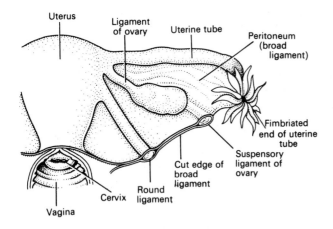

Uterus — Ligament of ovary — Uterine tube — Peritoneum (broad ligament) — Fimbriated end of uterine tube — Suspensory ligament of ovary — Cut edge of broad ligament — Round ligament — Cervix — Vagina

Figure 18.6 The main ligaments supporting the uterus. Only one side shown.

side of the uterus. They pass to the sides of the pelvis then through the *inguinal canal* to end by fusing with the labia majora.

Two uterosacral ligaments originate from the posterior walls of the cervix and vagina and extend backwards, one on each side of the rectum, to the sacrum.

Two transverse cervical ligaments (cardinal ligaments) extend from the sides of the cervix and vagina to the side walls of the pelvis.

The pubocervical fascia extends forward from the transverse cervical ligaments on each side of the bladder and is attached to the posterior surface of the pubic bones.

Functions

After puberty the uterus goes through a regular cycle of changes, the *menstrual cycle*, which prepares it to receive, nourish and protect a fertilised ovum. It provides the environment for the growing fetus, during the 40-week gestation period, at the end of which the baby is born. The cycle is usually regular, lasting between 26 and 30 days. If the ovum is not fertilised a new cycle begins with a short period of bleeding (menstruation).

If the ovum is fertilised the zygote embeds itself in the uterine wall which relaxes to accommodate the fetus as it grows. At the end of the gestation period *labour* begins and is concluded when the baby is born and the placenta extruded. During labour, the muscle of the fundus and body of the uterus contract intermittently and the cervix relaxes and dilates. As labour progresses the uterine contractions become stronger and more frequent. When the cervix is fully dilated the mother assists the birth of the baby by holding her breath and bearing down during the contractions.

Uterine tubes (Fallopian tubes)

The uterine tubes are about 10 cm long and extend from the sides of the uterus between the body and the fundus. They lie in the upper free border of the broad ligament and their trumpet-shaped lateral ends penetrate the posterior wall, opening into the peritoneal cavity close to the ovaries. The end of each tube has finger-like projections called *fimbriae*. The longest of these is the *ovarian fimbria* which is in close association with the ovary.

Structure

The uterine tubes have an outer covering of peritoneum (broad ligament), a middle layer of smooth muscle and are lined with ciliated epithelium.

Blood supply, lymph drainage and nerve supply

These are the same as for the uterus.

Function

The uterine tubes convey the ovum from the ovary to the uterus by peristalsis and ciliary movement. The mucus secreted by the lining membrane provides ideal conditions for movement of ova and spermatozoa. Fertilisation of the ovum usually takes place in the uterine tube, then the zygote is moved into the uterus.

Ovaries

The ovaries are the female gonads, or glands, and they lie in a shallow fossa on the lateral walls of the pelvis. They are 2.5 to 3.5 cm long, 2 cm wide and 1 cm thick. Each is attached to the upper part of the uterus by the *ovarian ligament* and to the back of the broad ligament by a broad band of tissue, the *mesovarium*. Blood vessels and nerves pass to the ovary in the mesovarium (Fig. 18.7).

Structure and functions

The ovaries have two layers of tissue.

The *medulla* lies in the centre and consists of fibrous tissue, blood vessels and nerves.

The cortex surrounds the medulla. It has a framework of connective tissue, or *stroma*, covered by *germinal epithelium*. It contains *ovarian follicles* in various stages of maturity, each of which contains an *ovum*. Before

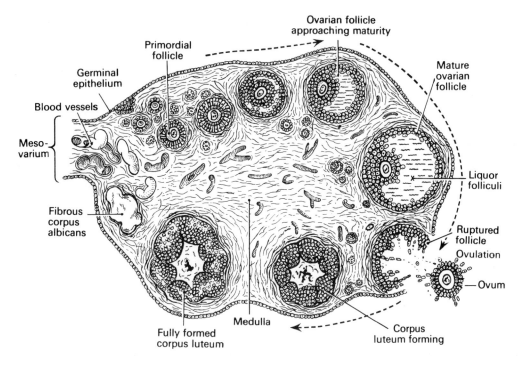

Figure 18.7 Diagram of a section of an ovary showing the stages of development of one ovarian follicle.

puberty the ovaries are inactive but the stroma already contains immature (primordial) follicles. During the childbearing years one ovarian follicle (*Graafian* follicle) matures, ruptures and releases its ovum into the peritoneal cavity. This is called *ovulation* and it occurs during each menstrual cycle (Fig. 18.7).

Maturation of the follicle is stimulated by *follicle stimulating hormone* (FSH) from the anterior pituitary. While maturing, the follicle lining cells produce the hormone *oestrogen*. After ovulation the follicle lining cells develop into the *corpus luteum* (yellow body), under the influence of the *luteinising hormone* (LH) from the anterior pituitary. The corpus luteum produces the hormone *progesterone*. If the ovum is fertilised it embeds itself in the wall of the uterus where it grows and develops and produces the hormone *human chorionic gonadotrophin* which stimulates the corpus luteum to continue secreting progesterone for the first 3 months of the pregnancy (Figs 18.8 and 18.9). If the ovum is not fertilised the corpus luteum degenerates and a new cycle begins with menstruation. At the site of the degenerate corpus luteum an inactive mass of fibrous tissue forms, called the *corpus albicans*. Sometimes more than one follicle matures at a time, releasing two or more ova in the same cycle. When this happens and the ova are fertilised the result is a multiple pregnancy.

Blood supply, lymph drainage and nerve supply

Arterial supply is by the *ovarian arteries* which branch

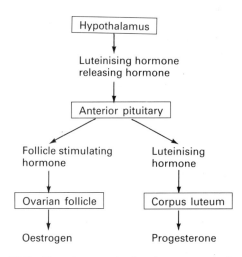

Figure 18.8 Female reproductive hormones and target tissues.

from the abdominal aorta just below the renal arteries.

Venous drainage is into a plexus of veins behind the uterus from which the ovarian veins arise. The right ovarian vein opens into the inferior vena cava and the left into the left renal vein.

Lymph drainage is to the lateral aortic and pre-aortic lymph nodes. The lymph vessels follow the same route as the arteries.

Nerve supply. The ovaries are supplied by parasympathetic nerves from the sacral outflow and sympathetic

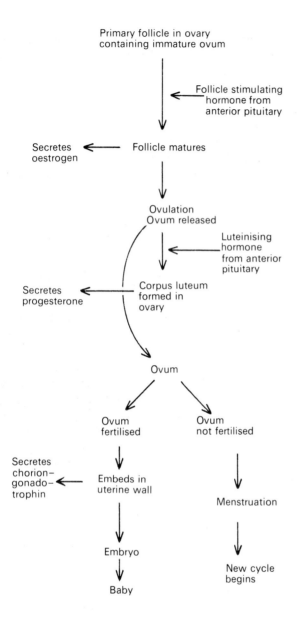

Figure 18.9 A summary of the stages of development of the ovum and the associated hormones.

nerves from the lumbar outflow. Their precise functions are not yet fully understood.

Puberty in the female

Puberty is the age at which the internal reproductive organs reach maturity. This is called the *menarche* which marks the beginning of the childbearing period. The ovaries are stimulated by the gonadotrophins from the anterior pituitary, the *follicle stimulating hormone* and the *luteinising hormone*.

The age of puberty varies between 10 and 14 years and a number of physical and psychological changes take place at this time:

- the uterus, the uterine tubes and the ovaries reach maturity
- the menstrual cycle and ovulation begin (menarche)
- the breasts develop and enlarge
- pubic and axillary hair begins to grow
- there is an increase in the rate of growth in height and widening of the pelvis
- there is an increase in the amount of fat deposited in the subcutaneous tissue, especially at the hips and breasts.

Menstrual cycle (Fig. 18.10)

This is a series of events, occurring regularly in females every 26 to 30 days throughout the childbearing period of about 36 years. The cycle consists of a series of changes that take place concurrently in the ovaries and uterine walls, stimulated by changes in the blood concentrations of hormones. Hormones secreted in the cycle are regulated by negative feedback mechanisms.

The *hypothalamus* secretes *luteinising hormone releasing hormone* (LHRH) which stimulates the anterior pituitary to secrete (see Table 9.1, p. 217):

- *follicle stimulating hormone* (FSH) which promotes the maturation of ovarian follicles and the secretion of *oestrogen*, leading to ovulation
- *luteinising hormone* (LH) which stimulates the development of corpus luteum and the secretion of *progesterone*.

The hypothalamus responds to changes in the blood levels of oestrogen and progesterone. It is depressed by high levels and stimulated when they are low.

The average length of the menstrual cycle is about 28 days. By convention the days of the cycle are numbered from the beginning of the *menstrual phase* of the menstrual cycle which usually lasts about 4 days. This is followed by the *proliferative phase* (about 10 days), then by the *secretory phase* (about 14 days).

Menstrual phase

When the ovum is not fertilised, the high level of progesterone in the blood inhibits the activity of the pituitary gland and the production of luteinising hormone is considerably reduced. The withdrawal of this hormone causes degeneration of the corpus luteum and thus progesterone production is decreased. About 14

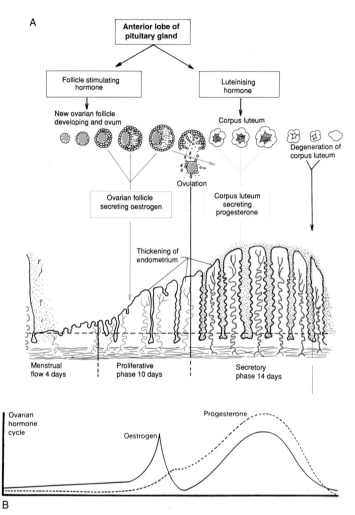

Figure 18.10 A. Diagram showing the endometrium at the various stages of the menstrual cycle. B. Changes in the hormonal levels during the cycle.

days after ovulation the lining of the uterus degenerates and breaks down and menstruation begins. The menstrual flow consists of the secretions from endometrial glands, endometrial cells, blood from the broken down capillaries and the unfertilised ovum.

When the amount of progesterone in the blood falls to a critical level another ovarian follicle is stimulated by the FSH and the proliferative phase begins.

Proliferative phase

At this stage an ovarian follicle, stimulated by FSH, is growing towards maturity and is producing *oestrogen*. Oestrogen stimulates the proliferation of the endometrium in preparation for the reception of a fertilised ovum. The endometrium becomes thicker by rapid cell

multiplication accompanied by an increase in the numbers of mucus-secreting glands and blood capillaries. This phase ends when *ovulation* occurs and oestrogen production declines.

Secretory phase

Immediately after ovulation, the lining cells of the ovarian follicle are stimulated by LH to develop the *corpus luteum*, which produces *progesterone*. Under the influence of progesterone the endometrium becomes oedematous and the secretory glands produce increased amounts of watery mucus. This is believed to assist the passage of the spermatozoa through the uterus to the uterine tubes where the ovum is usually fertilised. There is a similar increase in the secretion of watery mucus by the glands of the uterine tubes and by cervical glands which lubricate the vagina.

The ovum may survive in a fertilisable form for a very short time after ovulation, probably as little as 8 hours. The spermatozoa, deposited in the vagina during coitus, may be capable of fertilising the ovum for only about 24 hours although they may survive for several days. This means that the period in each cycle during which fertilisation can occur is relatively short. However, the date of ovulation cannot be predicted with certainty, even when cycles are regular.

If the ovum is not fertilised menstruation occurs and a new cycle begins.

If the ovum is fertilised there is no breakdown of the endometrium and no menstrual flow. The fertilised ovum (zygote) travels through the uterine tube to the uterus where it becomes embedded in the wall and produces the hormone *human chorionic gonadotrophin* (HCG) which is similar to anterior pituitary luteinising hormone. This hormone keeps the corpus luteum intact enabling it to continue to secrete progesterone for the first 3 to 4 months of the pregnancy, inhibiting the maturation of ovarian follicles (Fig. 18.9) During that time the *placenta* develops and produces oestrogen, progesterone and gonadotrophins. The placenta provides an indirect link between the circulation of the mother and that of the fetus. Through the placenta the fetus obtains nutritional materials, oxygen and antibodies and gets rid of carbon dioxide and other waste products.

Menopause (climacteric)

The *menopause* usually occurs between the ages of 45 and 55 years, marking the end of the childbearing period. It may occur suddenly or over a period of years, sometimes as long as 10 years. It is caused by the changes in the concentration of the sex hormones. The ovaries gradually become less responsive to the FSH and LH, and ovulation and the menstrual cycle become irregular, eventually ceasing. Several other phenomena may occur at the same time including:

- short-term unpredictable vasodilatation with flushing, sweating and palpitations, causing discomfort and disturbance of the normal sleep pattern
- shrinkage of the breasts
- axillary and pubic hair become sparse
- atrophy of the sex organs
- episodes of uncharacteristic behaviour sometimes occur, e.g. irritability, mood changes
- gradual thinning of the skin
- loss of bone mass that predisposes to osteoporosis (p. 394)
- slow increase in blood cholesterol levels that predisposes postmenopausal women to cardiovascular disorders.

Similar changes occur after bilateral irradiation or surgical removal of the ovaries.

Breasts or mammary glands

The breasts or mammary glands are accessory glands of the female reproductive system. They also exist in the male but only in a rudimentary form.

In the female the breasts are quite small until puberty. Thereafter they grow and develop to their mature size under the influence of oestrogen and progesterone. During pregnancy these hormones stimulate further growth. After the baby is born the hormone *prolactin* from the anterior pituitary stimulates the production of milk, and *oxytocin* from the posterior pituitary stimulates the release of milk in response to the stimulation of the nipple by the sucking baby.

Structure (Fig. 18.11)

The mammary glands consist of: glandular tissue, fibrous tissue and fatty tissue.

Each breast consists of about 20 lobes of *glandular tissue*, each lobe being made up of a number of lobules that radiate around the nipple. The lobules consist of a cluster of alveoli which open into small ducts and these unite to form large excretory ducts, called *lactiferous ducts*. The lactiferous ducts converge towards the centre of the breast where they form dilatations or

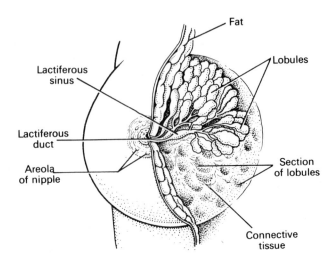

Figure 18.11   The breast.

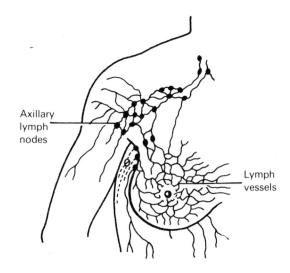

Figure 18.12   Lymph drainage from the breast.

reservoirs for milk. Leading from each dilatation, or *lactiferous sinus*, is a narrow duct which opens on to the surface at the nipple. Fibrous tissue supports the glandular tissue and ducts, and fat covers the surface of the gland and is found between the lobes.

The nipple is a small conical eminence at the centre of the breast surrounded by a pigmented area, the *areola*. On the surface of the areola there are numerous sebaceous glands (Montgomery's tubercles) which lubricate the nipple during lactation.

Blood supply, lymph drainage and nerve supply

Arterial blood supply. The breasts are supplied with blood from the thoracic branches of the axillary arteries and from the internal mammary and intercostal arteries.

Venous drainage. This describes an anastomotic circle round the base of the nipple from which branches carry the venous blood to the circumference and end in the axillary and mammary veins.

Lymph drainage (Fig. 18.12). This is mainly into the axillary lymph vessels and nodes. Lymph may drain through the internal mammary nodes if the superficial route is obstructed.

Nerve supply. The breasts are supplied by branches from the 4th, 5th and 6th thoracic nerves which contain sympathetic fibres. There are numerous somatic *sensory nerve endings* in the breast especially around the nipple. When these *touch receptors* are stimulated by sucking, impulses pass to the hypothalamus and the flow of the hormone oxytocin is increased, promoting the release of milk.

Function

Lactation. The mammary glands are active only during pregnancy and after the birth of a baby when they produce milk.

MALE REPRODUCTIVE SYSTEM

The male reproductive system consists of the following organs (Figs 18.13 and 18.14):

- 2 testes
- 2 epididymides } in the scrotum
- 2 deferent ducts (vas deferens)
- 2 spermatic cords
- 2 seminal vesicles
- 2 ejaculatory ducts
- 1 prostate gland
- 1 penis.

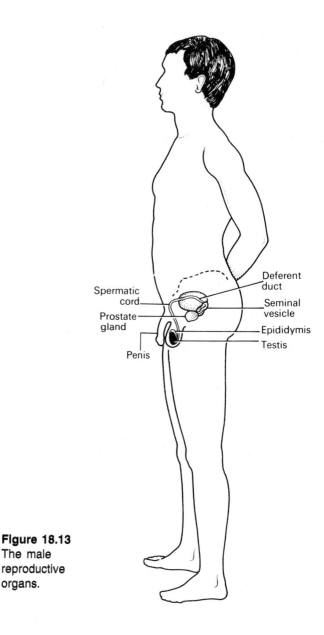

Figure 18.13
The male reproductive organs.

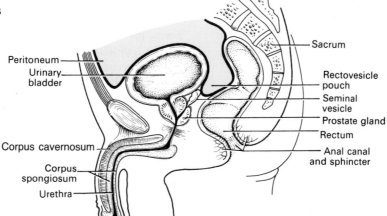

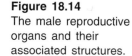

Figure 18.14
The male reproductive organs and their associated structures.

Scrotum

The scrotum is a pouch of deeply pigmented skin, fibrous and connective tissue and smooth muscle. It is divided into two compartments each of which contains one testis, one epididymis and the testicular end of a spermatic cord. It lies below the symphysis pubis, in front of the upper parts of the thighs and behind the penis.

Testes (Figs 18.15 and 18.16)

The testes are the reproductive glands of the male and are the equivalent of the ovaries in the female. They are about 4.5 cm long, 2.5 cm wide and 3 cm thick and are suspended in the scrotum by the spermatic cords. They are surrounded by three layers of tissue.

The tunica vaginalis is the outer covering of the testes and is a downgrowth of the abdominal and pelvic peritoneum. During early fetal life the testes develop in the lumbar region of the abdominal cavity just below the kidneys. They then descend into the scrotum taking with them coverings of peritoneum, blood and lymph vessels, nerves and the deferent duct. The peritoneum eventually surrounds the testes in the scrotum, becoming detached from the abdominal peritoneum. Descent of the testes into the scrotum should be complete by the 8th month of fetal life.

The tunica albuginea is a fibrous covering surrounding the testes situated under the tunica vaginalis. Ingrowths form septa dividing the glandular structure of the testes into *lobules*.

The tunica vasculosa consists of a network of capillaries supported by delicate connective tissue.

Structure of the testes

In each testis there are 200 to 300 lobules and within each lobule there are 1 to 4 convoluted loops composed of *germinal epithelial cells*, called *seminiferous tubules*. Between the tubules there are groups of *interstitial cells (of Leydig)* that secrete the hormone *testosterone* after puberty. At the upper pole of the testis the tubules combine to form a single tortuous tubule, the *epididymis*, which leaves the scrotum as the *deferent duct* (vas deferens) in the *spermatic cord*. Blood and lymph vessels pass to the testes in the spermatic cords.

Spermatic cords

There are *two spermatic cords*, one leading from each testis, consisting of:

- 1   testicular artery
- 1   testicular venous plexus
- lymph vessels
- 1   deferent duct (vas deferens)
- nerves.

The spermatic cord suspends the testis in the scrotum. It is composed of blood and lymph vessels, nerves and a deferent duct within a sheath of fibrous and connective tissue and smooth muscle. It passes through the inguinal canal. At the deep inguinal ring the structures within the cord diverge.

The testicular artery branches from the abdominal aorta, just below the renal arteries.

The testicular vein passes into the abdominal cavity. The left vein opens into the left renal vein and the right into the inferior vena cava.

The lymph drainage is through lymph nodes around the aorta.

The deferent duct is some 45 cm long. It passes upwards from the testis through the inguinal canal and ascends medially towards the posterior wall of the bladder where it is joined by the duct from the *seminal vesicle* to form the *ejaculatory duct* (Fig. 18.17).

The nerve supply is provided by branches from the 10th and 11th thoracic nerves.

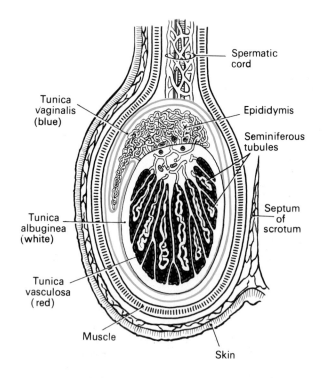

Figure 18.15   A section of testis and its coverings.

Seminal vesicles

The seminal vesicles are two small fibromuscular pouches lined with columnar epithelium, lying on the posterior aspect of the bladder (Fig. 18.18).

At its lower end each seminal vesicle opens into a short duct which joins with the corresponding deferent duct to form an ejaculatory duct. They secrete and expel a viscous fluid that helps to keep the spermatozoa alive.

Ejaculatory ducts

The ejaculatory ducts are two tubes about 2 cm long, each formed by the union of the duct from a seminal vesicle and a deferent duct. They pass through the prostate gland and join the prostatic urethra, carrying seminal fluid and spermatozoa to the urethra (Fig. 18.17).

The ejaculatory ducts are composed of the same layers of tissue as the seminal vesicles.

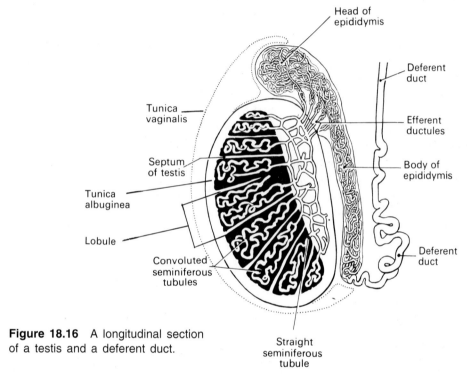

Figure 18.16   A longitudinal section of a testis and a deferent duct.

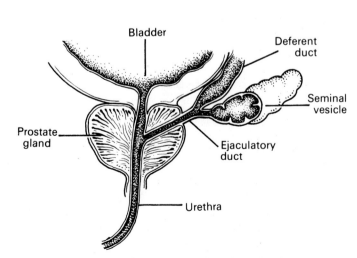

Figure 18.17   Section of the prostate gland and associated reproductive structures on one side.

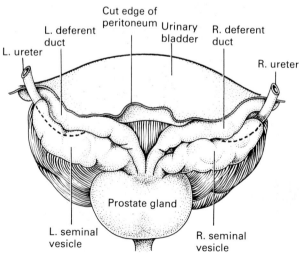

Figure 18.18   Structures associated with the prostate gland. Posterior view.

Prostate gland (Figs 18.17 and 18.18)

The prostate gland lies in the pelvic cavity in front of the rectum and behind the symphysis pubis, surrounding the first part of the urethra. It consists of an outer fibrous covering, a layer of smooth muscle and glandular substance composed of columnar epithelial cells. It secretes a thin lubricating fluid that passes into the urethra through numerous ducts.

Urethra and penis

Urethra

The male urethra provides a common pathway for the flow of urine and *semen*, the combined secretions of the male reproductive organs. It is about 19 to 20 cm long. It consists of three parts. The *prostatic urethra* originates at the urethral orifice of the bladder and passes through the prostate gland. The *membranous urethra* is the shortest and narrowest part that extends from the prostate gland to the bulb of the penis, after passing through the perineal membrane. The *spongiose* or *penile urethra* lies within the corpus spongiosum of the penis and terminates at the external urethral orifice in the *glans penis*.

There are two urethral sphincters. The *internal sphincter* consists of smooth muscle fibres at the neck of the bladder above the prostate gland. The *external sphincter* consists of striated muscle fibres surrounding the membranous part (see p. 347).

Penis (Fig. 18.19)

The penis has a *root* and a *body*. The root lies in the perineum and the body surrounds the urethra. It is formed by three cylindrical masses of *erectile tissue* and involuntary muscle. The erectile tissue is supported by fibrous tissue and covered with skin. It has a rich blood supply.

The two lateral columns are called the *corpora cavernosa* and the column between them, containing the urethra, is the *corpus spongiosum*. At its tip it is expanded into a triangular structure known as the *glans penis*. Just above the glans the skin is folded upon itself and forms a movable double layer, the *foreskin* or *prepuce*. Arterial blood is supplied by deep, dorsal and bulbar arteries of the penis which are branches from the internal pudendal arteries. A series of veins drain blood to the internal pudendal and internal iliac veins. The penis is supplied by autonomic and somatic nerves. Parasympathetic stimulation leads to engorgement with blood and erection of the penis.

Functions of the male reproductive system

As in the female, the male reproductive organs are stimulated by the *gonadotrophic hormones* from the anterior lobe of the pituitary gland (see Table 9.1).

The *follicle stimulating hormone* stimulates the *seminiferous tubules* of the testes to produce male germ cells, the spermatozoa (Fig. 18.20).

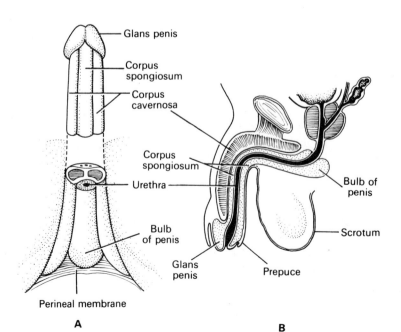

Figure 18.19 The penis.
A. Viewed from below.
B. Viewed from the side.

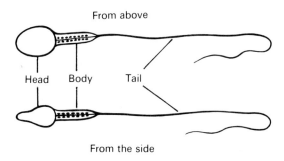

From above

Head | Body | Tail

From the side

Figure 18.20 A spermatozoon.

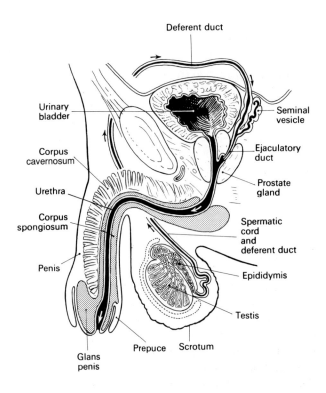

Figure 18.21 Section of the male reproductive organs. Arrows show the structures through which the spermatozoa pass.

The spermatozoa pass through the epididymis, deferent duct, seminal vesicle, ejaculatory duct and the urethra to be implanted in the female vagina during coitus.

In the epididymis and deferent duct the spermatozoa become more mature and are capable of independent movement through a liquid medium. An ejaculation usually consists of 2 to 5 ml of semen containing 40 to 100 million spermatozoa per ml. If they are not ejaculated, spermatozoa are reabsorbed by the seminiferous tubules (Fig. 18.21). The stored spermatozoa can retain their fertility for several months. During ejaculation the muscle in the walls of the deferent duct contracts, propelling the spermatozoa towards the urethra.

Successful spermatogenesis takes place at a temperature about 3°C lower than normal body temperature. This lower temperature is possible because the testes in the scrotum are covered by only a thin layer of tissue containing very little fat.

Semen is the fluid ejaculated from the urethra during coitus. It consists of:

- spermatozoa
- a viscid fluid which is secreted by the seminal vesicles and facilitates motility and contains the sugar fructose that helps to nourish the spermatozoa
- a thin lubricating fluid produced by the prostate gland
- mucus secreted by glands in the lining membrane of the urethra.

Puberty in the male

This occurs between the ages of 10 to 14 years. Luteinising hormone from the anterior lobe of the pi-

tuitary gland stimulates the *interstitial cells* of the testes to increase the production of *testosterone*. This hormone influences the development of the body to sexual maturity. The changes which occur at puberty are:

- growth of muscle and bone and a marked increase in height and weight
- enlargement of the larynx and deepening of the voice—it 'breaks'
- growth of hair on the face, axillae, chest, abdomen and pubis
- enlargement of the penis, scrotum and prostate gland
- maturation of the seminiferous tubules and production of spermatozoa
- the skin thickens and becomes more oily.

In the male, fertility and sexual ability tend to decline gradually with ageing. The secretion of testosterone gradually declines, usually at about 50 years of age. There is no period comparable to the menopause in the female.

DISEASES OF THE FEMALE REPRODUCTIVE SYSTEM

Inflammation

Infection of the reproductive system may be classified as:

- *Non-specific*, usually caused by a mixture of microbes, e.g. staphylococci, streptococci, coliform bacteria, *Clostridium perfringens (Cl. welchii)*
- *Specific*, caused by sexually transmitted microbes, the most common of which is *Neisseria gonorrhoeae*, *Trichomonas vaginalis*, chlamydia, herpes viruses, human immunodeficiency virus (HIV), hepatitis B.

Pelvic inflammatory disease (PID)

This infection may be specific or non-specific. It usually begins as vulvovaginitis, including the vulvar glands, then it may spread to the cervix, uterus, uterine tubes and ovaries. Upward spread is most common when microbes are present in the vagina before a surgical procedure, parturition or abortion, especially if some of the products of conception are retained.

Complications of PID include:

- infertility due to obstruction of uterine tubes
- peritonitis
- intestinal obstruction due to adhesions between the bowel and the uterus and/or uterine tubes
- bacteriaemia which may lead to meningitis, endocarditis, suppurative arthritis

- Bartholin's gland abscess or cyst formation if the duct is blocked.

Specific infections (venereal diseases)

In general, the microbes that cause sexually transmitted diseases:

- are unable to survive outside the body for long periods
- have no intermediate host
- produce lesions in the genital area which discharge the infecting microbes.

Gonorrhoea

This is the most commonly occurring venereal disease and affects men and women. It is caused by *Neisseria gonorrhoeae* which affects the mucosa of the reproductive and urinary tracts. In the male, suppurative urethritis occurs and the infection may spread to the prostate gland, epididymis and testes. In the female the infection may spread from vulvar glands, vagina and cervix to the body of the uterus, uterine tubes, ovaries and peritoneum. Healing by fibrosis in the female may cause obstruction of the uterine tubes, leading to infertility. In the male it may cause urethral stricture.

Non-venereal transmission of gonorrhoea may cause *neonatal ophthalmia* in babies born to infected mothers. The eyes are infected as the baby passes through the vagina.

Syphilis

This disease is caused by *Treponema pallidum*. There are three clearly marked stages although the third is now rarely seen in Britain. After an incubation period of several weeks, the *primary sore* (chancre) appears at the site of infection, e.g. the vulva, vagina, perineum, penis, round the mouth. In the female the

primary sore may be undetected if it is internal. After several weeks the chancre subsides spontaneously. *Secondary lesions* appear 3 to 4 months after infection. They consist of skin rashes and raised papules (condylomata lata) on the external genitalia and vaginal walls. These subside after several months and are followed by a latent period of a variable number of years. *Tertiary lesions* (gummas) develop in many organs and in a few cases the nervous system in involved, leading to general paralysis.

Sexual transmission occurs during the primary and secondary stages when discharge from lesions contains microbes. Congenital transmission occurs when microbes from an infected mother cross the placenta to the fetus often with fatal consequences. Accidental spread of infection may occur by blood transfusion if a donor's blood is taken during the incubation period after microbes have spread to the blood from the site of infection.

Trichomonas vaginalis

These *protozoa* cause acute vulvovaginitis. It is usually sexually transmitted and is commonly present in women with gonorrhoea.

Candidiasis

Candida albicans is the causative organism. It is a commensal in the vagina and causes infection (thrush) in some circumstances, e.g. in diabetes, malnutrition and general debility.

Acquired immune deficiency syndrome (AIDS) and hepatitis B infection

These viral conditions may be sexually transmitted but there are no local signs of infection. For a description of AIDS see page 80 and hepatitis B page 331.

Vulvar dystrophies

Atrophic dystrophy

This is thinning of vulvar epithelium and the formation of fibrous tissue, occurring after the menopause due to oestrogen withdrawal. It predisposes to infection, especially in debilitated women, and to malignant epithelial neoplasia.

Vulvar intra-epithelial neoplasia (VIN)

The extent of development of hyperplasia and dysplasia of cells of the skin of the vulva varies considerably. It is often associated with human papillomavirus infection. In the majority of cases the neoplasms are benign. Some VIN cases progress to invasive carcinoma while others regress spontaneously. In elderly women and immunosuppressed young women malignant tumours may develop which spread locally with early involvement of inguinal lymph nodes. Because of the anastomoses between lymph vessels on the two sides of the vulva, bilateral lymph node involvement is common.

Imperforate hymen

This is a congenital abnormality which may not be noticed until the onset of menstruation. Blood accumulates in the vagina, uterus and uterine tubes, and it may enter the peritoneal cavity and cause peritonitis. The uterine tubes may become obstructed by organised blood, leading to infertility.

Disorders of the cervix

Inflammation (cervicitis)

This occurs in most multiparous women and may be due to acute or chronic infection caused by specific or non-specific microbes. In non-specific infection there are several predisposing factors, e.g. trauma at childbirth, instruments used in gynaecological treatments, abnormal blood oestrogen levels, hypersecretion by cervical glands. In many cases the only indication of infection is excessive white vaginal discharge (leukorrhoea). Chronic inflammation may follow acute attacks or develop gradually, and may predispose to malignancy.

Cervical intra-epithelial neoplasia (CIN)

Dysplastic changes begin in the deepest layer of cervical epithelium, usually at the junction of the stratified squamous epithelium of the lower third of the cervical canal with the secretory epithelium of the upper two-thirds. The cell dysplasia may progress to involve the full thickness of epithelium, called *carcinoma-in-situ*. The cancer may develop further and spread locally to the vagina, uterine body and other pelvic structures. More widespread metastases occur late in the disease. All CIN cases do not develop to the cancerous stage but it is not possible to predict how far development will go, whether it will remain static or regress. Three degrees of dysplasia have been described, although clear distinction between them is not always possible:

- CIN 1 = mild dysplasia
- CIN 2 = moderate dysplasia
- CIN 3 = carcinoma-in-situ.

CIN 3 may progress to invasive carcinoma. Early spread is via lymph nodes and local spread is commonly to the uterus, vagina, bladder and rectum. In the late stages spread via the blood to the liver, lungs and bones may occur.

The disease takes 15 to 20 years to develop and it occurs mostly between 35 and 50 years of age. The carcinogens have not been identified but it has been suggested that herpes viruses and/or spermatozoal DNA may be involved. A high incidence is associated with some personal and social factors:

- early marriage and pregnancy
- a high number of pregnancies
- coitus beginning at an early age
- frequent coitus
- many sexual partners
- sexually transmitted disease
- low socio-economic status.

Disorders of the body of the uterus

Acute endometritis

This is usually caused by non-specific infection, following parturition or abortion, especially if fragments of membranes or placenta have been retained in the uterus. A variety of microbes may be involved, e.g. staphylococci, streptococci, *Escherichia coli, Pseudomonas*. The inflammation may subside after removal of retained products. The infection may spread to:

- myometrium, perimetrium and surrounding pelvic tissues which may lead to thrombosis of iliac veins

- uterine tubes, causing salpingitis, fibrosis, obstruction and infertility
- any of the above-mentioned areas, causing peritonitis and possibly adhesions.

Chronic endometritis

This may follow an acute attack or be due to spread of pelvic inflammatory disease. It may follow abortion or parturition and may be associated with chronic salpingitis, endometrial carcinoma or the use of intrauterine contraceptive devices.

Endometriosis

This is the growth of endometrial tissue outside the uterus, most commonly in the ovaries, uterine tubes and other pelvic structures. The ectopic tissue reacts to sex hormones as does uterine endometrium, causing menstrual-type bleeding and, in the ovaries, the formation of coloured cysts, 'chocolate cysts'. There is intermittent pain due to swelling, and recurrent haemorrhage causes fibrous tissue formation. Ovarian endometriosis may lead to pelvic inflammation, infertility and extensive pelvic adhesions, involving the ovaries, uterus, uterine ligaments and the bowel. The cause is not clear but it has been suggested that there may have been:

- abnormal cell differentiation in the fetus
- regurgitation of menstrual material through the uterine tubes
- spread of endometrial cells in lymph and blood during menstruation.

Adenomyosis

This is the growth of endometrium within the myometrium. The ectopic tissue may cause general or localised uterine enlargement. The lesions may cause dysmenorrhoea and irregular excessive bleeding, usually beginning between 40 and 50 years of age.

Endometrial hyperplasia

The hyperplasia may affect endometrial glands, causing cyst formation and/or focal hyperplasia of atypical cells. The focal type frequently undergo malignant change. Both types are associated with a sustained high blood oestrogen level which may be due to:

- failure of ovarian follicles to mature and release their ova
- oestrogen-secreting ovarian tumours
- prolonged oestrogen therapy.

Leiomyoma (fibroid, myoma)

These are very common, often multiple, benign tumours of myometrium. They are firm masses of smooth muscle encapsulated in compressed muscle fibres and they vary greatly in size. Large tumours may undergo degenerative changes if they outgrow their blood supply, leading to necrosis, fibrosis and calcification. They develop during the reproductive period and may be hormone dependent because they enlarge during pregnancy and when oral contraceptives are used. They tend to regress after the menopause. Large tumours may cause pelvic discomfort, frequency of micturition, menorrhagia, irregular bleeding, dysmenorrhoea and reduced fertility. Malignant change is rare.

Endometrial carcinoma

This occurs mainly in nulliparous women between 50 and 60 years of age. The cause is not known but there is some evidence that oestrogen may be involved. The incidence of carcinoma is increased when an oestrogen-secreting tumour is present and in women who are obese, hypertensive or diabetic, because they tend to have a high level of blood oestrogen. The tumour may develop as a diffuse mass, a localised plaque or a polyp and there is often ulceration and bleeding. Endometrium has no lymphatics so lymph spread is delayed until there is extensive local spread, involving other pelvic structures. Distant metastases, spread in blood or lymph, develop later, most commonly in the liver, lungs and bones. Invasion of the ureters leads to hydronephrosis and uraemia which is commonly the cause of death.

Disorders of the uterine tubes and ovaries

Acute salpingitis

This infection usually spreads from the uterus, and only occasionally from the peritoneal cavity. The outcome may be:

- uneventful recovery
- chronic inflammation, leading to fibrous tubal obstruction and infertility
- pus formation (*pyosalpinx*) and further spread to the ovaries and peritoneal cavity, leading to fibrous tubal obstruction, infertility and/or pelvic adhesions.

Ectopic pregnancy

This is the implantation of a fertilised ovum outside the uterus, most commonly in a uterine tube. As the fetus grows the tube ruptures and its contents enter the peritoneal cavity, causing acute inflammation (peritonitis) and possibly severe intraperitoneal haemorrhage.

Ovarian tumours

The majority of ovarian tumours are benign, usually occurring between 20 and 45 years of age. The remainder occur mostly between 45 and 65 years and are divided between borderline malignancy (low-grade cancer) and frank malignancy. There are three main types of cells involved: epithelial cells, germ cells and hormone-secreting cells (sex-cord stroma cells).

Epithelial cell tumours

Most of these are borderline or malignant tumours. They vary greatly in size from very large to quite small and some are partly cystic. Large tumours may cause pressure, leading to gastrointestinal disturbances, frequency of micturition, dysuria and ascites. Those suspended by a pedicle may twist, causing ischaemia, necrosis, haemorrhage or rupture of a cyst. The principal methods of spread are invasion of local and peritoneal structures. Later lymph- and blood-spread metastases may develop.

The prevalence is higher in developed societies and in the higher socio-economic groups. Pregnancy and suppression of ovulation by medicinal contraceptives, e.g. the oral contraceptive pill, may have a protective effect due to a reducton in the number of ovulatory menstrual cycles.

Germ cell ovarian tumours

These occur mainly in children and young adults and only a few are malignant. Benign *dermoid cysts* are the most common type. These are thick-walled cysts containing a variety of uncharacteristic tissues, e.g. hair, skin, epithelium, teeth. They are usually small and have a tendency to twist on a pedicle, causing ischaemia and necrosis.

Sex-cord stroma cell tumours

These cells are the precursors of the ovarian follicle lining cells, luteal cells and fibrous supporting cells. Mixed tumours develop, some of which secrete hormones. Oestrogen-secreting tumours cause precocious sexual development in children. In adults the excess oestrogen may cause endometrial hyperplasia, endometrial carcinoma, cystic disease of the breast or breast cancer. Androgen-secreting tumours occasionally develop, causing atrophy of the breast and genitalia and the development of male sex characteristics.

Metastatic ovarian tumours

The ovaries are a common site of metastatic spread from primary malignant tumours in other pelvic organs, the breast, stomach, pancreas and biliary tract.

Disorders of the breasts

Inflammation (mastitis)

Acute non-suppurative inflammation

This occurs during lactation and is associated with painful congestion and oedema of the breast. It is of hormonal origin.

Acute suppurative inflammation (pyogenic mastitis)

The microbes enter through a nipple abrasion caused by the infant sucking. The most common causative microbes are *Staphylococcus aureus* and *Streptococcus pyogenes* usually acquired by the infant while in hospital. The infection spreads along the mammary ducts of a lobe causing localised swelling and redness. If it does not resolve it can become chronic and an abscess may form.

Tumours

Benign tumours

Some are cystic and some solid and they usually occur in women nearing the menopause. They may originate from secretory cells, fibrous tissue or from ducts.

Malignant tumours

The most common types of tumour are usually painless lumps found in the upper outer quadrant of the breast. There is considerable fibrosis around the tumour that may cause retraction of the nipple and necrosis and ulceration of the overlying skin. It is increasingly common between 35 and 70 years.

Early spread beyond the breast is via lymph to the axillary and internal mammary nodes. Local invasion involves the pectoral muscles and the pleura. Blood-spread metastases may occur later in many organs and bones, especially lumbar and thoracic vertebrae. The causes of breast cancer are not known but it is known to occur more commonly in nulliparous women and those with early menarche and late menopause. Predisposing factors include:

- oestrogen excess. Normally there is cyclic proliferation of cells in the mammary ducts consistent with the menstrual rise and fall of oestrogen secretion. Excess oestrogen may cause abnormal cell proliferation and malignant change.
- familial tendencies. There may be genetic factors associated with susceptibility.
- viruses. It has been suggested that viruses may be involved although none has been identified so far.

DISEASES OF THE MALE REPRODUCTIVE SYSTEM

Classification of infection in the male is the same as in the female, i.e. *non-specific* and *specific* (p. 436). In addition to venereal diseases, non-specific infection of the testes (orchitis) may be caused by mumps viruses, blood-borne from the parotid glands.

Penis

Inflammation

Inflammation of the glans and prepuce may be caused by a specific or non-specific infection. In non-specific infections, or *balanitis*, lack of personal hygiene is an important predisposing factor, especially if *phimosis* is present, i.e. the orifice in the prepuce is too small to allow for its normal retraction. If the infection becomes chronic there may be fibrosis of the prepuce which increases the phimosis.

Urethra

Inflammation

Gonococcal urethritis is the most common specific infection. Non-specific infection may be spread from the bladder (cystitis) or be introduced during catheterisation, cystoscopy or surgery. Both types may spread throughout the system to the prostate, seminal vesicles, epididymis and testes. If infection becomes chronic, fibrosis may cause urethral stricture or obstruction, leading to retention of urine.

Epididymis and testes

Inflammation

Non-specific epididymitis and orchitis are usually due to spread of infection from the urethra, commonly following prostatectomy. The microbes may spread either through the deferent duct (vas deferens) or via lymph.

Specific epididymitis is usually caused by gonorrhoea spread from the urethra.

Orchitis is more commonly caused by mumps viruses, blood-borne from the parotid glands. Acute inflammation with oedema occurs about 1 week after the appearance of parotid swelling. The infection is usually unilateral but, if bilateral, severe damage to germinal epithelium of the seminiferous tubules may result in sterility.

Hydrocele

This is the most common form of scrotal swelling and is accumulation of serous fluid in the tunica vaginalis. The onset may be acute and painful or chronic. It may be congenital or be secondary to another disorder of the testis or epididymis.

Testicular tumours

Most testicular tumours are malignant. They occur in children and young adults in whom the affected testis has not descended or has been late in descending into the scrotum. The tumour tends to remain localised for a considerable time but eventually spreads in lymph to pelvic and abdominal lymph nodes, and more widely in blood. Occasionally hormone-secreting tumours develop and may cause precocious development in children.

Male infertility

This may be due to:

- endocrine disorders
- obstruction of the vas deferens
- failure of erection or ejaculation during intercourse
- surgical vasectomy
- suppression of spermatogenesis by, e.g. ionising radiation, chemotherapy and other drugs.

Prostate gland

Inflammation

Acute prostatitis is usually caused by non-specific infection, spread from the urethra or bladder, often following catheterisation, cystoscopy, urethral dilatation or surgery in which part of the gland is removed. Chronic infection may follow an acute attack, but it may develop insidiously and is not associated with known microbes. Fibrosis of the gland may occur during healing, causing urethral stricture or obstruction.

Benign prostatic enlargement

Hyperplastic nodules form around the urethra and may cause constriction or obstruction to the flow of urine, causing retention of urine. Urethral stricture may prevent the bladder emptying completely during micturition, predisposing to infection which may spread upwards and cause pyelonephritis and other complications. Prostatic enlargement is common in men over 50 years. The cause is not clear, but it may be an acceleration of the ageing process associated with the decline in androgen secretion which changes the androgen/oestrogen balance.

Malignant prostatic tumours

These are a relatively common cause of death in men over 50 years. The carcinogen is not known but changes in the androgen/oestrogen balance may be significant or viruses may be involved. Invasion of local tissues is widespread before lymph-spread metastases develop in pelvic and abdominal lymph nodes. Blood-spread metastases in bone are common and bone formation rather than bone destruction is a common feature. Lumbar vertebrae are a common site, possibly due to retrograde spread along the walls of veins. In many cases bone metastases are the first indication of malignant prostatic tumours.

Breast

Breast tissue in men consists of ducts and stroma only.

Gynaecomastia

This is proliferation of breast tissue in men. It usually affects one breast and is benign. It is common in adolescents and older men, and is often associated with:

- endocrine disorders, especially those associated with high oestrogen levels
- cirrhosis of the liver (p. 332)
- malnutrition
- some drugs, e.g. chlorpromazine, spironolactone, digoxin
- Klinefelter's syndrome, a genetic disorder in which there is testicular atrophy and absence of spermatogenesis.

Malignant tumours

These develop in a small number of men, usually in the older age groups.

Normal values

Note. *Some biological measures have been extracted from the text and listed here for easy reference. In some cases slightly different 'normals' may be found in other texts and used by different medical practitioners.*

Metric measures, units and SI symbols

Name	SI unit	Symbol
Length	metre	m
Mass	kilogram	kg
Amount of substance	mole	mol
Pressure	pascal	Pa
Energy	joule	J

Decimal multiples and submultiples of the units are formed by the use of standard prefixes.

Multiple	Prefix	Symbol	Submultiple	Prefix	Symbol
10^6	mega	M	10^{-1}	deci	d
10^3	kilo	k	10^{-2}	centi	c
10^2	hecto	h	10^{-3}	milli	m
10^1	deca	da	10^{-6}	micro	μ
			10^{-9}	nano	n
			10^{-12}	pico	p
			10^{-15}	femto	f

Hydrogen ion concentration (pH)

Neutral = 7   Acid = 0 to 7   Alkaline = 7 to 14

Normal pH of some body fluids

Blood	7.35 to 7.45
Saliva	5.4 to 7.5
Gastric juice	1.5 to 3.5
Bile	6.0 to 8.5
Urine	4.5 to 8.0

Some normal plasma levels in adults

Calcium	2.12 to 2.62 mmol/l	(8.5 to 10.5 mg/100ml)
Carbon dioxide	4.5 to 6 kPa	(34 to 46 mmHg)
Chloride	97 to 106 mmol/l	(97 to 106 mEq/l)
Cholesterol	3.6 to 6.7 mmol/l	(140 to 260 mg/100 ml)
Glucose	4.5 to 5.5 mmol/l	(60 to 100 mg/100 ml)
Oxygen	12 to 15 kPa	(90 to 110 mmHg)
Potassium	3.5 to 5 mmol/l	(3.5 to 5 mEq/l)
Sodium	135 to 143 mmol/l	(135 to 143 mEq/l)
Urea	2.5 to 6 mmol/l	(15 to 40 mg/100 ml)

Blood pressure

Normal adult 120/80 mmHg

Hypertension, i.e. above 'normal' maximum for age

20 years	140/90 mmHg
50 years	160/95 mmHg
75 years	170/105 mmHg

Pulse rate

At rest 60 to 80/min	
Sinus bradycardia	< 60/min
Sinus tachycardia	> 100/min

Respiration rate

At rest 15 to 18/min	
Tidal volume	500 ml
Dead space	150 ml
Alveolar ventilation	15 (500 − 150) = 5.25l/min

Blood count

Leukocytes	4	$\times 10^9$/l to 11	$\times 10^9$/l
Neutrophils	2.5	$\times 10^9$/l to 7.5	$\times 10^9$/l
Eosinophils	0.04	$\times 10^9$/l to 0.44	$\times 10^9$/l
Basophils	0.015	$\times 10^9$/l to 0.1	$\times 10^9$/l
Monocytes	0.2	$\times 10^9$/l to 0.8	$\times 10^9$/l
Lymphocytes	1.5	$\times 10^9$/l to 3.5	$\times 10^9$/l
Erythrocytes			
female	4.5	$\times 10^{12}$/l to 5	$\times 10^{12}$/l
male	4.5	$\times 10^{12}$/l to 6.5	$\times 10^{12}$/l
Thrombocytes	200	$\times 10^9$/l to 350	$\times 10^9$/l

Diet

Vitamins. Daily requirements see pp. 276 and 277

1 Calorie (C) = 4.182 kilojoules (kJ)
1 kilojoule approx. = 0.24 Calorie

Nutrients energy output	Proportion in diet
Carbohydrate 1g = 17kJ = 4C	55 to 75%
Protein 1g = 17kJ = 4C	10 to 15%
Fat 1g = 36kJ = 9C	15 to 30%

Urine

Specific gravity   1.020 to 1.030
Volume excreted   1000 to 1500 ml/day
Glucose in urine when blood level > 9 mmol/l
(180 mg/100ml)

Body temperature

Normal	36.8°C (98.4°F): axillary
Hypothermia	32°C (89.6°F): axillary
	35°C (95°F): core temperature
Death when below	25°C (77°F)

Cerebrospinal fluid pressure

Lying on the side   10 cm water

Intraocular pressure

1.3 to 2.6 kPa (10 to 20 mmHg)

Menstrual cycle

Duration 26 to 30 days

Menstruation	4 days
Proliferative phase	10 days
Secretory phase	14 days
Ovulation	about 14th day

Bibliography

Cooke E M 1991 Hare's bacteriology and immunity for nurses, 7th edn. Churchill Livingstone, Edinburgh

Cotton R E 1992 Lecture notes on pathology, 4th edn. Blackwell Scientific Publications, London

Department of Health 1991 Dietary reference values of food energy and nutrients for the UK: COMA report. HMSO, London

Duerdin B I, Reid T M S, Jewsbury J M, Turk 1993 Textbook of microbiology and parasitic infection. Hodder & Stoughton, London

Edwards C R W, Bouchier I A D (eds) 1991 Davidson's principles and practice of medicine, 16th edn. Churchill Livingstone, Edinburgh

Emery A E H, Mueller R F 1992 Elements of medical genetics, 8th edn. Churchill Livingstone, Edinburgh

Emslie-Smith D, Paterson C R, Scratcherd T, Read N W (eds) 1988 Textbook of physiology, 11th edn. Churchill Livingstone, Edinburgh

Forrest A P M, Carter D C, Macleod I B (eds) 1991 Principles and practice of surgery, 2nd edn. Churchill Livingstone, Edinburgh

Ganong W F 1991 Review of medical physiology, 15th edn. Prentice-Hall, London

Govan A D T, Macfarlane P S, Callander R 1991 Pathology illustrated, 3rd edn. Churchill Livingstone, Edinburgh

Guyton A C 1991 Textbook of medical physiology, 8th edn. Saunders, Philadelphia

Hinchliff S, Montague S (eds) 1988 Physiology for nursing practice. Baillière Tindall, London

Hinwood B 1993 A textbook of science for the health professions. Chapman & Hall, London

Lamb J F, Ingram C G, Johnston L A, Pitman R M 1991 Essentials of physiology, 3rd edn. Blackwell Scientific Publications, London

MacSween R N M, Whaley K (eds) 1992 Muir's textbook of pathology, 13th edn. Edward Arnold, London

Marieb E M 1992 Human anatomy and physiology, 2nd edn. Benjamin/Cummings Publishing, California

Merck manual of diagnosis and therapy 1992 16th edn. Merck Research Laboratories, New Jersey

Oh T E 1988 (ed) Intensive care manual, 3rd edn. Butterworths, Sydney

Rang H P, Dale M M 1995 Pharmacology, 3rd edn. Churchill Livingstone, Edinburgh

Rees J P, Trounce J R 1988 A new short textbook of medicine. Edward Arnold, London

Robbins S L, Conran R S, Ramzi S 1994 Pathological basis of disease, 5th edn. Saunders, Philadelphia

Rogers A W 1992 Textbook of anatomy. Churchill Livingstone, Edinburgh

Spector W G 1989 An introduction to general pathology, 3rd edn. Churchill Livingstone, Edinburgh

Tortora G J, Grabowski S R 1993 Principles of anatomy and physiology, 7th edn. HarperCollins, New York

Underwood J C E (ed) 1992 General and systematic pathology. Churchill Livingstone, Edinburgh

Vander A J, Sherman J H, Luciano D S 1990 Human physiology—the mechanisms of body function, 5th edn. McGraw Hill, New York

Weir D M, Stewart J 1993 Immunology, 7th edn. Churchill Livingstone, Edinburgh

West J B (ed) 1990 Best and Taytor's physiological basis of medical practice, 12th edn. Williams and Wilkins, Baltimore

Wheater P R, Burkitt H G, Daniels V G 1987 Functional histology, 2nd edn. Churchill Livingstone, Edinburgh

Whitney E N, Rolfes S R 1993 Understanding nutrition, 6th edn. West Publishing Company, Minneapolis

Williams P L, Warwick R, Dyson M, Bannister L H 1989 Gray's anatomy, 37th edn. Churchill Livingstone, Edinburgh

Index

Page numbers referring to anatomy and physiology are in ordinary type. Those referring to diseases are in italics. Page numbers in bold type refer to main discussions of anatomy and physiology. Those in bold italics refer to main discussions of diseases.